Methods in Toxicology

VOLUME 1

Part B
In Vitro Toxicity Indicators

Methods in Toxicology

Series Editors

Charles A. Tyson
Biochemical Toxicology Program
SRI International
Menlo Park, California

Hanspeter Witschi
Institute of Toxicology and Environmental Health
University of California, Davis

Volume 1A. *In Vitro* Biological Systems
Edited by Charles A. Tyson and John M. Frazier

Volume 1B. *In Vitro* Toxicity Indicators
Edited by Charles A. Tyson and John M. Frazier

Volume 2. Mitochondrial Dysfunction
Edited by Lawrence H. Lash and Dean P. Jones

Volume 3A. Male Reproductive Toxicology
Edited by Robert E. Chapin and Jerrold J. Heindel

Volume 3B. Female Reproductive Toxicology
Edited by Jerrold J. Heindel and Robert E. Chapin

Methods in Toxicology

VOLUME 1

Part B
In Vitro Toxicity Indicators

Edited by

Charles A. Tyson
Biochemical Toxicology Program
SRI International
Menlo Park, California

John M. Frazier
School of Hygiene and Public Health
The Johns Hopkins University
Baltimore, Maryland

Academic Press
A Division of Harcourt Brace & Company

San Diego New York Boston London Sydney Tokyo Toronto

This book is printed on acid-free paper. ♾

Academic Press, Inc.
525 B Street, Suite 1900, San Diego, California 92101-4495

United Kingdom Edition published by
Academic Press Limited
24–28 Oval Road, London NW1 7DX

International Standard Serial Number: 1063-3677

International Standard Book Number: 0-12- 461203-2 (Hardcover)

International Standard Book Number: 0-12- 461204-0 (Papercover)

PRINTED IN THE UNITED STATES OF AMERICA
94 95 96 97 98 99 EB 9 8 7 6 5 4 3 2 1

The editors express special thanks to Dr. Richard Recknagel in absentia. His enthusiasm and suggestions for improving the contents of this volume were graciously offered and gratefully accepted. Regrettably, Dr. Recknagel passed away before this volume was complete, but we remain forever in his debt for his constructive and positive contributions. We thank Dr. Recknagel for his care, cooperation, and expertise.

Contents

Section V

Functional Indices

Section VI

Biochemical Indices

Section VII

Lipid Peroxidation

Section VIII

Specialized Techniques

Contributors

Numbers in parentheses indicate the pages on which the authors' contributions begin.

Daniel Acosta (46), Department of Pharmacology and Toxicology, College of Pharmacy, The University of Texas, Austin, Texas 78712

Fernando Aguilar (237), Department of Carcinogenesis, Swiss Institute for Experimental Cancer Research, 1066 Epalinges/Lausanne, Switzerland

N. G. Anderson (463), Large Scale Biology Corporation, Rockville, Maryland 20850

N. L. Anderson (463), Large Scale Biology Corporation, Rockville, Maryland 20850

Mark J. Arends (228), Department of Pathology, CRC Laboratories, University of Edinburgh Medical School, Edinburgh EH8 9AG, Scotland, United Kingdom

Steven D. Aust (367), Biotechnology Center, Utah State University, Logan, Utah 84322

Thomas K. Baker (72), Department of Pharmacology and Toxicology, Division of Toxicology, Indiana University School of Medicine, Indianapolis, Indiana 46202

S. Banni (415), Dipartimento di Biologia Sperimentale, Sezione di Patologia Sperimentale, Universita di Cagliari, Cagliari, Italy

Giorgio Bellomo (58), Department of Experimental Medicine, and Oncology, Institute of General Pathology, Universita Degli Studi di Torino, 10125 Torino, Italy

Irene K. Berezesky (1), Department of Pathology, University of Maryland, School of Medicine, Baltimore, Maryland 21201

John M. Bond (438), Department of Cell Biology and Anatomy, Laboratories for Cell Biology, University of North Carolina at Chapel Hill, School of Medicine, Chapel Hill, North Carolina 27599

André B. Borle (315), Department of Cell Biology and Physiology, University of Pittsburgh, School of Medicine, Pittsburgh, Pennsylvania 15261

Alberto Boveris (384), Department of Biochemistry and Biophysics, School of Pharmacy and Biochemistry, University of Buenos Aires, 1113 Buenos Aires, Argentina

Enrique Cadenas (384), Institute for Toxicology, University of Southern California, Los Angeles, California 90033

Peter A. Cerutti (237), Department of Carcinogenesis, Swiss Institute for Experimental Cancer Research, 1066 Epalinges/Lausanne, Switzerland

Enrique Chacon (438), Department of Cell Biology and Anatomy, Laboratories for Cell Biology, University of North Carolina at Chapel Hill, School of Medicine, Chapel Hill, North Carolina 27599

Iih-Nan Chou (81), Departments of Microbiology and Pathology, Boston University School of Medicine, Boston, Massachusetts 02118

F. P. Corongiu (415), Dipartimento di Biologia Sperimentale, Sezione di Patologia Sperimentale, Universitá di Cagliari, Cagliari, Italy

Frank Dolbeare (178), Biology and Biotechnology Research Program, Lawrence Livermore National Laboratory, University of California, Livermore, California 94551

David L. Eaton (349), Department of Environmental Health, and Institute for Environmental Studies, University of Washington, Seattle, Washington 98195

Lars Ernster (33), Department of Biochemistry, Arrhenius Laboratories for Natural Sciences, Stockholm University, S-106 91 Stockholm, Sweden

R. Esquer-Blasco (463), Large Scale Biology Corporation, Rockville, Maryland 20850

Gregory L. Finch (279), Inhalation Toxicology Research Institute, Lovelace Biomedical and Environmental, Research Institute, Albuquerque, New Mexico 87185

Sue M. Ford (97), Toxicology Program, St. John's University, College of Pharmacy and Allied Health Professions, Jamaica, New York 11439

Evan P. Gallagher (349), Department of Environmental Health, and Institute for Environmental Studies, University of Washington, Seattle, Washington 98195

Sean R. Gallagher (164), Hoefer Scientific Instruments, San Francisco, California 94107

Cecilia Giulivi (384), Institute for Toxicology, University of Southern California, Los Angeles, California 90033

Eric A. Glende, Jr. (400), Department of Physiology and Biophysics, School of Medicine, Case Western Reserve University, Cleveland, Ohio 44106

Carlotta E. Groves (108), Department of Physiology, College of Medicine, University of Arizona, Tucson, Arizona 85724

Ian Harper (438), Department of Cell Biology and Anatomy, Laboratories for Cell Biology, University of North Carolina at Chapel Hill, School of Medicine, Chapel Hill, North Carolina 27599

Brian Herman (438), Department of Cell Biology and Anatomy, Laboratories for Cell Biology, University of North Carolina at Chapel Hill, School of Medicine, Chapel Hill, North Carolina 27599

Paul Hochstein (33), Institute for Toxicology, University of Southern California, Los Angeles, California 90033

Robert M. Hogg (228), Department of Pathology, CRC Laboratories, University of Edinburgh Medical School, Edinburgh EH8 9AG, Scotland, United Kingdom

Francesca Iosi (58), Laboratory of Ultrastructures, Istituto Superiore di Sanita, Roma, Italy

Dean P. Jones (140), Departments of Biochemistry and Pediatrics, and Winship Cancer Center, Emory University School of Medicine, Atlanta, Georgia 30322

Hermann Kappus (377), Department of Dermatology, Free University of Berlin, D-1000 Berlin 65, Germany

Terrance J. Kavanagh (349), Departments of Medicine and Environmental Health, University of Washington, Seattle, Washington 98195

V. Kefalas (50), Chemical Assessment Branch, National Occupational Health and Safety Commission, The University of Sydney, New South Wales 2001, Australia

James E. Klaunig (72), Department of Pharmacology and Toxicology, Division of Toxicology, Indiana University School of Medicine, Indianapolis, Indiana 46202

Richard G. Knowles (248), Biochemical Sciences, Wellcome Research Laboratories, Beckenham, Kent BR3 3BS, United Kingdom

Debra L. Laskin (431, 456), Department of Pharmacology and Toxicology, College of Pharmacy, Rutgers University, Piscataway, New Jersey 08855

Jeffrey D. Laskin (431), Department of Environmental and Community Medicine, UMDNJ-Robert Wood Johnson Medical School, Environmental and Occupational Health Sciences Institute, Piscataway, New Jersey 08854

John J. Lemasters (438), Department of Cell Biology and Anatomy, Laboratories for Cell Biology, University of North Carolina at Chapel Hill, School of Medicine, Chapel Hill, North Carolina 27599

Wande Li (81), Department of Microbiology, Boston University School of Medicine, Boston, Massachusetts 02118

William J. Lindblad (270), Department of Pharmaceutical Sciences, Wayne State University, Detroit, Michigan 48202

B. Lombardi (415), Department of Pathology, School of Medicine, University of Pittsburgh, Pittsburgh, Pennsylvania 15621

Walter Malorni (58), Laboratory of Ultrastructures, Istituto Superiore di Sanita, Roma, Italy

Sharon J. McGuinness (108), Department of Anesthesiology, College of Medicine, University of Arizona, Tucson, Arizona 85724

Michael J. Meredith (258), Department of Biochemistry, School of Dentistry, Oregon Health Sciences University, Portland, Oregon 97201

D. A. G. Mickle (407), Department of Clinical Biochemistry, The Toronto Hospital, Toronto, Ontario, Canada, M5G 2C4

Francesca Mirabelli (58), Department of Experimental Medicine, and Oncology, Institute of General Pathology, Universita Degli Studi di Torino, 10125 Torino, Italy

Leon Moore (121), Department of Pharmacology, Uniformed Services University of the Health Sciences, Bethesda, Maryland 20814

Sidney D. Nelson (340), Department of Medicinal Chemistry, University of Washington, Seattle, Washington 98195

Pierluigi Nicotera (23), Department of Toxicology, Karolinska Institutet, S-104-01 Stockholm, Sweden

Anna-Liisa Nieminen (438), Department of Cell Biology and Anatomy, Laboratories for Cell Biology, University of North Carolina at Chapel Hill, Chapel Hill, North Carolina 27599

Alistair Nunn (228), Department of Medicine, Royal Postgraduate Medical School, Hammersmith Hospital, London, England

Michael J. Olson (152), Biomedical Science Department, General Motors Corporation, NAO Research and Development Center, Warren, Michigan 48090

Stan Orrenius (23), Department of Toxicology, Karolinska Institutet, S-104-01 Stockholm, Sweden

Youngja Park (140), Department of Biochemistry, and Winship Cancer Center, Emory University School of Medicine, Atlanta, Georgia 30322

Chris I. Pogson (248), Biochemical Sciences, Wellcome Research Laboratories, Beckenham, Kent BR3 3BS, United Kingdom

Kurt Randerath (201), Department of Pharmacology, Baylor College of Medicine, Houston, Texas 77030

Richard O. Recknagel[1] (400), Department of Physiology and Biophysics, School of Medicine, Case Western Reserve University, Cleveland, Ohio 44106

M. Vijayaraj Reddy (201), Environmental and Health Sciences Laboratory, Mobil Oil Corporation, Princeton, New Jersey 08543

Jeffrey M. Reece (438), Department of Cell Biology and Anatomy, Laboratories for Cell Biology, University of North Carolina at Chapel Hill, School of Medicine, Chapel Hill, North Carolina 27599

Donald J. Reed (421), Department of Biochemistry and Biophysics, and Environmental Health Sciences Center, Oregon State University, Corvallis, Oregon 97331

Zbigniew Rymaszewski (164), Department of Internal Medicine, University of Cincinnati College of Medicine, Cincinnati, Ohio 45267

Rick G. Schnellmann (128), Department of Physiology and Pharmacology, College of Veterinary Medicine, The University of Georgia, Athens, Georgia 30602

Stephen B. Shears (328), Laboratory of Cellular and Molecular Pharmacology, National Institute of Environmental Health Sciences, Research Triangle Park, North Carolina 27709

Hilary V. Sheevers (108), Department of Pharmacology and Toxicology, College of Pharmacy, University of Arizona, Tucson, Arizona 85724

N. H. Stacey (50), Research and Scientific Division, National Occupational Health and Safety Commission, The University of Sydney, New South Wales 2001, Australia

Andrew P. Thomas (287), Department of Pathology and Cell Biology, Thomas Jefferson University, Philadelphia, Pennsylvania 19107

[1]Deceased.

Benjamin F. Trump (1), Department of Pathology, University of Maryland, School of Medicine and Maryland Institute for Emergency Medical Services Systems, Baltimore, Maryland 21201

Fulvio Ursini (384), Department of Chemistry, School of Food Science, University of Udine, I-34100 Udine, Italy

Mariapia Vairetti (58), Second Institute of Pharmacology, University of Pavia, Pavia, Italy

Martin Vanderlaan (178), Biology and Biotechnology Research Program, Lawrence Livermore National Laboratory, University of California, Livermore, California 94551

Alison A. Welder (46), Division of Medicinal Chemistry and Pharmacodynamics, College of Pharmacy, The University of Oklahoma Health Sciences Center, Oklahoma City, Oklahoma 73190

Vincent L. Wilson (216), Molecular Genetics/Oncology, The Children's Hospital, University of Colorado School of Medicine, Denver, Colorado 80218

Andrew H. Wyllie (228), Department of Pathology, CRC Laboratories, University of Edinburgh Medical School, Edinburgh EH8 9AG, Scotland, United Kingdom

Tak Yee Aw (140), Department of Physiology and Biophysics, Louisiana State University Medical Center, Shreveport, Louisiana 71130

Glen B. Zamansky (81), Department of Microbiology, Boston University School of Medicine, Boston, Massachusetts 02118

Preface

In vitro technology has advanced so rapidly in recent years that now such technology is an accepted and valued research option for solving toxicological problems. Volume 1A, the inaugural volume in the *Methods in Toxicology* series, is a compilation of *in vitro* biological systems that are valuable tools for toxicologists in the field. Volume 1B is the sequel, covering toxicity indicators for use in conjunction with such *in vitro* systems, primarily for detecting and investigating cytotoxic injury.

In Volume 1B we have departed slightly from the format used in 1A. Section I, Perspectives, consists of three chapters instead of the usual, single introductory chapter to the volume. These Perspectives chapters were written by recognized authorities in the field to provide overviews of toxicity mechanisms that are of current interest to many researchers. The main goal of these chapters is to stimulate thought and provide a framework of reference for the toxicologist in formulating a hypothesis and designing experiments for the research problem at hand.

The remaining chapters describe diverse methods for detecting and monitoring critical events within cells that can occur as a result of a cytotoxic challenge. The chapters are arranged in the following sections based on sites of probable cytotoxicant action and types of response: Section II, Membrane Integrity and Function; Section III, Energy Metabolism; Section IV, DNA-Related Indices; Section V, Functional Indices; Section VI, Biochemical Indices; and Section VII, Lipid Peroxidation. Section VIII covers several specialized techniques that are also of interest and value but do not fall into the other categories.

In general, the chapters in Sections II through VIII review methods available for mechanistic studies and screening tests using *in vitro* systems and offer guidance on their selection. The chapters themselves vary in content. Some chapters are essentially reviews in cases where the choice of available indicators is the central issue (e.g., fluorescent indicators) and guidance for the reader is needed while others chapters address cases where the methods have already been well described and updated material and a theoretical treatment were considered to be of most value (e.g., chemiluminescence). Other chapters follow the traditional format for describing methods and procedures and are more detailed and limited in scope.

Decisions on how to focus each chapter were often made at the urging of Editors and Publisher and were not necessarily based on the desire of the writer. In these cases, we express our appreciation for their cooperation, as well as for the care and expertise of the authors and we hope the beneficiary is the reader. Finally, we thank Noriko Tyson and Barbara Frazier, without whose patience, sacrifice, and support this work and the preceding volume could not have been completed.

As a result of time pressure and other constraints, some important methodologies were not included in this volume. We recognize their importance and trust that they will be included in future volumes of *Methods in Toxicology* along with new methods that are being developed in this rapidly expanding field.

Charles A. Tyson and John M. Frazier

1

Cellular and Molecular Pathobiology of Reversible and Irreversible Injury

Benjamin F. Trump and Irene K. Berezesky

INTRODUCTION

The purpose of this chapter is to review the characteristics of reversible and irreversible injury to mammalian cells. It is of the utmost importance to consider this problem in detail, because the understanding of such reactions represents the basis of diagnosing reactions to toxic injury, and represents a reliable guide to the underlying mechanisms involved. Cell injury and cell death represent the fundamental basis of mammalian disease processes, and therefore constitute major problems in pathobiology. Cell death represents a major event in both normal and abnormal biology, as it is involved in the pathogenesis of disease (e.g., necrosis), in normal differentiation and development (e.g., programmed cell death), in aging, and in the killing of cells for the treatment of disease by chemotherapy, radiotherapy, and surgery.

DEFINITIONS

Cell Injury

Cell injury is defined as the result of a chemical or physical stimulus, either in excess or in deficiency, that transiently or permanently alters the homeostasis of the cell (Fig. 1). There is obviously a gray, and philosophically indeterminate, zone between physiological and pathological stimuli. From the standpoint of the cell, however, it must be recognized that in either case the stimulus may lead to altered homeostasis and ultimately cell death, which itself can be physiological or pathological from the point of view of the organism.

Classification of Injurious Stimuli

For many purposes stimuli may be classified as accidental (i.e., occurring as a result of environmental perturbations), either immediately, as in the case of acute chemical toxicity, or over a longer period, as in nutritional abnormalities which lead to atherosclerosis, and ultimately thrombosis and infarction. Other types

METHODS IN TOXICOLOGY, Volume 1B

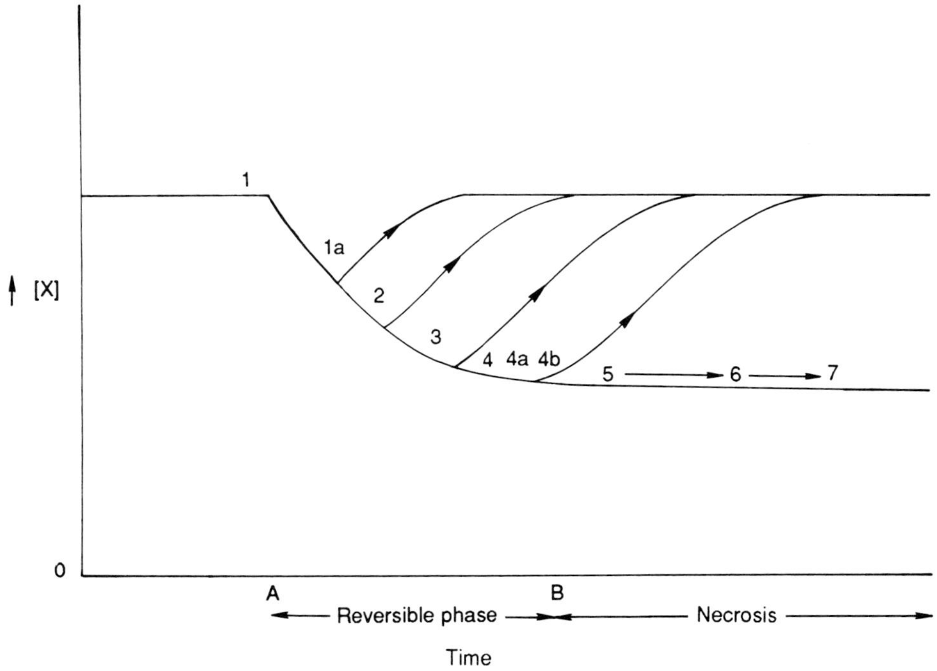

Figure 1 The sequence of events following application of an injury at point A. Either of two phases then takes place: a reversible phase or an irreversible phase (necrosis); the point of cell death is indicated by B. Arabic numerals along the curve refer to the stages of cell injury, which are reversible through stages 4a,b. Stages 5, 6, and 7 are irreversible, and may contain mitochondrial calcifications. Along the ordinate, the [x] indicates the concentration of a vital metabolite such as ATP. [Modified from Trump and Arstila (12) with the permission of Oxford University Press.]

can be regarded as "programmed" (1). These are stimuli which represent part of the normal physiology of the cell, as a part of development, normal turnover (as in the gastrointestinal tract), normal terminal differentiation [as in the case of keratinization in the skin (2)], or apoptosis resulting from alterations in hormone levels (3).

Responses to Injury

The disease process represents the response of cells to injury (Fig. 1). These responses are complex and form patterns of altered structure and function by which diseases are defined and understood. Responses to injury can be classified

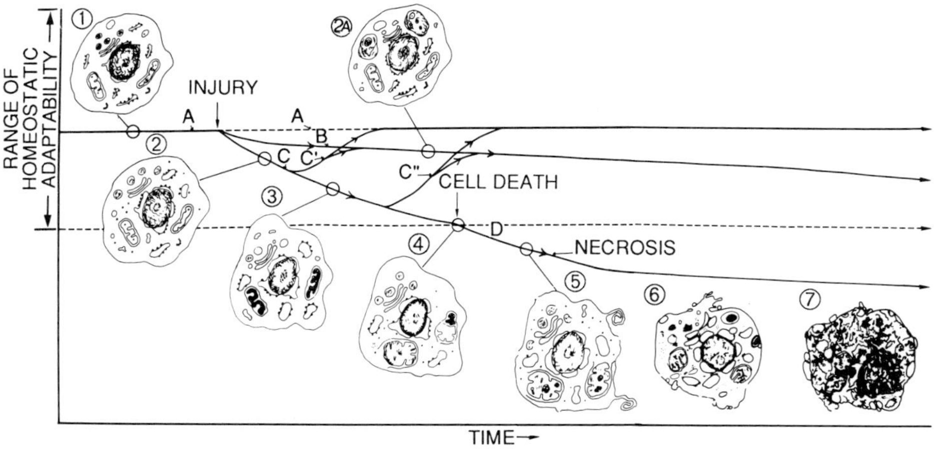

Figure 2 The stages of cell injury as described in the text. Stage 1 depicts a cell in a normal steady state (curve A). At the arrow, an injury is applied that may be acutely lethal or sublethal. In the case of a lethal injury, the cell loses homeostatic ability along curve C. Prior to the point of cell death, however, recovery can occur if the injurious stimulus is removed. Such recovery may then proceed along curve C′ or curve C″. Note that incomplete recovery during the reversible phases after lethal injury might also result in a new steady state, depicted by the right-hand limb of curves C′ and C″. [Modified from Trump and Arstila (12) with the permission of Oxford University Press.]

as reversible (i.e., the cell enters a temporary or long-term altered steady state, which does not lead to cell death) or irreversible, implying that the cell has passed a "point of no return" (4) and dies, undergoing various types of responses known as necrosis, apoptosis, and terminal differentiation. Figures 2–10 illustrate these responses (i.e., stages) and are discussed and referenced below.

Reversible Responses

Such responses may represent the early phase of irreversible injury (e.g., on the pathway leading to cell death, lasting from minutes to a few hours) or may be sustained, often called cellular adaptations, in which the cell achieves longer-term new steady states. Examples of this include hypertrophy of the endoplasmic reticulum (ER) following drugs and chemicals, which induce the cytochrome P450 system, or fatty metamorphosis (e.g., in hepatocytes following inhibition of protein synthesis). It has become evident in recent years that changes that occur during the reversible phase following a lethal injury, including ion deregulation and induction of immediate-early genes, may be responsible for such cells reentering the mitotic cycle, resulting in regeneration.

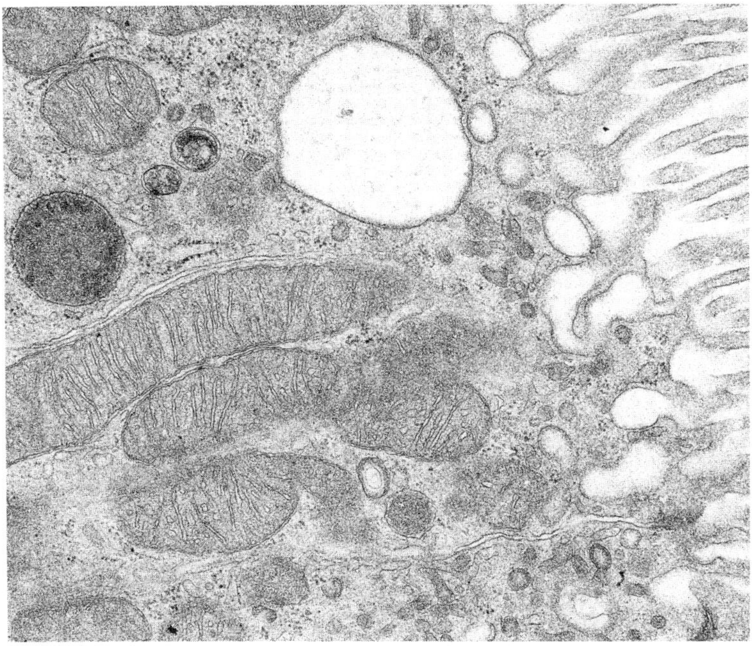

Figure 3 Transmission electron micrograph (TEM) of a portion of a stage 1 control proximal convoluted tubule (PCT) cell from a rat kidney *in vivo.* [Reproduced with permission from Trump *et al.* (26).]

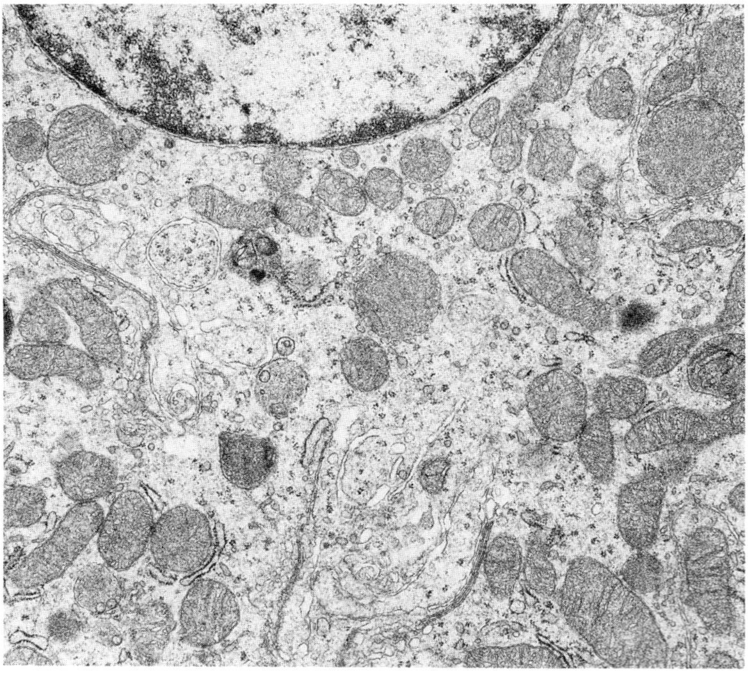

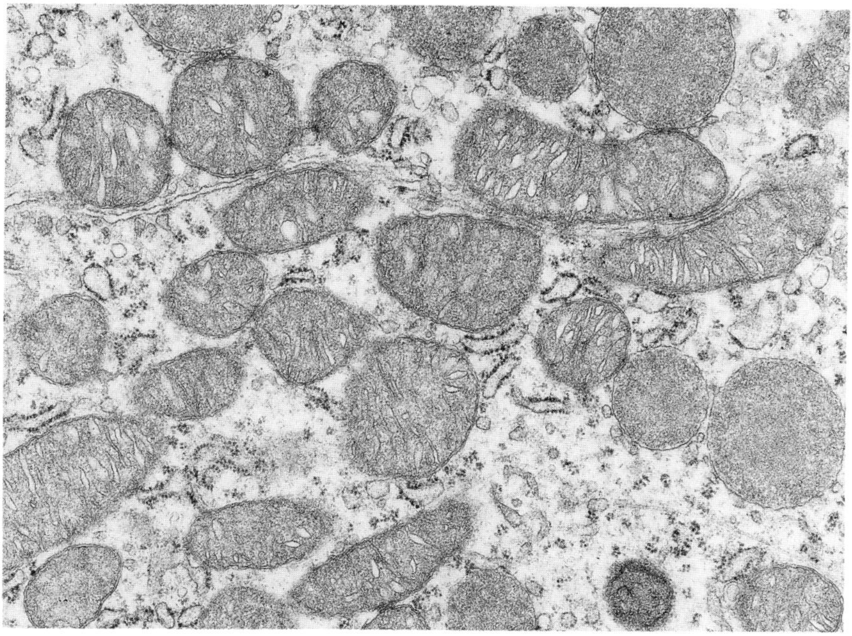

Figure 5 TEM of a portion of a stage 3 rat PCT cell following 15 min of *in vivo* ischemia. Note condensed mitochondria and slightly dilated ER. [Reproduced with permission from Trump *et al.* (26).]

Irreversible Responses

Irreversible responses refer to the cellular changes that occur following the "point of no return" and lead to equilibration with the environment. In this phase the changes are principally degradative, leading to interruption of membrane continuity and to the hydrolysis of phospholipids, proteins, and nucleic acids. The principal types of irreversible responses are necrosis, apoptosis, and terminal differentiation. As discussed below, in necrosis the organelles undergo a sequence of changes in the cell, beginning with changes in compartment volume, such as the cytosol, ER, and mitochondria, and ending with interruption of cell membrane continuity, formation of dense aggregates and/or calcifications in the mitochondria, and karyolysis.

In apoptosis (1,5) the earliest changes consist of cytoplasmic and nuclear blebbing, cell shrinkage, nuclear chromatin condensation and fragmentation,

Figure 4 TEM of a portion of a stage 2 PCT cell following 15 min of *in vivo* ischemia induced by clamping of the renal artery. Note slight enlargement or dilatation of the rough ER. [Reproduced with permission from Glaumann *et al.* (27).]

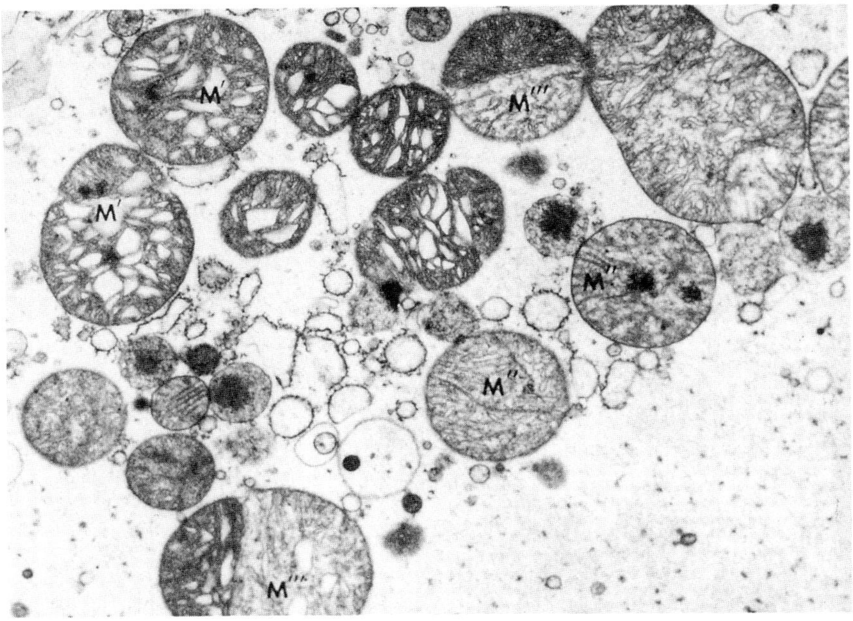

Figure 6 TEM of a portion of a rat PCT cell from a renal cortical slice incubated in Robinson's buffer at 4°C for 48 hr, illustrating three types of mitochondria. In the first type (M′) the matrix is markedly condensed, with expansion of intracristal spaces and flocculent densities. In the second type (M″) the inner compartments are expanded and contain flocculent densities. In the third type (M‴) both types of changes are present in the same mitochondrion, indicative of stage 4. [Reproduced with permission from Trump *et al.* (28).]

and often the early onset of DNA double-strand breaks in internucleosomal regions, giving the characteristic so-called "ladder" pattern in acrylamide gels. Ultimately, fragmentation of the entire cell occurs with sloughing or phagocytosis of the fragments. At the time of fragmentation, the cell fragments appear to be viable and then later to die, either in the phagolysosomal system of the phagocytizing cell or in the extracellular space.

In terminal differentiation, thus far best studied in the skin, the cells undergo progressive shrinkage, accumulation of intermediate filaments, which often become cross-linked, and karyolysis of the nuclei.

METHODS FOR DETERMINING REVERSIBLE AND IRREVERSIBLE RESPONSES TO INJURY

A number of methods have been used to define reversible or irreversible cell injury *in vivo* or *in vitro.* These methods vary in their ease of application and sensitivity and are briefly described below.

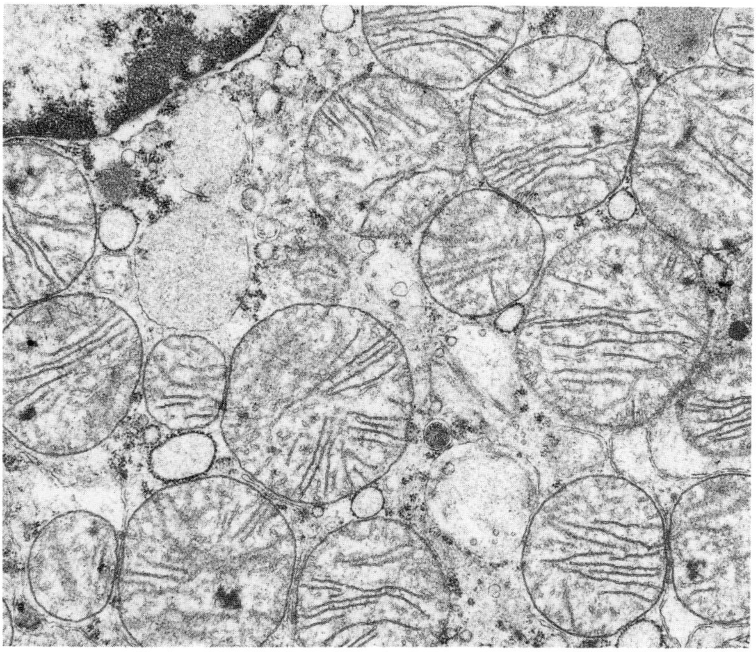

Figure 7 TEM of a portion of a stage 4b rat PCT cell following 60 min of *in vivo* ischemia. Note swollen mitochondria, some of which contain small dense aggregates. [Reproduced with permission from Glaumann *et al.* (27).]

Vital Dyes

These methods are based on the principle that many charged dyes are unable to penetrate and stain viable cells. Following loss of irreversibility, and therefore of plasma membrane integrity, these dyes enter the cell and stain both the nucleus and the cytoplasm. In the past the most commonly applied dyes, including trypan blue, erythrosin, and nigrosin, had chromophores which were visualized by absorption. More recently, sensitivity of detection and quantitation have been improved through the use of fluorescent dyes, such as propidium iodide, the iodoacetamides, the bromoacetamides, and 4′,6-diamidino-2-phenylindole HCl (DAPI), which bind to nuclear DNA (6). For *in vitro* studies these methods appear to be the most reliable for estimating viability and can be utilized in conjunction with other fluorescent dyes (e.g., Fura 2, which measures $[Ca^{2+}]_i$) to measure intracellular ions. Another principle recently used as a screening assay employs dyes, such as neutral red, which are normally taken up by the cells and stored in lysosomes (7). Following lethal injury, the dye is released into the extracellular fluid. By utilizing this assay in conjunction with microtiter plates and plate readers, it is now possible to screen large numbers of cells quantitatively

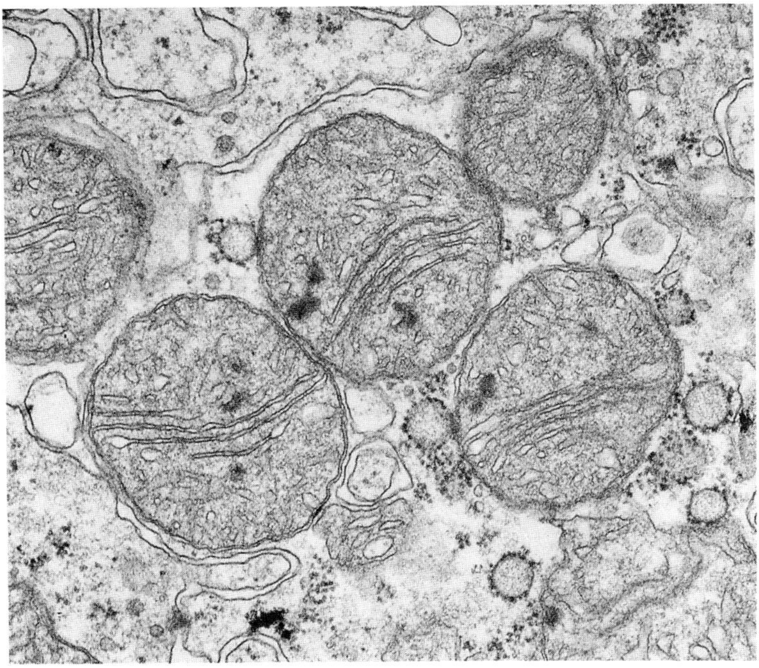

Figure 8 TEM of a portion of a stage 5 rat PCT cell following 120 min of *in vivo* ischemia. All mitochondria exhibit marked swelling and most contain large flocculent densities, the hallmark of irreversibility. [Reproduced with permission from Trump *et al.* (26).]

in a rapid fashion. Similar use of fluorescence combined with automotive plate readers has also been used for fluorescent vital dyes, such as propidium iodide.

Enzyme Release

Release of enzymes, especially from the cytosol, but also in some cases from lysosomes, constitutes another assay both *in vivo* and *in vitro.* The same principle, namely, interruption of plasma membrane continuity as mentioned for vital dyes, applies here. Such enzymes include lactate dehydrogenase, creatine kinase, SGPT, and SGOT.[1] These methods can be applied *in vivo,* and the use of isoenzymes may permit some estimation of specific organ involvement. Although such methods are readily quantitated, they are population based, and it now appears that release is readily possible from sublethally altered cells, probably due

[1] SGPT, Serum glutamic–oxaloacetic transaminase; SGOT, serum glutamate pyruvate transaminase.

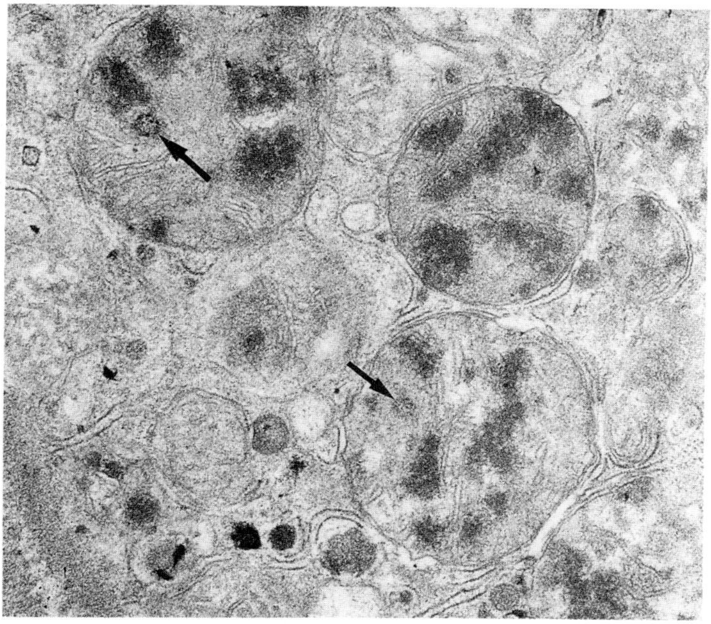

Figure 9 TEM of a portion of a stage 5c rat PCT cell following 120 min of *in vivo* ischemia followed by 24 hr of reflow. Note the swollen mitochondria with large flocculent densities, some of which contain calcifications (arrows). [Reproduced with permission from Trump *et al.* (26).]

to cytoplasmic blebbing, with pinching off of the blebs, and release of the enzyme to the cell remaining viable (8).

Chromium Release

Release of ^{51}Cr, prebound to the cell plasma membrane, has been used to estimate plasma membrane irreversible damage. However, this method has been shown to have several disadvantages in hepatocyte suspensions (9), and therefore has recently been superseded by fluorescence methods (10), which may or may not be reliable alternatives.

Morphology

Morphological techniques are extremely valuable methods for assessing the presence and type of reversible and irreversible injury. Because of numerous detailed studies correlating morphology with the other methods mentioned above,

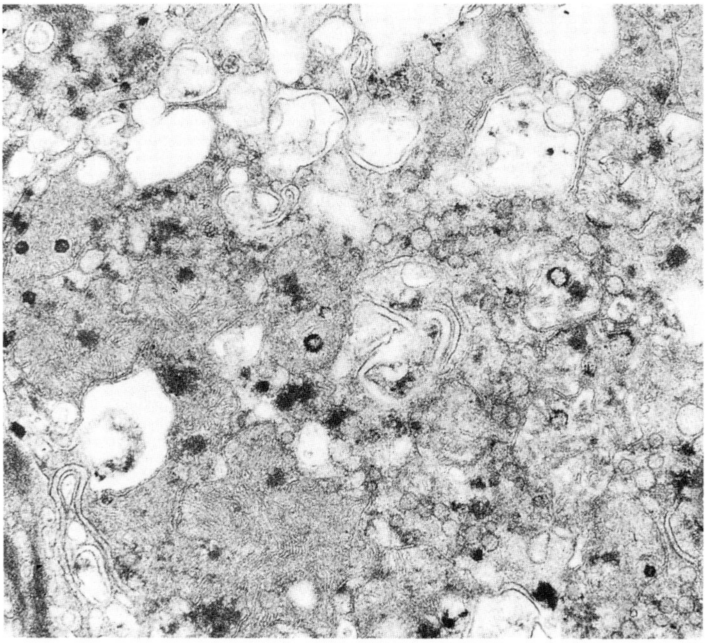

Figure 10 TEM of a portion of a stage 7 rat PCT cell following 60 min of *in vivo* ischemia followed by 24 hr of reflow. Disrupted organelles are seen with swollen mitochondria containing flocculent densities and some calcifications. [Reproduced with permission from Glaumann and Trump (31), Studies on the pathogenesis of ischemic cell injury. III. Morphological changes of the proximal pars recta tubules (P_3) of the rat kidney made ischemic *in vivo. Virchows Arch. B* **19**, 303–323 (1975).]

it is now possible to define the extent, distribution, and type of prelethal and lethal injury by light and electron microscopy. Light-microscopic studies of fixed and embedded tissues can readily estimate the amount of distribution of irreversible injury in any organ; however, in general, changes—such as increased eosinophilia, nuclear chromatin clumping and karyolysis, karyorrhexis, and pyknosis—are relatively late, but still provide essential information in many investigations.

Electron-microscopic criteria, as based on our classification of ultrastructural alterations into various stages (4,11–13) (e.g., the presence of flocculent densities and/or calcifications in mitochondria and interruptions in cell membrane continuity) (Fig. 2), can serve as excellent markers of cell death. Figures 3 through 10 illustrate some of these stages, and detailed descriptions are given in the legends.

Changes in Intracellular Ions

Ion deregulation, particularly intracellular ionized calcium ($[Ca^{2+}]_i$), has been found to play a pivotal role both in the initiation (reversible) and maintenance

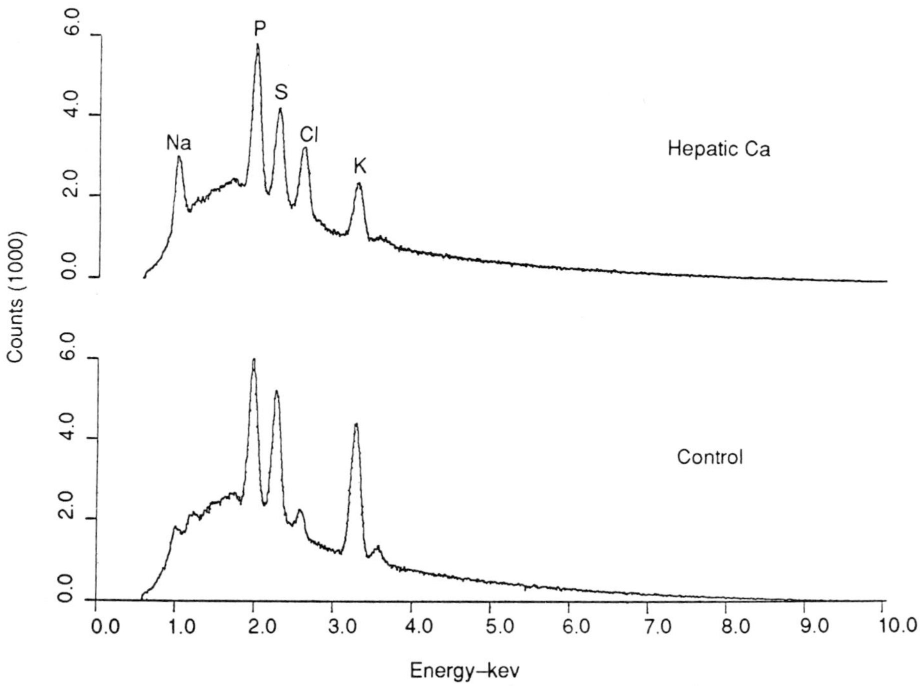

Figure 11 Typical energy-dispersive X-ray microanalysis spectra taken over freeze-dried 5-μm cryosections of control and tumor livers from mice following 75 weeks of dietary exposure to 0.4% (w/w) safrole in corn oil. Note the increases in sodium and chlorine and the decrease in potassium in the tumor. Calcium is also increased, but its small peak is obscured by the K β-peak. [Reproduced with permission from Trump *et al.* (29).]

(reversible–irreversible) phases of cell injury (14–19). Therefore, characterization of these ions is very important. Methods such as atomic absorption and energy-dispersive X-ray microanalysis (Fig. 11) have been widely used in the past to indicate early, usually reversible, cell injury through the measurement of decreases in total K^+, increases in Na^+ and Cl^-, and increases in cell water. Such changes in ion and cell water levels are often correlated with decreased ATP concentration, all occur early, and all are good indicators of reversible cell injury. Thus, when they are correlated with various methods such as the vital dye assays mentioned above, one can estimate the time course of reversible and then irreversible injury. This area has been greatly facilitated in recent years by the development of fluorescent probes, such as Fura 2 (20), for the measurement of $[Ca^{2+}]_i$ in single living cells grown in culture (Figs. 12–17). Similar probes have also been developed for $[Na^+]_i$, $[K^+]_i$, $[Mg^{2+}]_i$, and pH_i. These fluorescent dyes can also be used to estimate cell death following irreversible injury, as they are rapidly lost from dead cells.

Figures 12–15 Ratioed digital imaging fluorescence microscopy images displayed in pseudocolor to indicate $[Ca^{2+}]_i$ concentrations ranging from ~100 nm (color ramp blue) to >2 μM (color ramp white). Fura 2 images were captured at 340- and 380-nm excitation wavelengths, using a filter cube to eliminate transmission below 420 nm and allowing emission at 510 ± 20 nm.

Figure 12 (a–d) Ratioed images of a Fura 2-loaded rat primary tubule epithelial (PTE) cell and PTE cells after treatment with xanthine/xanthine oxidase (500 μM/10 mU/ml) in normal (1.37 mM) calcium in the cell medium. Note the gradual rise in $[Ca^{2+}]_i$, which then becomes quite high by 40 min. (a) 0 time; (b) 10 min; (c) 20 min; (d) 40 min. [Reproduced with permission from Swann *et al.* (30).]

Figure 13 (a–d) Ratioed images of a Fura 2-loaded cultured rat control hepatocyte and hepatocytes treated with KCN (25 mM) and iodoacetic acid (IAA) (1 mM) in normal (1.37 mM) calcium to mimic chemical ischemia. $[Ca^{2+}]_i$ rises at different times in different cells. When $[Ca^{2+}]_i$ reaches ~300 nm, bleb formation occurs. By 14 min, $[Ca^{2+}]_i$ reaches its maximum and blebs are obvious. (a) 0 time; (b) 5 min; (c) 7.5 min; (d) 14 min. [Reproduced with permission from B. F. Trump, I. K. Berezesky, and M. W. Smith, *in* "Methods in Toxicology" (D. P. Jones and L. H. Lash, eds.), Vol. 2, pp. 337–353. Academic Press, San Diego, 1993.]

Figure 14 (a–f) Ratioed images of a Fura 2-loaded rabbit primary cultured PTE control cell and PTE cells treated with 50 μM $HgCl_2$ in normal (1.37 mM) calcium. $[Ca^{2+}]_i$ rises steadily and by 14 min is high and blebs are present. (a) 0 time; (b) 12 min; (c) 14.75 min; (d) 16 min. Images (e) and (f) are gray-tone fluorescent images acquired at 340-nm excitation, demonstrating Fura 2 distribution and clearly illustrating the presence of blebs. (e) 14.75 min; (f) 16 min. [Reproduced with permission from M. W. Smith, P. C. Phelps, and B. F. Trump, Cytosolic Ca^{2+} deregulation and blebbing after $HgCl_2$ injury to cultured rabbit proximal tubule cells as determined by digital imaging microscopy. *Proc. Natl. Acad. Sci. U.S.A.* **88,** 4926–4930 (1991).]

Figure 15 (a–f) Ratioed images of Fura 2-loaded human colon adenocarcinoma (LYc5) control cells and cells after exposure to 6 μM ionomycin. (Results of peak $[Ca^{2+}]_i$ elevation are used for calibrating $[Ca^{2+}]_i$ by insertion as R_{max} in the Grynkiewicz (20) equation.) $[Ca^{2+}]_i$ rises rapidly and approaches maximum at 6 min. Blebs are also present at 6 min and increase in size with time. (a) 0 time; (b) 1 min; (c) 6 min; (d) 15 min. Images (e) and (f) are phase-contrast images taken at 7.5 and 20 min, respectively, and show the presence of numerous blebs. (Courtesy of P. C. Phelps.)

Figure 16 Rat PTE cells loaded with rhodamine-123. Cells were viewed with a Zeiss photomicroscope III adapted for epifluorescence using a fluorescein isothiocyanate (FITC) filter set. (a) Control cells showing highly fluorescent strandlike mitochondria. 690×. (b) Cells following 18-min exposure to 50 μM $HgCl_2$ in normal (1.37 mM) calcium. Mitochondria continue to retain rhodamine-123, and therefore to maintain their membrane potential; however, their shape is altered and appears globular. 430×. [Reproduced with permission from Trump *et al.* (18).]

(*legends continue*)

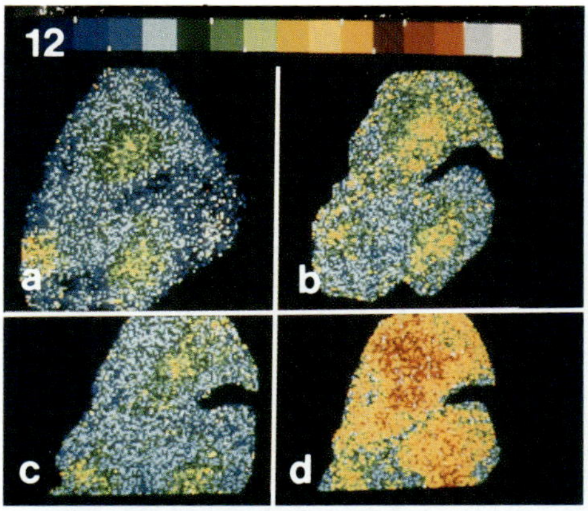
12
a
b
c
d

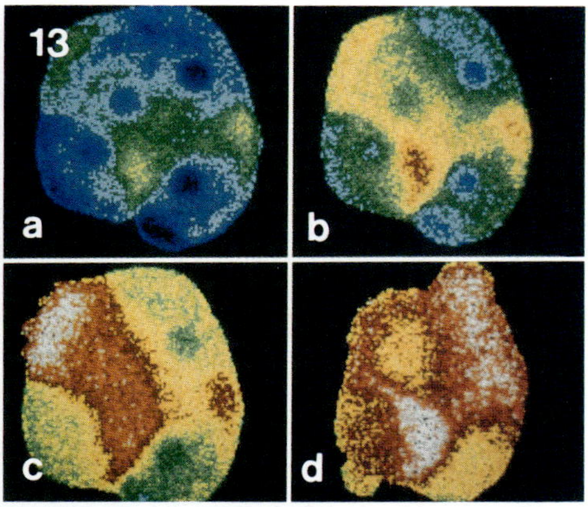
13
a
b
c
d

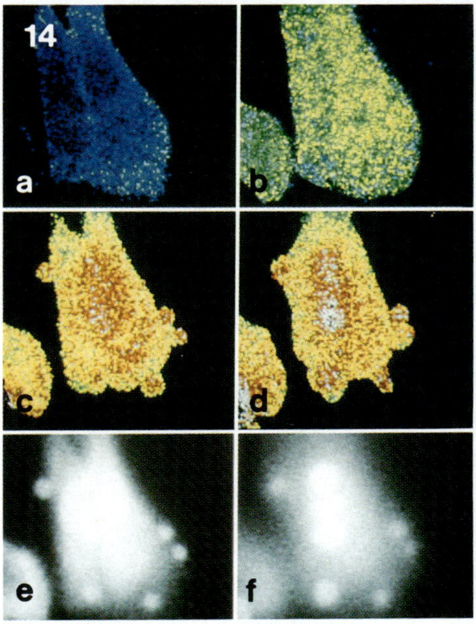
14
a
b
c
d
e
f

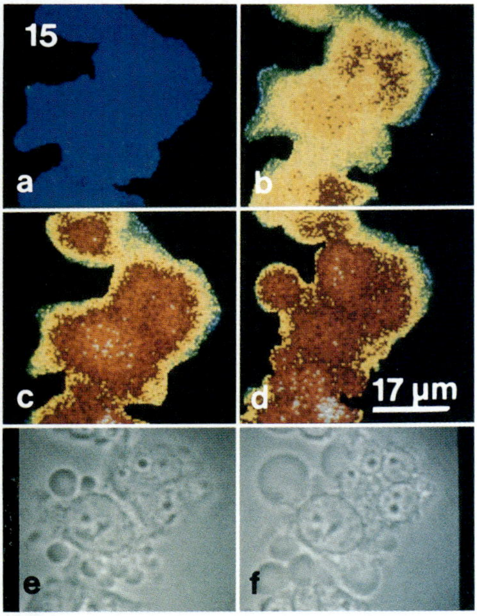
15
a
b
c
d
17 µm
e
f

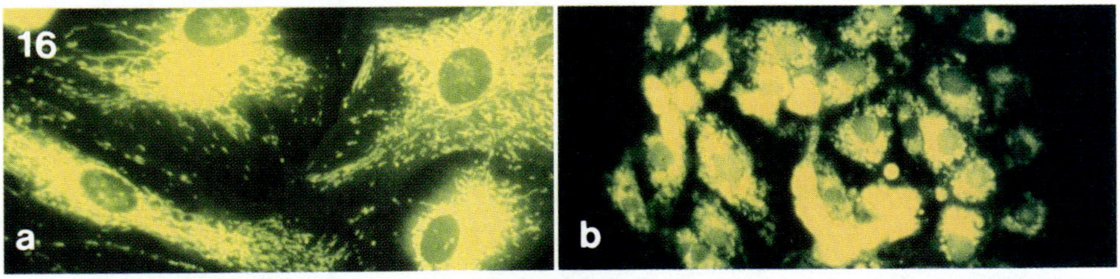
16
a
b

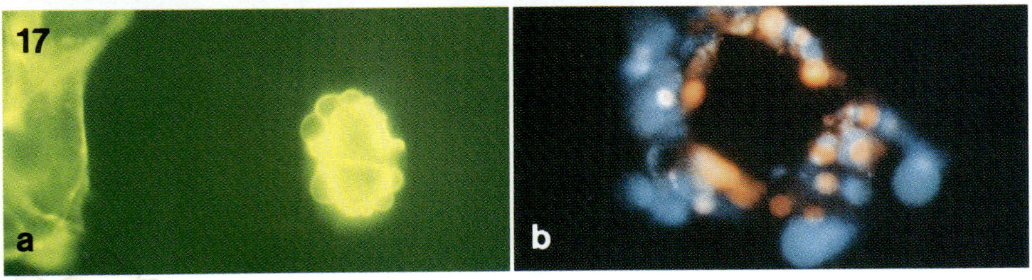
17
a
b

Cell Replication

Methods for measuring cell replication have been widely used in certain areas of investigation, including studies of the effects of radiation therapy and chemotherapy. These are based on estimating the rates of cell replication, including clonal growth rate. Growth rates have the advantage of being readily quantifiable and can yield dose–response curves; however, they suffer from the false assumption that cells that are unable to divide are irreversibly injured, which is clearly not the case. Many cells, including neurons and adult cardiac myocytes, are quite viable but are unable to divide. Thus, these methods should not be used to estimate cell death, but cytostasis produced by various conditions.

SUBCELLULAR CHARACTERISTICS OF REVERSIBLE INJURY

A variety of organelle structural and functional changes have been identified as reversible injury. These range from changes found in the prelethal phase after a lethal injury, such as a chemical toxin or ischemia, to chronic changes representing new steady states or cellular adaptations. In this and the following sections, we discuss some of the principal changes; obviously, space constraints preclude a thorough description of any one category.

Plasma Membrane

The plasma membrane and surrounding cytoplasm undergo many conformational changes. Among the most striking in the prelethal phase is the formation of cytoplasmic blebs (8), which occur around the cellular periphery in cells in suspension or along free margins, such as lumens *in vivo* (Figs. 18 and 19). These are associated with changes in the underlying cytoskeleton, including actin, actin-binding proteins, and tubulin (Fig. 17a) (21). The blebs increase in

Figure 17 Rat PTE cells stained with fluorescein phalloidin after 6-min exposure to 100 μM $HgCl_2$ in normal (1.37 mM) calcium. Cells were viewed with a Zeiss photomicroscope III adapted for epifluorescence using a FITC filter set. (a) No actin filaments are seen in the cytoplasm or the interior of the blebs; however, there is a clear band of fluorescent staining around each cell and their blebs. 700 ×. [Reproduced with permission from Elliget *et al.* (21).] (b) Rat PTE cells preloaded with Fura 2 in the presence of propidium iodide 40 min after exposure to 50 μM $HgCl_2$ in normal (1.37 mM) calcium. Cells were viewed with a Zeiss photomicroscope III adapted for epifluorescence using a broad-band ultraviolet filter set. The blue staining represents Fura 2 in the cells or blebs, and the orange staining represents dead cells which have taken up propidium iodide. 690 ×. [Reproduced with permission from Trump *et al.* (18).]

size, often seal off at the base, and detach into the extracellular space. Many other types of prelethal changes in the plasma membrane, such as microvilli distortion, and changes in basal and laminal infoldings are also commonly observed.

Endoplasmic Reticulum and Golgi Apparatus

In prelethal acute injury these organelle systems undergo changes in volume with dilatation of the cisternae. This dilatation can be so extreme as to cause large vacuoles in the cytoplasm (e.g., the hydropic changes seen after acute carbon tetrachloride hepatic toxicity) and is usually associated with loss of polysome patterns and detachment of ribosomes from the ER surface. The Golgi apparatus can undergo similar changes, including dispersion of saccules. Some of these changes are associated with ion redistribution; others, with defective

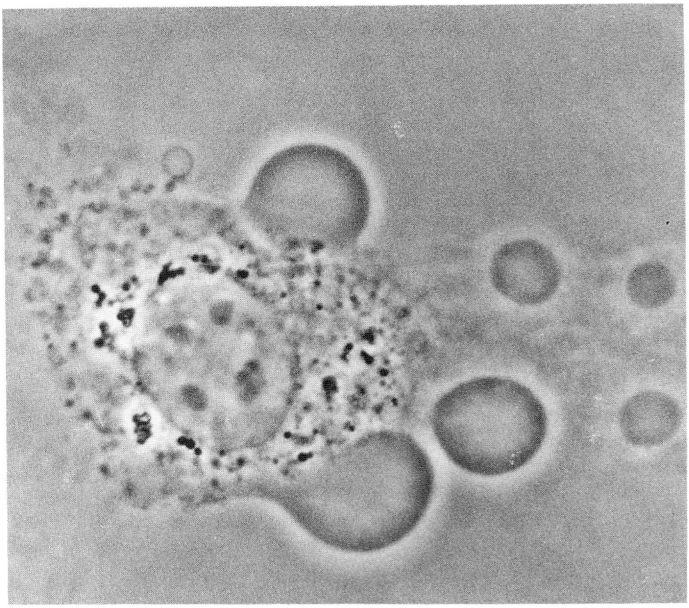

Figure 18 Phase-contrast micrograph of a JB6 keratinocyte (clone 41) *in vitro* following exposure to $10^{-4}M$ sodium lauryl sulfate for 15 min. Note the early bleb formation at its periphery. Mitochondria are rounded and there is nuclear clumping. 1700×. [Reproduced with permission from P. T. Jain, M. J. Fitzpatrick, P. C. Phelps, I. K. Berezesky, and B. F. Trump, *Toxicol. Pathol.* **20,** 394–404, 1992.]

protein synthesis. One commonly observed adaptive change of the ER, which is prelethal or nonlethal, is the pronounced hypertrophy seen after cytochrome P-450 induction.

Cytoskeleton

Alterations in the cytoskeleton are undoubtedly very important in prelethal injury, resulting in cytoplasmic blebbing as mentioned above, in redistribution of membrane proteins, and in changes in organelle mobility. Such changes may also be involved in transmembrane signaling and control of gene expression.

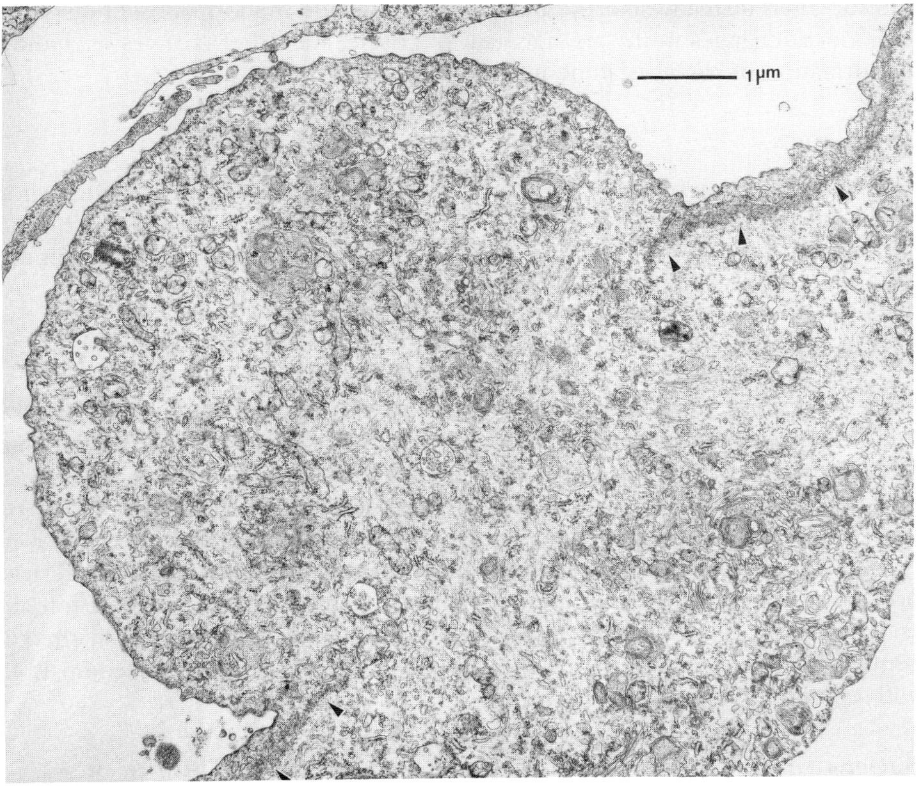

Figure 19 TEM of a rabbit primary PTE monolayer culture cell exposed *in vitro* to 50 μM $HgCl_2$ for 3 min at 37°C with low Ca^{2+} in the medium. Bands of fine filaments resembling actin are present at the border edges of a bleb (arrowheads). 28,000×. (Courtesy of P. C. Phelps.)

Cytosol

Expansion and dilution of the cytosol are commonly observed in the early phases associated with changes in Na^+ and water content.

Mitochondria

Changes in mitochondrial structure and function occur early during the reversible phase. These include loss of mitochondrial matrix granules, condensation of the matrix (see Fig. 5), and swelling involving the inner compartment. Such changes are associated with decreased levels of ATP synthesis, but maintenance of mitochondrial membrane potential is preserved. These changes are readily reversed, as is the ATP depletion, following removal of the injury. Chronic altered steady states of mitochondria include the formation of megamitochondria, changes in the arrangement of cristae, and other changes, including the formation of paracrystalline intramatrical inclusions.

Peroxisomes

Early changes in peroxisomal structure and function include swelling and pallor of the peroxisomal matrix. Again, these are readily reversed. Among the chronic adaptive changes resulting from toxic injury is proliferation of peroxisomes, which may have a role in preneoplasia and oxidative stress.

Lysosomes

Many reversible changes in lysosomes have been described. Following prelethal injury the lysosomes become pale, slightly swollen, and more fragile upon tissue homogenization, representing an early indicator of injury. Furthermore, loss of lysosomal enzymes, such as *N*-acetylglucosaminidase in the urine from the proximal tubule, can represent signs of early prelethal injury. Chronic changes in lysosomes commonly involve lysosomal overload, either with watery materials, producing vacuoles (as in administration of mannitol, sucrose, or nitrilotriacetate in the kidney), or with protein, forming hyaline droplets (as in the recently characterized hyaline droplet nephropathy). All of these are compatible with continued cell survival.

Nucleus

Early reversible changes in nuclear morphology consist of chromatin clumping and clearing of the nuclear matrix. This occurs during the early stages of both necrosis and apoptosis. Such changes can be associated with single- or double-strand breaks at internucleosomal regions, being characteristic of the pattern described as apoptosis. At this time in reversibly injured cells or in the prelethal phase, there is increased expression of immediate-early genes, such as c-*fos,* c-*jun,* and c-*myc* (22–24), followed later by stress genes such as *hsp70* (24) and metallothionein.

SUBCELLULAR CHARACTERISTICS OF IRREVERSIBLE INJURY

The following alterations are characteristics of irreversible injury. These may vary to some extent with cell type and injury; however, a remarkable similarity exists among most mammalian cell types. Furthermore, the details of the progression vary between apoptosis and necrosis, as discussed further below.

Plasma Membrane

After the stage of blebbing, mentioned in the discussion of the reversible phase, a variety of changes occur in the configuration and integrity of the cell membrane. Characteristic of the early period of irreversible injury is the presence of multiple interruptions in the continuity of the cell membrane. This is associated with distortion of specializations, such as microvilli. Later in the necrotic phase, myelin figures and whorls, formed by derivatization of the plasmalemma, can be observed. At this stage the plasma membrane is freely permeable to vital dyes or to escape of cytosolic enzymes.

Endoplasmic Reticulum and Golgi Apparatus

Dilatation of the ER often continues, but is now associated with extensive fragmentation and vesiculation. Ultimately, the rough ER becomes entirely free of polysomes. The Golgi apparatus continues to disintegrate, ultimately becoming indistinguishable from ER fragments (see Fig. 7).

Cytoskeleton

Destabilization of virtually all elements of the cytoskeleton occurs, including actin, actin-associated proteins, tubulin, and intermediate filaments. In addition, detachment from cell membrane proteins occurs and marked changes in relationships of cell shape are evident. In the case of terminal differentiation, especially in the skin, new types of intermediate filaments with keratin of high molecular weight occur; this is associated with cross-linking and formation of cross-linked envelopes at the cell periphery. This appears to be the mechanism by which these cells can retain shape and not undergo lysis following death, due to stabilization of these envelopes through the transglutamase reaction at the cell periphery.

Mitochondria

At this phase the swollen mitochondria undergo a major alteration in the matrix, including the formation of flocculent densities and/or calcifications (see Figs. 8–10). The latter represent precipitates of calcium phosphate, first amorphous and then crystalline, in the form of hydroxyapatite. The flocculent densities are enlarged amorphous aggregates of denatured protein in the mitochondrial matrix (25) and signal the "point of no return." This is an extremely important morphological criterion which occurs at the time of cell death. Mitochondrial calcification, which is an active process, occurs only in types of injury that do not primarily interfere with mitochondrial membrane potential, such as damage to the plasma membrane. These include $HgCl_2$ or carbon tetrachloride toxicity, activation of complement, or mechanical trauma (for reviews see Refs. 11–13).

Peroxisomes

Peroxisomes continue to swell and ultimately lyse, with disappearance of the central core in organs such as the liver and the kidney. This is associated with modification of peroxisomal enzymes, including catalase.

Lysosomes

Lysosomal swelling continues, with clarification of the matrix and remarkable fragility. Ultimately, lysosomal enzymes are released, resulting in further degradation in other cytoplasmic, as well as nuclear, compartments.

Nucleus

The nuclear changes continue to progress, in some cases leading to total degradation of chromatin, so-called "karyolysis," seen in necrosis and apoptosis. There is condensation, compaction (pyknosis), or fragmentation (karyorrhexis).

CONCLUSIONS

As mentioned earlier, there are many cellular, subcellular, and molecular changes that occur during the course of sublethal and lethal injury. Of particular emphasis in this chapter are those that follow an acute injury that is destined to be lethal. Such an injury can lead to a variety of early and reversible changes, but also ultimately to cell death.

At the present time cell death is considered to be immediate or delayed. Examples of immediate cell death are rapid freezing, chemical fixation (e.g., glutaraldehyde or osmium tetroxide), or mechanical damage (e.g., tissue homogenization). These types of cell killing are normally not seen *in vivo;* however, they are induced by the observer to perform morphological or biochemical analyses.

It is delayed cell death that is usually observed following toxicity *in vivo.* This category includes necrosis, apoptosis followed by necrosis, and terminal differentiation. Each of these types of cell death is characterized by irreversible loss of plasma membrane continuity, resulting in the release of cytosolic enzymes, and in the uptake of so-called "vital dyes," such as trypan blue, nigrosin, and propidium iodide. In the case of necrosis or apoptosis followed by necrosis, the cells eventually undergo lysis and degradation. In the case of terminal differentiation, especially in the skin, the process of terminal differentiation is accompanied by cross-linking of intermediate filaments, forming a resistant barrier beneath the plasma membrane, which prevents lysis. In the case of other cells exhibiting terminal differentiation and ultimately cell death, such as the polymorphonuclear leukocyte, the ciliated cell in the respiratory epithelium, and the neuron, the ultimate process of cell death at the present time appears similar to the changes described with necrosis.

Ion deregulation, especially that of $[Ca^{2+}]_i$, has been shown to play a pivotal role and is involved in several types of cell death and differentiation, though in slightly different ways. As illustrated in Fig. 20, which diagrammatically represents the possible effects of such deregulation based on data obtained not only in our own laboratory but also in those of other investigators, deregulation of $[Ca^{2+}]_i$ can initiate a variety of intracellular changes. These include, but are not limited to, alterations of the cytoskeleton and cytoskeletal membrane interactions, which are key to blebbing in the early events in a variety of types of lethal injury, including those that lead to necrosis as well as apoptosis; deterioration of intracellular membranes, especially those of the inner mitochondrial membrane, leading to loss of mitochondrial membrane potential and irreversible loss of oxidative phosphorylation; and finally, interruption of plasma membrane continuity and function immediately preceding cell death.

In the case of terminal differentiation of keratinocytes, increased $[Ca^{2+}]_i$ appears to be important not only in the initiation of the process, but also in the terminal stages of intermediate filament cross-linking through the transglutaminase reaction. It is also important to note that some of the prelethal cellular changes are responsible for promoting differentiation, either temporary or permanent, or regeneration. In the latter case a sequence of signals must be involved, first leading to cell division, and later to redifferentiation. We have identified some of the events, including calcium-mediated gene activation of immediate-early genes, such as c-*fos,* c-*jun,* and c-*myc* (22–24), which may be involved with later signalling events leading toward cell division in some cases or toward cell differentiation in others (23). Furthermore, the same signals appear to initiate the transcription of genes such as *hsp70* (24) and metallothionein, which permit protection of the cell against further injury.

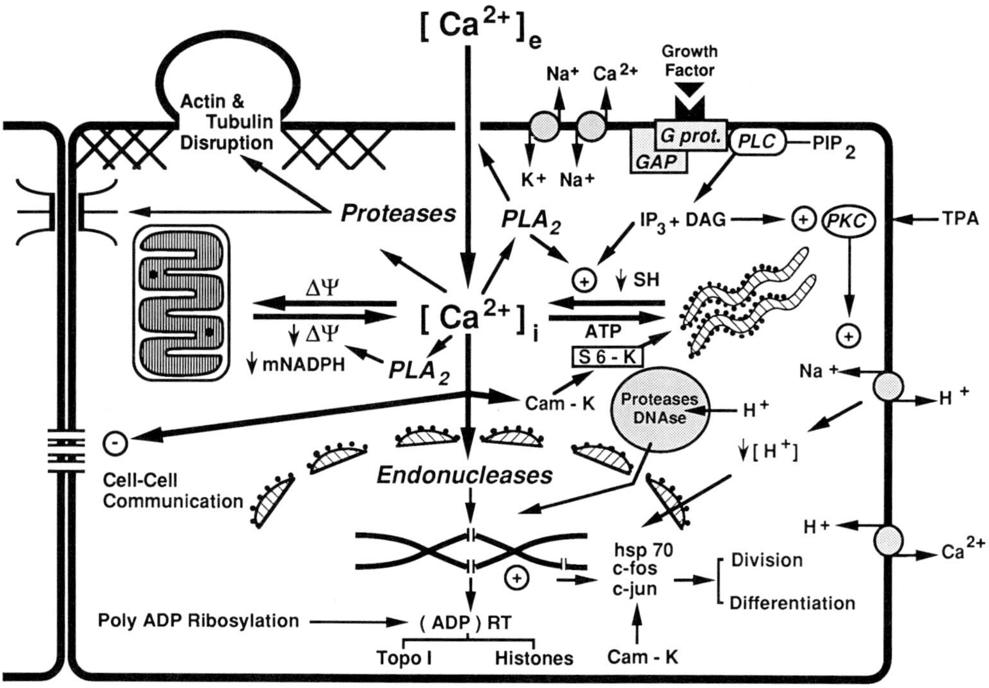

Figure 20 Representation of a cell illustrating our current working hypothesis concerning the role of $[Ca^{2+}]_i$ in cell injury (see text for details). GAP, G protein-activating protein; PLC, phospholipase C; PIP_2, phosphoinositol diphosphate; PLA_2, phospholipase A_2; IP_3, inositol triphosphate; DAG, diacylglycerol; PKC, protein kinase C; TPA, tetradecanoyl phorbol acetate; SH, sulfhydryls; S6-K, S6-kinase; Cam-K, calmodulin-kinase; RT, ribosyltransferase; Topo I, topoisomerase I; $\Delta\Psi$, membrane potential. [Reproduced with permission from Trump *et al.* (19).]

SUMMARY

Acute cell injury is followed by a sequence of events, some of which lead to cell death, while others are compatible with continued cell survival. Several types of cell death can be recognized, which are in two principal categories: immediate and delayed cell death. The cellular reactions to injury described above can be used to characterize reversible versus irreversible injury and to determine the type of cell death. In some cases the changes allow statements to be made concerning mechanisms. There is also a considerable body of data indicating that the initiation and progression of prelethal and lethal cell injury are based on the deregulation of $[Ca^{2+}]_i$, namely, that increases in $[Ca^{2+}]_i$ stimulate a sequence of events involving phospholipases, proteases, and endonucleases and that increased $[Ca^{2+}]_i$ is also capable of initiating immediate-early and stress gene expression.

Although much more experimentation is needed for clarification of these phenomena, such deregulation not only results in both the initiation (reversible) and maintenance (reversible–irreversible) phases of cell injury, but also relates to cell toxicity, cell injury, cell death, cell division, and cell differentiation.

ACKNOWLEDGMENTS

This work was supported by grants from the National Institutes of Health (DK15440) and the U.S. Navy, Office of Naval Research (N00014–91–J–1863). This is contribution No. 3271 from the Cellular Pathobiology Laboratory, University of Maryland School of Medicine, Baltimore.

REFERENCES

1. M. J. Arends and A. H. Wyllie, *Int. Rev. Exp. Pathol.* **32,** 223 (1991).
2. S. Yuspa, H. Hennings, R. Tucker, S. Jaken, A. Kilkenny, and D. Roop, *Ann. N.Y Acad. Sci.* **548,** 191 (1988).
3. A. H. Wyllie, *in* "Cell Death in Biology and Pathology" (I. D. Bowen and R. A. Lockshin, eds.), pp. 9–84. Chapman & Hall, London, 1981.
4. B. F. Trump and F. L. Ginn, *in* "Methods and Achievements in Experimental Pathology" (E. Bajusz and G. Jasmin, eds.), Vol. IV, pp. 1–29. Karger, Basel, 1969.
5. B. F. Trump and I. K. Berezesky, *Curr. Opin. Cell Biol.* **4,** 227 (1992).
6. R. P. Haugland, "Molecular Probes: Handbook of Fluorescent Probes and Research Chemicals." Molecular Probes, Eugene, Oregon, 1992.
7. E. Borenfreund and J. A. Puerner, *Toxicol. Lett.* **24,** 119 (1985).
8. P. C. Phelps, M. W. Smith, and B. F. Trump, *Lab. Invest.* **60,** 630 (1989).
9. C. A. Tyson and C. E. Green, "The Isolated Hepatocyte," pp. 119–130. Academic Press, Orlando, Florida, 1987.
10. M. Provinciali, G. DiStefano, and N. Fabris, *J. Immunol. Methods* **155,** 19 (1992).
11. B. F. Trump, B. P. Croker, Jr., and W. J. Mergner, *in* "Cell Membranes: Biological and Pathological Aspects" (G. W. Richter and D. G. Scarpelli, eds.), pp. 84–128. Williams & Wilkins, Baltimore, 1971.
12. B. F. Trump and A. U. Arstila, *in* "Principles of Pathobiology" (M. F. LaVia and R. B. Hill, Jr., eds.), pp. 9–95. Oxford University Press, New York, 1975.
13. B. F. Trump and I. K. Berezesky, *in* "Drug Metabolism and Drug Toxicity" (J. R. Mitchell and M. G. Horning, eds.), pp. 261–300. Raven, New York, 1984.
14. B. F. Trump, I. K. Berezesky, and P. C. Phelps, *Scanning Electron Microsc.* **2,** 434 (1981).
15. B. F. Trump and I. K. Berezesky, *Surv. Synth. Pathol. Res.* **4,** 248 (1985).
16. B. F. Trump and I. K. Berezesky, *Carcinogenesis* **8,** 1027 (1987).
17. B. F. Trump and I. K. Berezesky, *Comments Toxicol.* **3,** 47 (1989).
18. B. F. Trump, I. K. Berezesky, M. W. Smith, P. C. Phelps, and K. A. Elliget, *Toxicol. Appl. Pharmacol.* **97,** 6 (1989).
19. B. F. Trump, T. W. Jones, K. A. Elliget, M. W. Smith, P. C. Phelps, A. Maki, and I. K. Berezesky, *Renal Failure* **12,** 183 (1990).

20. G. Grynkiewicz, M. Poenie, and R. Y. Tsien, *J. Biol. Chem.* **260,** 3440 (1985).
21. K. A. Elliget, P. C. Phelps, and B. F. Trump, *Cell Biol. Toxicol.* **7,** 263 (1991).
22. A. Maki, I. K. Berezesky, J. Fargnoli, N. J. Holbrook, and B. F. Trump, *FASEB J.* **6,** 919 (1992).
23. P. A. Cerutti and B. F. Trump, *Cancer Cells* **3,** 1 (1991).
24. N. Yamamoto, A. Maki, J. D. Swann, I. K. Berezesky, and B. F. Trump, *Renal Failure* **15,** 163 (1993).
25. Y. Collan, E. M. McDowell, and B. F. Trump, *Virchows Arch. B* **35,** 189 (1981).
26. B. F. Trump, I. K. Berezesky, K. U. Laiho, A. R. Osornio, W. J. Mergner, and M. W. Smith, *Scanning Electron Microsc.* **3,** 437 (1980).
27. B. Glaumann, H. Glaumann, I. K. Berezesky, and B. F. Trump, *Virchows Arch. B* **24,** 1 (1977).
28. B. F. Trump, J. M. Strum, and R. E. Bulger, *Virchows Arch. B* **16,** 1 (1974).
29. B. F. Trump, I. K. Berezesky, R. E. Pendergrass, S. H. Chang, R. E. Bulger, and W. J. Mergner, *Scanning Electron Microsc.* **2,** 1027 (1978).
30. J. D. Swann, M. W. Smith, P. C. Phelps, A. Maki, I. K. Berezesky, and B. F. Trump, *Toxicol. Pathol.* **19,** 128 (1991).
31. B. Glaumann and B. F. Trump, *Virchows Arch. B.* **19,** 303 (1975).

2 Molecular Mechanisms of Toxic Cell Death: An Overview

Pierluigi Nicotera and Sten Orrenius

INTRODUCTION

The interaction between toxicants and cell systems *in vitro* can result in the activation of a number of adverse reactions which can lead to cell death. Often, a cytotoxic reaction has a distinct threshold of activation which may differ among various cell types. Thus, it is tempting to speculate that, in a given system, the contribution of a cytotoxic mechanism is a function of its threshold of activation and the dose of the toxicant. However, in many instances more than one cytotoxic pathway is operative at the same time. The issue is further complicated by the tendency to generalize the role of a cytotoxic pathway based on studies in a single *in vitro* system. For example, cells which depend strictly on growth factors for survival are easily affected by agents which interfere with growth stimulation. In contrast, cells which can survive *in vitro* without trophic factors do not display the same sensitivity to this cytotoxic effect. Further, different cytotoxic mechanisms can also be recruited, depending on the dose of the toxicant. An example of this is the opposite effects of increasing levels of oxidation on protein kinase C activity: Exposure to mild oxidative stress can result in protein kinase C activation and cell proliferation, whereas the inhibition of protein kinase C activity at higher oxidant levels may promote cell death (see below).

After these few introductory notes of caution, we would like to draw the reader's attention to the fact that our knowledge of the molecular mechanisms involved in toxic cell killing has increased considerably in recent years. The understanding that physiological mechanisms can be responsible for the killing of cells exposed to toxic agents and the elucidation of the mechanisms involved in intracellular signal transduetion has emphasized the importance of possible interference of toxicants at low doses with cell signaling systems. Furthermore, the finding that an endogenous cell death program can be activated by an imbalance in cell signaling has indicated that interactions between toxicants and cell signaling systems may have implications for aging and carcinogenesis.

During the past several years we have studied the role of several cytotoxic mechanisms in cell killing. These include cytoskeletal alterations, mitochondrial dysfunction and energy deprivation, thiol modification, and perturbation of in-

METHODS IN TOXICOLOGY, Volume 1B

tracellular Ca^{2+} homeostasis with subsequent activation of degradative enzymes. More recently, we have become particularly interested in cytotoxic mechanisms activated as a consequence of an impairment of cell signaling. We have examined the potential implications of disturbances of intracellular Ca^{2+} signaling, such as those resulting from alteration of Ca^{2+} transport and from Ca^{2+} overload. Furthermore, we have devoted particular attention to the multiple signaling pathways which appear to be involved in the activation of programmed cell death, or apoptosis, in various experimental systems. Here, we give a brief overview of some of these mechanisms and their involvement in cell killing by toxic agents.

DISRUPTION OF CYTOSKELETAL ARCHITECTURE IN TOXIC CELL KILLING

One of the early events in cell injury caused by a variety of toxic conditions is the appearance of multiple surface protrusions, often referred to as "blebs" (1). The pathophysiology of bleb formation has not been fully elucidated, as several mechanisms probably participate independently, but it is generally accepted that a disruption of cytoskeletal organisation and of plasma membrane–cytoskeleton interaction plays a critical role. This is supported by the ultrastructural evidence of a marked reorganization of several cytoskeletal elements which accompanies the appearance of plasma membrane blebs (2) and by the demonstration that well-known cytoskeletal toxins, such as cytochalasins and phalloidin, cause bleb formation in a variety of cell types (3). A number of investigations have clearly demonstrated the importance of various Ca^{2+}-dependent events in the control of cytoskeletal organisation and function. Ca^{2+}-dependent cytoskeletal alterations include modification of the association between actin and actin-binding proteins, disturbances of microtubule organisation, and Ca^{2+}-dependent proteolysis of actin-binding proteins (4,5).

However, other mechanisms of cytoskeletal damage and bleb formation have also been implied in chemical injury. ATP depletion is probably sufficient to cause depolymerization of actin (6), breakdown of the actomyosin network (7), and a change in the lipid order of the plasma membrane (8). Oxidative stress induced by diamide or menadione in hepatocytes has been shown to cause the oxidation of thiol groups in actin and other cytoskeletal proteins, which results in the formation of protein aggregates and in the relocalization of microfilaments, generating weak sites in the periphery of the cell for potential bleb formation (9).

Finally, it is becoming clear that disturbances in protein phosphorylation may affect cytoskeletal structure. Several cytoskeletal proteins are substrates for phosphorylation catalyzed by kinases, and it has recently been reported that inhibition of cytoskeletal protein dephosphorylation can lead to rapid microfilament reorganization and blebbing in hepatocytes (10). These studies also suggested that an altered balance of protein kinase/protein phosphatase activity can result in abnormal phosphorylation of cytoskeletal, and possibly other, proteins, ultimately leading to cell death. Calyculin A, another inhibitor of protein phosphatases, has been found to cause enhanced phosphorylation of vimentin and 20-kDa myosin light chain in 3T3 fibroblasts and to promote their detachment from the substratum (11), providing further support for this proposal.

Several methodologies have been used in the study of cytoskeletal alterations induced by chemical toxicants, including isolation of cytoskeletal components and immunocytochemical investigations, light and electron microscopy, and, more recently, confocal microscopy.

MITOCHONDRIAL DAMAGE AND ENERGY DEPLETION

Work from several laboratories has indicated that mitochondrial damage may represent a common event in cell injury caused by a variety of toxic agents. Mitochondrial damage is initially manifested by a decrease in the mitochondrial membrane potential followed by ATP depletion. Protons are constantly pumped from the matrix into the intermembrane space in the mitochondria of living cells (12). Since the inner mitochondrial membrane is relatively impermeable to anions, a considerable proportion of the energy resulting from the proton concentration gradient is stored as membrane electric potential (13). The proton gradient and the transmembrane potential represent the electrochemical forces that are used for ATP synthesis as well as for other metabolic activities, including the maintenance of Ca^{2+} homeostasis within mitochondria. Ca^{2+} can be actively transported into mitochondria via an electrophoretic uniporter. The driving force for the continuous Ca^{2+} pumping is provided by the transmembrane potential. However, studies performed in isolated mitochondria have demonstrated that during Ca^{2+} uptake the membrane potential decreases and the extent of the decrease is proportional to the amount of Ca^{2+} taken up by the mitochondria (14).

Thus, it appears that, under conditions which cause massive amounts of Ca^{2+} to accumulate in the mitochondria, their membrane potential would collapse. This has been confirmed recently by studies in which isolated rat hepatocytes were incubated with sodium orthovanadate to inhibit the endoplasmic reticular and plasma membrane Ca^{2+} translocases. Under these conditions the cytosolic Ca^{2+} level increases and large amounts of Ca^{2+} are accumulated in the mitochondria (15). Concomitantly, the membrane potential decreases to an extent proportional to the amount of Ca^{2+} accumulated, and ATP depletion invariably follows. Other studies in which cells were exposed to the Ca^{2+} ionophore, ionomycin, or permeabilized with digitonin in the presence of Ca^{2+} have recently demonstrated that intracellular Ca^{2+} overload can cause the collapse of the mitochondrial membrane potential (16).

The existence of different Ca^{2+} uptake and release pathways in mitochondria provides a basis for Ca^{2+} cycling (14). This process continuously utilizes energy which is primarily generated by proton pumping from the matrix into the intermembrane space. Since the inner mitochondrial membrane is relatively impermeable to anions, a considerable portion of the energy resulting from the proton concentration gradient is stored as membrane electric potential. A number of investigations, using mitochondria isolated from different sources, have demonstrated that the oxidation of intramitochondrial NAD(P)H can activate the release route and accelerate Ca^{2+} cycling across the mitochondrial membrane. This condition is associated with a decrease in the mitochondrial membrane potential that parallels the rate of Ca^{2+} cycling.

An interesting aspect of the relationship between the mitochondrial membrane potential and intracellular free Ca^{2+} level is that mitochondrial toxins can cause a toxic increase in the cytosolic Ca^{2+} concentration. Due to the energy requirement of the various Ca^{2+} transport systems which control Ca^{2+} homeostasis, it is easy to understand that mitochondrial dysfunction and subsequent ATP depletion will invariably result in the disruption of intracellular Ca^{2+} homeostasis. Thus, treatment of cultured rat hepatocytes with the uncoupler protonophore, CCCP,[1] causes an early transient increase in the cytosolic Ca^{2+} concentration, which single-cell studies revealed to be restricted to the peripheral regions of the cell and which is likely result of Ca^{2+} release from mitochondrial stores (16).

However, at these early time points (0–5 min), the intracellular concentration of ATP and the ATP:ADP ratio are still high enough to allow the plasma membrane and the endoplasmic reticular Ca^{2+}-ATPases to function in lowering the cytosolic Ca^{2+} concentration. Later, when the intracellular ATP concentration has fallen to very low levels and the ATP-dependent Ca^{2+} pumps are no longer functional, the intracellular Ca^{2+} concentration increases to toxic levels, which can potentially trigger a series of Ca^{2+}-dependent events, ultimately leading to cell death.

GLUTATHIONE AND PROTEIN THIOL MODIFICATIONS

Alkylating agents and free radicals, including species derived from molecular oxygen, can induce a perturbation of cellular redox balance. Both nonenzymatic and enzymatic defence mechanisms normally protect cells from excessive oxidation. However, when these cellular defense systems are overwhelmed, a condition known as oxidative stress is brought about. Under extreme conditions oxidative injury can result in acute cell death, which is preceded by loss of glutathione (GSH) and by protein thiol oxidation. This can, in turn, result in

[1] CCCP, carbonylcyanide-3-chlorophenylhydrazone.

lipid peroxidation, inhibition of glycolysis, and cytoskeletal alterations (see above), which may eventually affect a host of cellular functions.

Thiol modification by active oxygen species can also play a role in modulating the binding of various agonists to receptors as well as the activity of enzymes involved in signal transduction, including G proteins and phospholipases (17). In addition, both oxidants and antioxidants can directly modulate kinase activities, such as protein kinase C activation (18,19), which may result in disturbances of cell growth. Effects on thiol groups in nuclear proteins may affect gene expression and DNA repair.

Ca^{2+} OVERLOAD AND ACTIVATION OF Ca^{2+}-DEPENDENT CATABOLIC PROCESSES

The role of Ca^{2+} as intracellular regulator of many physiological processes is now well established. On the other hand, during the past several years it has also become clear that Ca^{2+} can play a determinant role in a variety of pathological process. Disturbances of the mechanisms which regulate intracellular Ca^{2+} homeostasis are often early events in the development of irreversible cell injury (20). Thus, it was proposed that intracellular Ca^{2+} accumulation may be a common step in the development of cytotoxicity.

Normally, intracellular Ca^{2+} homeostasis is controlled by the concerted operation of plasma membrane Ca^{2+} translocases and intracellular compartmentalization systems. Disturbances of these processes during cell injury can result in enchanced Ca^{2+} influx, release of Ca^{2+} from intracellular stores, and inhibition of Ca^{2+} extrusion at the plasma membrane, which can lead to an uncontrolled rise in the intracellular Ca^{2+} concentration. Such sustained increases in intracellular Ca^{2+} will obliterate the transient Ca^{2+} responses normally caused by hormone stimulation, compromise mitochondrial function and cytoskeletal organization, and, ultimately, activate degradative process. Since Ca^{2+} is an activator of several enzymes involved in the catabolism of proteins, phospholipids, and nucleic acids, a sustained increase in the cytosolic free Ca^{2+} concentration above the physiological level can potentially result in an uncontrolled breakdown of macromolecules of vital importance for the maintenance of cell structure and function.

The involvement of Ca^{2+}-activated catabolic processes in cytotoxicity has been suggested by several studies (for a review, see Ref. 20). Thus, Ca^{2+}-activated proteolysis seems to play a role in the toxicity of oxidents in liver and in cardiomyocytes exposed to venom toxins, as well as in Ca^{2+} overload in neural cells. Although little is known about preferential substrates of Ca^{2+}-activated proteases, the observation that, under certain conditions, leupeptin can prevent the appearance of plasma membrane blebs caused by toxic agents (5) suggests that cytoskeletal proteins or cytoskeletal anchoring integral proteins could be degraded by the Ca^{2+}-dependent proteases (see also "Disruption of Cytoskeletal Architecture in Toxic Cell Killing").

Ca^{2+}-dependent phospholipases are involved in a number of physiological cell functions. For example, phospholipase A_2 has been implicated in the detoxification of phospholipid hydroperoxides because of its ability to release fatty acids from peroxidized membranes (21). However, phospholipase A_2 activity is Ca^{2+} and calmodulin dependent and is thus susceptible to stimulation following an increase in the intracellular Ca^{2+} concentration. When the increase in Ca^{2+} is sustained, the activation of phospholipase A_2 would result in extensive membrane breakdown and in the generation of toxic metabolites. Ca^{2+}-dependent activation of phospholipase A_2 has been detected during ischemic and anoxic injury and has been associated with cytotoxicity caused by carbon tetrachloride and quinoneimines in hepatocytes, by the toxin pyrularia thionin in 3T3 fibroblasts, and by Ca^{2+} ionophores in alveolar epithelial cells (see Ref. 20 and references therein).

More recently, it has become apparent that Ca^{2+} overload may also result in DNA degradation. This includes single-strand breakage (22) as well as the endonuclease-mediated cleavage of DNA in cells undergoing apoptosis (23). Finally, Ca^{2+} overload may also stimulate other enzymatic processes that result in DNA damage. Elevated Ca^{2+} levels can lock topoisomerase II in a form that cleaves, but does not religate, DNA, and topoisomerase II-mediate DNA fragmentation has been implicated in the cytotoxic action of some anticancer drugs (24).

APOPTOSIS

The term "apoptosis" is used to define a characteristic mode of cell death which occurs in many instances of programmed cell deletion during development and in adult cells (23). Apoptosis is characterized by morphological changes such as plasma membrane and nuclear membrane blebbing, organelle relocation and compaction, and chromatin condensation. A well-recognized biochemical end point associated with this process is the cleavage of DNA in fragments of multiples of ~200, which is mediated by a Ca^{2+}- and Mg^{2+}-dependent endonuclease activity. Endonuclease activation has been observed in the killing of target cells by cytotoxic T lymphocytes and natural killer cells and the death of thymocytes exposed to glucocorticoids or to an antibody to the CD3–T cell receptor complex (see Ref. 20 and references therein). Ca^{2}-dependent endonuclease activation has also been detected in thymocytes treated with toxic agents, including 2,3,7,8-tetrachlorodibenzo-*p*-dioxin and tributylin, and in tumor cells exposed to endogenous cytotolytic agents such as tumor necrosis factor α.

Although intracellular Ca^{2+} overload seems to trigger endonuclease activation in many systems, other observations suggest that the signaling involved in the induction of apoptosis is more complex and that additional mechanisms are involved. Thus, in some experimental models apoptosis can occur in the absence of detectable increases in intracellular Ca^{2+}. Moreover, studies in our laboratory and others have indicated that stimulation of protein kinase C activity by phorbol esters or growth factors can prevent DNA fragmentation also in the presence of high Ca^{2+} levels.

More recently, we have shown that agents known to modify chromatin structure (i.e., polyamines, namely, spermine) can prevent DNA fragmentation and apoptosis in thymocytes exposed to glucocorticoids, Ca^{2+} ionophores, or organotin compounds (25). The mechanism responsible for the inhibition of DNA fragmentation appears to be related to the ability of the polyamines to modify the chromatin structure. Conversely, agents which cause chromatin unfolding seem to stimulate DNA fragmentation, and polyamine-depleted cells appear to be more susceptible to the onset of apoptosis. This suggests that the endonuclease-mediated internucleosomal cleavage is secondary to chromatin decondensation or local reduction in histone–DNA interaction. Thus, changes in chromatin structure may play a determinant role in the triggering of apoptosis. Since Ca^{2+}, other ions, and a variety of growth stimuli are known to influence chromatin conformation, it is conceivable that disturbances in ion signals, or rather an imbalance of several signaling systems, is necessary to stimulate predisposed cells toward apoptosis.

ALTERATIONS IN CELL SIGNALING: Ca^{2+} SIGNALS

The inability of cells to respond to Ca^{2+}-mobilizing hormones can be the consequence of the selective depletion of the intracellular agonist-sensitive Ca^{2+} pool by compounds such as 2,5-di-(*tert*-butyl)-1,4-benzohydroquinone (26) or bromotrichloromethane (27). Also, G_p, the transducing G protein for inositol 1,4,5-trisphosphate-generating receptors, is susceptible to inactivation by thiol-oxidizing agents. Finally, prolonged increases in the intracellular Ca^{2+} concentration may obliterate the Ca^{2+} transients normally evoked by physiological agonists, thereby resulting in an impairment of cell signaling.

As discussed above, in contrast to the situations in which oxidants appear to block the cell signaling machinery at concentrations that are lethal to the cell, it has recently become clear that low levels of oxidants can have quite the opposite effect. This is exemplified by our recent studies in neuroadrenergic PC-12 cells exposed to $HgCl_2$ in which we found that treatment with low $HgCl_2$ concentrations (50–300 nM) enhanced the intracellular Ca^{2+} signals elicited by agonists or depolarization and potentiated nerve growth factor-induced cell differentiation. Conversely, at higher concentrations (2–5 μM), $HgCl_2$ caused a concentration-dependent increase in the cytosolic Ca^{2+} level and rapidly resulted in cell death (28).

An intriguing example of cytotoxic mechanisms activated via physiological Ca^{2+} signals has recently been provided by Snyder and co-workers (29), who have characterized the molecular structure and some of the properties and functions of nitric oxide (NO) synthase. In addition to its role as intracellular messenger in neuronal and endothelial cells, NO is also important in macrophage cytotoxicity and may be toxic to neurons. The constitutive NO synthase in the brain has an absolute requirement for the Ca^{2+}-binding protein, calmodulin. Thus, intracellular Ca^{2+} elevation mediated by the glutamatergic pathway can stimulate NO production. Interestingly, Snyder and co-workers have found that the neural NO synthase is responsible for their well-known NADPH diaphorase activity and suggested that the NADPH diaphorase-containing neurons are more resistant to ischemic injury mediated through glutamate receptor stimulation. Hence, while neurons containing NO synthase may be protected from the cytotoxicity caused by glutamate receptor stimulation, the generation of NO triggered by the intracellular Ca^{2+} increase in these neurons may be lethal to neighboring cells (see Ref. 29 and references therein).

PROTEIN KINASE C AND GROWTH STIMULATION

As mentioned above, different levels of oxidants may exert dissimilar effects on signal transduction. For example, low levels of oxidants are known to stimulate cell proliferation and can lead to tumor promotion, as suggested by work from Cerutti's laboratory (30). Studies in our laboratory have shown that exposure of rat hepatocytes to low levels of oxidants can result in a rapid increase in protein kinase C activity (18). This increase is due to the oxidative modification of the protein, most likely through a modification of the thiol/disulfide balance of the enzyme. The involvement of thiol residues in the activation phenomenon is strongly supported by the finding that partially purified protein kinase C from rat brain could be activated using low concentrations of glutathione disulfide in a glutathione redox buffer.

These observations suggest that, while more selective mechanisms may be involved in low-oxidant toxicity and in carcinogenesis, multiple acutely cytotoxic mechanisms may be recruited in a dose-dependent fashion under conditions of pronounced oxidative stress. The selective dose-dependent activation of different mechanisms for proliferation and cell death caused by oxidants is exemplified by our recent studies on the effects of the redox-cycling quinone, 2,3-dimethoxy-1,4-naphthoquinone (DMNQ), in RINm5F cells, a rat insulinoma cell line. At a concentration of 10 μM, DMNQ stimulated RINm5F cell proliferation, whereas at marginally higher concentrations of DMNQ (30 μM), cell growth was inhibited and a portion of the cell population underwent apoptosis. Finally, at 100 μM concentration, DMNQ caused GSH and ATP depletion, Ca^{2+} overload, and necrotic cell death (31). Resuming the proliferative stimulus by pretreatment with phorbol esters prevented the activation of the death program in cells treated with 30 μM DMNQ. This suggests that appropriate proliferative signals may counteract the oxidant-mediated inhibition of protein kinase C.

CONCLUSIONS

Recent studies have established a number of potentially lethal reactions which can all result in irreversible alterations compromising cell survival. In this opening overview we have outlined some of the mechanisms which have received much attention during the last few years. Far from being a comprehensive review of all proposed cytotoxic mechanisms, this introduction aimed to provide a guide for the intricate debate on the cause of cell death.

REFERENCES

1. S. A. Jewell, G. Bellomo, H. Thor, S. Orrenius, and M. T. Smith, *Science* **217,** 1257 (1982).
2. W. Malorni, F. Iosi, F. Mirabelli, and G. Bellomo, *Chem.–Biol. Interact.* **80,** 217 (1991).
3. A. Naramota, S. Ohno, K. Furuta, N. Itoh, K. Nakazawa, M. Nakano, and H. Shigematsu, *Hepatology* **13,** 222 (1991).
4. P. C. Phelps, M. W. Smith, and B. F. Trump, *Lab. Invest.* **60,** 630 (1989).
5. F. Mirabelli, A. Salis, M. Vairetti, G. Bellomo, H. Thor, and S. Orrenius, *Arch. Biochem. Biophys.* **270,** (1989).
6. A. L. Nieminen, G. J. Gores, Y. Tanaka, B. Herman, and J. J. Lemasters, *Cell Calcium* **9,** 237 (1988).
7. A. Weeds, *Nature (London)* **296,** 811 (1982).
8. K. Florine-Casteel, J. J. Lemasters, and B. Herman, *FASEB J.* **5,** 2078 (1991).
9. F. Mirabelli, A. Salis, V. Marinoni, G. Finardi, G. Bellemo, H. Thor, and S. Orrenius, *Arch. Biochem. Biophys.* **264,** 261 (1988).
10. J. E. Eriksson, J. G. Paatero, J. A. Meriluoto, G. A. Codd, G. E. N. Kass, P. Nicotera, and S. Orrenius, *Exp. Cell Res.* **185,** 86 (1989).
11. L. Chartier, L. L. Rankin, R. E. Allen, Y. Kato, N. Fusetani, H. Karaki, S. Watabe, and D. J. Harsthorne, *Cell Motil. Cytoskeleton* **18,** 26 (1991).
12. R. C. Prince, *Trends Biochem. Sci.* **13,** 159 (1988).
13. L. B. Chen, *Annu. Rev. Cell Biol.* **4,** 155 (1988).
14. T. E. Gunther and D. R. Pfeiffer, *Am. J. Physiol.* **258,** C755 (1990).
15. P. Richelmi, F. Mirabelli, A. Salis, G. Finardi, F. Berte, and G. Bellomo, *Toxicology* **57,** 29 (1989).
16. G. Bellomo, R. Fulceri, E. Albano, A. Gamberucci, A. Pompella, M. Parola, and A. Benedetti, *Cell Calcium* **12,** 335 (1991).
17. G. Bellomo, H. Thor, and S. Orrenius, *J. Biol. Chem.* **262,** 1530 (1987).

18. G. E. N. Kass, S. K. Duddy, and S. Orrenius, *Biochem. J.* **260,** 499 (1989).
19. D. Boscoboinik, A. Szewczyk, and A. Azzi, *Arch. Biochem. Biophys.* **286,** 264 (1991).
20. P. Nicotera, G. Bellomo and S. Orrenius, *Annu. Rev. Pharmacol. Toxicol.* **32,** 449 (1992).
21. F. J. G. M. Van Kuijk, A. Sevanian, G. J. Handelman, and E. A. Dratz, *Trends Biochem. Sci.* **12,** 31 (1987).
22. J. M. Dypbukt, H. Thor, and P. Nicotera, *Free Radical Res. Commun.* **8,** 347 (1990).
23. M. J. Arends, R. G. Morris, and A. H. Wyllie, *Am. J. Pathol.* **136,** 593 (1990).
24. A. Udvardy, P. Schedl, M. Sander, and T. Hsieh, *J. Mol. Biol.* **191,** 231 (1986).
25. B. Brüne, P. Hartzell, P. Nicotera, and S. Orrenius, *Exp. Cell Res.* **195,** 323 (1991).
26. G. E. N. Kass, S. Duddy, and S. Orrenius, *J. Biol. Chem.* **264,** 15192 (1989).
27. A. Benedetti, P. Graf, R. Fulceri, A. Romani, and H. Sies, *Biochem. Pharmacol.* **38,** 1799 (1989).
28. A. Rossi, L. Manzo, S. Orrenius, M. Vahter, and P. Nicotera, *Pharmacol. Toxicol.* **68,** 424 (1991).
29. D. S. Bredt, P. M. Hwang, C. E. Glatt, C. Lowenstein, R. R. Reed, and S. H. Snyder, *Nature (London)* **351,** 714 (1991).
30. R. Larsson, and P. Cerutti, *J. Biol. Chem.* **263,** 17452 (1988).
31. J. M. Dypbukt, M. Ankarcrona, M. Burkitt, K. Ström, S. Orrenius, and P. Nicotera, submitted for publication (1994).

3 Membrane Lipid Peroxidation: Cellular Mechanisms and Toxicological Implications

Lars Ernster and Paul Hochstein

INTRODUCTION

The peroxidation of lipids is one of the earliest recognized and most extensively investigated manifestations of oxygen activation and toxicity in biology. Over the years this subject has been reviewed in numerous articles, monographs, and conference proceedings (see Refs. 1–7). In this chapter we give a brief historical survey of this field of research and a description of some current concepts and perspectives of the machanisms and implications of lipid peroxidation as it occurs in biological membranes and other complex lipid structures.

BACKGROUND

Interest in research relating to lipid peroxidation dates back to 1820 (Table I), less than 50 years after the discovery of oxygen and its role in respiration and photosynthesis. de Saussure observed that walnut oil exposed to air increases its weight and becomes ill smelling. Berzelius suggested that this phenomenon, just as the self-ignition of wood upon lubrication with linseed oil, might be due to autoxidation.

Experiments by Fahrion in the early 1900s suggested that unsaturation is an essential feature of molecules that undergo autoxidation, and in 1923 Meyerhof demonstrated that sulfhydryl compounds may catalyze the autoxidation of unsaturated lipids (8). At about this time, vitamin E was discovered by Evans and Bishop (9), and its antioxidant properties were subsequently described by several investigators (10–12). The sequence of reactions now generally recognized to account for the peroxidation of polyunsaturated fatty acids, including the involvement of free radicals, was clarified within a few years. The events briefly described above provided the framework for our current concepts of the involvement of lipid peroxidation in toxicological reactions.

In 1932 Andre and Hou (13) discovered soybean lipoxygenase, the first reported instance of an enzyme catalyzing lipid peroxidation. The subsequent elu-

METHODS IN TOXICOLOGY, Volume 1B

Table I Biochemistry of Lipid Peroxidation: Some Historical Landmarks[a]

Year	Finding	Investigators
1820	Oils increase in weight in air due to autoxidation?	de Saussure, Berzelius
1904–1912	Unsaturation essential for autoxidation	Fahrion
1922	Discovery of vitamin E	Evans and Bishop
1923	Sulfhydryl compounds initiate autoxidation of lipids	Meyerhof
1932	Discovery of soybean lipoxygenase	Andre and Hou
1941–1954	Role of free radicals in fatty acid peroxidation	Farmer *et al.*, Bateman, Bolland Gee *et al.*
1943–1947	Characterization of soybean lipoxidase	Balls *et al.*, Cosby and Sumner Theorell *et al.*
1948	Development of TBA test for lipid peroxidation	Bernheim *et al.*
1959–1963	Nonenzymatic lipid peroxidation in biological membranes; prevention by vitamin E	Ottolenghi, Tappel and Zalkin, Thiel and Huff, Hunter *et al.*
1963	Enzymatically induced lipid peroxidation	Hochstein and Ernster
1964	Prostaglandin biosynthesis	Bergström *et al.*, van Dorp *et al.*

[a] TBA, Thiobarbituric acid. From Ref. 5.

cidation of the "arachidonic acid cascade," which leads to the biosynthesis of prostaglandins, thromboxanes, leukotrienes, and related bioregulators, opened a new chapter in biochemistry. The lipoxygenases involved in these latter processes act on unesterified fatty acids and do not attack the complex phospholipids of biological membranes.

Membrane lipid peroxidation was first described between 1959 and 1963, using isolated mitochondria and microsomes as subcellular membrane preparations and added hematin, ascorbate, or sulfhydryl compounds as nonenzymatic initiators (see Ref. 3). The process was assayed by the thiobarbituric acid (TBA) reaction described by Bernheim *et al.* (14) for the detection of malondialdehyde (MDA). The latter is one of many reactive breakdown products of lipid peroxides. Despite several limitations (6), the measurement of TBA-reactive substances continues to be a simple and useful tool for detecting the extent of lipid peroxidation both *in vitro* and *in vivo.*

In 1963 Hochstein and Ernster (15) reported an enzymatically induced peroxidation of endogenous lipids in liver microsomal preparations. NADPH and ADP were essential components of the system. The reaction was proposed to involve the enzyme known at that time as TPNH cytochrome *c* reductase (later identified as NADPH–cytochrome P-450 reductase) and to proceed through an ADP–Fe^{3+}–O_2^- (perferryl) complex (Fig. 1). The source of iron in this first re-

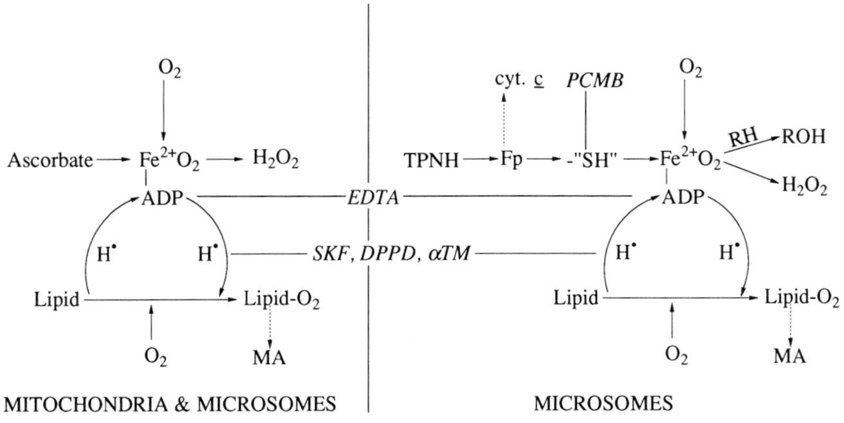

Figure 1 Schematic representation of lipid peroxidation linked to ascorbate or TPNH oxidation in microsomes and mitochondria. MA, malonyldialdehyde; TPNH (NADPH), reduced triphosphopyridine nucleotide; SKF (SKF525A), diethylaminomethyl-diphenylpropylacetate; DPPD, diphenylphenylenediamine; αTM, 2-(3-hydroxy-3-methylcarboxypental)-3,5,6-trimethylbenzoquinone; PCMB, *p*-chloromercuribenzoate; cyt. c, cytochrome *c*; F_p, TPNH cytochrome *c* reductase. (From Ref. 15.)

port was not specified, but was assumed to be related to the terminal catalyst of the "mixed-function oxidase" subsequently identified by Sato *et al.* (16) as cytochrome P-450. It soon emerged that, in addition to endogenous catalysts, lipid peroxidation requiring NADPH and ADP also required exogenous iron. Iron was present as a contaminant of commercial preparations of ADP (and other nucleoside di- and triphosphates or inorganic pyrophosphates) used in these early experiments (17). Mitochondria were also shown to exhibit and ADP-activated lipid peroxidation, although this did not occur with NADPH as an electron donor (15); rather, a nonenzymatic reductant such as ascorbate was essential. Again, the reaction was assumed to involve endogenous iron of unspecified identity. Exogenous iron as an ADP contaminant was obviously also present in this system.

The occurrence of enzymatically induced lipid peroxidation was soon confirmed in several laboratories, and served during the following years as a useful system for studying membrane lipid peroxidation (18). These studies were extended to include experiments with submitochondrial particles and liposomes in combination with various redox systems in the presence of either added iron chelates or heme and nonheme iron proteins (19–21). Much of our current knowledge of the mechanisms of lipid peroxidation originates from these types of investigations. For this reason, we focus the following discussion on the insights derived from such research. Some implications of this information will be considered as they apply to intact cells and organisms under physiological and pathological conditions.

GENERAL MECHANISMS

The well-established sequence of reactions involved in the peroxidation of polyunsaturated fatty acids is illustrated in Fig. 2. The initial steps include the abstraction of a hydrogen atom from a fatty acid containing at least two methylene-interrupted double bonds (LH), giving rise to a carbon-centered free radical (L·) along with a concomitant rearrangement of the double bonds (diene conjugation). This is followed by an interaction of L· with molecular oxygen to form a peroxy radical (LOO·). The latter can then abstract a hydrogen atom either from an adjacent LH, thereby inducing a propagation reaction, or from another hydrogen donor (e.g., an antioxidant). In both instances a fatty acid hydroperoxide (LOOH) is formed.

Lipid hydroperoxides can undergo other reactions not illustrated in Fig. 2. They may be reoxidized to LOO·. Such an event will reinitiate peroxidation reactions by propagation. They may also be reduced to alkoxy radicals (LO·), which can again reinitiate fatty acid peroxidation through hydrogen abstraction from an adjacent LH. This process is sometimes referred as "branching" and may result in the formation of an alcohol (LOH) as the end product. Fatty acid hydroperoxides may also be enzymatically reduced directly to alcohols. Other end products can be formed through fragmentation reactions to yield MDA and other aldehydes, ketones, ethers, alcohols, and hydrocarbons. Peroxidation can

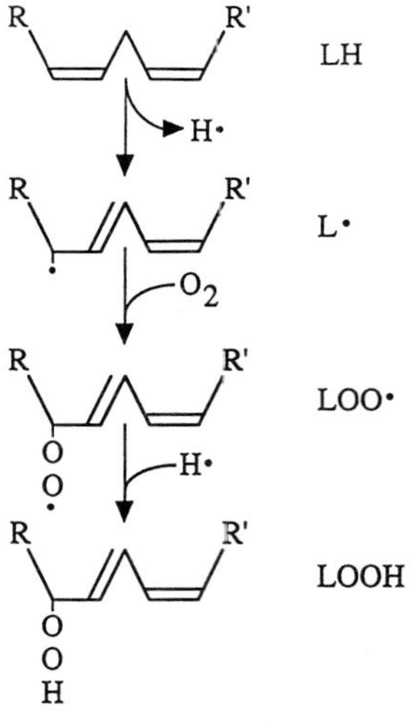

Figure 2 Reaction sequence involved in lipid peroxidation.

also be terminated through the interaction of two fatty acid radicals to form products such as LL, LOL, and LOOL.

In the following section we briefly consider the mechanisms of some of the above reactions as they occur in membrane phospholipids, with special reference to the roles of iron, iron chelators, and enzymes.

ROLE OF IRON

It is generally accepted that, in most instances of membrane lipid peroxidation, iron (or another transition metal, such as copper) is involved. Such metals participate in both the initiation and reinitiation phases of the process (6) as well as in the breakdown of lipid peroxides (22). In the initiation phase, the role of transition metals is generally believed to be the activation of oxygen to a species (Table II) that has the ability to abstract a hydrogen atom from LH. In addition to the perferryl radical, originally proposed in 1963 (15), the ferryl and hydroxyl radicals have also been considered as potential initiators (6). Although the latter two species may be more active than the perferryl radical, their involvement in enzymatic lipid peroxidation in microsomes is unlikely in view of the insensitivity of the process to catalase, which removes the H_2O_2 necessary for the formation of these species. The process is also insensitive to high concentrations of mannitol that quench hydroxyl radicals. Of course, these radicals may be involved in the initiatioin of lipid peroxidation in other systems—for example, in the presence of a Fenton reagent, that is, H_2O_2, in combination with nonprotein or protein-bound ferrous iron (6).

A "ferrous–ferric-oxygen" complex has also been suggested as an initiating species (23). This idea is based on the observations (24) that Fe^{3+} maximally stimulates Fe^{2+}-induced lipid peroxidation in liposomes at equal concentrations of their two valence states. A similar effect has been observed in microsomes (25). However, as pointed out by Ursini *et al.* (26), an alternative explanation for this phenomenon is that Fe^{3+} thermodynamically counteracts the dissociation of $Fe^{3+}–O_2^-$ into Fe^{3+} and O_2^-. Such an effect would increase the steady-state concentration of the initiating perferryl species.

Table II Some Potential Initiators of Lipid Peroxidation[a]

Perferryl species	$Fe^{2+}O_2 \Leftrightarrow Fe^{3+}O_2^{\cdot -}$
Ferryl species	$[FeOH]^{3+}$ or $[FeO]^{2+}$
Ferrous–ferric-oxygen complex	$Fe^{2+}–O_2–Fe^{3+}$
Hydroxyl radical	$HO \cdot$

[a] From Ref. 5.

The superoxide anion radical (O_2^-) is generally thought not to be able to initiate lipid peroxidation. On the other hand, singlet oxygen ($^1O_2$) can also initiate lipid peroxidation (27). Its formation from O_2 does not require the participation of a transition metal, but it is formed at the expense of light energy in the presence of a suitable sensitizer (e.g., chlorophyll or porphyrins). Membrane lipid peroxidation caused by singlet oxygen may be of special interest in plant and animal tissues exposed to light, such as the skin or the eye. The formation of hydroxyl radicals (OH ·), which have the potential to initiate the peroxidation of lipids, may also take place in the absense of transition metals, through the radiolysis of water.

ROLE OF IRON CHELATORS

Iron chelators play a central role in the initiation of lipid peroxidation. The effect of ADP in promoting NADPH-dependent microsomal peroxidation was shortly found to be shared by other nucleoside di- and triphosphates and, within a limited concentration range, by inorganic pyrophosphate (15). It was proposed that all of these substances act in their capacity to chelate iron. Late, this list was extended to include oxalate, malonate, and 8-hydroxyquinoline (25). On the other hand, the cyanide, *o*-phenanthroline, and EDTA chelates of iron were inactive; EDTA even inhibited the ADP–Fe^{3+}-initiated reaction. Unchelated Fe^{3+} in combination with NADPH was also inactive, but was active in the presence of ascorbate as the reducing agent. These findings suggested that the complexing agent was required for rendering Fe^{3+} into a form enzymatically reducible by NADPH, rather than by simpling maintaining it in solution.

More recent studies (26) indicate that, in order to be able to initiate NADPH-dependent microsomal lipid peroxidation, an Fe^{3+} complex must fulfill three criteria: (a) reducibility by NADPH; (b) reactivity of the reduced complex with oxygen; and (c) the formation of a relatively stable perferryl radical (i.e., one that does not readily dissociate into Fe^{3+} and O_2^-). It was this last criterion that was proposed to explain the stimulation of Fe^{2+} -induced lipid peroxidation by Fe^{3+} (26). As illustrated in Table III, unchelated iron (Fe^{3+} and H_2O) and the desferrioxamine chelate of Fe^{3+} do not meet criterion (a); the cyanide complex and the *o*-phenanthroline complex fail to fulfill criterion (b) and the EDTA and the inorganic pyrophosphate (PP_i) chelates do not fulfill criterion (c). Thus, these chelates are unable to initiate NADPH-dependent lipid peroxidation. Conversely, the ADP (and other nucleoside di- and triphosphates) as well as the malonate and oxalate chelates, which initiate lipid peroxidation, meet all three criteria. Moreover, a combination of unchelated Fe^{3+} with either the EDTA or the PP_i chelates does initiate lipid peroxidation, apparently due to the fact that these chelates are reduced by NADPH, and the reduced chelates can then reduce unchelated Fe^{3+}, which in turn initiates lipid peroxidation.

Table III Conditions Determining the Capacity of Various Fe^{3+} Chelates to Initiate NADPH-Linked Lipid Peroxidation[a]

Chelate	Reducibility by NADPH	Reactivity with O_2	Stability of perferryl radical	Initiation of lipid peroxidation
Fe^{3+}–H_2O	−	−	+	−
Fe^{3+}–CN	+	−		−
Fe^{3+}–*o*-phenanthroline	+	−		−
Fe^{3+}–desferrioxamine	−			−
Fe^{3+}–EDTA	+	+	−	−
Fe^{3+}–PP_i	+	+	−	−
Fe^{3+}–ADP	+	+	+	+
Fe^{3+}–ATP	+	+	+	+
Fe^{3+}–oxalate	+	+	+	+
Fe^{3+}–malonate	+	+	+	+
Fe^{3+}–H_2O + Fe^{3+}–EDTA	+	+	+	+
Fe^{3+}–H_2O + Fe^{3+}–PP_i	+	+	+	+

[a] From Ref. 26.

An unresolved issue with respect to hydrophilic perferryl radicals concerns their ability to reach the sites in membranes where polyunsaturated fatty acids are located. Sevanian *et al.* (28) have shown, with liposomes consisting of phosphatidylcholine and phosphatidylethanolamine, that the addition of a critical amount of deoxycholate is necessary to permit the initiation of peroxidation by ADP–Fe^{3+} in the presence of ascorbate. In addition, unpublished experiments (1992) by Dr. Mary Lou Wratten at the Institute for Toxicology of the University of Southern California have demonstrated that the incorporation of cardiolipin into phosphatidylcholine liposomes overcomes the requirement for deoxycholate (see Ref. 5). It remains to be determined whether this is due to the formation of "inverted micelles" by cardiolipin, which would result in fatty acid moieties exposed to the surface; or, alternatively to a binding of the perferryl radical to the negatively charged headgroup of the phospholipid and a consequent change in membrane conformation. Perhaps both factors are involved. In any event, it is clear that the physical state and phospholipid composition of membranes are crucial determinants for the initiation of lipid peroxidation.

ROLE OF ENZYMES

There is some confusion in the literature with regard to the terms "enzymatic" and "enzymatically induced" lipid peroxidation (6,27). The former term refers to reactions catalyzed by enzymes acting directly on polyunsaturated fatty acids, primarily arachidonic acid (29). The reactions catalyzed by such enzymes are regio- and stereospecific, and, as previously indicated, they act on unesterified fatty acids, not on phospholipids. In contrast, "enzymatically induced" lipid peroxidation refers to an enzyme(s) catalyzing the reduction of certain electron acceptors, notably iron, present in the form of various chelates or in heme or nonheme proteins. These chelates can in turn initiate or propagate lipid peroxidation. These latter enzymes may play an important role in membrane lipid peroxidation which results in cellular injury *in vivo* and should not be regarded as artifacts.

In the case of microsomes, it is accepted that the reduction of various Fe^{3+} chelates proceeds through NADPH–cytochrome P-450 reductase. This notion is in accordance with the original suggestion by Hochstein and Ernster (15,30) and has been substantiated by Aust and colleagues (31,32), who demonstrated that antibodies raised against this enzyme inhibited NADPH-dependent lipid peroxidation. They also showed that the purified enzyme, when incorporated into liposomes, permitted NADPH to initiate lipid peroxidation, but in that case cytochrome P-450 was also required for the reaction. The available data indicate that cytochrome P-450 can act in both its oxidized and reduced forms (24,28), converting LOOH to LOO· or LO·, respectively, thus promoting reinitiation and subsequent propagation and "branching." Other experiments indicating a multiple role for cytochrome P-450 in lipid peroxidation have been reported from the laboratories of Coon (33) and Ingelman-Sundberg (34).

These concepts are summarized in schematic form in Fig. 3. The scheme also includes the potential role of the enzyme phospholipid hydroperoxide glutathione peroxidase, first described by Ursini *et al.* in 1985 (35), in the process of lipid peroxidation. This enzyme functions in association with various membranes to catalyze the reduction of LOOH to LOH, hence circumventing the formation of LO·.

Finally, it should be noted that, in addition to the pathways described above, microsomal lipid peroxidation has also been shown to occur in the presence of NADH, rather than NADPH, and an iron chelate (36). The maximal velocity and the requirement for a suitable iron chelator is the same as in the case of NADPH, but the concentration of iron needed for half-maximal velocity is about 10 times higher. The reaction apparently proceeds via NADH–cytochrome b_5 reductase, in accordance with an earlier proposal by Bidlack *et al.* (37). Furthermore, enzymatically induced lipid peroxidation has also been demonstrated in submitochondrial particles, using NADH or NADPH in combination with ADP–Fe^{3+} (21). These reactions have been shown to proceed via NADH: ubiquinone oxido reductase (complex I) of the respiratory chain (21), although through different pathways of NADH and NADPH (38).

It is striking that in all studies quoted above, exogenous iron in the form of a suitable chelate has been an absolute requirement for lipid peroxidation. This is remarkable in that both microsomes and mitochondria contain large amounts of

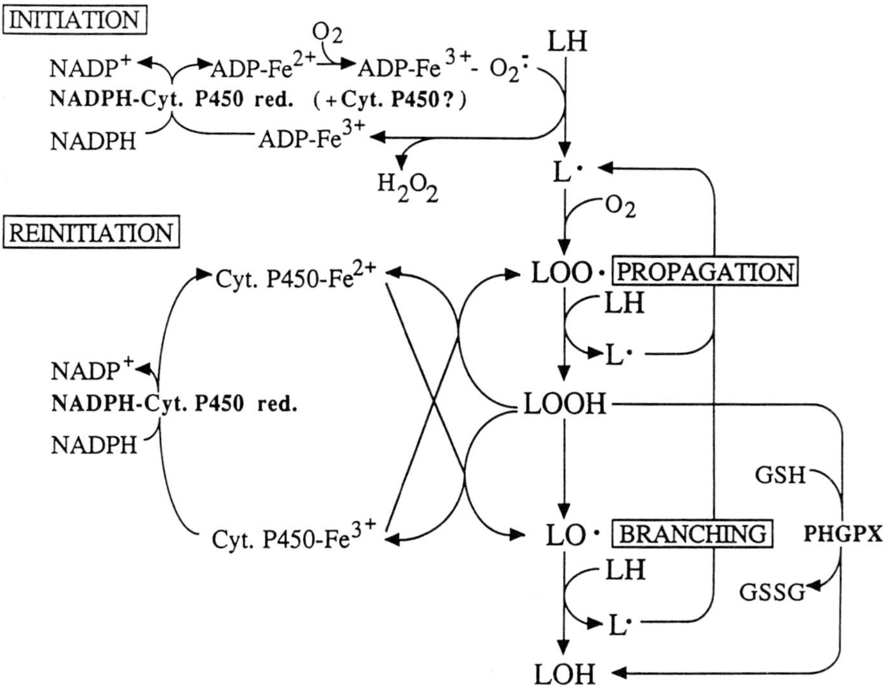

Figure 3 Reactions involved in enzymatically induced lipid peroxidation. Cyt. P450-Fe^{3+} or Fe^{2+}, Cytochrome P-450, oxidized or reduced form, respectively; PHGPX, phospholipid hydroperoxide glutathione peroxidase. (From Ref. 5.)

protein-bound iron as redox catalysts, which can be reduced by the same NADPH or NADH-linked flavoproteins as those involved in the reduction of the iron chelates involved in lipid peroxidation. However, these iron-containing proteins do not induce lipid peroxidation, with the notable exception of the ethanol-inducible species of cytochrome P-450 (33,34). Hatefi and Hanstein (39) have shown that chaotropic agents can modify heme and nonheme iron proteins so as to permit them to induce lipid peroxidation. It seems likely that several of the iron-containing catalysts of microsomes and mitochondria might be potential initiators of lipid peroxidation if their chemical structure or their physical relationship to other membrane components were to be altered.

OCCURRENCE OF MEMBRANE LIPID PEROXIDATION *IN VIVO*

Although most of the paramenters usually used to demonstrate membrane lipid peroxidation *in vivo,* including MDA formation, increased diene conjugation, occurrence of lipid hydroperoxides, or deposition of lipofuscin granules, may have their shortcomings, the accumulated evidence strongly supports the conclusion that the process indeed does occur. This concept is susbstantiated by the increase in these parameters under conditions of diminished antioxidant status (e.g., in vitamin E deficiency) (40). In fact, it is possible that what we see under physiological conditions is only the tip of the iceberg and that, in pathological states, when antioxidant mechanisms might be overwhelmed, lipid peroxidation may be far greater than normally found. The question therefore is not whether, but now, this occurs.

It appears likely that those mechanisms that involve membrane NAD(P)H reductases in combination with ADP–Fe^{3+} might serve as potential initiators. They require "free" iron, (i.e., nonprotein bound) in the micromolar range, and ADP or other nucleoside di- or triphosphates at below-millimolar concentrations; the latter levels are those which occur *in vivo.* Although the question of the concentration of "free" iron *in vivo* is controversial, these levels may increase in the presence of superoxide anion radicals which have the potential to release iron from ferritin (41). Such increases might be important in the injury associated with ischemic (42) and inflammatory diseases (43).

Ascorbate in the presence of iron is a potential nonenzymatic initiator of membrane lipid peroxidation. However, it is well known that it can act as both as a pro- and an antioxidant (see Ref. 44), depending on its concentration relative to that of vitamin E. Thus, while ascorbate is an essential factor in the intestinal absorption of iron, intake of ascorbate and iron together may set the stage for lipid peroxidation, unless adequately compensated by vitamin E.

Most membrane-bound heme and nonheme iron proteins are remarkably inert in generating agents that can initiate lipid peroxidation. Exceptions are certain species of cytochrome P-450 which can produce oxygen radicals even in the absence of substrate (45), as well as other species involved in the oxidation of carbon tetrachloride (46) or various polycyclic hydrocarbons (47). As indicated above, still other iron proteins may become active in inducing lipid peroxidation upon modification by chaotropes (48) and ongoing lipid peroxidation (49). Finally, it should be mentioned that heme proteins such as myoglobin and hemoglobin can initiate lipid peroxidation when they are oxidized by hydrogen peroxidate to their hypervalent forms (50). These forms have the capacity to generate singlet oxygen (51). It is of interest that in these instances ascorbate acts as antioxidant, apparently by reducing the iron in these proteins to the ferrous state (52).

CONSEQUENCES OF MEMBRANE LIPID PEROXIDATION

The most common consequences of membrane lipid peroxidation involve the perturbation of essential organellar and cellular membrane functions. These include transport processes, maintenance of ion and metabolite gradients, and receptor-mediated signal transduction. Lipid peroxidation can also cause damage to DNA and proteins. In the case of DNA, this can take place through oxidation of DNA bases, primarily guanine (53), by lipid peroxy or alkoxy radicals (54). In addition, covalent binding of certain breakdown products (e.g., MDA) results in strand breaks and cross-linking (54). The latter can also damage proteins and lead to the formation of lipofuscin aggregates (55). Oxidative damage to DNA is especially extensive in mitochondria (56) and may be responsible for mitochondrial DNA deletions found in certain degenerative diseases and with aging (57). There is increasing evidence that oxidative damage to DNA *in vivo* is mediated by the products of lipid peroxidation (58,59). It is noteworthy that oxidative damage to proteins shows a striking increase with age (60).

CONCLUSIONS

Lipid peroxidation seems to be a fact of life. The basic conditions in order for it to occur are present in most animal cells, even under physiological conditions. This is due to the abundance of iron and other transition metals and of systems that can mobilize these metals and use them for the generation of reactive species of oxygen. These species can attack lipids and, directly or indirectly, almost all biological constituents. In this sense, oxygen and lipid peroxidation represent an inherent challenge to aerobic life.

To meet this challenge, aerobic organisms are equipped with a battery of mechanisms to protect themselves from such effects. In animal cells these defense mechanisms consist partly of antioxidant enzymes, whose levels can often be regulated to meet actual needs. In addition, antioxidant substances, in the form either of vitamins such as the tocopherols, carotenoids, and ascorbate or of molecules such as ubiquinol and glutathione, play an essential role in cellular protective mechanisms (see Refs. 5 and 44).

We have not discussed these antioxidant systems in this brief review. However, it is abundantly clear that they must play a critical role, not only in protecting normal cells against endogenous free radical injury, but also in providing for effective protection against a host of exogenous toxic agents whose effects are mediated through the generation of such oxidants. These systems, along with various endogenous repair mechanisms, represent a first line of the coordinated cellular defenses against oxygen toxicity in general and lipid peroxidation in particular.

ACKNOWLEDGMENTS

This review is partly based on an opening lecture by L.E. at the Fifth International Congress on Oxygen Radicals, Kyoto, Japan, November 17–21, 1991 (Ref. 5). We thank our colleagues, particularly Enrique Cadenas, Patrik Forsmark, Alex Sevanian, Fulvio Ursini, and Mary Lou Wratten, for stimulating discussions. Research from our laboratories has been supported by the National Institutes of Health, the American Heart Association (Los Angeles Chapter), the Swedish Medical and Natural Science Research Councils, the Swedish Cancer Society, and the Bank of Sweden Tercentenary Research Foundation.

REFERENCES

1. S. Bergström and R. T. Holman, *Adv. Enzymol.* **8,** 425 (1948).
2. A. L. Tappel, *Vitam. Horm. (N.Y.)* **20,** 563 (1961).
3. T. A. Barber and F. Bernheim, *Adv. Gerontol. Res.* **2,** 355 (1967).
4. K. Yagi (ed.), "Lipid Peroxides in Biology and Medicine." Academic Press, New York, 1982.
5. L. Ernster, *in* "Active Oxygens, Lipid Peroxides and Antioxidants" (K. Yagi, ed.), pp. 1–38. Japan Sci. Soc. Press, Tokyo and CRC Press, Boca Raton, Florida, 1993.
6. B. Halliwell and J. M. C. Gutteridge, *in* "Methods in Enzymology" (L. Packer and A. N. Glazer, eds.), Vol. 186, p. 1. Academic Press, San Diego, 1990.
7. A Sevanian and P. Hochstein, *Annu. Rev. Nutr.* **5,** 365 (1985).
8. O. Meyerhof, Pfluegers *Arch. Gesamte Physiol.* **200,** 1 (1923).
9. H. M. Evans and K. S. Bishop, *Science* **56,** 650 (1922).
10. K. U. Ingold, *Chem. Rev.* **61,** 653 (1961).
11. A. L. Tappel, *in* "The Enzymes" (P. D. Boyer, ed.) Vol. 8, p. 355. Academic Press, New York, 1962.
12. G. W. Burton and K. U. Ingold, *Acc. Chem. Res.* **19,** 194 (1989).
13. E. Andre and K. W. Hou, *Comptes Rendus* **194,** 645 (1932).
14. F. Bernheim, M. L. C. Bernheim, and K. M. Wilber, *J. Biol. Chem.* **174,** 254 (1948).
15. P. Hochstein and L. Ernster, *Biochem. Biophys. Res. Commun.* **12,** 388 (1963).
16. R. Sato, T. Omura, and H. Nishibayashi, *in* "Oxidases and Related Redox Systems" (T. E. King, H. S. Mason, and M. Mrrison, eds.), p. 861. Wiley, New York, 1965.
17. P. Hochstein, K. Nordenbrand, and L. Ernster, *Biochem. Biophys. Res. Commun.* **14,** 323 (1964).
18. T. F. Slater, *Biochem. J.* **222,** 1 (1984).
19. A. Bindoli, *Free Radicals Biol. Med.* **5,** 247 (1988).
20. S. N. Chatterjee and S. Agarwal, *Free Radicals Biol. Med.* **4,** 51 (1988).
21. K. Takeshige, R. Takayananagi, and S. Minakami, *Biochem. J.* **192,** 861 (1980).
22. M. Lieberman and P. Hochstein, *Science* **152,** 213 (1966).
23. G. Minotti and S. D. Aust, *J. Biochem. Chem.* **262,** 1098 (1987).
24. M. Tien and S. D. Aust, *in* "Lipid Peroxides in Biology and Medicine" (K. Yagi, ed.), p. 23., Academic Press, New York 1982.
25. L. Ernster, K. Nordenbrand, and S. Orrenius, *in* "Lipid Peroxides in Biology and Medicine" (K. Yagi, ed.) p. 55., Academic Press, New York 1982.
26. F. Ursini, M. Maiorino, P. Hochstein, and L. Ernster, *Free Radicals Biol. Med.* **63,** 31 (1989).
27. B. Halliwell and J. M. C. Gutteridge, "Free Radicals in Biology and Medicine" 2nd ed. Clarendon, Oxford, 1989.
28. A. Sevanian, K. Nordenbrand, K. Kim, L. Ernster, and P. Hochstein, *Free Radicals Biol. Med.* **8,** 145 (1990).

29. S. Yamamato, *Free Radicals. Biol. Med.* **10,** 149 (1991).
30. P. Hochstein and L. Ernster, *in* "Ciba Foundation Symposium on Cellular Injury" (A. V. A. de Reuck and J. Knight, eds.), p. 123. Churchill, London, 1964.
31. T. C. Pederson, J. A. Buese, and S. D. Aust, *J. Biol. Chem.* **248,** 7134 (1973).
32. T. C. Pederson and S. D. Aust, *Biochim. Biophys. Acta* **385,** 232 (1975).
33. A. D. N. Vaz, E. S. Roberts, and M. J. Coon, *Proc. Natl. Acad. Sci. U.S.A.* **87,** 5499 (1990).
34. M. Ingelman-Sundberg and G. Ekström, *in* "Biological Free Radical Formation and Antioxidants" (F. Ursini and E. Cadenas, eds.), p. 43. CLEUP, Padua, Italy, 1992.
35. F. Ursini, M. Maiorino, and C. Gregolin, *Biochim. Biophys. Acta* **839,** 62 (1985).
36. P. Hochstein and S. K. Jain, *Fed. Proc., Fed. Am. Soc. Exp. Biol.* **40,** 183 (1981).
37. W. R. Bidlack, R. T. Okita, and P. Hochstein, *Biochem. Biophys. Res. Commun.* **53,** 459 (1973).
38. M. Glinn, L. Ernster, and C. P. Lee, *Arch. Biochem. Biophys.* **290,** 57 (1991).
39. Y. Hatefi and W. G. Hanstein, *Biochemistry,* **12,** 3515 (1973).
40. A. L. Tappel and H. Zalkin, *Nature (London)* **185,** 35 (1960).
41. P. Biemond, H. G. Van Eijk, A. J. G. Swaak, and J. F. Koster, *J. Clin. Invest.* **73,** 1576 (1984).
42. J. M. McCord, *N. Engl. J. Med.* **312,** 159 (1985).
43. B. M. Babior, *Adv. Enzymol.* **65,** 49 (1992).
44. L. Ernster, P. Forsmark, and K. Nordenbrand, *BioFactors* **3,** 241 (1992).
45. E. T. Morgan, D. R. Koop, and M. J. Coon, *J. Biol. Chem.* **257,** 13951 (1982).
46. F. P. Corongiu, G. Poli, M. U. Dianzani, K. H. Cheesman, and T. F. Slater, *Chem.–Biol. Interact.* **59,** 147 (1986).
47. L. J. Marnett, *Carcinogenesis* **820,** 1365 (1987).
48. Y. Hatefi and W. G. Hanstein, *Arch. Biochem. Biophys.* **138,** 73 (1970).
49. H. Narabayashi, K. Takeshige, and S. Minakami, *Biochem. J.* **202,** 97 (1982).
50. D. Galaris, A. Sevanian, E. Cadenas, and P. Hochstein, *Arch. Biochem. Biophys.* **281,** 163 (1990).
51. D. Galaris, D. Mira, A. Sevanian, E. Cadenas, and P. Hochstein, *Arch. Biochem. Biophys.* **262,** 221 (1988).
52. D. Galaris, E. Cadenas, and P. Hochstein, *Arc. Biochem. Biophys.* **273,** 497 (1989).
53. H. Kasai and S. Nishimura, *Environ. Health Perspect.* **67,** 111 (1988).
54. J. W. Park and R. A. Floyd, *Free Radicals Biol. Med.* **12,** 245 (1992).
55. U. T. Brunk and R. S. Sohal, *in* "Membrane Lipid Oxidation" (C. Vigo Pelfrey, ed.), Vol. 2, p. 191. CRC Press, Boca Raton, Florida, 1991.
56. C. Richter, J. W. Park, and B. N. Ames, *Proc. Nat. Acad. Sci. U.S.A.* **85,** 6465 (1988).
57. A. W. Linnane, S. Marzuki, T. Ozawa, and M. Tanaka, *Lancet* **1,** 642 (1989).
58. A. M. Hruszkewycz and D. S. Bergtold, *Mutat. Res.* **244,** 123 (1990).
59. J. R. Zhang and A. Sevanian, *Biochim. Biophys. Acta* **1085,** 159 (1991).
60. E. R. Stadtman and C. N. Oliver, *J. Biol. Chem.* **226,** 2005 (1991).

4 Enzyme Leakage as an Indicator of Cytotoxicity in Cultured Cells

Allison A. Welder and Daniel Acosta

INTRODUCTION

In developing cell culture models for evaluating the toxic effects of xenobiotics to organ systems, essential requirements include utilization of inexpensive, reliable, reproducible, and rapid methods to assess toxicity. Leakage of cytoplasmic enzymes from injured cells into the culture medium has proven to be useful for the evaluation of early or late cytotoxicity in primary cultures obtaind from various primary organ systems including the heart, liver, and kidney (1,2). Cytotoxicity has been effectively determined by these assays after treatment with therapeutic agents (1), environmental chemicals (1), drugs of abuse (3,4), and conditions of hypoxia/ischemia (1,5). Specifically, this method assays the integrity of the plasma membrane to retain cellular enzymes (1,2,6).

Lactate dehydrogenase (LDH) is an ubiquitous enzyme among vertebrate organisms and carries out the following cytoplasmic enzyme reaction:

$$NAD^+ + \text{lactate} \rightleftharpoons NADH + \text{pyruvate}$$

The enzyme activity is typically measured spectrophotmetrically at 340 nm by following either the oxidation of NADH with pyruvate (decrease in absorbance) or reduction of NAD^+ with lactate (increase in absorbance) at rates producing a change in absorbance of 0.05 to 0.1 per min (6–8). Under standard conditions one unit of enzyme catalyses the oxidation of NADH or reduction of NAD^+ at 1 μmol-min (7). Since there is no evidence that cells actively secrete LDH, LDH release from the cell has been and is continuing to be used as a manifestation of cellular injury (1,2). Its release into the medium surrounding the cell cultures after exposure to a xenobiotic is quantitated and correlated to the breakdown in the permeability of the cell barrier, the plasma membrane (1,2).

MATERIALS/REAGENTS

0.1 M Phosphate Buffer

Prepare 0. 1 *M* phosphate buffer by adding 2.1761 g/liter KH_2PO_4 (potassium phosphate monobasic; Fisher Cat. No. P285–500, Fairlawn, NJ) and 22.4658

METHODS IN TOXICOLOGY, Volume 1B

g/liter $Na_2HPO_4 \cdot 7H_2O$ (sodium phosphate dibasic heptahydrate; Mallinckrodt Cat. No. 7782–85–6, Paris, KY) to 500 ml of double-distilled deionized water. Stir until all of the powder is dissolved and then add distilled deionized water to a total volume of 1000 ml in a volumetric flask (6,8).

NADH Solution

Prepare NADH (β-nicotinamide adenine dinucleotide, reduced form; Sigma Cat. No. N–8129, St. Louis, MO) solution (2.5 mg/ml) in 10 ml of 0.1 *M* phosphate buffer in a volumetric flask and place on ice. Prepare this solution fresh daily (6,8).

Pyruvic Acid Solution

Prepare sodium pyruvate (α-ketopropionic acid; 2-oxopropanoic acid; Sigma Cat. No. P–2256) solution (1 mg/ml) in 25 ml of 0.1 *M* phosphate buffer in a volumetric flask and place on ice. This solution should be prepared fresh daily (6,8).

PROCEDURES

Treatment of Cultures with Chemicals, Drugs, or Toxicants

Water-soluble agents are dissolved in the desired culture medium or balanced salt solution. Agents which are not soluble in water are dissolved in ethanol, dimethyl sulfoxide, or propylene glycol. The cultures are then exposed to the desired concentrations of agent for the desired periods. Control cultures are treated in the same fashion as the agent-treated cultures without the agent and serum (6).

Obtaining Samples for Lactate Dehydrogenase (LDH) Determination

Both LDH released from the cells in culture and the amount remaining in the cells (cellular LDH) can be quantitated. At the periods of injury evaluation, a 100-μl sample of medium is taken from each control and drug-treated culture and placed in a 13 × 100-mm test tube, which is maintained on ice for the evaluation of LDH released by the cells into the surrounding medium. Cellular LDH is determined at the last time point of injury evaluation by pouring off the remaining medium and adding 1 ml of 0.1 *M* phosphate buffer to the cultures and scraping the monolayer of cells off of each dish with a Teflon scraper. The buffer containing the cells is transferred to a 13 × 100-mm test tube using a Pasteur pipette. The contents of each of these test tubes (maintained on ice) is sonicated with a Fisher Sonic Dismembrator (Model 300) for 10 sec at a relative output of 0.4 to release all LDH from the cells. A 100-μl sample is taken from each tube and placed in a clean 13 × 100-mm test tube maintained on ice for the determination of cellular LDH (6,8).

Basically, the same procedure can be used with cell suspensions by taking two equal volumes, one for assay of LDH in the supernatant after centifugation of the cells and the second for total LDH in the vial after lysing the cells first with 1% Triton X-100. In the latter case the cells and debris are removed by centrifugation for 3 min at 1200 *g*, and the supernatant is assayed for total LDH. Cellular LDH can be determined by the difference, if desired (9).

LDH Assay Procedure

To each 13 × 100-mm test tube containing the 100-μl sample obtained as described above are added 0.2 ml of NADH solution, 0.2 ml of sodium pyruvate solution, and 2.5 ml of warm (37°C) 0.1 *M* phosphate buffer. The contents are vortexed for 5 sec and the solution is transferred to a 4.0-ml cuvette. The cuvette is placed into a Shimadzu (Kyoto, ultraviolet Japan) 160 *A* spectrophotometer (temperature controlled with an automatic positioner) at a temperature of 30°C. Absorbance readings are taken at 1-min intervals for 4 min at a wavelength of 340 nm (6,8).

LDH Calculations

Calculate the mean ΔA per minute for the 4 min measured. Calculate LDH units per milliliter by the following formula: U LDH/ml $= \Delta A \times D \times F$, where D is the dilution factor (10,000) and F is a temperature factor of 1.16 at 30°C (5). Values can then be expressed as the percentage of the total cellular LDH (total LDH = released LDH + cellular LDH) (6,8).

COMMENTS

LDH is exclusively a cytosolic enzyme and its leakage from cultured cells is correlated with cell membrane injury, but does not always lead to irreversible cell injury. For example, when cell cultures were allowed to recover after exposure to conditions of ischemia (5) and treatment with a polyene macrolide antibiotic (10), the cells recovered. In both instances varying amounts of LDH leaked out of the cells due to acute membrane permeability changes without long-range toxicity and cell death (5,10). Therefore, differences of opinion exist addressing the actual meaning of LDH release (2). It has been suggested to represent reversible graded increases in plasma membrane permeability (2).

In comparison, the LDH assay is much less subjective and time consuming (when large numbers of samples are to be analyzed, they may be stored for 24–

48 hr at 4°C and analyzed in a multicell reader or centrifugal analyzer if these apparatuses are available) in ascertaining cell damage than using subjective staining procedures with dyes such as trypan blue (1,2,6). Nevertheless, the LDH assay has some disadvantages. It may be partly inactivated by the xenobiotic tested or by freezing (2). In situations in which injury is minimal and reversible, LDH leakage would most likely be better assessed by measuring other cellular functions, such as ion flux (1,2).

ACKNOWLEDGMENTS

Research support for this work was provided in part by the National Institute on Drug Abuse First Independent Research Support Award (DA-05699) and a research grant from the Presbyterian Health Foundation of Oklahoma City awarded to A.A.W. D.A. is a Burroughs Wellcome Scholar in Toxicology.

REFERENCES

1. D. Acosta, E. M. B. Sorensen, D. C. Anuforo, D. B. Mitchell, K. Ramos, K. Santone, and M. A. Smith, *In Vitro Cell. Dev. Biol.* **21**, 495 (1985).
2. C. J. Danpure, *Cell Biochem. Funct.* **2**, 144 (1984).
3. A. A. Welder, *in* "Cellular and Molecular Toxicology and in Vitro Toxicology" (D. Acosta, ed.), p. 121. CRC Press, Boca Raton, Florida, 1990.
4. R. B. Melchert, T. J. Herron, and A. A. Welder, *Med. Sci. Sports Exercise* **24**, 206 (1992).
5. D. Acosta, M. Puckett, and R. McMillin, *In Vitro* **14**, 728 (1978).
6. D. B. Mitchell, K. S. Santone, and D. Acosta, *J. Tissue Cult. Methods* **6**, 113 (1980).
7. C. L. Market, *Cell Biochem. Funct.* **2**, 131 (1984).
8. R. J. Henry, N. Chiamori, O. J. Golub, and S. Berkman, *Am. J. Clin. Pathol.* **30**, 149 (1960).
9. C. A. Tyson and C. E. Green, *in* "The Isolated Hepatocyte" (E. J. Raukman and G. M. Padilla, eds.), p. 119. Academic Press, San Diego, 1987.
10. P. B. Fisher, V. Bryson, and C. P. Schaffner, *J. Cell. Physiol.* **97**, 345 (1978).

5 Cellular K^+

V. Kefalas and N. H. Stacey

INTRODUCTION

Potassium ion leakage may indicate interference with transport sites such as the Na^+–K^+ pump (1). Actual damage to the membranes also results in potassium loss from the cell to the external milieu. This can be an extensive and usually irreversible change, and loss of K^+ has been used to estimate cell toxicity and death.

In 1975 Baur *et al.* (2) reported membrane potential as well as intracellular Na^+ and K^+ concentrations to be the most sensitive criteria of viability in isolated hepatocytes. This was supported by a comprehensive comparative study with other parameters for estimating cell viability/toxicity by Stacey and Klaassen (3). The benefits of using K^+ as a parameter were reviewed by Klaassen and Stacey (4). Over the ensuing years intracellular levels of K^+ have been used as indicators of viability and toxicity in various *in vitro* preparations of hepatocytes and other cells.

This chapter covers the measurement of intracellular K^+ as an indicator of disruption of membrane integrity. Only the materials and reagents used for estimating intracellular K^+ in isolated hepatocytes using a rapid centrifugal filtration technique and analysis by flame photometry are provided in detail below. Also included throughout the chapter are various alternatives, with references provided for the studies using other methods, should the reader wish to establish other techniques.

MATERIALS, EQUIPMENT, AND REAGENTS

Rapid Centrifugal Filtration with Silicon Oil

Microcentrifuge (Microfuge B, Beckman, Palo Alto, CA)
Microfuge tubes, polypropylene (400 μl)
Autopipettes (200 and 100 μl)
Eppendorf multipipette (Eppendorf Inc., Fremont, CA) (15–100 μl, for silicon oil)
Perchloric acid: Available as a 70% solution. Dilute with distilled water as required. Store at room temperature until needed.
Silicon oil: A final specific gravity of 1.02 is achieved by mixing equal parts

METHODS IN TOXICOLOGY, Volume 1B

of Dow Corning 550 fluid [*d* (density) 1.06, Cat. No. 6546] and Dow Corning 556 fluid (*d* = 0.98, Cat. No. 6517). In Australia this product is packed and distributed by Ajax Chemicals (Sydney). Similar oils are available from other sources.

Sample Preparation and Flame Photometry

Flame photometer and pump (Corning 405 flame photometer and Corning 850 air compressor, Corning Ltd., Halstead, Essex, England)
Disposable microbeakers (5 ml) and rack
Volumetric flasks (100 and 1000 ml)
Scalpel and cutting board, or tube cutter (Resco, Detroit, MI)
Diluent (Corning 460/405) diluted 1 : 1000 with distilled water in a 1000-ml volumetric flask
Flame photometer standard (Corning 80 m*M* potassium) diluted 1 : 1000 with distilled water in a 100 ml volumetric flask

PROCEDURE

The leakage of K^+ from hepatocytes may be estimated by determining the intracellular concentration of K^+ or this ion in the extracellular medium. Sample preparation is dictated by whether extra- or intracellular K^+ is to be measured and also by which type of *in vitro* system—suspension, monolayer culture, or tissue slices—is used. These different *in vitro* systems are dealt with separately below. It is our experience that it is preferable to determine intracellular concentrations, as these are higher than in the extracellular medium and give more reproducible results.

Cell Suspension

Measurement of K^+ in the Extracellular Medium

Various cell types, including rat hepatocytes (5,6) and human red blood cells (7), may be used in suspension and be in need of estimation of viability. There are currently two main methods of separating hepatocytes in suspension from the surrounding media. The first involves centrifuging the suspension at 200–300 *g* for 1–3 min (depending on the method), washing (using further centrifugation) the cell pellet in an isotonic K^+-free solution, and then lysing the cell pellet. The lysates are then ready for analysis. Any of the following solutions may be used:

Washing Solutions

Cold 140 m*M* choline chloride/10 m*M* HEPES, pH 7.4 (8)
Cold 154 m*M* choline chloride, pH 7.4 (9)

0.9% NaCl (10)
0.32 *M* sucrose, pH 7.4 (11)
50 m*M* Tris–HCL, pH 7.4 (12)

Lysing Solutions

7% Perchloric acid (PCA) (13)
3% PCA (12,14)
HNO_3, concentration not given (11)
6% Trichloroacetic acid (10)
Water (8)

The second method, which is preferred and therefore described in detail, is rapid centrifugal filtration. The cell suspension is layered over an "oil" layer and then centrifuged. Due to the greater density of the cells, they pass through the oil, leaving the culture medium on top. The rapid centrifugal filtration method used in our laboratory is a modification of that used by Baur *et al.* (2).

Into a 400-μl Eppendorf tube place 100 μl of 6% PCA and overlay it with at least 50 μl of silicon oil (d = 1.02). Note that this should be done before the actual experiment. At the time of the experiment, carefully add 100–200 μl of cell suspension containing 1.4–2 $\times$ 10^6 cells/ml from the experimental flask and centrifuge for ~10 sec at top speed in a microcentrifuge (Beckman Microfuge B). During the rapid spin, cells plus adherent fluid enter the PCA layer in 1–2 sec and are immediately lysed and precipitated (as shown in Fig. 1). These

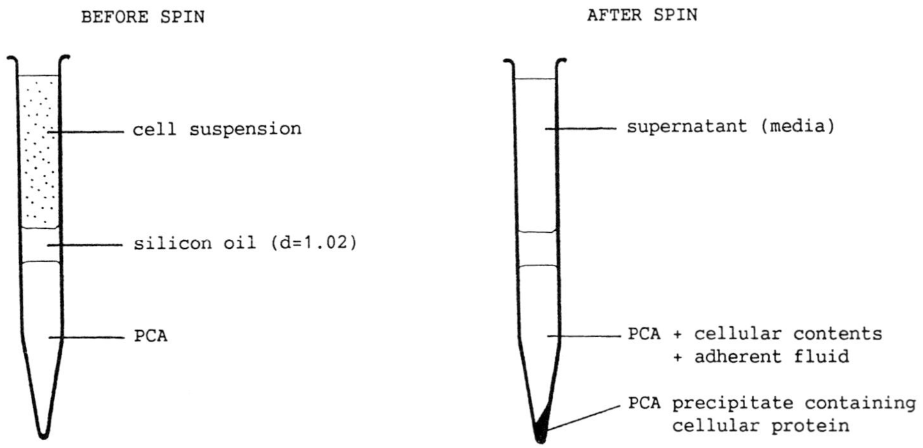

Figure 1 Rapid centrifugal filtration with silicon oil—cellular distribution before and after centrifugation. PCA, Perchloric acid.

samples can now be either stored (~1 week at room temperature; longer at 4°C) or immediately prepared for analysis.

Fariss *et al.* (15) described a rapid centrifugal method similar to that of Baur *et al.* (2) using dibutyl phthalate (d = 1.046) instead of silicon oil layered over 10% PCA (d = 1.06). This is detailed in Chapter 36, by Reed.

Other separation liquids, such as bromodecane (16) and bromododecane (16,17), have been used for centrifugal filtration. However, silicon oil and dibutyl phthalate have proved most popular for *in vitro* studies with hepatocytes.

Sample Preparation and Analysis

Microfuge tubes (400 μl) containing the lysed and precipitated hepatocytes in PCA from the microcentrifugation step are simply cut just below the oil layer with a scalpel or a tube cutter. For analysis using a flame photometer (Corning 405), a 50-μl aliquot of the PCA layer is immediately taken and diluted 1:20 with diluent in a microbeaker. The flame photometer is calibrated with the Corning standard and the zero diluent standard (the instrument response is linear within this range) and the samples are read. Other flame photometric procedures may involve the use of internal standards (18) or a standard curve (19). Corrections are made for any dilution factors and the percentage of viable cells at the onset of the experiment. Results are usually expressed in our studies as either μmol/g wet weight (determined gravimetrically from the parent cell suspension) or μmol/mg protein. The protein content is estimated from a duplicate microfuge tube containing 3*M* KOH instead of PCA, by the Lowry method (20). Concentrations may alternatively be expressed as nmol/1 million cells by estimating the DNA content of the PCA pellet (15,19), or as a percentage of total cell K^+. Total cell K^+ estimates by other laboratories have been made in aliquots of cell suspension which have been sonicated (21) or deproteinized with 30% trichloroacetic acid (5 parts suspension to 1 part acid) (22), followed by centrifugation and analysis of the supernatant.

Cultured Cells

Cellular K^+ levels have also been determined in hepatocyte cultures in other laboratories as an estimate of toxicity. The methods used are outlined below.

Sendelbach *et al.* (23) described a method for estimating intracellular K^+ concentrations in primary rat hepatocyte cultures. Medium is removed from 60-mm culture dishes containing primary cultures on Vitrogen-100 (Collagen Corp., Palo Alto, CA) and the cultured cells are rinsed twice with a phosphate buffer (200 m*M* NaCl, 0.34 m*M* $Na_2HPO_4 \cdot 7H_2O$, 8.5 m*M* Tris, 10 m*M* EGTA, free acid) and twice with isotonic saline. The EGTA prohibits K^+ leakage (24).

Two milliliters of Tris–HCl (10 m*M*, pH 7.4, 25°C) is added to the dishes, which are then scraped with a rubber policeman. The suspension is sonicated for 10 sec at 4°C with a cell disrupter (Model W-10, Heat Systems, Plainview, NY). Aliquots are centrifuged for 60 sec in a microcentrifuge (Beckman). Analysis is then carried out on the supernatant.

The method of Harman and Fischer (25) involves removal of the hepatocytes from a collagen membrane by adding purified collagenase (50 U) to each plate for 15 min. The resultant cell suspension is pipetted into a test tube and stored on ice. A 1.5-ml aliquot of suspension is taken and centrifuged at 50 *g* for 2 min. Protein is precipitated by resuspending the cell pellet in 1 ml of 3% metaphosphoric acid and centrifuging at 5000 rpm for 15 min. The supernatant is then ready for analysis.

A far more expedient method, however, is that of Bruschi and Priestly (26), which measures the K^+ that has leaked into the medium, rather than the intracellular concentration. Quite simply, medium is diluted and the ion concentration is then measured, using a K^+-sensitive electrode.

Liver Slices

Sipes *et al.* (27) and Weiss and Putney (28) described methods of estimating K^+ in rat liver slices. Both methods first require the liver slices to be blotted and weighed after incubation. Sipes *et al.* (27) then sonicated the slices (10 pulses, Model 350, Branson Sonic Power, Danbury, CT) and added 70% PCA to precipitate the protein. After centrifuging for 5 min in a microcentrifuge (Beckman), the supernatant was assayed by flame photometry. Weiss and Putney (28) dried the tissue overnight (100°C), followed by ashing over the next night (500–600°C), solubilizing with 0.1 *M* HCl and 0.01 *M* $SrCl_2$ and then assaying for K^+.

COMMENTS

Other Detection Methods for K^+

Besides flame photometry, other methods, such as atomic absorption spectrometry (29) and K^+ electrodes, have been used to measure levels of this ion. Furthermore, a fabricated double-barreled microelectrode has been used to determine K^+ in liver slices (30,31).

Rapid Cell Separation Using Silicon Oil

The silicon oil separation method provides a rapid way of separating cells from medium, thus making it possible to process a greater number of samples as compared to other separation methods. Additionally, after separation the supernatant in the top layer may be used for the measurement of other toxicity markers, such as release of cellular enzymes, as well as indices of biochemical perturbations.

The density of silicon oil is critical. It must be greater than that of the incubation medium used, but lower than that of the PCA or the cells themselves. However, the effective density range is quite large. In our laboratory we have found that oil densities between 1.02 and 1.033 are effective for hepatocytes. Appropriate centrifugation conditions for other cell types with unknown densities can be determined empirically.

Sainsbury *et al.* (32) showed that silicon oil with a density of 1.03 was adequate in preventing any solute loss from isolated hepatocytes during the separation. Likewise, Fariss *et al.* (15) reported that intracellular contents were unaffected by rapid centrifugation through dibutyl phthalate. They also checked the completeness of separation of viable and nonviable cells from a sample of isolated hepatocytes. By substituting 36% (v/v) Percoll in Hanks' salt solution (d = 1.06) for PCA, it was found that only viable hepatocytes pelleted in the Percoll layer.

Rapid centrifugation techniques with silicon oil (2,33) and brominated hydrocarbons (16) do not separate viable from nonviable cells at the densities described. However, nonviable cells have lost the majority of their K^+ and do not contribute significantly to the total amount of intracellular K^+, making the silicon oil method suitable for the estimation of that entity. When measuring other end points, the presence of nonviable cells may not be desirable, particularly if the investigator is interested in processes bringing about cell injury, rather than cell death. In this case the dibutyl phthalate filtration method of Fariss *et al.* (15) should be considered (Fig. 2). As only viable cells pass through the dibutyl phthalate at density 1.046, the number of cells in the PCA will differ for each sample. To compensate for these differences, each sample is later assayed for

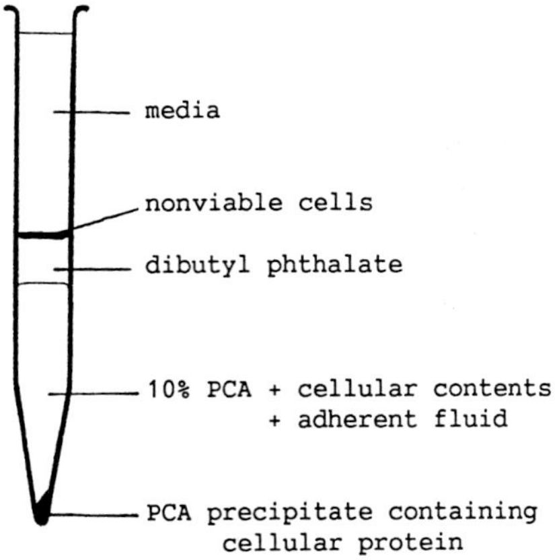

Figure 2 Rapid centrifugal filtration with dibutyl phthalate—cellular distribution after centrifugation. PCA, Perchloric acid.

DNA or for protein content. As this method measures only K^+ in viable cells, it cannot be applied in and of itself as an estimate of cell death in a population of cells.

Analysis by Flame Photometry

Occasionally, unexpected off-scale readings may result. These may be attributed to contaminated microbeakers. It is important not to touch the inside surface or allow any material to enter the microbeaker. For this reason samples should be prepared just prior to reading or should be stored covered in an isolated area. Silicon oil present in the sample mix may also cause this problem.

Microbeakers are recommended when using a sampling probe for flame photometry. Empirically, we have observed that with other-shaped vessels (tubes and flasks) K^+ is often not distributed evenly throughout the sample.

REFERENCES

1. J. W. Bridges, D. J. Benford, and S. A. Hubbard, *in* "Cellular Systems for Toxicity Testing" (G. M. Williams, V. C. Dunkel, and V. A. Ray, eds.), p. 42. New York Academy of Sciences, New York, 1983.
2. H. Baur, S. Kasperek, and E. Pfaff, *Hoppe-Seyler's Z. Physiol. Chem. Bd.* **356,** 827 (1975).
3. N. H. Stacey and C. D. Klaassen, *Toxicol. Appl. Pharmacol.* **58,** 8 (1981).
4. C. D. Klaassen and N. H. Stacey, *in* "Toxicology of the Liver" (G. Plaa and W. R. Hewitt, eds.), p. 147. Raven, New York, 1982.
5. M. Frimmer and R. Kroker, *Naunyn-Schmiedeberg's Arch. Pharmacol.* **278,** 285 (1973).
6. T. Capiod, B. Berthon, J. Poggioli, G. M. Burgess, and M. Claret, *FEBS Lett.* **141,** 49 (1982).
7. A. Sanchez, J. Garcia-Sancho, and B. Herreros, *FEBS Lett.* **110,** 65 (1980).
8. A. Binet and J. Bolard, *Biochem, J.* **253,** 435 (1988).
9. J. W. Edmondson and N. U. Bang, *Am. J. Physiol.* **241,** C3 (1981).
10. O. Barnabei, G. Leghissa, and V. Tomasi, *Biochim. Biophys. Acta* **362,** 316 (1974).
11. F. Medzhiradsky and M. J. Marks, *Biochem. Med.* **13,** 164 (1975).
12. A. B. DiRenzo, A. J. Gandolfi, S. D. Brooks, and K. Brendel, *Drug Chem. Toxicol.* **8,** 207 (1985).
13. M. L. Berger, H. Bhatt, B. Combes, and R. W. Estabrook, *Hepatology,* **6,** 36 (1986).
14. N. Stacey and B. G. Priestly, *Toxicol. Appl. Pharmacol.* **45,** 29 (1978).
15. M. W. Fariss, M. K. Brown, J. A. Schmitz, and D. J. Reed, *Toxicol. Appl. Pharmacol.* **79,** 283 (1985).
16. C. Cornell, *Anal. Biochem.* **102,** 326 (1980).
17. A. Noda, T. Sendo, K. Ohno, H. Noda, and S. Goto, *Chem. Pharm. Bull.* **35,** 2538 (1987).
18. G. F. Rush, M. Ripple, and R. Chenery, *J. Pharmacol. Exp. Ther.* **233,** 741 (1985).

19. T. M. O'Hara, J. F. Borzelleca, E. C. Clarke, M. A. Sheppard, and L. W. Condie, Jr., *Fundam. Appl. Toxicol.* **13,** 605 (1989).
20. O. H. Lowry, N. J. Rosebrough, A. L. Farr, and R. J. Randall, *J. Biol. Chem.* **193,** 265 (1951).
21. W. M. Bracken and C. D. Klaassen, *J. Toxicol. Environ. Health* **22,** 163 (1987).
22. E. Albano, G. Poli, E. Chiarpotto, N. D'Anelli, and M. U. Dianzani, *Pharmacology,* **9,** 961 (1981).
23. L. E. Sendelbach, W. M. Bracken, and C. D. Klaassen, *Toxicology* **55,** 83 (1989).
24. G. A. Pascoe and D. J. Reed, *Free Radicals Biol. Med.* **6,** 209 (1989).
25. A. W. Harman and L. J. Fischer, *Toxicol. Appl. Pharmacol.* **71,** 330 (1983).
26. S. A. Bruschi and B. G. Priestly, *Toxicol. in Vitro* **4,** 743 (1990).
27. I. G. Sipes, R. L. Fisher, P. F. Smith, E. R. Stine, A. J. Gandolfi, and K. Brendel, *Arch. Toxicol.* **11,** 20 (1987).
28. S. J. Weiss and J. W. Putney, Jr., *J. Pharmacol. Exp. Ther.* **207,** 669 (1978).
29. C. E. Thomas and D. J. Reed, *J. Pharmacol. Exp. Ther.* **245,** 493 (1988).
30. M. Fujimoto and T. Kubota, *J. Physiol. (London)* **26,** 631 (1976).
31. K. Okada, S. Yamada, Y. Kawashima, F. Kitade, K. Okajimo, and M. Fujimoto, *Cancer Res.* **40,** 1663 (1980).
32. G. M. Sainsbury, M. Stubbs, R. Hems, and H. A. Krebs, *Biochem. J.* **180,** 685 (1979).
33. N. H. Stacey, L. R. Cantilena, and C. D. Klaassen, *Toxicol. Appl. Pharmacol.* **53,** 470 (1980).

6

Morphological and Biochemical Investigations on Plasma Membrane Blebbing during Cell Injury

Giorgio Bellomo, Francesca Mirabelli, Mariapia Vairetti, Francesca Iosi, and Walter Malorni

INTRODUCTION

An early event in cell injury caused by toxic agents is the appearance of multiple surface protrusions, often referred to as "blebs" (Fig. 1). Bleb formation has been described both *in vitro* and *in vivo* after exposure of animals, tissues, or cells to a variety of toxic conditions (1–4). Once formed, the blebs can be reabsorbed, some of them can merge to form a larger bleb, they can be "pinched-off," or, following the rupture of the surrounding membrane, they can release their content into the extracellular medium (5). Bleb rupture has therefore been proposed as the predominant mechanism for the release of intracellular enzymes into plasma following tissue injury.

The biochemical and structural alterations underlying plasma membrane blebbing have not yet been clarified in detail. However, it is generally accepted that damage to cytoskeletal structure and organization occurs under these conditions. This assumption is supported by the demonstration that two cytoskeletal toxins, cytochalasin B and phalloidin, which interfere with the polymerization status of actin, cause bleb formation (6). Several biochemical mechanisms have been proposed to play a crucial role in inducing cytoskeletal alterations during toxic cell injury. They include direct interaction of the toxin with cytoskeletal structures (6), mitochondrial damage and ATP depletion (7), and disruption of thiol and calcium ion homeostasis (2,8).

Many different types of surface blebs have been recognized, and a sophisticated scoring system, composed of six different stages based on the diameter of the largest bleb(s) on each cell relative to the diameter of the cell itself, has been proposed (4). For example, the toxicity of several sulfhydryl reagents to isolated rat hepatocytes has been shown to cause two major types of cell blebbing, arbitrarily named types A and B (9). Type A blebbing is characterized by the appearance of numerous protrusions on the hepatocyte surface, while type B blebbing is characterized by the presence of a single large bleb arising from the whole surface of the cell, which also appears swollen. Type A blebbing is

METHODS IN TOXICOLOGY, Volume 1B

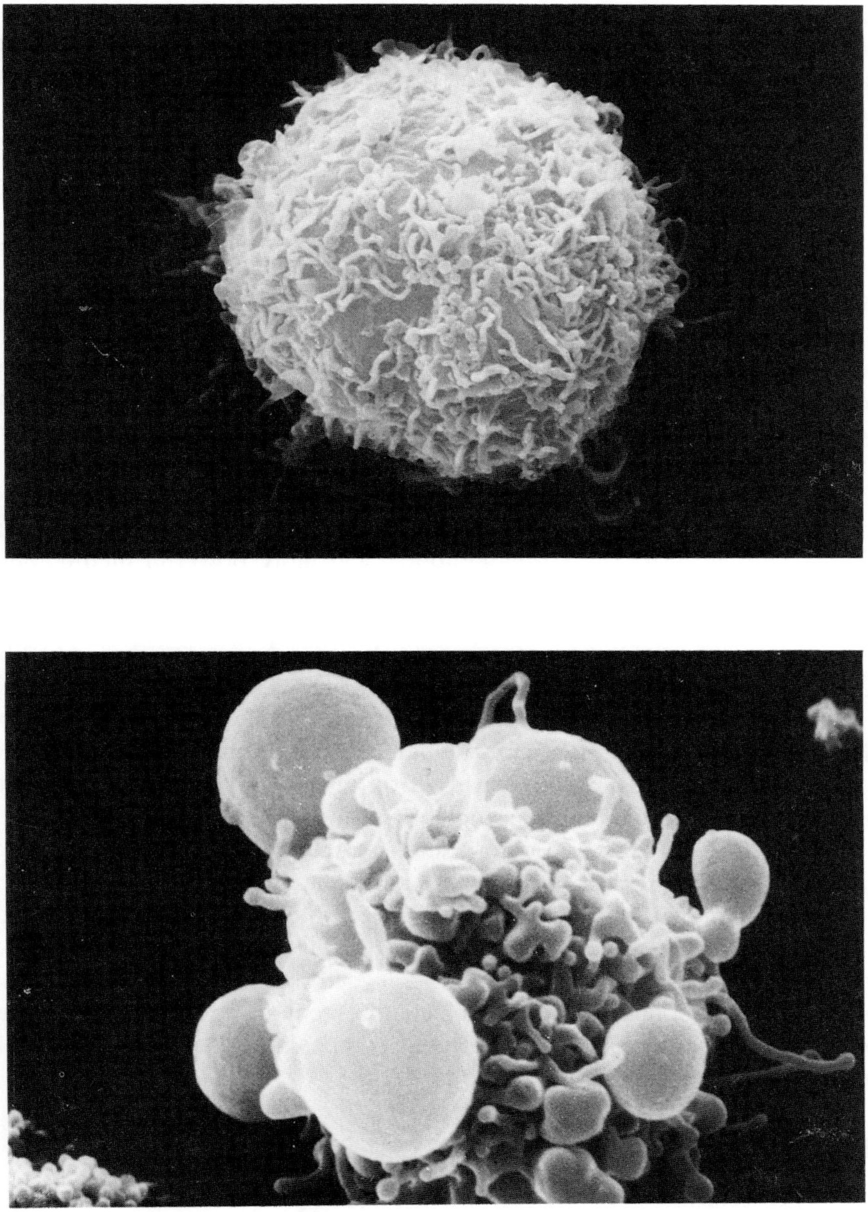

Figure 1 Scanning electron microscopy of a THP cell undergoing blebbing following exposure to the toxic redox-cycling compound menadione (2-methyl-1,4-naphthoquinone). THP cells were incubated without (top) or with (bottom) 200 μM menadione in Krebs–Henseleit buffer supplemented with 25 mM HEPES (pH 7.4) for 60 min.

caused by sulfhydryl reagents able to cross the plasma membrane, irrespective of their mechanism of action (oxidation or alkylation); type B blebbing is caused by agents unable to cross the plasma membrane and exclusively acting on the cell surface (Fig. 1).

However, since the pathophysiological mechanisms of bleb formation are still unclear, these scoring systems have a mere phenomenological significance, and any correlation to the specificity of the toxic agent used or to the biochemical alterations underlying the morphological changes is, at present, only speculative.

Our laboratories have been engaged in the last few years in investigating the ultrastructural and biochemical events associated with bleb formation. The first approach to studying plasma membrane blebbing is the quantitation of the phenomenon, and this can be investigated by light microscopy as the percentage of cells exhibiting multiple surface protrusions. In particular, experiments can be performed in freshly isolated or cultured cells growing in suspension or in monolayer. However, adherent cells undergoing blebbing can remain attached to the culture dish or can be released in the culture medium, and furthermore, the blebbing phenomenon can be minimal and hardly detected by light-microscopic analysis. Therefore, additional and more powerful methodologies, such as scanning electron microscopy, should be used.

Another crucial point in clarifying the mechanisms of bleb formation is the identification of subcellular and structural alterations occurring during blebbing. Among them, particularly relevant are the modifications of intracellular organelle trafficking and distribution, and changes in membrane protein expression and in their association with submembrane structures. Morphological data can be obtained with transmission electron microscopy and scanning electron microscopy of freeze-fractured samples.

Moreover, disturbances in cytoskeleton structure and function are likely involved in the pathogenesis of bleb formation (6). It thus appears critical to investigate the organization of cytoskeletal fibers in cells undergoing blebbing following exposure to toxic compounds or conditions. This can be done with immunocytochemical localization of some cytoskeletal proteins by means of monoclonal antibodies or other specific fluorescent stains (10–12) as well as by biochemical investigation of the protein composition of different cytoskeletal fractions isolated from cells (13–18).

METHODOLOGIES FOR INVESTIGATING CELL BLEBBING

Light Microscopy

Sample Preparation

Light-microscopic analyses can be done using fresh (unfixed) or fixed cells. The procedure for unfixed cells does not require specific sample preparation. Cells in suspension can be concentrated by low-speed (200 *g* for 5 min) centrifugation and then resuspended in a small amount of incubation medium [phosphate-buffered saline (PBS) (pH 7.4) or Krebs–Henseleit medium supplemented with 25 m*M* HEPES (pH 7.4) at a density of 1–2 × 10^6 cells/ml]. Cells growing on tissue culture dishes can be directly analyzed in their culture medium. For fixation, cells in suspension (10^6 cells/ml) are resuspended in ice-cold 3.7% formaldehyde solution in PBS for 10 min, and adherent cells attached to glass coverslips are covered with the same formaldehyde solution for the same period. Morphological analysis is subsequently performed using a light microscope (a Nikon Diaphot with a 40× objective is used in our laboratories).

Comments

Surface blebbing in freshly isolated cells in suspension can be easily quantitated by phase-contrast microscopy. A typical example is reported in Fig. 2 that refers to experiments performed with isolated rat hepatocytes incubated with the redox compound 2-methyl-1,4-naphthoquinone (menadione). Menadione metabolism is associated with the production of considerable amounts of oxygen-reactive species that attack different molecular targets, finally leading to irreversible damage and cytotoxicity (19). At different time points during the incubation procedure, samples of the cell suspension are taken for the simultaneous quantitation of cell blebbing and trypan blue uptake (as an index of increased plasma membrane permeability and cell death) (20). A comparative analysis of menadione-induced surface blebbing in various cell types is reported

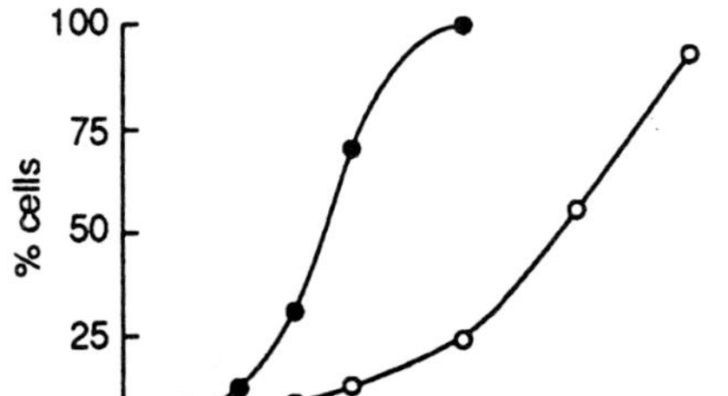

Figure 2 Surface blebbing and cytotoxicity induced by 2-methyl-1,4-naphthoquinone (menadione) metabolism in isolated rat hepatocytes. Rat hepatocytes were incubated with 0.2 m*M* menadione, and at the indicated time points the percentage of cells exhibiting multiple surface protrusions (●) or taking up trypan blue (○) was evaluated.

Table I Surface Blebbing Caused by 2-Methyl-1,4-naphthoquinone in Freshly Isolated and Cultured Cells[a]

Cell type	Blebbing (%)[b]
Rat hepatocytes (freshly isolated)[c]	100
Rat hepatocytes (primary cultures)	88
A431	48
BT-20	52
CG5	42
GH3	64
HeLa	65
HEp2	55
K562[d]	90
LoVo	48
McCoy	68
THP[3]	93

[a] The indicated cell types were incubated for 60 min (freshly isolated rat hepatocytes) or for 120 min (other cell types) with 200 μM menadione in Ca^{2+}- (1.3 mM) and Mg^{2+}- (1 mM) supplemented phosphate-buffered saline before quantitation of blebbing. For further experimental details see Ref. 15.

[b] Surface blebbing was expressed as the percentage of the cells exhibiting multiple surface protrusions, as detected by phase-contrast microscopy.

[c] Freshly isolated cells maintained in suspension.

[d] Cells grown in suspension.

in Table I. An additional interesting feature of light-microscopic analysis is the possibility of performing time course experiments on single living cells to investigate the appearance and the fate of surface blebs.

The quantitation of surface blebbing in adherent cells by light microscopy has two major drawbacks. First, the investigation on substrate-adherent cells challenged with toxic compounds may lead to an underestimation of the percentage of cells exhibiting blebbing, since these cells detach from the substrate and are released in the incubation medium. One possible way to treat this problem is to quantitate the time course of the percentage of adherent and detached cells that are blebbed. Such an approach will give estimations that are both sensitive (since blebbing in adherent cells usually occurs before their detachment) and comprehensive (since the percentage of blebbing in adherent plus detached cells represents the total amount of blebbed cells). Additionally, the conventional light-microscopic analysis of attached cells may neglect some of the cells exhibiting blebs exclusively at the top surface of the cell, and thus more detailed morphological analyses (such as scanning electron microscopy) could be helpful.

Scanning Electron Microscopy

Sample Preparation

Cell monolayers (or cells in suspension seeded on polylysine-coated coverslips) are fixed with 2.5% glutaraldehyde in 100 m*M* cacodylate buffer (pH 7.4) for 30 min at room temperature. After postfixation in unbuffered 1% OsO_4 for 30 min, cells are dehydrated through graded ethanols, and critical point dried in CO_2. The critical point drying technique provides a much better means of avoiding the damaging effects of surface tension forces than does air-drying. The specimen is transferred into a closed pressure vessel, where it is first infiltrated and surrounded by liquid CO_2. The temperature and the pressure within the vessel are then raised above the critical values, at which point (the critical point) the liquid and gas phases have the same density. After passing the critical point, the pressure is slowly reduced so that the recondensation of the fluid through adiabatic cooling is avoided. The specimens are then coated with a conducting layer to inhibit charging. Sputter coating by gold has the advantage of requiring only a low-pressure vacuum (0.1 torr) and has been proven to be satisfactory for observation. The samples are examined with the scanning electron microscope (Cambridge 360 and Philips 515 are the two models used in our laboratories).

Comments

In addition to the visualization of surface blebbing, scanning electron microscopy can be used to detect changes in microvilli arrangement accompanied by surface smoothing, an alteration that often precedes extensive blebbing (10).

Transmission Electron Microscopy (Ultrathin Sections)

Sample Preparation

Cell monolayers (typically in 25-cm^2 tissue culture flasks or 6-cm-diameter tissue culture dishes) as well as cells in suspension ($1–2 \times 10^6$ cells), recovered from the incubation medium by low-speed centrifugation, are fixed in 1.5% glutaraldehyde in 50 m*M* cacodylate buffer (pH 7.4) for 20 min at room temperature, washed twice in the same buffer, postfixed in unbuffered 1% OsO_4, dehydrated in ascending grades of ethanol (15 min for each wash), and embedded in agar 100. In particular, cell monolayers are embedded directly in the culture flasks by sequential steps, with increasing resin concentration. Cells in suspension are first collected in beems and treated in the same manner as described for adherent cells. Ultrathin sections are obtained with an LKB Ultratome microtome and are stained with a saturated aqueous solution of uranyl acetate for 10 min, followed by a 3% aqueous solution of lead citrate for 20 min (10). Specimens are examined with Zeiss electron microscope EM10C or EM902, using a voltage of 60–100 kV.

Comments

Cells with blebs often display several morphological markers of injury preceding cell death (e.g., mitochondrial swelling, dilated vesicles, and clumping of chromatin). As concerns bleb formation, the initial short and large protrusions can follow two distinct fates. The surrounding membrane can disrupt, thus releasing intracellular constituents into the extracellular medium. Alternatively, the bleb undergoes a progressive basal narrowing, giving rise to the formation of a thin cytoplasmic bridge. Subsequent detachment of the bleb from the cell body can often occur, with the remaining membrane apparently upright in its structure (10).

The analysis of subcellular organelle distribution in the matrix of blebs formed under various toxic conditions led to the identification of two different types of blebs, namely, zeiotic and potocytotic blebs (4). Zeiotic blebs contain organelles such as mitochondria, lysosomes, endoplasmic reticulum, Golgi cisternae, and even nuclear fragments or DNA clumps. This type if bleb is frequently present in cells undergoing apoptosis (21). Potocytotic blebs are generally void of organelles and contain only amorphous cytoplasmic material and free ribosomes. They usually appear in cells undergoing necrosis. The pathophysiological mechanisms underlying the different types of blebs are not fully clarified, but the integrity of cortical cytoskeleton is thought to be critical in preventing the migration of cytoplasmic organelles to the bleb matrix.

Transmission Electron Microscopy (Freeze-Fracturing)

Sample Preparation

Cells in suspension are collected by low-speed centrifugation and are usually fixed with 2.5% glutaraldehyde in phosphate buffer (0.13 *M*, pH 7.2) for 20 min at 37°C. After fixation the medium is decanted and the cell pellet is resuspended in the same PBS containing 25% glycerol as cryoprotectant and incubated at room temperature for 30 min. Cells recovered by low-speed centrifugation are put on specific carriers (provided by Balzers) and quickly frozen in Freon 22 partially solidified by cooling with liquid nitrogen. The mounted carriers are then transferred into a Balzers freeze-etch unit, cleaved at −100°C at a pressure of 2–4 × 10^{-7} mbar, fractured with the appropriate knife, shadowed with a 25-

nm film of platinum–carbon (at an angle of 45°), and replicated with a 20-nm film of carbon (at an angle of 90°). The thickness of the deposit can be evaluated by means of a quartz crystal film monitor. Cells are then digested from the replica with bleach, mounted on 300-mesh grids, and examined with the electron microscope specified above (10).

Comments

This technique allows detection of the presence, distribution, and density of intramembrane particles (IMPs) (which represent membrane proteins) on both exoplasmic and protoplasmic fracture faces. In addition, when the fracture occurs across the cell, organelle membrane proteins and ultrastructure of mitochondria and nuclear pores can also be observed (4,10).

Different patterns of IMP distribution have been detected in membrane blebs formed in cells exposed, for example, to oxidants. In particular, randomly distributed membrane proteins were observed in small blebs, while clusters of IMPs mainly located at the base of the bleb were often observed in large bulb-like structures (10,22).

Fluorescence Microscopy (Immunocytochemical Visualization of Cytoskeletal Proteins)

Sample Preparation

Immunocytochemical investigations on the organization and distribution of cytoskeletal proteins can be performed in both substrate-adherent cells and cells in suspension. Adherent cells are grown on 13-mm-diameter glass coverslips in separated wells (5×10^4 cells per well) of six-well tissue culture plates (obtained from Flow Laboratories) and processed as described below. Cells in suspension can be seeded on glass coverslips coated with 0.01% polylysine or centrifuged using a cytocentrifuge.

For detection of actin, α-actinin, vinculin, tubulin, and microtubule-associated proteins, cells grown on coverslips are fixed in 3.7% formaldehyde in PBS (pH 7.4) for 10 min at room temperature. After washing in PBS, cells are permeabilized with 0.2% Triton X-100 in PBS for 5 min at room temperature. For detection of intermediate filament proteins, cells on coverslips are fixed for 5 min with absolute methanol at room temperature, followed by immersion in cold (−20°C) acetone 5–10 sec.

Incubation with specific monoclonal or polyclonal antibodies for the protein of interest is then performed at 37°C for 30 min in a humidified atmosphere. We usually use a 1 : 64 dilution of the polyclonal serum and a 1 : 200 dilution of monoclonal antibody in PBS. The coverslips are then extensively washed (usually three subsequent washes by immersion for 5 min in PBS) to remove unbound antibody and subsequently incubated with fluorescein- or rhodamine-linked secondary antibodies at a dilution of 1 : 100 at 37°C for 30 min in the dark and in a humidified atmosphere. For actin staining, a 0.3–1 μM solution of fluorescein–phalloidid can be used. This compound selectively binds polymerized actin and allows direct localization of actin filaments in fixed cells. Finally, coverslips are extensively washed in PBS to remove unbound secondary antibody, and thus, to decrease unspecific fluorescence, the coverslips are mounted with 50% glycerol in PBS and observed with an epifluorescence microscope. Mounted samples can be stored in the dark at 4°C for several days.

Comments

A potential use of this methodology, in addition to detecting single cytoskeletal fibers, is in investigation of the association between different cytoskeletal elements. For example, actin microfilaments can be visualized with fluorescein–phalloidin, and α-actinin and vinculin (two actin-binding proteins) can be detected using monoclonal antibodies and rhodamine-conjugated second antibodies, in the same cell undergoing blebbing (G. Bellomo, unpublished observations).

Fluorescence Microscopy (Immunochemical Detection of Surface Proteins)

Sample Preparation

Cells grown on glass coverslips (adherent cells) or seeded on polylysine (0.01%)-coated glass coverslips (cells in suspension, obtained after low-speed centrifugation) are first fixed in ice-cold 3.7% formaldehyde in PBS for 10 min to retain a well-preserved morphology, followed, when needed, by treatment with 0.2% Triton X-100 in PBS in order to permeabilize the plasma membrane and to detect intracellular molecules. Fixed cells are then incubated with monoclonal or polyclonal antibodies specific for receptors or membrane proteins, at 4°C for 45 min, washed three times with ice-cold PBS to remove unbound antibody, and then incubated with fluorescein- or rhodamine-linked second antibodies for 45 min at 4°C (12). Coverslips are extensively washed in PBS to remove unbound secondary antibody, mounted with 50% glycerol in PBS, and observed with an epifluorescence microscope. Mounted samples can be stored in the dark at 4°C for several days.

Comments

In addition to the described methodology, the availability of fluorescein-linked lectins from *Triticum vulgaris* (WGA), *Ulex europeus* (UEA), and *Phaseolus vulgaris* (PNA) that specifically bind to *N*-acetylglucosamine. L-fucose, and galactose, respectively, have made possible the detection of surface glycoproteins carrying the indicated carbohydrates.

The results of a study performed to investigate alterations occurring in the expression of some surface molecules in epithelial cells exposed to the oxident menadione are reported in Table II (10).

Biochemical Analysis of Cytoskeletal Proteins

Sample Preparation

The preparation of cytoskeletal fractions from freshly isolated as well as cultured cells is mainly based on the use of buffers containing nonionic detergents such as Triton X-100 or NP-40 that solubilize most of the nonstructural proteins, leaving cytoskeletal and nuclear matrix structures intact. Briefly, 1–5 $\times$ 10^7 cells are collected from the incubation medium by low-speed centrifugation and resuspended in 5 ml of an ice-cold extraction buffer containing 40 m*M* KCl, 5 m*M* $MgCl_2$, 5 m*M* EGTA, 1% Triton X-100, and 50 m*M* Tris-HCl (pH 7.4). After incubation on ice for 30 min, the suspension is centrifuged at 4000 *g* for 20 min and the pellet is washed twice in the same medium. This fraction is highly enriched in actin, actin-binding proteins, intermediate filament proteins, and histones (13).

The whole cytoskeletal fraction can be further subfractionated using the following procedure. The pellet obtained after Triton X-100 extraction is resuspended in a buffer containing 1 *M* KCl, 5 m*M* $MgCl_2$, 5 m*M* EGTA, 50 m*M* Tris/HCl pH 7.4 and incubated for 30 min at room temperature. The suspension is then centrifuged at 4.000 *g* for 20 min and the pellet washed twice in the same medium. This treatment solubilizes most of the filamentous actin and of the microfilament-associated proteins, leaving intact the intermediate filament-

Table II Expression of Surface Molecule on the Bleb Membrane and on the Unaffected Membrane of 2-Methyl-1, 4-naphthoquinone-Treated Cells[a]

Surface molecule	Bleb membrane	Unaffected membrane
Fibronectin	−	+
Sialoproteins	−	+
Collagen IV receptor	−	+
β_2-Microglobulin	−	+
EGF receptor	+	+

[a] CG5 cells were incubated with 200 μM menadione for 120 min and then processed for immunocytochemical localization of surface proteins as described in the text. For further experimental details see Ref. 12. EGF, Epidermal growth factor.

nuclear matrix scaffold (14). The pellet obtained after incubation in KCl medium is then solubilized in 8 *M* urea, 1 m*M* EGTA, 1 m*M* phenyl-methyl-sulfonyl-fluoride, 0.1 m*M* $MgCl_2$, 20 m*M* Tris-HCl (pH 7.4) for 60 min at room temperature with occasional stirring. The clear solubilized fraction (obtained after centrifugation at 4000 *g* for 20 min) is dialyzed overnight against 500 vol of 150 m*M* KCl, 2 m*M* dithiothreitol, 0.1 m*M* EGTA, 0.2 m*M* phenyl-methyl-sulfonyl-fluoride, 5 m*M* $MgCl_2$, and 25 m*M* imidazole (pH 7.1). At the end of the dialysis, the whitish flocculent material formed is collected by centrifugation at 2500 *g* for 20 min. This fraction is highly enriched in intermediate filament polypeptides and practically devoid of microfilament or nuclear matrix proteins (15). The polypeptides remaining in the solution after dialysis are precipitated with 60% cold acetone and are enriched in lamins and nuclear matrix proteins (16).

Polyacrylamide Gel Electrophoresis

Polyacrylamide gel electrophoresis (PAGE) is performed in 10–15% vertical gradient slab gels (1.5–2 mm thick) by the procedure described by Laemmli (17). Gels are fixed and stained for 2–4 hours with 20% methanol, 7.5% acetic acid, and 0.05% Coomassie brilliant blue and destained in 20% methanol and 7.5% acetic acid until background staining is negligible (usually 20 hr, with repetitive changes of the destaining solution).

For immunological detection of cytoskeletal proteins, samples are first analyzed as described above, then, after rinsing the gel in PBS, the proteins are electrophoretically transferred to a sheet of nitrocellulose membrane. Thereafter, unreacted groups are blocked by treatment with 3% bovine serum albumin in PBS. The nitrocellulose sheet is then incubated for 12 hr with monoclonal antibodies for the cytoskeletal protein of interest at a conventional dilution of 1 : 2000–1 : 4000. The incubation with the peroxidase-conjugated secondary antibody and the following detection are done essentially as described by Towbin *et al.* (18).

To specifically detect oxidative changes in cytoskeletal proteins, we developed a specific two-dimensional PAGE procedure in which samples are analyzed under nonreducing conditions (without dithiothreitol or β-mercaptoethanol) in the first dimension, then reduced, alkylated, and analyzed under reducing conditions in the second dimension. Specifically, the lane to be analyzed in the second dimension is excised from the gel and incubated with 10 m*M* β-mercaptoethanol in PBS at 60°C for 30 min, followed by 25 m*M* *N*-ethylmaleimide at 60°C for an additional 30 min. The treated lane is then placed horizontally on top of a new slab gel and subjected to a new (second-dimension) electrophoresis. The fixation and staining procedures are identical to those described before. Using this technique, it is possible to detect, in the second dimension, polypeptides that originate from the reductive cleavage of oxidatively cross-linked protein aggregates (13).

MECHANISMS OF OXIDATIVE STRESS-INDUCED MEMBRANE BLEBBING

The techniques described in the previous sections have been used in our laboratories to investigate the morphological and biochemical alterations associated with cellular injury caused by oxidative, stress, and the results obtained are briefly summarized here.

The term "oxidative stress" is generally used to describe a condition in which the balance between prooxidants and antioxidants is shifted in favor of the former (23). It can be mimicked *in vitro* using experimental conditions in which considerable amounts of oxygen-reactive species (superoxide anion free radical, hydrogen peroxide, and hydroxyl radical) are produced during the biotransformation of certain drugs and xenobiotics. Among these, quinones (24) have been extensively investigated in our laboratories and have been demonstrated to cause cytotoxicity via activation of several molecular mechanisms, including direct and indirect damage to cytoskeletal structures (10,12,22). Surface blebbing is a typical feature of quinone-induced cell injury, and extensive plasma membrane blebbing always precedes cell death. The experimental protocols used in understanding the biochemical and morphological bases of cytoskeletal alterations and bleb formation during oxidative stress are summarized in Fig. 3.

In time course experiments it was demonstrated that oxidation of soluble and protein thiols as well as ATP depletion and an increase in cytosolic free Ca^{2+} occurred before and were mechanistically linked to either blebbing and cell death (2). Investigations performed using PAGE analysis of the cytoskeletal fraction extracted from oxidative stress-challenged cells have revealed the oxidation of critical sulfhydryl groups in the actin molecule, leading to the formation of dimers and polymers of actin (13). These findings have been confirmed by immunocytochemical studies on microfilament distribution in a variety of cultured cells, showing the presence of clumps and patches of actin localized in discrete regions of the cell, with several portions of the plasma membrane apparently not anchored to the microfilament network (12).

The dissociation of actin filaments from the anchoring domains in the inner surface of the plasma membrane has been confirmed by the biochemical demonstration of a consistent loss of some actin-binding proteins (α-actinin, ABP, and vinculin) from the cytoskeletal fraction isolated from treated cells (25). This loss was apparently due to an nonphysiological increase in cytosolic free Ca^{2+} concentration that has been shown to directly dissociate α-actinin and to activate a Ca^{2+}-dependent protease cleaving other actin-binding proteins (25).

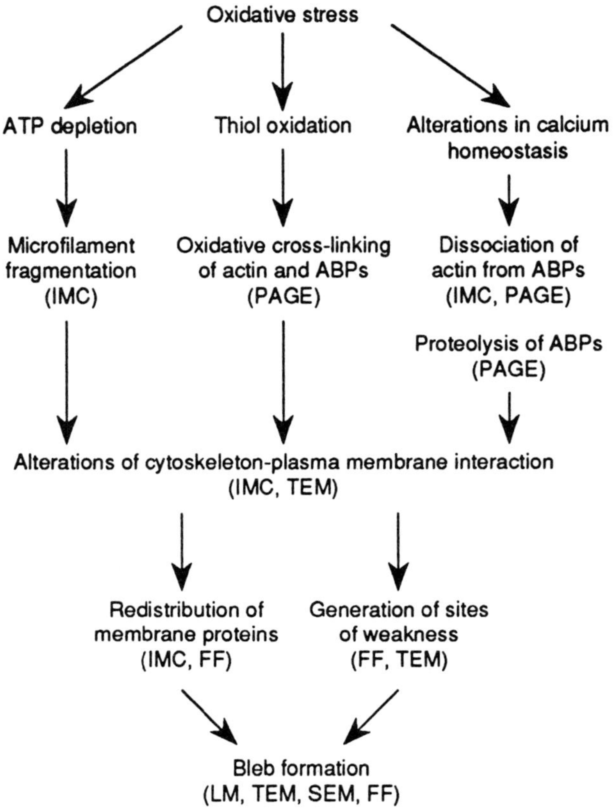

Figure 3 Mechanisms underlying surface blebbing during oxidative stress and morphological and biochemical methods to investigate them. ABPs, Actin-binding proteins; IMC, immunocytochemistry; PAGE, polyacrylamide gel electrophoresis; TEM, transmission electron microscopy; FF, freeze-fracture and electron microscopic analysis; LM, light microscopy; SEM, scanning electron microscopy.

The oxidation- and Ca^{2+}-dependent mechanisms generated sites of weakness where the plasma membrane was not anchored to the submembrane cytoskeletal network. In these sites a redistribution of intramembrane proteins took place (as demonstrated by electron-microscopic analysis of freeze-fractured samples) (10) and progressive protrusions of plasma membrane were formed, leading to the generation of blebs, whose rupture precipitated cell death.

ACNOWLEDGMENTS

The work described here has been supported by grants from Consiglio Nazionale delle Ricerche (Special Project Biologia e Patologia del Ca^{2+}) and from Ministero dell'Università e della Ricerca Scientifica e Tecnologica.

REFERENCES

1. J. J. Lemasters, S. Ji, and R. G. Thurman, *Science* **213,** 661 (1981).
2. S. A. Jewell, G. Bellomo, H. Thor, S. Orrenius, and M. T. Smith, *Science* **217,** 1257 (1982).
3. T. Sato, J. Tanaka, and J. Kono, *Lab. Invest.* **47,** 304 (1982).
4. M. J. Borelli, R. L. L. Wong, and W. C. Dewey, *J. Cell. Physiol.* **126,** 181 (1986).
5. W. M. Frederiks, G. L. Myagkaga, K. S. Bosh, G. M. Fronik, H. Veen, I. M. C. Vogel, and J. James, *Histochemistry* **78,** 459 (1983).
6. D. A. M. Mesland, G. Los, and H. Spiele, *Exp. Cell Res.* **135,** 431 (1981).
7. J. J. Lemasters, J. D. DiGiuseppi, A. L. Nieminen, and B. Herman, *Nature (London)* **325,** 78 (1987).
8. G. Bellomo and S. Orrenius, *Hepatology* **5,** 876 (1985).
9. F. Mirabelli, A. Salis, M. Vairetti, P. Crinò, G. Finardi, P. Richelmi, and G. Bellomo, *Med. Biol. Environ.* **16,** 187 (1988).
10. W. Malorni, F. Iosi, F. Mirabelli, and G. Bellomo, *Chem.–Biol. Interact.* **80,** 217 (1991).
11. G. Bellomo, F. Mirabelli, A. Salis, M. Vairetti, P. Richelmi, G. Finardi, H. Thor, and S. Orrenius, *Ann. N. Y. Acad. Sci.* **551,** 128 (1988).
12. G. Bellomo, F. Mirabelli, M. Vairetti, F. Iosi, and W. Malorni, *J. Cell. Physiol.* **143,** 118 (1990).
13. F. Mirabelli, A. Salis, V. Marinoni, G. Finardi, G. Bellomo, H. Thor, and S. Orrenius, *Arch. Biochem. Biophys.* **264,** 261 (1988).
14. M. Staufenbiel and W. Deppert, *J. Cell Biol.* **98,** 1886 (1984).
15. M. Vairetti, F. Mirabelli, P. Richelmi, and G. Bellomo, *Med. Biol. Environ.* **17,** 327 (1989).
16. E. Fey, and S. Penman, *Proc. Natl. Acad. Sci. U.S.A.* **85,** 121 (1988).
17. U. K. Laemmli, *Nature (London)* **227,** 680 (1970).
18. H. Towbin, T. Staehelin, and J. Gordon, *Proc. Natl. Acad. Sci. U.S.A.* **76,** 4350 (1979).
19. D. DiMonte, G. Bellomo, H. Thor, P. Nicotera, and S. Orrenius, *Arch. Biochem. Biophys.* **235,** 343 (1984).
20. F. Mirabelli, A. Salis, M. Perotti, F. Taddei, G. Bellomo, and S. Orrenius, *Biochem. Pharmacol.* **37,** 3423 (1987).
21. A. H. Willie, J. F. R. Kerr, and A. R. Currie, *Int. Rev. Cytol.* **68,** 251 (1980).
22. G. Bellomo, F. Mirabelli, P. Richelmi, W. Malorni, F. Iosi, and S. Orrenius, *Free Radical Res. Commun.* **8,** 391 (1990).
23. H. Sies (ed.), "Oxidative Stress," Academic Press, Orlando, Florida, 1986.
24. H. Thor, M. T. Smith, P. Hartzell, G. Bellomo, S. A. Jewell, and S. Orrenius, *J. Biol. Chem.* **257,** 12419 (1982).
25. F. Mirabelli, A. Salis, M. Vairetti, G. Bellomo, H. Thor, and S. Orrenius, *Arch. Biochem. Biophys.* **270,** 478 (1989).

7 Morphological Evaluation of Gap Junctional Intercellular Communication

James E. Klaunig and Thomas K. Baker

INTRODUCTION

This chapter focuses on the measurement of the function of the gap junction and the alteration of this function following exposure to xenobiotic chemicals in cultured cells (1,2). The gap junction is an important plasma membrane organelle (3). It serves as a regulated conduit for the intercellular exchange of low-molecular-weight water-soluble molecules in a tissue (4). The maintenance of the integrity of gap junctional intercellular communication appears to be important and required for the correct functioning of the cell, including electrical coupling, maintenance of homeostasis, and normal embryogenesis (5–7).

The importance of the gap junction in normal cell physiology also makes it a target for the toxic effects of a number of chemicals (8,9). Blockage of gap junctional intercellular communication by toxic agents has been implicated in the induction of arrhythmic disturbances in cardiac and smooth muscle, in the stages of cancer promotion and progression, and in ischemic injury (10–12). While the mechanism(s) by which toxic chemicals may modulate gap junction intercellular communication remains to be fully defined, there are several distinct stages in the process of formation of gap junctions and activation of gap junction function which may be targets for interference and inhibition by toxic agents (Fig. 1). Toxic chemicals may interfere with either the formation of the gap junction protein and/or the opening and closing of the gap junction channel (13). Toxicants may affect the transcription, translation, and/or incorporation of the gap junction protein into the plasma membrane. Interference at any of these stages may result in the failure of the cell to produce a functional gap junction channel. In addition, it appears that once the channel is formed, modulation of the opening and closing of the gap junction channel can be effected by both normal cellular control mechanisms (e.g., phosphorylation, calcium, and hydrogen ion concentration) and toxicants. (14). While a number of methods are available to assess functional intercellular communication in cultured cells, we restrict our discussion to the use of fluorescent dye transfer (dye coupling) in this chapter (10,15).

METHODS IN TOXICOLOGY, Volume 1B

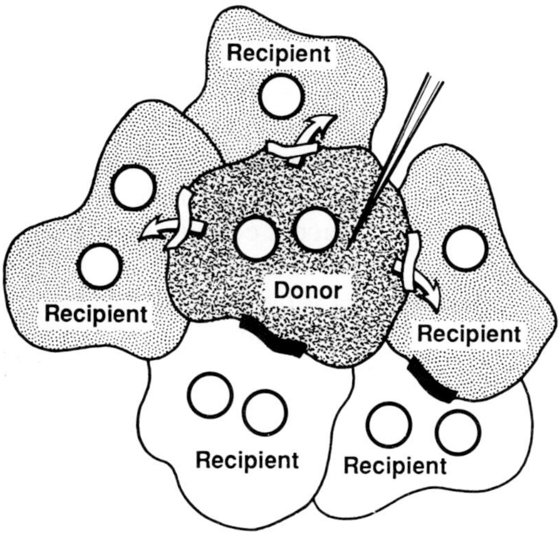

Figure 1 The formation and maintenance of functioning gap junctional intercellular communication are dependent on several steps involving both the formation of the gap junction protein and the maintenance of an open gap junctional pore. Gap junction protein synthesis is controlled by the transcription of the gene (step A) and formation of mRNA. Translation of the mRNA code to protein (step B) occurs and the gap junction protein is packaged and incorporated into the plasma membrane (step C). The maintenance of a functional gap junction is also dependent on cellular processes, including phosphorylation, intracellular free calcium concentration, and intracellular pH (step E). Gap junction protein is also routinely degraded (step D). Toxic agents may interact at any of these steps, resulting in a noncommunicating cell.

Gap junctional intercellular communication can be detected in an instantaneous and timely manner by visualizing the transfer of fluorescent dyes between adjacent cells (12,16). This process is referred to as dye coupling. In the use of dye coupling, the fluorescent dye usually either carboxyfluorescein or Lucifer yellow CH is microinjected into one cell and dye spread to adjacent cells is quantitated. If gap junctions are blocked, dye flow will not be seen (using a fluorescent microscope) between the injected cell and the adjacent touching cell. If gap junctional intercellular communication is intact, the fluorescent dye will rapidly transfer through the gap junctions of the inject "donor" to the neighboring adjacent cells. The normal unimpeded transfer of microinjected dye is quick (within seconds). Dye transfer can easily be quantitiated and scored with a fluorescent microscope. Advanced imaging systems have also been incorporated to allow for finite quantitation of the amount of dye spread between the cells (17).

In addition to the microinjection approach, techniques involving scrape loading and photobleaching have also been utilized. In the scrape-loading method a confluent cell culture is scraped with a razor blade or a rubber policeman in the presence of the fluorescent dye in the culture medium. The cells along the scraped edge pick up the dye (probably the result of transient damage and subsequent repair to their plasma membrane). Once the dye is incorporated into the cells, it can further diffuse to adjacent cells if gap junctions are present (18). Scrape loading is a quick method for assessing dye spread in confluent cultures. Its use is diminished by the fact that it does not appear to work well in primary cultured cells and is often difficult to quantitate. More recently, a third method of fluorescent dye transfer has been employed using photobleaching (19). In the photobleaching technique all cells in the culture are loaded with a fluorescent dye that can transfer through gap junctions. A single cell (target cell) in the culture is selected and photobleached by a laser. After the fluorescent dye in the target cell is photobleached, dye from adjacent cells in the culture will diffuse back into the photobleached target cell if the gap junctions are functional. This technique requires the use of sophisticated and expensive laser photobleaching equipment, potentially preventing its widespread application to most research laboratories.

After considering the various techniques, we have adapted the microinjection dye-coupling method in our laboratory and have successfully examined the effects of toxic agents on gap junctional intercellular communication in several cell types, with particular emphasis on hepatocytes (1,9,10,15,20). For this discussion primary cultured hepatocytes serve as our cell culture model, since these cells have been previously shown to have the needed metabolic functions to metabolize and detoxify many chemical toxicants and these cells readily express gap junctions and exhibit gap junctional intercellular communication once they are placed in primary culture (20,21). Dye coupling following microinjection is also applicable to other cell types in both primary and secondary cultures.

MATERIALS

The following materials are required for the evaluation of gap junctional intercellular communication by dye coupling using the microinjection technique.

Reagents

All reagents should be of the highest quality obtainable. Specific vendors are noted only for purpose of example.

Mg- and Ca- free Hanks' balanced salt solution (MCF-HBSS) (cat. No. H-2387, Sigma, St. Louis, MO)

Sodium bicarbonate (Sigma)

EGTA (Cat. No. E-4378, Sigma)
HEPES (Cat. No. H-7006 Sigma)
Leibowitz (L-15) medium (Cat. L-4386, Sigma),
Dextrose (Cat. No. D-4902, Fisher, Fairlawn, NJ)
Fetal bovine serum (FBS) (Cat. No. A-1115-L, HyClone, Logan, UT)
Gentamicin sulfate (Cat. No. G-1264, Sigma)
Dexmethasone (Cat. No. D-4902, Sigma)
Lucifer yellow CH (Cat. No. L-0259, Sigma)
Lithium chlorine (Cat. No. L121-100, Fisher)
Collagenase D (Cat. No. 1088-882, Boehringer Mannheim, Indianapolis, IN)
Sigma Diagnostics lactate dehydrogenase (LDH) Cat. No. 228-UV, Sigma)

Solutions

9.5 g (one bottle) of MCF-HBSS, 350 mg of $NaHCO_3$ 190 mg of EGTA, and 2.6 g of HEPES is added to 800 ml of ultrapure 18-MΩ water from a Milli-Q UF Plus water purification system (Millipore, Bedford, MA). The solution is mixed on a magnetic stir plate for 10 min. Adjust the pH to 7.2 with 1 N HCl or 1 N NaOH. Bring the final volume to 1 liter with ultrapure water in a volumetric flask. Sterile-filter using a Gelman acrocap 0.2-μm filter (Cat. No. 09-730-266, Fisher), attached to a Masterflex peristaltic pump (Model 7520-25, Cole-Parmer, Niles, IL). The sterile medium is collected and stored in 500-ml sterilized glass medium bottles.

14.8 g (one bottle) of L-15 medium and 1 g of dextrose is added to 800 ml of ultrapure 18-MΩ water from a Milli-Q UF Plus water purification system. The solution is mixed on a magnetic stir plate for 10 min. Adjust the pH to 7.2 with 1 N HCl or 1 N NaOH. Bring the final volume to 1 liter with ultrapure water in a volumetric flask. Sterile-filter using a Gelman acrocap 0.2-μm filter attached to a Masterlfex peristaltic pump. The sterile medium is collected and stored in 500-ml sterilized glass medium bottles.

Complete L-15 of culture medium combines 500 ml of stock of L-15 solution with 50 ml of FBS, 100 μl 1×10^6 *M* dexamethasone, and 500 μg of 25 μg/ml gentamicin sulfate. Gently mix the solution by swirling. Store at 4°C.

Lithium chloride (0.1 *M* solution): Store at room temperature.

Lucifer yellow CH dye for dye coupling (5% Lucifer yellow in a 0.1 *M* LiCl solution): Store at room temperature in the dark.

Equipment

Masterflex pump
Masterflex pump head, (Cat. No. 7013-21, Cole-Parmer)

Masterflex Tygon tubing (Cat. No. 6409-13, Cole-Parmer)
Baker class II HEPA-filtered biological cabinet (Cat. No. SG. 400, DayStar, Indianapolis, IN)
ESPEC incubator with CO_2 capabilities (Cat. No. BNA-211, DayStar)
PuL-1 pipette puller (Cat. No. PUL-1 E, World Precision Instruments, Sarasota, FL)
Nikon Diaphot–TMB inverted phase-contrast microscope with epifluorescene equipment (Fryer, Carpentersville, IL)
Narashige MO-388 joystick hydraulic micromanipulator (Fryer)
Narashige MM-188 three-dimensional motor drive course manipulator (Fryer)
COBAS Mira S transfer analyzer (Syntex, San Jose, CA)

PROCEDURE

Hepatocyte Isolation

Hepatocytes are isolated from rodent liver using a two-step portal vein perfusion (22). (MCF-HBSS) is perfused through the liver for 6–8 min to clear the organ of blood using a Masterflex peristaltic pump. Immediately following this L-15 medium plus dextrose containing 0.5 mg/ml collagenase is perfused through the liver for 18–20 min. The temperature of the perfusate is maintained at 37°C. Following completion of the perfusion, the liver is excised and placed in a dish containing L-15 culture medium and 0.5 mg/ml collagenase (37°C) under a sterile laminar flow hood, where it is carefully minced for cellular separation. Once minced, the liver suspension containing both cells and tissue is pipetted 10 times with a 25-ml wide-bore pipette in the collagenase solution. The resulting cell suspension is filtered through sterile gauze and centrifuged at 20 *g* for 5 min at 20°C. The supernatant containing the nonviable cells is removed, leaving a pellet of predominantly viable cells. This viable cell pellet is resuspended in fresh complete L-15 medium. The number and viability of the hepatocytes are determined by trypan blue dye exclusion using a hemocytometer under a light microscope (3). The cells are plated on 60-mm culture dishes containing 5 ml of complete L-15 medium at a density of 1×10^6. The hepatocytes are incubated at 37°C, at 90% humidity and 100% air atmosphere for 3 hr, allowing for cell attachment. Following the attachment period the medium is removed and replaced with fresh complete L-15 medium. The cultures are returned to the incubator. After 18 hr the medium is removed and replaced with 5 ml of complete L-15 medium (23).

Measurement of Cytolethality

It is important that, to fully assess the effects of toxic agents on gap junctional intercellular communication in cell cultures, the exposure of the cells be performed in a dose–response manner. Persuant to this, it is also important that initial studies (prior to the measurement of the gap junctional intercellular communication) be performed to assess the cytolethality of the toxic compound in question. To this end, a dose–response analysis of the cytolethality of each compound being tested should be performed. Studies in our laboratory have shown that with primary hepatocyte cultures, two measurements of cytolethality, LDH leakage and trypan blue dye exclusion, have proved to be reliable, sensitive, and easy assays to perform.

LDH Leakage

In performing the LDH leakage assay, primary hepatocyte cultures are treated with each toxicant at selected concentrations and for selected durations. We routinely use concentrations of 10, 5, 1, 0.5, 0.1, 0.05, 0.01, 0.005 and 0.001 m*M* along with a control at durations of 2, 4, 24, and 48 hr in initial range-finding cytolethality studies. (Subsequent studies may be performed to narrow the concentrations and durations of exposure to be examined based on results of the range-finding studies.) Triplicate cultures (60-mm dishes) are treated with each concentration of the compound for each duration. After the treatment period 200 μl of medium is removed from each treated culture dish and placed in COBAS autosampler tubes for determination of LDH using a COBAS Mira S transfer analyzer and Roche LDH reagents. Results are reported as U/liter. After taking each medium sample, the remaining culture is treated with Triton X-100 (10% in ultrapure water). The dishes are then placed on a rocker for 30 min, ensuring total cell death by the Triton X-100. After Triton X-100 treatment 200 μl of medium is removed and the total LDH content of the cultured cells is determined with the COBAS transfer analyzer. The LDH leakage induced from the toxicant treatment is expressed as the LDH content in the medium of the dish divided by the Triton X-100-treated cell LDH medium sample times 100. This ratio, when compared to the untreated control sample, is taken to indicate the percentage of cell death due to the cytolethality of the toxic compound (24).

Trypan Blue Dye Exclusion Measurement

If the toxicant used in the study interferes with the LDH enzyme reaction, such as peroxide-containing compounds that actively remove H from NADH, then an alternate method of cell viability must be performed. One such alternate method is the trypan blue dye exclusion method (23). Triplicate dishes of cultured hepatocytes are treated as described above with each toxic compound in a dose-dependent manner. Following the treatment regimen the cells are washed by letting them set in fresh serum-free L-15 medium in the 37°C incubator for 10 min. Each culture is then treated with 5 ml of serum-free L-

15 medium containing 0.2 ml of 0.4% trypan blue dye. After setting for 5 min at 36.5°C, the viable (trypan blue-excluding cells) and nonviable (trypan blue-staining cells) are counted in 25 0.25-mm^2 reticle fields per 60-mm culture dish under an inverted phase-contrast microscope at 100X magnification. Triplicate dishes are examined for each concentration of toxicant at each duration of exposure along with appropriate control cultures. The viable and nonviable cells in each dish are counted and the percentage of viable to total cells is calculated as a measurement of cytolethality.

Measurement of Gap Junctional Intercellular Communication

Gap junctional intercellular communication is determined in primary culture hepatocytes following iontophoretic injection of Lucifer yellow CH. Each chemical to be examined for its effect on dye coupling should be examined at several concentrations and for various times of exposure based on the cytolethality results, including concentrations of each compound below those that produce cell death. Microelectrode injection needles were pulled from 1.5-mm-diameter single-barrel glass Kwik-Fil capillaries (World Precision Instruments), using a World Precision PUL-1 micropipette puller. The tip opening diameter is measured through tip resistance to be 1 μm (25). Using a binocular dissecting scope, the pipettes are initially loaded with 5 μl of 5% Lucifer yellow CH and backfilled with LiCl. The injection pipettes must be made fresh before each injection period. The pipette is secured to the Narashige manipulator. The injection micropipette is located in the microscope field of view at 200X and maneuvered slowly to the cell of interest using the Narashige manipulators until the tip pierces the plasma membrane at a glancing angle. A current of 3 nA is then placed into the micropipette, forcing the Lucifer yellow CH into the cell cytoplasm. Injection continues for 15–30 sec. Five minutes after injection, the cell that was injected (referred to as the donor cell) is viewed with the fluorescence microscope and the amount of dye coupling is scored. Dye coupling is quantitated by counting both the number of cells (recipients) that contact the donor cell that express dye coupling to them and the number of recipients that do not show dye coupling with the donor cell. The percentage of dye coupling is determined by dividing the number of coupled recipients by the total number of recipients (both coupled and uncoupled) (Fig. 2). Enough donor cells are microinjected so that 50–75 recipients can be evaluated per culture dish. Triplicate dishes should be examined for each concentration and duration of toxicant examined.

COMMENTS

It has become apparent that a number of cellular organelles are targets for the interaction and modification by toxic agents in subcytolethal concentrations. One such target organelle, the gap junction, is important in normal cellular

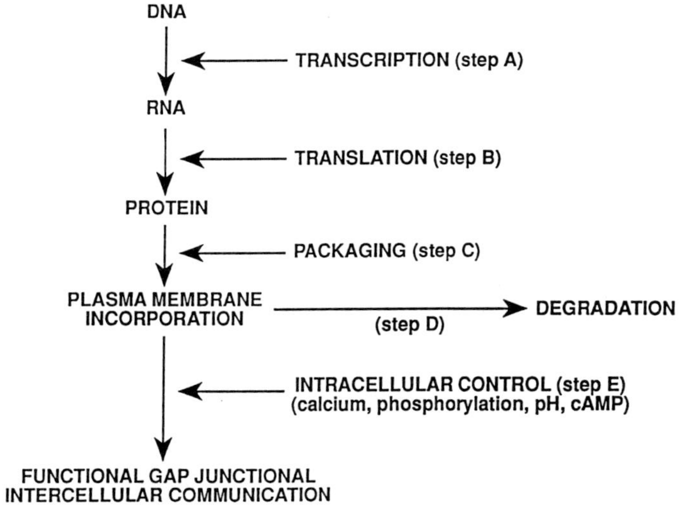

Figure 2 This diagram depicts what may be seen during the iontophoretic injection of a cultured hepatocyte with Lucifer yellow CH. The donor hepatocyte (darkly shadowed in the center has been injected. The adjacent recipient cells (lightly shadowed) represent cells that received dye transfer. These cells are dye coupled. The recipient cells that lack shadowing illustrate recipient cells that did not dye couple. Therefore, three of the five recipient cells shown here are dye coupled, while the remaining two are not, thus exhibiting 60% dye coupling.

physiology. Modification in gap junction structure and function has been shown in a number of toxicological events and processes, including ischemia, neoplasia, and teratogenesis (17). Accurate and reproducible measurement of the function of this organelle following exposure to toxic agents is required to fully assess the importance of the gap junction in cell toxicity. The method described above is a relatively easy, reproducible, and inexpensive means for the measurement of gap junctional intercellular communication. While we have limited our discussion to cultured hepatocytes, the methodology of dye coupling is readily applicable to other cell types in both primary and secondary cultures.

REFERENCES

1. J. E. Klaunig, R. J. Ruch, and C. M. Weghorst, *In Vitro Toxicol.* **3,** 91 (1990).
2. R. J. Ruch and J. E. Klaunig, *Cancer Res.* **48,** 2519 (1988).
3. J. P. Rexel and M. Karnovsky, *J. Cell Biol.* **33,** C7, (1967).
4. J. L. Flagg-Newton, I. Simpson, and W. R. Loewenstein, *Science* **205,** 404 (1979).
5. S. Caveney, *Annu. Rev. Physiol.* **47,** 319, (1985).
6. W. R. Loewenstein, *Physiol. Rev.* **61,** 829 (1981).

7. B. Rose and R. Rick, *J. Membr. Biol.* **44,** 377 (1978).
8. J. E. Klaunig and R. J. Ruch *Lab. Invest.* **62,** 135 (1990).
9. R. J. Ruch, J. E. Klaunig, and M. A. Pereira, *Toxicol. Appl. Pharmacol.* **87,** 111 (1986).
10. W. E. Estape W. C. DeMello, *Cell Biol. Int. Rep.* **7,** 91 (1983).
11. J. D. Pitts, and M. E. Finbow, *J. Cell Sci., Suppl.* **4,** 239 (1986).
12. C. M. Weghorst and J. E. Klaunig, *Toxicologist* **8,** 194 (1988).
13. D. C. Spray and M. V. L. Bennett, *Annu. Rev. Physiol.* **47,** 281 (1985).
14. C. M. Jone, C. M. Erickson, J. E. Trosko, M. Netzloff, and C. C. Chang, *Teratogen. Carcinogen. Mutagen.* **5,** 379 (1985).
15. E. L. Hertzberg, and R. G. Johnson "Gap Junctions." Liss, New York, 1987.
16. J. E. Klaunig and R. J. Rich, *Lab. Invest.* **62/2,** 135 (1990).
17. M. H. El-Fouly, J. E. Trosko, and C. C. Chang, *Exp. Cell Res.* **168,** 422 (1987).
18. M. H. Wade, J. E. Trosko, and M. Schindle, **232,** 429 (1986).
19. J. E. Klaunig, P. J. Goldblatt, D. E. Hinton, M. M. Lipsky, J. Chacko, and B. F. Trump, *In Vitro* **17,** 913 (1981).
20. D. D. Haberlach, "The Imaging Workshop Manual," Version 1.2, pp. 2–89. 1992.
21. R. J. Ruch, and J. E. Klaunig, *Cell Biol. Toxicol.* **2**(4), 469 (1987).
22. J. E. Klaunig, P. J. Goldblatt, D. E. Hinton, M. M. Lipsky, and B. F. Trump, *In Vitro* **17,** 826 (1981).
23. S. A. Gross, B. Subhanker, and J. E. Klaunig, *Proc. Soc. Exp. Biol. Med.* **190,** 163 (1990).
24. M. B. A. Djamgoz, "Principles of Microelectrode Techniques," p. 27. Orlean, Middlesex, England, 1983.
25. J. D. Pitts, E. Kam, and D. Morgan, (E. L. Hertzberg and R. G. Johnson, eds.), pp. 397–409. Liss, 1987.

8 Fluorescence Microscopic Examination of Cytoskeletal Elements

Iih-Nan Chou, Wande Li, and Glen B. Zamansky

INTRODUCTION

The cytoskeleton refers to an extensive, highly organized, three-dimensional network of filamentous structures in the cytoplasm of eukaryotic cells. It is composed of three major structural elements, namely, microtubules (MTs), intermediate filaments (IFs), and microfilaments (MFs) (1). Each cytoskeletal element consists of polymers of protein subunits. For MTs and MFs a dynamic equilibrium exists between subunits and their polymers (1). The cytoskeleton is responsible for the maintenance of cellular architecture and internal organization, in addition to providing an essential scaffolding on which metabolic processes occur. It is also important in regulating cell shape, motility, migration, transport, cell division, and other cellular processes (1,2). Intricately distributed patterns of MTs, IFs, and MFs, have been visualized in fibroblasts, endothelial and epithelial cells, lymphocytes, etc., from different species by fluorescence microscopy (1,3–5).

Many toxic substances are known to interact with cytoskeletal elements (6). For example, colchicine, a potent mitotic inhibitor, selectively inhibits MT assembly, whereas cytochalasins, a family of toxic mold metabolites which inhibit cytokinesis, depolymerize MFs (1). Diphtheria toxin disrupts the vimentin IFs of monkey kidney CV-1 cells (7). It should be noted that many environmentally hazardous agents also can act on the cytoskeleton. They include metals (As, Cd, Co, Cr, Ni, etc.) (8), mineral fibers (asbestos) (9), pesticides (kepone) (10), herbicides (2,4-D, 2,4,5-T, and paraquat), and others (11–13). Different toxic agents cause different patterns of damage to the cytoskeleton. Therefore, cytoskeletal perturbation may be an important indicator of cellular injury upon insult by a toxic chemical.

We describe here the fluorescence microscopic methodology to visualize the alterations in cytoskeletal organization of (1) 3T3 mouse cells, (2) human skin fibroblasts, and (3) human epidermal keratinocytes exposed to various toxic agents under appropriate culture conditions. The protocols used contain several modifications (8,10–15) of the procedures described by Solomon *et al.* (16) and Wang *et al.* (17).

METHODS IN TOXICOLOGY, Volume 1B

MATERIALS AND REAGENTS

Phosphate-buffered saline (PBS): 150 m*M* NaCl and 5 m*M* KCl, in 10 m*M* $NaPO_4$ buffer (pH 7.4)

PM2G MT stabilizing buffer (pH 6.9): 0.1 *M* PIPES, 1 m*M* $MgSO_4$, 2 *M* glycerol, and 2 m*M* EGTA, adjusted with NaOH to the desired pH

Solution A: 10 m*M* glucose, 3 m*M* KCl, 130 m*M* NaCl, 1 m*M* Na_2HPO_4, and 30 m*M* HEPES (pH 7.4)

3.7% Formaldehyde, freshly diluted from a 37% stock with the PM2G buffer

0.1 *M* l-glycine in PBS (pH 7.4)

0.3% Nonidet P40 (NP40), a nonionic detergent from Sigma (St. Louis, MO), freshly diluted in PBS

Rabbit antitubulin antiserum (as a primary antibody), obtained from Polysciences (Warrington, PA)

Rabbit antikeratin antiserum (as a primary antibody), obtained from Biomedical Technologies (Stoughton, MA)

Rhodamine-conjugated goat anti-rabbit immunoglobulin G (IgG) (as the secondary antibody), obtained from Organon-Teknika (Malvern, PA)

N-(7-nitrobenz-2-oxa-1,3-diazol-4-yl) (NBD)–phallacidin in methanol (as a direct labeling agent for F-actin), from Molecular Probes (Eugene, OR)

Gelvatol mounting solution (see below for preparation procedure)

Glass coverslips (No. 1 thickness, 12 × 12 mm, from Bradford Scientific, Epping, NH) and slides for mounting coverslips

PROCEDURES

Swiss 3T3 Cells

Preparation of Cells

Swiss 3T3 mouse cells are plated at 3×10^4 cells per 35-mm-diameter dish, each containing two glass coverslips in 2 ml of Dulbecco's modified Eagle's medium (DMEM) (GIBCO, Grand Island, NY) supplemented with 10% fetal bovine serum (FBS). After incubation for 24 hr, the medium is removed and cell growth is arrested by incubation in 2 ml of DMEM containing 0.3% FBS for 72 hr. The medium is changed again and the flattened quiescent cells, which are ideal for microscopic examination, are used for experiments (18).

Extraction of the Cytoskeleton

All procedures for extracting and staining the cytoskeleton are carried out at room temperature with prewarmed reagents (11,18). For cells grown on coverslips placed in a 35-mm plate, all washings, extractions, and fixations are done with 2 ml of appropriate solutions. 3T3 cells on coverslips are washed gently twice with PBS and once with PM2G. They are fixed with 3.7% formaldehyde in PM2G for 30 min, washed in PBS for 5 min, and incubated in 0.1 *M* glycine in PBS for 5 min. The cells are extracted for 10 min with 0.3% NP40 in PBS, and then washed twice with PBS. This detergent-extracted cytoskeleton can now be fluorescently stained, or, if necessary, the coverslips can be stored in PBS at 4°C for 1–2 days before staining.

Fluorescent Double-Staining of MTs and MFs

MTs and MFs are labeled by indirect immunofluorescence and direct fluorescence techniques, respectively. When preparing staining reagents, the total volume should be calculated such that it is sufficient for 2 or three extra coverslips. The extra volume is needed to compensate for loss or incomplete recovery during preparation and staining steps. To reconstitute NBD–phallacidin with the primary antibody, an aliquot of NBD–phallacidin (stored at −20°C), equivalent to 10 μl per coverslip as recommended by the supplier, is removed using a needle coupled to a syringe and placed in a glass tube. The solution is evaporated to dryness under a gentle stream of air and the tube is held on ice. A vial of frozen (−80°C) rabbit antitubulin antibody is thawed quickly in 37°C water, diluted with PBS to provide 20 μl of diluted antibody solution per coverslip, and microcentrifuged at 4°C for 10 min. The supernatant is transferred to the glass tube containing "dry" NBD-phallacidin, and the reconstituted NBD–phallacidin/primary antibody solution is mixed by gently shaking the tube and then kept on ice. To prepare a diluted secondary antibody solution, a vial of frozen (−80°C) rhodamine-conjugated goat anti-rabbit antibody is thawed quickly and an aliquot is diluted with PBS to provide 20 μl per coverslip. After microcentrifugation at 4°C, the supernatant is removed to a clean microfuge tube and kept on ice.

A coverslip containing extracted cytoskeleton is removed from a plate using a pair of fine-tipped forceps, and the excess PBS is drained by touching a corner to the edge of a paper towel. The coverslip is carefully placed in a covered chamber (e.g., a 150-mm dish) containing a piece of moistened filter paper and overlaid with 20 μl of the NBD–phallacidin/primary antibody mixture. This step is repeated until all coverslips are processed. The filter paper is moistened, if necessary, by slowly adding drops of distilled water using a Pasteur pipette. The chamber is incubated at 37°C in a humidified incubator for 30 min. During incubation coverslips should be checked and, if necessary, another 20 μl of the NBD-phallacidin/primary antibody mixture may be added. After incubation one coverslip is removed and the excess antibody solution is drained as described above. The coverslip is washed thoroughly by dipping it five times into each of five beakers containing 50 ml of PBS. It is important to remember which side the cells are on. The coverslip is drained, placed back in the moistened chamber, and overlaid with 20 μl of the secondary antibody. This step is repeated until all coverslips are done. The filter paper is moistened and the chamber is then incubated at 37°C for another 30 min. Coverslips are washed thoroughly with *fresh* PBS as described above and finally with double-distilled water to desalt. Coverslips are drained of excess water and mounted *cell side down* on glass slides with the aid of a small drop of Gelvatol mounting solution.

To prepare the Gelvatol mounting solution, 20 g of Gelvatol 20/30 (Monsanto, St. Louis, MO) is added to 80 ml of PBS and, after stirring for 16 hr at room temperature, 40 ml of glycerol is added and the mixture is stirred for at least 16 hr. After centrifugation at 17,210 *g* for 15 min, the viscous supernatant is aliquoted into glass vials and stored at 4°C. The slides are stored flat at 4°C for at least 24 hr and then examined under a Nikon Optiphot fluorescence microscope (Nikon Inc. Instrument Group, Garden City, NY) equipped with an epifluorescence attachment and a Nikon Microflex UFX automatic exposure system. All photographs are taken at the same magnification using a Nikon Plan Apochromat oil objective (40×) with Kodak (Rochester, NY) Tri-X pan film (ASA 400). The film is actually exposed at ASA 800 and "push"-developed to an effective rating of ASA 1600 to enhance the contrast (11).

Human Skin Fibroblasts

Preparation of Cells and Cytoskeletal Elements

It should be noted that the procedure for preparing human skin fibroblasts is different from that for 3T3 cells. We routinely maintain cultures of human skin fibroblasts (Coriell Institute for Medical Research, Camden, NJ) in Eagle's minimum essential medium supplemented with 10% FBS, 0.9 g/liter D-glucose, 0.66 mg/l sodium pyruvate, 110 U/ml penicillin, and 110 μg/ml streptomycin sulfate. To harvest cells for inoculating experimental cultures, confluent stock cultures are washed two times with PBS and exposed to PBS containing 0.25% trypsin for ~10 sec. The trypsin-containing solution is then removed and the culture flask is incubated at 37°C for 1–2 min. Trypsinized cells are then resuspended in medium containing 10% FBS. Cells are diluted in medium to a density of 7000 cells/cm^2 for inoculation of 35-mm dishes containing one or two coverslips. Cultures on coverslips are allowed to grow 1–3 days prior to exposure to the agent of interest. In order to avoid obscuring the visualization of cytoskeletal elements, it is important that the cultures not be allowed to become too dense.

The fixation and extraction of cells and the staining of MTs and/or MFs are performed as described above for 3T3 cells.

Human Epidermal Keratinocytes

Several approaches are now available for culturing human epidermal keratinocytes and maintaining features characteristic of these cells in the normal epidermal epithelium. In our laboratories we have taken advantage of a Ca^{2+}-regulated culture system originally described by Boyce and Ham (19). Proliferation of keratinocytes is maintained using a modified MCDB153 medium (Clonetics, San Diego, CA) containing 0.15 m*M* $CaCl_2$ and supplemented with 0.1 ng/ml human recombinant epidermal growth factor, 5 μg/ml insulin, 0.5 μg/ml hydrocortisone, 0.4% (v/v) bovine pituitary extract, 50 μg/ml gentamicin, and 0.5 μg/ml amphotericin B (low-Ca^{2+} medium). Terminal differentiation—characterized by the formation of desmosomes, cellular stratification, increased transglutaminase activity, and the synthesis of cornified envelopes—is induced by switching cells into medium containing 1–2 m*M* Ca^{2+} (high-Ca^{2+} medium). An early effect of this Ca^{2+} switch is a dramatic reorganization of the cytoskeleton (14). Thus, this culture system permits studies of the effects of physical and chemical agents on the organization of the cytoskeleton in proliferating cells and/or the effects on the ability of the cells to reorganize their cytoskeletons and differentiate upon Ca^{2+} stimulation.

Preparation of Cells

We routinely maintain keratinocytes (Clonetics) in low-Ca^{2+} medium at 37°C in an atmosphere of 95% air : 5% CO_2. Cultures are inoculated into plastic culture flasks at densities between 2500 and 10,000 cells/cm^2. Fresh medium is added to the cultures 1 day later and every other day thereafter. Upon becoming approximately 50% confluent, the cultures appear to remain healthiest if fresh medium is added daily. Cells should be harvested and used for inoculating experiments or for serial passaging prior to reaching confluency.

Cells may be removed from their plastic growth surface by rinsing the cultures with solution A and incubating the cultures at room temperature for 1 min in solution A containing 0.025% trypsin and 0.01% EDTA (1 ml per T-25 flask). This solution is removed, and the closed flask is maintained at room temperature to continue the trypsinization process for an additional 3–4 min. Micro-

---

Figure 1 Distinct cytoskeletal injuries induced by metal compounds and the herbicide paraquat. Quiescent Swiss 3T3 cells were exposed to various toxic agents under conditions as indicated and processed for fluorescent double-staining for visualization of both microtubules (A, C, E, G, I, K, M, and O) and microfilaments (B, D, F, H, J, L, N, and P) in the same cells. (A and B) Control cells are presented; the metal-treated cells are shown as follows: (C and D) 100 μM $NaAsO_2$ for 3 hr; (E and F) 400 μM $NaAsO_2$ for 1.5 hr; (G and H) 75 μM $CdCl_2$ for 1.5 hr; (I and J), 100 μM $CoSO_4$ for 16 hr; (K and L), 1.5 m*M* $NiSO_4$ for 20 hr; (M and N), 100 μM K_2CrO_4 for 8 hr; and the paraquat-treated cells are shown (O and P): 1.25 m*M* for 20 hr. (Sections A–N reprinted by permission of Academic Press, Inc., from "Distinct Cytoskeletal Injuries Induced by As, Cd, Co, Cr, and Ni Compounds" by I.-N. Chou, *Biomed. Environ. Sci.* **2**, 358–365, copyright © 1989 by Academic Press, Inc., and Sections O and P from "Paraquat-Induced Cytoskeletal Injury in Cultured Cells" by W. Li, Y. Zhao, and I.-N. Chou, *Toxicol. Appl. Pharmacol.* **91**, 96–109, copyright © 1987 by Academic Press, Inc.)

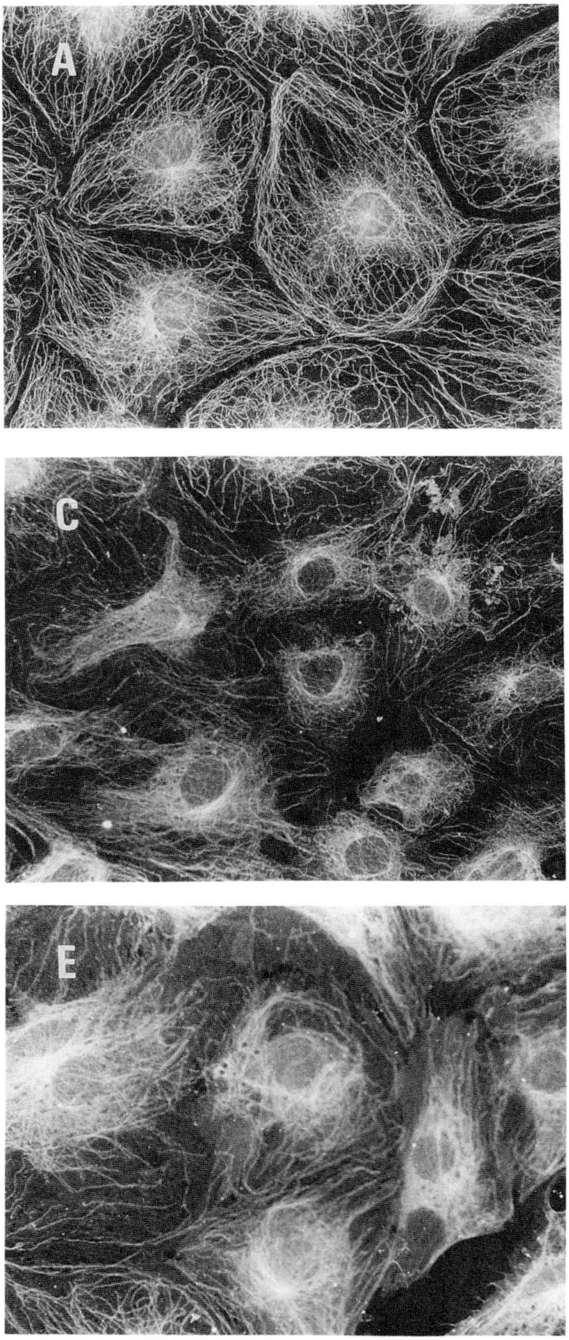

Figure 1 (*continued*)

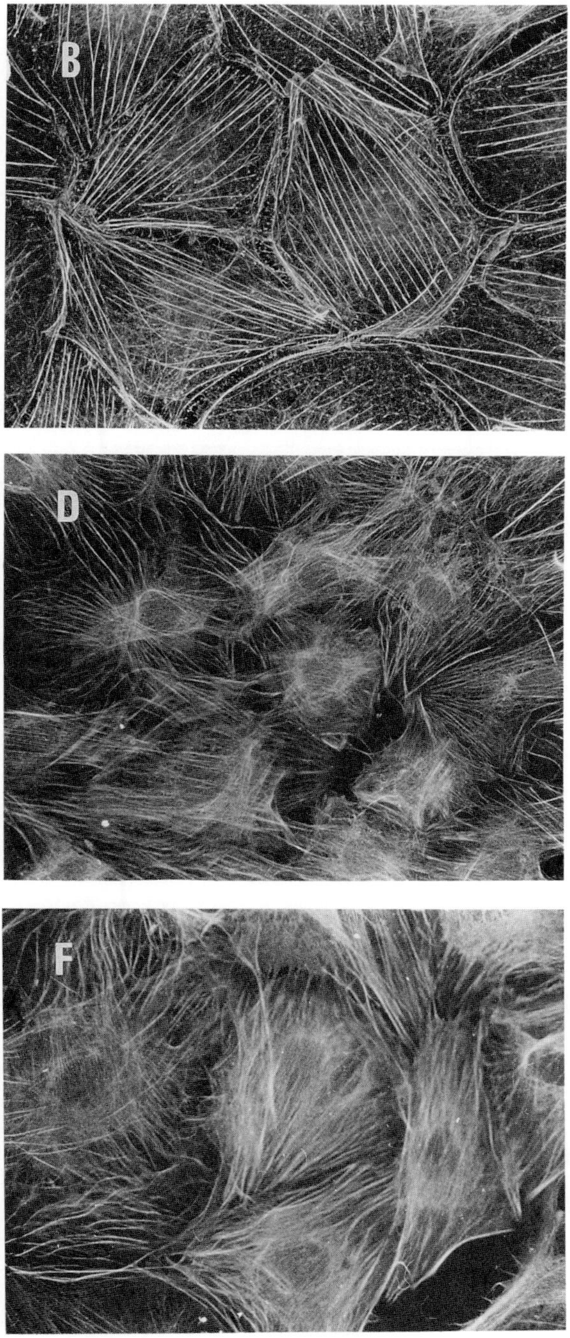

Figure 1 (*continued*)

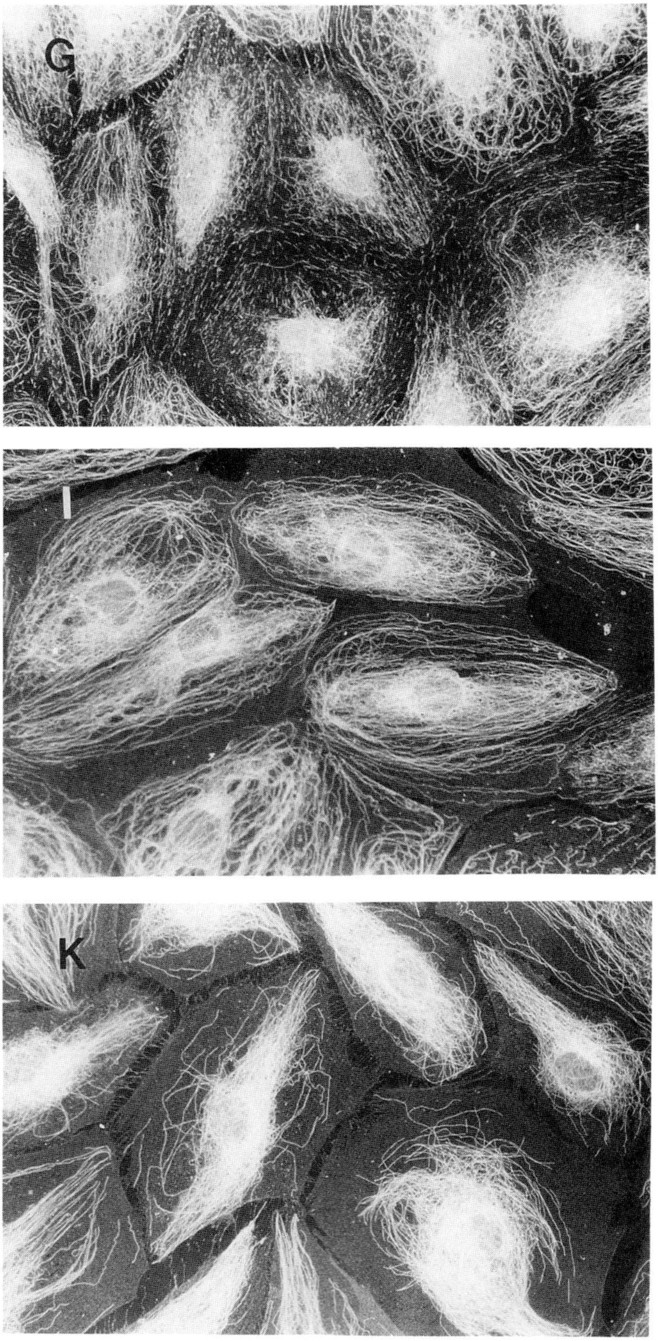

Figure 1 (*continued*)

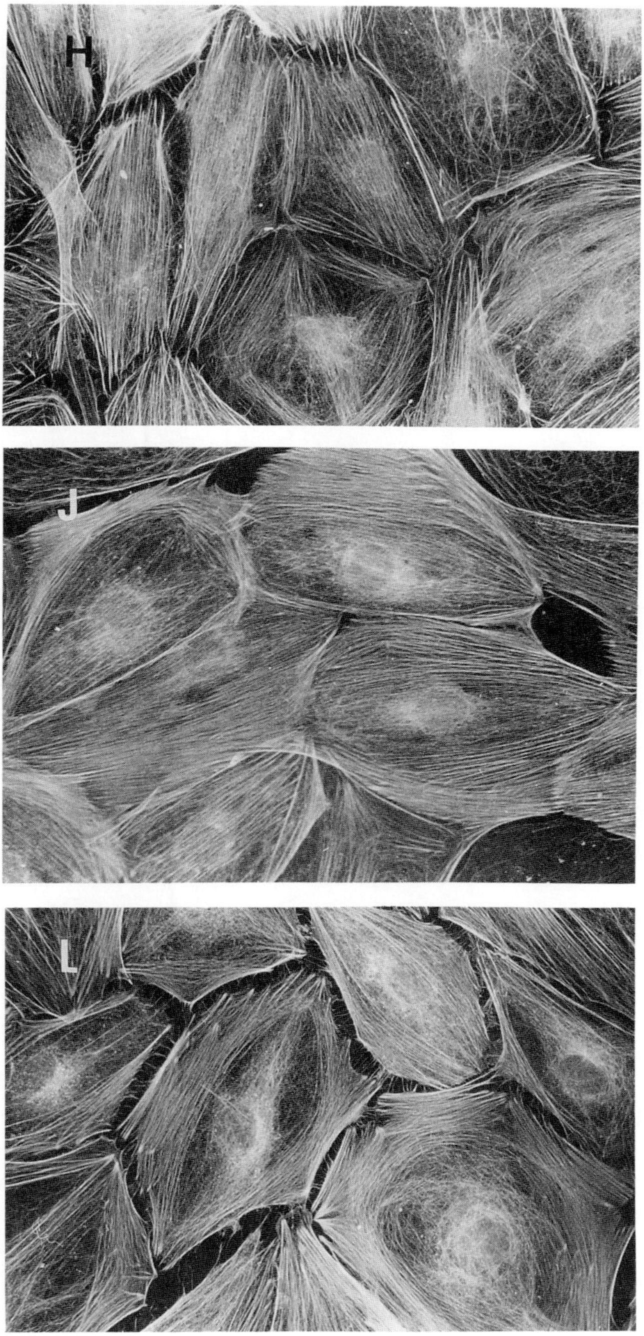

Figure 1 (*continued*)

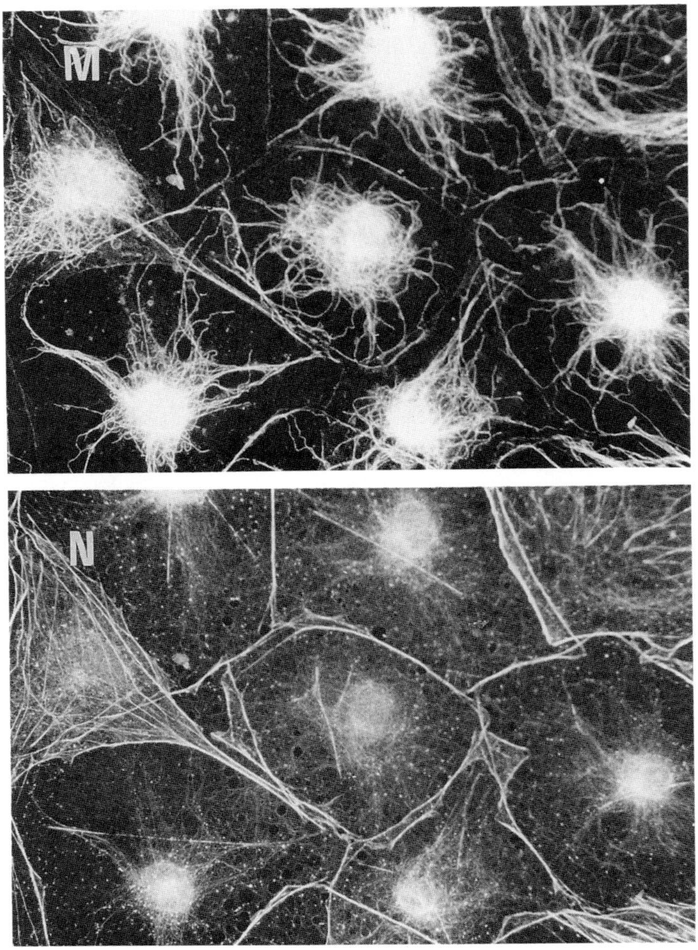

Figure 1 *(continued)*

scopic examination of the rounding and detaching cells is helpful in determining when to end the trypsinization. Following trypsinization the cells are resuspended in solution A containing 15% FBS, and the cells are pelleted by centrifugation. The pellet is then resuspended in medium. For experiments 35-mm dishes containing glass coverslips (prepared as described below) are inoculated in 2 ml of low-Ca^{2+} medium at a density of 5000 cells/cm^2. Culture media are changed as discussed earlier and cultures are allowed to grow for 4–5 days prior to exposure to the agent of interest. Drug exposure can be administered for the entire time in low- or high-Ca^{2+} medium, or exposure can be initiated in low-Ca^{2+} medium and continued in high-Ca^{2+} medium, depending on the purpose of the study.

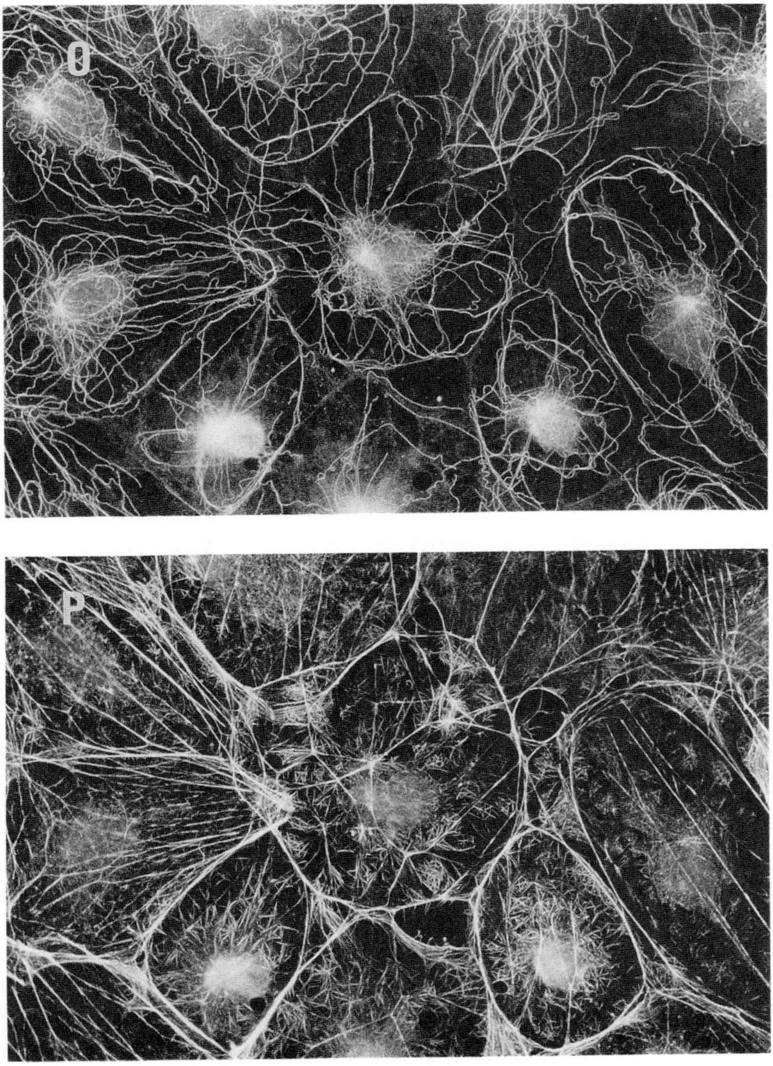

Figure 1 (*continued*)

Extraction of the Cytoskeleton

Following exposure to the agent of interest, cultures are washed twice with solution A containing the same concentration of Ca^{2+} as used in the experiment. Cells in which MTs and/or MFs are to be stained can then be fixed and extracted as described for 3T3 cells. However, a different protocol is required for cells in which the keratin IFs are to be stained, since antikeratin antibodies do not usually bind to keratin filaments in formaldehyde-fixed cells (14,20). Therefore, following the solution A rinses, cultures are fixed for 5 min at −20°C in precooled (−20°C) methanol. The coverslips are then rinsed once with cold distilled water (4°C) and twice with cold PBS. Coverslips may then be stored in PBS at 4°C until staining.

Immunofluorescence Staining of Keratin IFs

Staining of MTs and/or MFs can be performed in formaldehyde-fixed and NP40-extracted cells as described for 3T3 cells. For the staining of keratin IFs methanol-fixed coverslips are covered with 20 μl of rabbit antikeratin IgG antibodies for 30 min at 37°C in a humidified chamber. Coverslips are then washed with PBS and incubated for 15 min with 20 μl of 10% normal goat serum in PBS to block nonspecific binding of secondary antibodies. Following another wash with PBS, coverslips are incubated for 30 min with 20 μl of goat anti-rabbit IgG antibodies conjugated to rhodamine. Coverslips are then washed with PBS and mounted onto glass slides as described above.

Double-labeling of keratin filaments and MFs or MTs is accomplished using appropriate primary and secondary antibodies, provided that the primary antibodies have been screened for their ability to bind to their antigen in methanol-fixed cells.

COMMENTS

1. Growth-arrested Swiss 3T3 cells provide an excellent model for cytoskeletal studies because of their flattened polygon-shaped morphology with well-defined boundaries (18). These properties greatly facilitate the fluorescence microscopic examination of cytoskeletal elements. A typical pattern of MT and MF organization in control 3T3 cells is shown in Fig. 1. Growth-arrested cells contain an intricate network of MTs which emanate from a brightly stained organizing center localized in the perinuclear area to the cell periphery. The characteristic wavy and curving morphology of MTs is quite uniform among a population of cells examined. In contrast, MFs are usually less uniform and often variable in their morphology and distribution. Most cells contain thick long cables of actin filaments resembling stress fibers, in addition to nu-

Figure 2 The organization of the cytoskeleton in keratinocytes maintained in low-Ca^{2+} medium (A–C) or switched into high Ca^{2+} medium for 4 hr (D–F). Keratin intermediate filaments (A and D), microtubules (B and E), and microfilaments (C and F) were stained. (Reprinted by permission of Elsevier Science Publishing Company Inc., from "An Immunofluorescence Study of the Calcium Induced Coordinated Reorganization of Microfilaments, Keratin Intermediate Filaments, and Microtubules in Cultured Human Epidermal Keratinocytes" by G. B. Zamansky, U. Nguyen, and I.-N. Chou, *J. Invest. Dermatol* 97, 985–994, copyright © 1991 by The Society for Investigative Dermatology, Inc.)

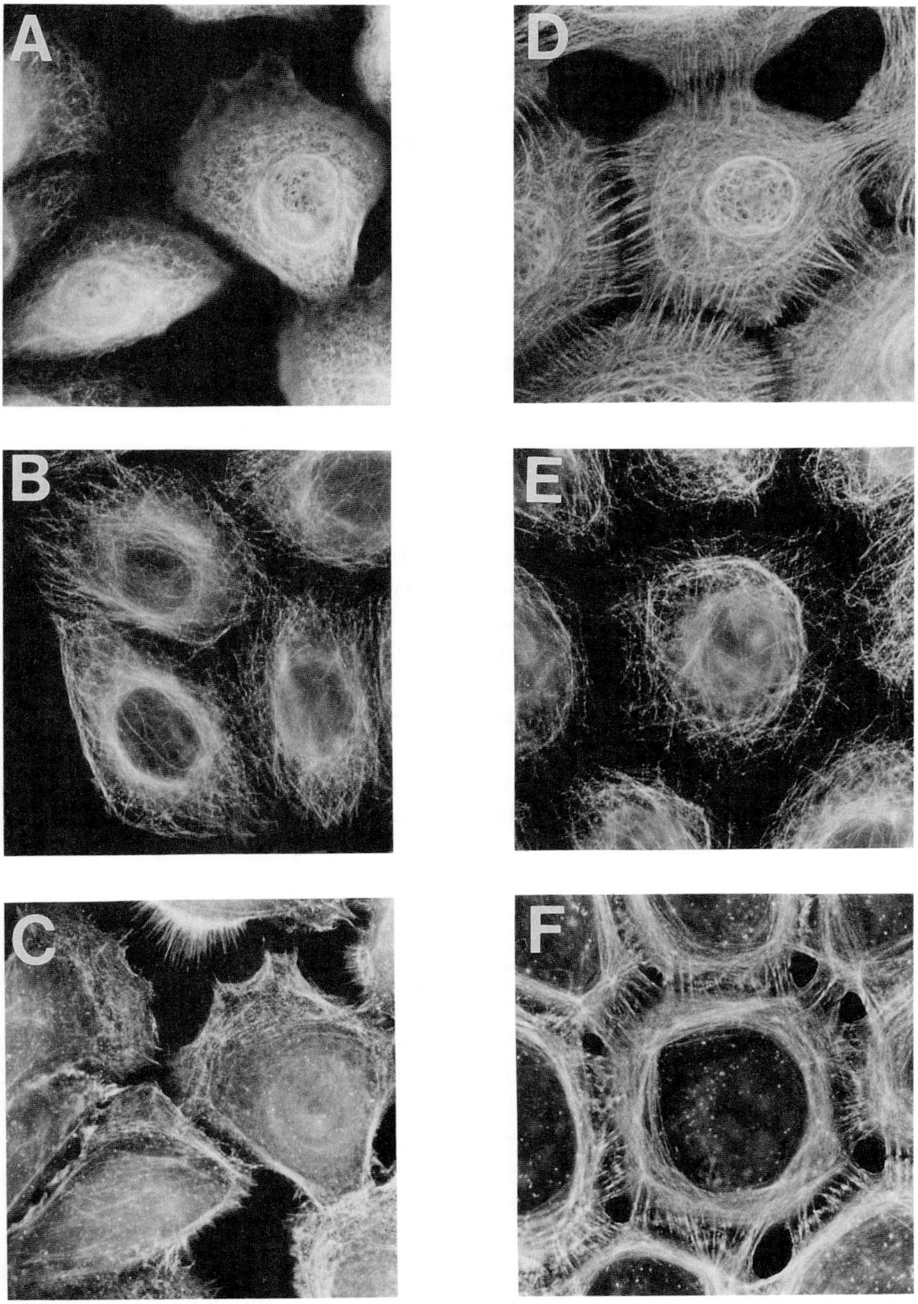
A
B
C
D
E
F

merous thinner filaments. However, a small population of cells may lack such conspicuous cables and contain only finer fibers. Nevertheless, both thick actin cables and thinner filaments are readily recognized by NBD–phallacidin. The stress fibers often span the entire cytoplasm.

2. The appearance of MFs, MTs, and keratin IFs in keratinocyte cultures maintained in low-Ca^{2+} medium or switched into high-Ca^{2+} medium for 4 hr is shown in Fig. 2. These protocols have also been used to study the cytoskeleton in keratinocyte cultures exposed to cytochalasin D, demecolcine, and ultraviolet radiation (14,15,21).

3. Coverslips should be cleaned thoroughly by washing with double distilled water 10 times and then with 95% ethanol three times. They are stored in 95% ethanol in a sealed container (e.g., a beaker). Coverslips can be picked up conveniently using a sterile Pasteur pipette connected through a flask to a vacuum outlet in the hood (pour out ethanol first) and released easily onto a culture dish by pinching the connecting tubing. When finished, ethanol is returned to the coverslip container.

4. For the cells described in this chapter, incubation with 0.3% NP40 for 10 min is sufficient to extract the cytoskeleton. However, the concentration of NP40 and the length of extraction may vary with cell types. Aliquots of 15% NP40 in PBS are stored at −20°C and diluted to 0.3% before use.

5. Each antibody preparation must be tested at different dilutions prior to its use in staining experiments. It is essential that optimal dilutions of both the primary and secondary antibodies be used in combination to give the best staining results.

6. Different lots of antibodies raised against the identical cytoskeletal protein may require variations in the fixation protocol because of differences in the epitope to which particular antibodies bind. It is therefore useful to pretest antibodies in cells fixed using more than one fixation protocol. It should also be pointed out that phallacidin and other phalloidin derivatives do not bind to actin in methanol-fixed cells.

7. Monoclonal antibodies may be substituted for the polyclonal primary antibodies or phallacidin. However, this will require using the appropriate secondary antibodies. When staining two cytoskeletal elements in the same cells, it will be necessary for the primary antibodies to be from animal species which differ sufficiently to prevent individual fluorochrome-conjugated secondary antibodies from binding to both primary antibodies.

8. During antibody staining it is important to drain and apply stain to one coverslip prior to draining the next coverslip in order to avoid drying. Drying out will result in poor staining quality.

9. To mount coverslips onto a slide, it is convenient and efficient to obtain a small drop of viscous Gelvatol by first shallowly dipping one end (the smoothend) of a small glass rod into the Gelvatol mounting solution, followed

by gently touching the surface of a clean glass slide. Excess of Gelvatol should be avoided. We routinely mount three coverslips onto a slide.

10. Our studies have demonstrated that the cytoskeletal morphology is very sensitive to a variety of toxicants. As shown in Fig. 1, 3T3 cells treated with different agents (e.g., metals and herbicides) exhibit different patterns of injury in their cytoskeletal organization.

REFERENCES

1. B. Alberts, D. Bray, J. Lewis, M. Raff, K. Roberts, and J. D. Watson, "Molecular Biology of the Cell," p. 549. Garland, New York, 1983.
2. K. Porter, *J. Cell Biol.* **99,** 1S (1984).
3. E. C. Raff, *Int. Rev. Cytol.* **59,** 1 (1979).
4. S. Penman, A. Fulton, D. Capco, A. Ben-Zeév, S. Wittlesberger, and C. F. Tse, *Cold Spring Harbor Symp. Quant. Biol.* **46,** 1013 (1982).
5. B. Anand and I.-N. Chou, *J. Biol. Chem.* **267,** 10716 (1992).
6. T. W. Clarkson, P. R. Sager and T. L. M. Syversen (eds.), "The Cytoskeleton, a Target for Toxic Agents." Plenum, New York, 1986.
7. A. H. Sharpe, L. B. Chen, J. R. Murphy and B. N. Fields, *Proc. Natl. Acad. Sci. U.S.A.* **77,** 7267 (1980).
8. I.-N. Chou, *Biomed. Environ. Sci.* **2,** 358 (1989).
9. A. B. Brody, L. H. Hill, T. W. Hesterberg, J. C. Barrett, and K. B. Adler, *in* "The Cytoskeleton, a Target for Toxic Agents" (T. W. Clarkson, P. R. Sager, and T. L. M. Syversen, eds.), p. 221. Plenum, New York, 1986.
10. W. Li, Y. Zhao, and I.-N. Chou, *Fed. Proc., Fed. Am. Soc. Exp. Biol.* **46,** 1323 (1987).
11. Y. Zhao, W. Li, and I.-N. Chou, *J. Toxicol. Environ. Health* **20,** 11 (1987).
12. W. Li, Y. Zhao, and I.-N. Chou, *Toxicol. Appl. Pharmacol.* **91,** 96 (1987).
13. G. B. Zamansky and I.-N. Chou, *J. Invest. Dermatol.* **89,** 603 (1987).
14. G. B. Zamansky, U. Nguyen, and I.-N. Chou, *J. Invest. Dermatol.* **97,** 985 (1991).
15. G.B. Zamansky, U. Nguyen, and I.-N. Chou, *Cell Motil. Cytoskeleton* **22,** 296 (1992).
16. F. Solomon, M. Magendantz, and A. Salzman, *Cell* **18,** 431 (1979).
17. K. Wang, J. R. Feramisco, and J. F. Ash, *in* "Methods in Enzymology" (D. W. Frederiksen and L. W. Cunningham, eds.), Vol. 85, p. 514. Academic Press, New York, 1982.
18. I.-N. Chou and J. P. Shaw, *Cell Biol. Int. Rep.* **8,** 441 (1984).
19. S. T. Boyce and R. G. Ham, *J. Invest. Dermatol.* **81,** 33s (1983).
20. M. Osborne, W. W. Franke, and K. Weber, *Proc. Natl. Acad. Sci. U.S.A.* **74,** 2490 (1977).
21. G. B. Zamansky and I.-N. Chou, *Photochem. Photobiol.* **52,** 903 (1990).

9 Energy Coupled Na^+ Cotransport

Sue M. Ford

INTRODUCTION

The gradient hypothesis of membrane transport was proposed and developed by Crane to explain the dependence of intestinal glucose transport on the presence of sodium (1,2). This principle has been recognized to be a fundamental mechanism for the biological transport of many solutes. Potential energy in the form of a transmembrane gradient of one compound can be harnessed to promote the uptake of another by coupling the the two processes in a single transport system. This process facilitates the entry of molecules such as hexoses, amino acids, and phosphate into a variety of cells, as well as the reabsorption of these compounds by the kidneys and the intestines.

The substrate for which the favorable gradient is established is the "driver" molecule, and may move in either the same direction as the cotransported agent (symport) or in the opposite direction (antiport or exchange). The rate of translocation in either case depends on the transmembrane concentration gradient of both species. Transport may also depend on the transmembrane electrical potential and/or the pH gradient (3). Apart from their potential energy contribution, some driver molecules affect the rate of transport of the cosubstrate by allosteric or other mechanisms. Consequently, it is often difficult to distinguish the energy-based contributions of Na^+, H^+, and other driver species from the mechanistic effects (3).

Sodium-dependent cotransport is an example of secondary active transport (2,4). The Na^+ gradient is established by the primary active transporter, which is the Na^+, K^+-ATPase (Na^+ pump) in the plasma membrane (Fig. 1). During the activity of the pump, ATP is hydrolyzed with the extrusion of three intracellular Na^+ ions in exchange for two extracellular K^+ ions. Na^+ cotransport thus requires cellular energy to establish and maintain the gradient. The magnitude of the gradient depends on the balance between the rate of influx of the solute and the rate of efflux by transport systems or by "leakage." The activity of the pump and the low Na^+ and K^+ conductances of most plasma membranes maintain intracellular concentrations of Na^+ and K^+ at 5 and 140 m*M* in the presence of external concentrations of 140 and 5 m*M*, respectively. By using the potential energy stored in this Na^+ gradient, solutes accumulated by cotransport can attain intracellular levels greater than those possible by simple diffusion.

METHODS IN TOXICOLOGY, Volume 1B

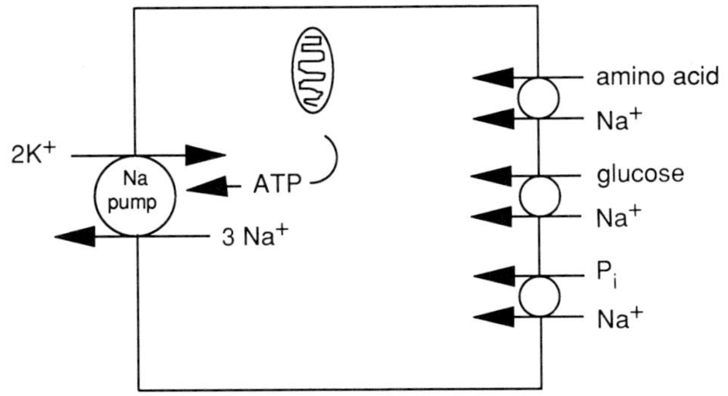

Figure 1 Sodium-dependent cotransport of amino acids, hexoses, and phosphate. The inwardly-directed Na^+ gradient created by the active Na^+ pump provides the potential energy for accumulation of cotransported solutes.

Na^+-dependent cotransport systems depend on the integrity of the plasma membrane, as well as that of Na^+, K^+-ATPase and energy-supplying pathways. Due to such complexity, they represent a possible target for toxicants. This chapter describes the general procedures for assessing Na^+-dependent cotransport and considers problems specific to amino acid, hexose, and phosphate transport.

MATERIALS AND REAGENTS

Transport Media

These are physiological buffers used during the uptake experiments and contain the radiolabeled amino acid substrate. Typical buffers are listed in Table I. The solutions are prepared using high-purity deioinized water. Insofar as the cells will not be cultured in this medium, tissue culture-tested reagents are not necessary and analytical-grade chemicals suitable for physiological or biochemical studies can be used. It is advisable to prepare concentrated stock solutions (10×) of the components and mix these immediately before use. This facilitates determining the optimal buffer composition and prevents the precipitation of calcium salts during storage that would occur with the complete admixture.

Radiolabeled Transport Substrates

Transported substrates are generally added to the media at 0.2–2.0 μCi/ml (Table I). Amino acids and hexoses labeled with ^{14}C or ^{3}H, and $[^{32}P]$-H_3PO_4 are readily available from suppliers of radiochemicals.

Table I Composition of Typical Transport Buffers.

	$+Na^+$		$-Na^+$	
	$+HCO_3^=$	$-HCO_3^=$	$+HCO_3^=$	$-HCO_3^=$
Buffer (m*M*)				
NaCl	137	137	—	—
KCl	5.4	5.4	5.4	5.4
KH_2PO_4	0.1	0.1	0.1	0.1
$MgSO_4$	1.2	1.2	1.2	1.2
$CaCl_2$	2.8	2.8	2.8	2.8
$NaHCO_3$[a]	14	—	—	—
$KHCO_3$[a] or $ChHCO_3$[a,b]	—	—	14	—
HEPES or Tris	—	14	—	14
ChCl[c]	—	—	137	137
Unlabeled substrate[d]	0–0.2	0–0.2	0–0.2	0–0.2
Radiolabeled substrate (μCi/ml)[d]	0.2–2	0.2–2	0.2–2	0.2–2

[a] Buffers with bicarbonate concentrations of 14 m*M* must be adjusted to pH 7.4 with 5% CO_2.
[b] Choline bicarbonate.
[c] Choline chloride.
[d] Transport substrate (amino acid, hexose, or PO_4).

Rinse Buffer

A second buffer is used at 37°C to rinse culture media from the cells prior to the experiment and later (at 4°C) to terminate the uptake process. This solution usually is similar in composition to the transport medium, but the radiolabeled species (and the Na^+ in some cases) should be omitted.

PROCEDURES

Basic Protocol

The volumes of reagents presented here are for 35-mm dishes and should be adjusted proportionately for larger or smaller vessels. For very short uptake periods (<5 min) the experiment can be done at room temperature or the samples can be placed on a temperature-controlled surface, such as a slide warmer. For longer experiments the samples should be maintained at 37°C and gently shaken at ~100 rpm. A Dubnoff metabolic incubator (Precision Scientific Inc., Chicago, IL) provides the required temperature, shaking action, and gaseous atmosphere; a platform can be taped together from multiwell dish parts to secure the culture plates and flasks in the instrument. Alternatively, a rocker platform placed directly in a tissue culture incubator is suitable.

The cells are washed two or three times with 1–2 ml of warm rinse buffer to remove the culture medium. To initiate uptake, the transport buffer (2 ml) containing the labeled substrate is added and the samples are placed in a temperature-controlled environment at 37° with 5% CO_2 (if bicarbonate buffers are used). When establishing the sodium dependence of the transport, parallel samples are tested with Na^+-free buffer. After the samples are incubated for the desired interval, the transport buffer is aspirated and the samples are quickly rinsed two to four times with chilled rinse buffer to stop the uptake and to remove extracellular radioactivity. The cells are solubilized in 1.0–1.5 ml of 0.1 N NaOH or a detergent-containing solution (e.g., 0.5% Triton X-100), or are extracted with 10% trichloroacetic acid. Aliquots of the resulting solutions are assayed for radioactivity by appropriate scintillation methods and also for protein or DNA content. Transport experiments with suspended cells are terminated by dilution of the suspension with cold rinse medium and rapid centrifugation, after which the supernatant is aspirated and the cells are digested as above. Alternatively, the diluted suspension is poured onto a membrane (e.g., 45 μm) in a filtration manifold with a low vacuum (500 torr), and the filters with the cells are dissolved and counted as above.

COMMENTS

Buffer Composition and Handling

Bicarbonate buffers must be bubbled with CO_2 to the desired pH and kept tightly covered on ice until needed. If it is necessary to hold the solution at 37° for a prolonged period during an experiment, the buffer should be maintained in an atmosphere with the appropriate pCO_2 to prevent pH changes and precipitation of calcium salts. For short incubation periods in a non-CO_2 atmosphere, bicarbonate can be replaced by HEPES or Tris. However, bicarbonate is indirectly involved in certain transport systems and should not be omitted in such cases. Transport inhibitors or unlabeled substrates might be added to the rinse buffer to prevent efflux at the end of the experiment. This should be done with caution since these substances promote extrusion of some substrates from the cell (5).

Cells

Transport experiments can be done with attached or suspended cells, with a few differences in the procedure. Cells that form monolayers are used *in situ* to avoid the membrane damage that occurs when the cells are removed from the growth surface (5). Access of medium components to the bottom side of attached cells might be limited, although this can be used to advantage when studying apical transport processes. For epithelial cells, in particular, it is important that they are confluent and attached to a surface, because the tight junctions between the cells maintain the polarized distribution of transporters and Na^+, K^+-ATPase. Cells can be grown on permeable substrata such as collagen disks or membrane filters to study the transcellular transport of a solute. Although this should allow the more physiological development of cultured epithelial cells, we have observed greater uptake of some substrates by cells cultured on plastic. The confluence of cells grown on transparent substrata is checked visually with a microscope. For cells grown on opaque filters, indirect confirmation of confluence can be made by staining representative filters (0.1% crystal violet in 20% methanol) (6), measuring the transepithelial resistance (7), or assessing the ability of the monolayer to prevent movement of radiolabeled inulin across the cell layer (7).

Confirmation of Sodium Dependence

Elimination of the external Na^+ will prevent Na^+-dependent cotransport; any uptake occurring under this condition represents leakage into the cell or uptake by Na^+-independent facilitated diffusion. The need for Na^+ as a driver ion can be substantiated by replacing NaCl and other Na^+ salts in the transport buffer with *N*-methyl-D-glucamine, mannitol, or the chloride salts of choline, Li^+, K^+, Cs^+, or NH_4^+. The substitution should maintain the osmolality of the solution at the same value as the Na^+-containing solution.

Inhibition of Na^+, K^+-ATPase by the specific inhibitor ouabain can be used to diminish the inwardly directed Na^+ gradient. However, there are significant species variations in response to ouabain; for example, Na^+, K^+-ATPase in the rat kidney is especially insensitive compared to those of other species (8). Other factors to consider in the use of ouabain include the time necessary for the drug to penetrate to the Na^+, K^+-ATPase on the basolateral side of the cell, as well as possible toxic effects of the compound. Consequently, Na^+ deprivation is the most direct and effective way to demonstrate Na^+ dependence of transport, typically producing 75–90% inhibition of phosphate uptake compared to ~35% for ouabain (9). Ionophores (e.g., gramicidin) can also be used to dissipate the electrochemical gradient of Na^+ and confirm its role in cotransport (10,11).

In the same way that Na^+ in the buffer stimulates uptake of Na^+-dependent substrates, the presence of the substrate will stimulate uptake of Na^+. This can be demonstrated by an increase in $^{22}Na^+$ uptake from the medium when the substrate is added. Alternatively, the current of Na^+ ions across a monolayer in the presence or absence of the cosubstrate can be assessed by the electrophysiological measurement of short-circuit current, which is the amount of external current needed to offset the movement of Na^+ (12,13).

Confirmation of Energy Dependence

The need of cotransport systems for cellular energy can be examined by manipulating the experimental buffer to increase or decrease intracellular ATP (14–16). It is possible to examine the contribution of particular metabolic pathways with suitable inhibitors. Glycolysis can be inhibited with iodoacetamide or iodoacetate (0.5 m*M*), whereas mitochondrial ATP production is sensitive to cyanide (2 m*M*), 2,4-dinitrophenol (0.5 m*M*) (9,15,17), rotenone (10 μM) (16), FCCP[1] (7 μM) (18), or incubation in an anaerobic atmosphere (e.g., 5% CO_2/95% N_2). Care must be taken when using an inhibitor to ensure that it does not affect the transporter itself or the cell membrane at the concentration used. For example, high concentrations of iodoacetate (1 m*M*) increase the membrane permeability to inorganic phosphate (Pi) and other small molecules (19).

Hexose Transport

Several subsets of hexose transporters have been identified, differing in their specificity, requirement for Na^+, and responsiveness to modulating factors such as hormones and substrate deprivation (20,21). Glucose can be used as a model; however, it may be metabolized, and, for some cell types, is not a good substrate for the Na^+-dependent hexose transporter (22). More frequently, nonmetabolizable glucose analogs labeled with ^{14}C or ^{3}H are used, including 2-deoxy-D-glucose (2-DDOG) and α-methylglucoside (AMG; methyl-α-D-glucopyranoside). AMG is a frequent choice, as it competes with glucose for Na^+-dependent transport, yet unlike glucose does not enter or exit cells by Na^+-independent pathways (8). 6-Deoxy-D-glucose (6-DOG) is a potent inhibitor of AMG transport (23). 2-DOG can be transported into the cell and phosphorylated, but it is not metabolized further in some (24) but not all (25) cells. 3-*O*-Methylglucose (3-OMG) enters cells primarily by a passive carrier-mediated pathway but cannot be phosphorylated (26); at its equilibrium concentration 3-OMG can be useful for measuring intracellular volume (27).

The Na^+-dependent and -independent pathways of glucose accumulation respond differently to the inhibitors phlorizin (phloridzin), phloretin (21), and cytochalasin B (28). The sensitivity of hexose uptake to these compounds can be used to confirm the Na^+-dependence of the transport. Phlorizin is an effective competitive inhibitor of Na^+-dependent transport at low concentrations (1–10 μM), whereas phloretin and cytochalasin B (10–15 μM) inhibit the non-sodium-dependent facilitated transport of glucose. It should be noted that phlorizin impairs several aspects of cell metabolism at higher concentrations ($\geq$1 m*M*) (29).

[1] FCCP, Carbonyl cyanide *p*-trifluoromethoxyphenylthydrazone.

Amino Acid Transport

Amino acids and amino acid derivatives enter cells by multiple systems differing in substrate specificity and Na^+-requirement. The major transporters identified for mammalian cells in culture are the alanine-preferring system A, the leucine-preferring system L, and system ASC, which transports alanine, serine, and cysteine (30–32). System A, which transports alanine, α-aminoisobutyric acid (AIB), serine, proline, and glycine, is Na^+dependent. In contrast, system L has greater affinity for the branched chain and aromatic amino acids but does not require sodium. Some amino acids (e.g., methionine and those with long straight hydrocarbon side chains) have a high affinity for both A and L; consequently, there are Na^+-dependent and -independent components of transport for these amino acids. System A appears to be more sensitive than system L to hormones (30), while factors that arrest cell growth (e.g., approach to confluence, serum depletion, and inhibition of protein synthesis) decrease the activity of system A and increase that of system L (33). The above systems have a wide distribution among cell types; other Na^+-dependent amino acid transport systems have been identified in specific cells (31,34).

The nonmetabolizable amino acid analog AIB is frequently used to assess uptake by system A. Alternatively, the nonmetabolizable amino acids D-aspartate (for the acidic system) (35) and cycloleucine (for systems L and ASC) are common choices. The amino acid transport systems differ significantly from one another in rate of initial uptake, time course, and Na^+ dependence, even for the same cell line, so that these parameters should be delineated for each experimental model.

Phosphate Transport

Labeled inorganic phosphate is available as the sodium salt, $Na_2H[^{32}P]O_4$ (14), as well as other forms (e.g., $H_3[^{32}P]O_4$ and $K_2H[^{32}P]O_4$) for studies with Na^+-free media (8). Phosphate uptake can be competitively inhibited with phosphate analogs such as arsenate (1 m*M*) (3,17,36,37) or derivatives of phosphonocarboxylic acid (36), such as phosphonoformic acid (1–2 m*M*). The rate of P_i transport depends on the P_i content of the buffer (38,39). Cellular uptake of P_i differs between the monobasic and dibasic forms in some cell lines (5), but not others (18). Consequently, the intra- and extracellular pH, by altering the ratio of mono- to dibasic phosphate, will affect the transport behavior of P_i in some cases. This factor should be considered when it is possible that the experimental treatment will alter the pH. Phosphate accumulation by many cultured cells is responsive to the same factors that influence P_i transport *in vivo,* including parathyroid hormone and phosphate depletion (40).

Use of Na^+ Cotransport in Toxicology Studies

The stoichiometries of energy and Na^+ dependence differ among the transporters, as does the requirement for additional driver ions (4). Furthermore, the behavior of the transport systems often varies markedly among the cell culture models. Before using a cotransport process as an end point for toxicity studies, the particular system under investigation should be validated by determining its Na^+ requirement, time course of transport, and response to specific inhibitors. For example, we have found that aspartic acid accumulation by LLC-PK_1 cells is much more rapid than that of AIB and also reaches a maximum earlier (15 min). Thereafter, the accumulation decreases until the intracellular levels are equal to that of the Na^+-independent component of uptake at 120 min. AIB accumulation, on the other hand, continues steadily and at a lower rate for up to 120 min. Thus, the time frame for studying the uptake of these two amino acids will be markedly different.

When using transport as an end point in toxicity studies, the possible effects of the treatment on cell volume should be considered. The total amount of the substrate accumulated during a given interval is influenced not only by the membrane properties, but also by the cell volume. It is possible that accumulation of a substrate may be greater following exposure to a particular toxicant, due not to a greater intracellular concentration, but rather to an increase in cell volume. Measurement of the volume of cultured cells can be accomplished by comparing the behavior of passively distributed compounds (e.g., 3-OMG, or $[^3H]H_2O$) with that of extracellular markers (16,23,27).

Characterization of transport systems generally relies on the use of substrates radiolabeled with ^{14}C, ^3H, or ^{32}P. The metabolic fate of functional groups on the transported species should be considered in the choice and location of the ^{14}C or ^3H label for amino acids or glucose. In cases where intracellular metabolism of the transported species could be rapid and thereby change the concentration gradient for transport, it might be necessary to ascertain the intracellular fate of the radiolabel during the period of the experiment (30). If the metabolism of a substrate subsequent to transport is altered by the experimental treatment, it would be possible to observe a change in the accumulation of the molecule without a direct effect on the transporter. Amino acids, in particular, have several metabolic options; for example, it is important, with protocols involving long incubations, to establish that incorporation into proteins is negligible (11). Otherwise, a toxic effect on protein synthesis could be misconstrued as an impairment of transport. In some cases the rate of phosphorylation of 2-DOG may be rate limiting for transport, rather than its translocation across the membrane, and transported phosphorus may be metabolized in several ways, including incorporation into ATP or ADP.

The presence of intracellular pools of a substrate can stimulate or inhibit transport. Many membrane transporters can operate bidirectionally, depending on the relative intra- and extracellular concentrations of the transported species. For example, system A substrates present in the cytoplasm stimulate the uptake of extracellular radiolabeled AIB from the medium (31), whereas depletion of other amino acids accomplishes the same effect (31,33,41,42). It is probable that such differences in transport behavior represent uptake of AIB by several transporters. Conversely, intracellular pools of other substrates decrease the rates of uptake, possibly by reducing the transmembrane gradient (30,33).

The composition of the transport media can influence the rate of uptake of the transported molecule. Substrates transported by separate Na^+-dependent systems may compete with each other for Na^+. Such interaction could be of concern, for example, if glucose is included in the medium to provide an energy substrate for amino acid (11) or phosphate transport studies, or when phosphate is used as a buffer. The intra- or extracellular pH influences several transport processes. H^+ can alter the ionic form of amino acids (11) or phosphate, thereby changing the proportion of the transported species. The pH of the media can also become important under certain conditions (12). The activity of the Na^+/H^+ antiporter, which transports H^+ out of and Na^+ into the cell, may complicate results for some cell types.

The growth stage of cells affects transport, often by influencing the size and utilization of the intracellular pools of a substrate. The effect of confluence varies among transporters (5,8,30,33,43). Generally, amino acid uptake is greatest during active proliferation; this effect appears to be due to the size and composition of the pools during this stage (33). On the other hand, hexose transport, as measured by AMG accumulation, is greater in confluent cultures (23). Hexose, amino acid, and phosphate transporters are modulated by hormones and growth factors so that variations in these components in the growth medium (e.g., the serum) may be important. These transport systems also respond to deprivation of the substrate by increasing the number of transporters, thereby increasing the rate of uptake (39,40,44–47).

Polarized epithelia provide special opportunities for transport studies. For such cells, hexoses accumulate by Na^+-dependent pathways on the apical (brush border) side of the cell and exit by Na^+-independent facilitated diffusion on the basolateral side. Amino acids also enter the cells by different mechanisms on the apical and basolateral sides. Cells from several sources (e.g., renal or intestinal cells) can be grown on porous substrata, thus allowing independent access to the basolateral and apical membranes. This provides many possibilities for toxicant exposure, as well as localization of a lesion to either side of the cell. Several companies (e.g., Millipore, Whatman, and Falcon) provide prefabricated membrane filter devices that accommodate treatment of cells in six- or 24-well dishes (48).

REFERENCES

1. R. K. Crane, *Rev. Physiol. Biochem. Pharmacol.* **78,** 101 (1977).
2. E. Heinz and P. Geck, *Kidney Int.* **36,** 334 (1989).
3. J. P. Wehrle and P. L. Pedersen, *J. Membr. Biol.* **111,** 199 (1989).
4. D. M. Scott, *BioEssays* **7,** 71 (1987).
5. C. A. Rabito, *Miner. Electrolyte Metab.* **12,** 32 (1986).
6. S. M. Ford, P. D. Williams, S. Grassl, and P. D. Holohan, *Am. J. Physiol.* **259,** C103 (1990).
7. M. J. Palmoski, B. A. Masters, S. M. Ford, and O. P. Flint, *J. Tissue. Cult. Methods.* **13,** 169 (1991).
8. C. Clerici, P. Soler, and G. Saumon, *Biochim. Biophys. Acta* **1063,** 27 (1991).
9. B. Escoubet, K. Djabali, and C. Amiel, *Am. J. Physiol.* **256,** C322 (1989).
10. J. C. Chen, J. L. Stevebs, A. L. Trifillis, and T. W. Jones, *Toxicol. Appl. Pharmacol.* **103,** 463 (1990).
11. J. A. Schafer and D. W. Barfuss, *Am. J. Physiol.* **238,** F335 (1980).
12. A. Gupta and J. L. Renfro, *Am. J. Physiol.* **260,** R704 (1991).
13. L. Mandel and R. S. Balaban, *Am. J. Physiol.* **240,** F357 (1981).
14. M. B. De Young and A. Scarpa, *Am. J. Physiol.* **260,** C1182 (1991).
15. C. Rea and S. Segal, *Kidney Int.* **2,** 101 (1972).
16. N. Tessitore, L. M. Sakhrani, and S. G. Massry, *Am. J. Physiol.* **251,** C120 (1986).
17. M. A. Waqar, J. Seto, S. D. Chung, S. Hiller-Grohol, and M. Taub, *J. Cell. Physiol.* **124,** 411 (1985).
18. J. Biber, C. D. A. Brown, and H. Murer, *Biochim. Biophys. Acta* **735,** 325 (1983).
19. S. A. Kempson, K. J. Kunkler, and H. Murer, *Physiologist* **32,** 212 (1989).
20. M. Silverman, *Annu. Rev. Biochem.* **60,** 757 (1991).
21. M. Silverman, *Biochim. Biophys. Acta* **457,** 303 (1976).
22. K. Malström, G. Stange, and H. Murer, *Biochim. Biophys. Acta* **902,** 269 (1988).
23. J. M. Mullin, J. Weibel, L. Diamond, and A. Kleinzeller, *J. Cell. Physiol.* **104,** 375 (1980).
24. A. Klip, T. Ramlal, P. J. Bilan, L. Lam, and L. A. Leiter, *Endocrinology (Baltimore)* **130,** 2535 (1992).
25. J. S. Kerr, J. Reicherter, and A. B. Fisher, *Am. J. Physiol.* **243,** C14 (1982).
26. J. M. Mullin, L. M. Kofeldt, L. M. Russo, M. M. Hagee, and A. H. Dantzig, *Am. J. Physiol.* **31,** F480 (1992).
27. B. States, R. Reynolds, J. Lee, and S. Segal, *In Vitro Cell. Dev. Biol.* **26,** 105 (1990).
28. A. Klip, W. J. Logan, and G. Li, *Biochim. Biophys. Acta* **687,** 265 (1982).
29. S. Segal, A. A. Blair, and L. E. Rosenberg, *Biochim. Biophys. Acta* **71,** 676 (1963).
30. D. L. Oxender, M. Lee, P. A. Moore, and G. Cecchini, *J. Biol. Chem.* **252,** 2675 (1977).
31. M. A. Shotwell, M. S. Kilberg, and D. L. Oxender, *Biochim. Biophys. Acta* **737,** 267 (1983).
32. M. K. Patterson, Jr., "Growth, Nutrition, and Metabolism of Cells in Culture" (G. H. Rothblatt and V. J. Cristofolo, eds.), Vol. 1. Academic Press, New York, 1972.
33. D. L. Oxender, M. Lee, and G. Cecchini, *J. Biol. Chem.* **252,** 2680 (1977).

34. P. Boerner, M. Evans-Layng, H. S. Ü, and M. H. Saier, Jr., *J. Biol. Chem.* **261,** 13957 (1986).
35. C. A. Rabito and M. V. Karish, *J. Biol. Chem.* **258,** 2543 (1983).
36. M. Szczepanska-Konkel, A. N. K. Yusufi, M. VanScoy, S. K. Webster, and T. P. Dousa, *J. Biol. Chem.* **261,** 6375 (1986).
37. M. L. Chen, R. S. King, and H. J. Armbrecht, *J. Cell. Physiol.* **143,** 488 (1990).
38. C. L. Bell, H. S. Tenenhouse, and C. R. Scriver, *In Vitro Cell. Dev. Biol.* **24,** 683 (1988).
39. M. Jahan and P. J. Butterworth, *Biochem. J.* **252,** 105 (1988).
40. J. Caverzasio, C. D. A. Brown, J. Biber, J. P. Bonjour, and H. Murer, *Am. J. Physiol.* **248,** F122 (1985).
41. P. I. Karl, K. L. Alpy, and S. E. Fisher, *Am. J. Physiol.* **31,** C834 (1992).
42. D. S. Kelley and V. R. Potter, *J. Biol. Chem.* **353,** 9009 (1978).
43. K. Amsler and J. S. Cook, *Am. J. Physiol.* **242,** C94 (1982).
44. H. C. Haspel, E. W. Wilk, M. J. Birnbaum, S. W. Cushman, and O. M. Rosen, *J. Biol. Chem.* **261,** 6778 (1986).
45. A. Moran, R. J. Turner, and J. S. Handler, *J. Biol. Chem.* **258,** 15087 (1983).
46. A. Moran, R. J. Turner, and J. S. Handler, *J. Biol. Chem.* **258,** 15067 (1983).
47. E. Wertheimer, S. Sasson, and E. Cerasi, *J. Cell. Physiol.* **143,** 330 (1990).
48. S. M. Ford and P. D. Williams, "In Vitro Methods of Toxicology" (R. R. Watson, ed.), p. 123. CRC Press, Boca Raton, Florida, 1992).

10 Renal Organic Ion Transport

Carlotta E. Groves, Hilary V. Sheevers, and Sharon J. McGuinness

INTRODUCTION

Numerous organs in the body work to excrete, secrete, and absorb a variety of substances, especially ions. One of the principal organs associated with organic ion transport is the kidney. Renal organic cation and anion secretion is responsible for the excretion of many endogenous and exogenous compounds and is one of the major lines of defense against potentially toxic agents. Impaired renal excretion of xenobiotics and metabolites can lead to their accumulation in the body, resulting in potentially toxic effects.

During net secretion, organic ions cross the peritubular and apical membranes of the proximal tubule using specific transport systems. Several contraluminal transport systems for organic anions have been reported, for example: (1) Na^+–dicarboxylate cotransport, (2) sulfate–HCO_3 exchange, and (3) *p*-aminohippuric acid (PAH)–dicarboxylate exchange (1). The PAH transport system secretes many endogenous compounds, such as urate and glucuronide conjugates (2). Pharmacologically active compounds such as sulfonamides, salicylates, penicillins, and cephalosporins also utilize this system. Secretion of PAH exhibits interspecies variation, which is an important consideration in cross-species comparisons. For example, in the rat the S_2 and S_3 segments of the proximal tubule show equal PAH uptake activity, although in the rabbit the S_2 segment seems more active than the S_1 and S_3 segments (3,4).

The transport route for the active transcellular secretion of organic cations is separate from the organic anion system. The organic cation substrates are typically primary, secondary, tertiary, or quaternary amines. Transported substrates include choline, acetylcholine, dopamine, histamine, and plant alkaloids introduced through diet (5) and the pharmacologically active compounds amiloride, cimetidine, morphine, and procainamide. Organic cations also show heterogeneity of transport, but in at least one species (rabbit), and in contrast to organic anions, the pattern of secretion is $S_1 \geq S_2 > S_3$ (6). The organic cation prototypes tetraethylammonium (TEA) and *N*-methylnicotinamide are commonly used in the study of this transport system.

METHODS IN TOXICOLOGY, Volume 1B

The measurement of organic ion transport is a powerful and useful tool in renal toxicology. Numerous techniques have been used in the study of organic ion transport. Clearance studies using the whole animal or the isolated perfused kidney have been used to provide general information on the renal handling of a substance. However, the transport site within the nephron cannot be localized using these techniques. In addition, extrarenal and renal medullary processes may alter renal substrate handling. To overcome some of these difficulties, renal cortical slices have been utilized extensively to examine organic ion transport. Advantages of slices include maintenance of renal cortical structural integrity similar to that *in vivo* and the absence of extracortical effects. However, the presence of a heterogeneous cell population in renal slices may circumvent precisely defining the transport site within the nephron. Since organic ion transport is localized in the renal proximal tubule, these tubules in suspension have been used to examine this process because suspensions provide a more homogeneous cell population. Since access to the luminal surface in renal cortical slices and tubule suspensions appears to be limited (7), the information gained is limited primarily to basolateral membrane transport. Access to the basolateral membrane is greater in tubule suspensions than in renal slices, allowing for more rapid organic ion uptake.

Two *in vitro* systems, renal slices and suspensions of renal proximal tubules, have been applied to the study of organic ion transport and to the toxicity testing of two organic cations, 1-benzylquinolinium (1-BQ) and celiptium. The scope of the application of these methods in this chapter is limited to organic cations, to demonstrate in detail how to examine ion transport.

MATERIALS AND REAGENTS

Materials for Renal Slices

Heptanoic acid, (2-hydroxyethyl)-1-piperazineethanesulfonic acid (HEPES, free acid, and sodium salt), and Dulbecco's modified Eagle's medium/Ham's F-12 50:50 mix with 15 m*M* HEPES and L-glutamate, without sodium bicarbonate and phenol red (DME/F-12) were purchased from Sigma (St. Louis, MO). The organic cation TEA and the organic anion PAH were purchased from Aldrich (Milwaukee, WI). ^3H_2O was purchased from ICN (Irvine, CA; 40 μCi/ml). [^{14}C]TEA (specific activity, 56 mCi/mmol) and [^{14}C]PAH (specific activity, 42 mCi/mmol) were purchased from Wizard Laboratories (Davis, CA) and New England Nuclear (NEN)–Dupont (Boston, MA), respectively. Tissue solubilizer (Solvable) and scintillation cocktail (Ecolite) were from NEN–DuPont and ICN, respectively. 1-BQ and celiptium were provided by Dr. Stephen H. Wright (University of Arizona and Pasteur Merieux, France).

Materials for Renal Tubules

Heptanoic acid, deoxyribonuclease (type I), penicillin G (sodium salt), Percoll, bovine serum albumin (BSA; fraction V), HEPES, and DME F-12 medium were purchased from Sigma. Collagenase (class I) and deferoxamine were obtained from Worthington (Freehold, NJ) and Ciba (Summit, NJ), respectively. The *n*-tetraalkylammonium compounds tetramethylammonium (TMA), TEA, tetrapropylammonium (TPrA), tetrabutylammonium, (TBA), and tetrapentylammonium (TPeA) were purchased from Aldrich. ^3H_2O was purchased from ICN (40 μCi/ml). [^{14}C]TEA (specific activity, 56 mCi/mmol) was purchased from Wizard Laboratories. Tissue solubilizer (Solvable) and scintillation cocktail (Ecolite) were also used.

Renal Slice Reagents

Krebs–HEPES buffer with the following additions—132 m*M* NaCl, 10 m*M*-$NaC_2H_3O_2$; 4.8 m*M* KCl, 1.2 m*M* KH_2PO_4, 2.5 m*M* $CaCl_2$, 1.2 m*M* $MgSO_4$, 13 m*M* HEPES acid, and 13 m*M* HEPES sodium—was used in the slicing procedure. The buffer was gassed with 95% O_2/5% CO_2 and adjusted to pH 7.4 with NaOH while bubbling. Renal slices were incubated in DME-F12 medium with the addition of 2 m*M* heptanoic acid. The medium was heated to 37°C and gassed with 95% O_2/5% CO_2, and the pH was adjusted to 7.4 with NaOH. If experiments beyond 8 hr were necessary, penicillin (4 mg/ml) and streptomycin (24 U/ml) were used to avoid bacterial contamination. Note: Addition of these antibiotics may decrease organic anion transport.

Isolated Tubule Reagents

DME/F-12 medium with the following additions—15 m*M* $NaHCO_3$, 2 m*M* heptanoic acid, and 100 u/ml penicillin G—was dissolved in 800–900 ml of deionized water. The medium was adjusted to pH 7.4 at 4°C with NaOH and brought to 1 liter with deionized Water. Double-concentration (2×) DME-F12 medium was prepared by diluting a 1-liter vial (or 15.6 g) of DME/F-12 into 400 ml of deionized water. The pH was adjusted to 7.4 at 4°C with NaOH and the medium was brought to a final volume of 500 ml. The incubation buffer was a modified Krebs–Henseleit solution containing 1 m*M* L-alanine, 5 m*M* dextrose, 2 m*M* heptanoic acid, 4 m*M* lactate, 5 m*M* malate, 115 m*M* NaCl, 15 m*M* NaHCO3, 5 m*M* KCl, 2 m*M* NaH_2PO_4, 1 m*M* $MgSO_4$, 1 m*M* $CaCl_2$, and 10 m*M* HEPES. To prepare the incubation buffer, all reagents except $CaCl_2$ were dissolved in an appropriate volume of deionized water and the solution was bubbled with 95% O_2/5% CO_2 for 5 min. $CaCl_2$ was then added to the buffer while bubbling. The buffer was adjusted to pH 7.4 at 37°C with NaOH while bubbling and brought to volume with deionized water. To prepare the Percoll gradient (unformed) for tubule isolation, 40 ml of 2 × DME/F-12 was mixed with 40 ml of Percoll (adjust to pH 7.4 at 4°C with 1 N HCl). Enzymatic digestion medium was prepared by diluting 150 U/ml collagenase (class I), 70 U/ml deoxyribonuclease, 0.2% BSA and 1 m*M* deferoxamine into 25 ml of DME/F-12 and kept on ice until used.

Transport Reagents

Tissue:Medium Ratio

The TEA solution, for organic cation uptake studies, consisted of equal parts of TEA (1 m*M*), [^{14}C]TEA (4 μCi/ml), and $^{3}H_2O$ (40 μCi/ml) diluted in deionized water. The PAH solution, for anion uptake studies, consisted of equal parts of PAH (1 m*M*), [^{14}C]PAH (4 μCi/ml), and $^{3}H_2O$ (40 μCi/ml) diluted in deionized water. To measure organic ion uptake, PAH or TEA transport solution (36 μl) was added to 1.6 ml of Krebs–HEPES buffer in 20-ml scintillation vials.

Organic Ion Uptake, Kinetics, and Efflux

[^{14}C]TEA (in ethanol) was diluted to 0.1 μCi or 0.4 μCi/ml with deionized water. The organic cations TPeA, TBA, TPrA, TEA, and TMA were diluted to the appropriate concentration in incubation buffer.

PROCEDURES

Renal Slices

Preparation

Renal slices were prepared from New Zealand White rabbits (1.5–2.0 kg) using a Krumdieck mechanical tissue slicer (Alabama Reseach and Development, Munford, AL) (8). Rabbits were killed by injection of an overdose of sodium pentobarbital (~3 ml of a 64.8 mg/ml solution), and the kidneys were removed, decapsulated, and placed in ice-cold Krebs–HEPES buffer (9). The kidney was cored with a custom-made stainless steel tube (0.012-inch wall, 6-mm inner dimension) sharpened on one end and rapidly rotated on a drill press. The kidney can also be cored using a hand-held biopsy punch (Acuderm, Ft. Lauderdale, FL). The biopsy punch gives lower-quality cores, but is an inexpensive method for preliminary studies. Six cores (6 mm) were removed along the corticopapillary axis. Cores were trimmed of medullary tissue, placed in ice-cold Krebs–HEPES buffer in a Krumdieck mechanical tissue slicer and cut perpendicular to their tubular axis. In the tissue slicer, the cores were held in a well below a weighted piston and an automatic arm pulled the core across a vibrating microtome blade; the slice was automatically delivered to a glass holding vessel.

Incubation Systems

Slices were exposed to the test compound (i.e., 1-BQ or celiptium) in an *in vitro* incubation system modified from a version detailed by Ruegg *et al.* (10). The system consisted of 16 Teflon vessels (2 × 3 inches) which hold a 20-ml volume of DME-F12 medium containing the appropriate concentration of the test compound. Up to six slices rested on a stainless steel screen in the center of the vessel. The screen was supported in the center by stainless steel tubing. A 23-gauge needle protruded into the middle of each Teflon vessel and provided constant 95% O_2/5% CO_2 atmosphere to the slices. The Teflon vessels were in a solid block of aluminum (9 × 9 inches) which was channeled with copper tubing and connected to a recirculating water bath to maintain the temperature at 37°C. At timed intervals slices were removed and blotted dry, and organic ion uptake was evaluated as described below.

Organic Ion Uptake

To measure uptake of radiolabeled organic ion, a second incubation system was utilized to minimize the use of [^{14}C]-TEA or [^{14}C]PAH (11). PAH or TEA transport buffer (36 μl) was added to 1.6 ml of Krebs–HEPES buffer in 20-ml scintillation vials. Three to five slices were placed on stainless steel screens circumvented by stainless steel rings and placed in the vials. Slices were oxygenated (95% O_2/5% CO_2) immediately prior to attaching a screw-top lid and placed for 40 min on a heated roller system (37°C) to constantly bathe the slices in medium. Preliminary studies had shown that steady-state accumulation of TEA and PAH was reached by 40 min. Accumulation was terminated by removing each slice with forceps from the medium, blotting dry on a paper towel, and placing each slice in a 1.5-ml microfuge tube containing 0.5 ml of tissue solubilizer (Solvable). The TEA or PAH medium was saved for later analysis. The solubilized slice (0.5 ml) was transferred to scintillation vials that contained 5 ml of liquid scintillation fluid. Media samples (50 μl) were added to vials containing 5 ml of scintillation fluid and 450 μl Solvable. The ^{14}C-labeled substrates were counted and expressed as a ratio of the ^3H_2O counts in each sample. Since a ratio of the radiolabels was measured in both the slice and the buffer, no correction was needed for the difference in tissue versus buffer volumes used in the assay. Accumulation of radiolabeled organic ion was expressed as:

$$\frac{^{14}\text{C cpm in tissue}}{^{3}\text{H cpm}} \div \frac{^{14}\text{C cpm in media}}{^{3}\text{H cpm}} \qquad (1)$$

A slice:media ratio greater than 1 indicates tissue accumulation of the organic ion.

Renal Proximal Tubules in Suspension

Isolation and Incubation

Renal proximal tubules were isolated from male or female New Zealand White rabbits (1.5–2.0 kg) according to the methods of Vinay *et al.* (12), as modified by Dickman and Mandel (13) and Groves *et al.* (14). Briefly, this method involves collagenase digestion of the renal cortex followed by differential centrifugation in 50% Percoll. A butterfly catheter was inserted into the ear vein and heparin (3000 U) was injected, followed by an overdose of sodium pentobarbital (~3 ml of a 64.8 mg/ml solution) to kill the rabbit. Kidneys were rapidly excised, decapsulated, and placed in ice-cold DME/F-12 medium. The renal cortex was cut away from the medulla with a No. 20 scalpel blade, minced with two razor blades into ~1-mm cubes, and suspended in enzymatic digestion media. Tissue was digested in an orbital shaking water bath (200 rpm) at 37°C under a 95% O_2/5% CO_2 atmosphere (30 ml/min flow rate) for 20–30 min. The suspension was filtered through a 253-μM Nitex Swiss nylon monofilament screening fabric (Tetko, Los Angeles, CA) to remove undigested tissue. The filtered tissue was transferred to two 50-ml conical tubes and spun for 2 min at 50 *g* at 4°C to rinse the tissue. The supernatant was aspirated by vacuum suction; the tissue was resuspended in DME/F-12 medium and rinsed two additional times with DME/F-12. The proximal tubules were isolated on a Percoll gradient (50% Percoll and 50% 2×DME/F-12, pH 7.4) at 37,000 *g* for 30 min at 4°C. The lower band, composed of proximal tubules, was removed with a Pasteur pipette, rinsed once with DME/F-12 medium, and followed by two rinses with incubation buffer. Tubules were resuspended at a protein concentration of 1–5 mg/ml (as determined by standard protein assay) in incubation buffer. During all experiments with tubule suspensions described below, an appropriate volume (5–10 ml) of tubule suspensions was preincubated for 15 min in Erlenmeyer flasks at 37°C in an orbital shaking water bath (150 rpm) under an atmosphere of 95% O_2/5% CO_2 [10–15 ml/min flow rate as adjusted using a Gilman flowmeter (VWR, Phoenix, Az)].

Tubule:Medium Ratio

Tubule suspensions (3–5 mg/ml) were preincubated with the test drug. At timed intervals the tubules were transferred to 15-ml polypropylene tubes, pelleted at 50*g* and resuspended in fresh incubation buffer without drug. [^{14}C]PAH or [^{14}C]TEA substrate mixtures (36 μl) were added to 1.6 ml of tubule suspension and incubated for 30 min at 37°C under an atmosphere of 95% air/5% CO_2 with shaking (200 rpm). Preliminary studies showed that steady-state TEA or PAH accumulation was reached within 30 min. Accumulation was terminated by centrifuging 0.5 ml of the suspension through 0.4 ml of a 2:1 dibutylphthalate:diotylphthalate oil layer (in a 1.5-ml microfuge tube) at

14,000 *g* for 60 sec. The upper medium layer was removed with a Pasteur pipette and saved and the tube above the oil layer was washed twice with deionized water to remove residual radiolabel. The oil layer was removed and discarded. The tubule pellet was solubilized in 0.5 ml of Solvable. The solubilized pellet was transferred to scintillation vials containing 5 ml of liquid scintillation cocktail. Media samples were treated in the following manner: media (50 μl) and Solvable (450 μl) were added to scintillation vials containing 5 ml of scintillation cocktail. The samples were counted and the accumulation of radiolabeled organic ion was expressed as described by Eq. (1).

Peritubular Organic Ion Uptake

Following preincubation of tubule suspensions as described above in "Isolation and Incubation," [^{14}C]TEA (0.1 μCi/ml) alone or [^{14}C]TEA with unlabeled organic cation was added to the suspension. At timed intervals 0.5-ml aliquots of suspension were removed and added to a 15-ml polypropylene tube containing 5 ml of ice-cold incubation buffer to stop transport. Samples were immediately centrifuged at 1480 *g* for 20–30 sec to pellet was the suspension. The supernatant fraction was aspirated and the pellet was rinsed a second time with ice-cold incubation buffer. The pellet was dissolved in 0.5 ml of 1 N NaOH and aliquots were taken for liquid scintillation counting.

Kinetics

Following preincubation, a 0.5-ml aliquot of tubule suspension was pipetted into a 15-ml polypropylene tube. A 0.5-ml aliquot of incubation buffer containing [^{14}C]TEA (0.4 μCi/ml) and varying concentrations of the unlabeled *n*-tetraalkylammonium compounds were added to 0.5 ml of tubule suspension. After 30 sec 5 ml of ice-cold TPeA (1 m*M*) in incubation buffer was added to stop uptake, and the tubules were pelleted and prepared for radiolabel counting as described above. Note: once cold TPeA (1 m*M*) has been added to stop transport, samples can sit on ice for ~5–10 min with no net loss of accumulated substrate.

Efflux Studies

Following preincubation, [^{14}C]TEA (0.1 μCi/ml) was added to tubule suspensions and incubation was continued for 30 min. In addition, a 15-ml polypropylene tube containing 4.5 ml of the unlabeled *n*-tetraalkylammonium compounds at a saturating concentration (that concentration which produces maximal inhibition of TEA uptake as determined by preliminary studies) was also preincubated at 37°C for 15 min. Efflux of accumulated TEA from the preloaded tubules was determined as follows: an aliquot (0.5 ml) of the tubule suspension was removed and added to 5 ml of ice-cold 1 m*M* TPeA to establish tubule TEA content at time zero of the efflux period. An aliquot (0.5 ml) was also added to tubes containing 4.5 ml of an unlabeled *n*-tetraalkylammonium compound or incubation buffer alone and incubation was continued for 5–10 min. The reaction was terminated by the addition of 5 ml of ice-cold TPeA (1 m*M*) and the tubule pellets were prepared for radiolabel counting as described above.

COMMENTS

Results and Analysis

The ability of a compound to inhibit organic cation TEA and organic anion PAH accumulation is commonly used both *in vivo* and *in vitro* to assess nephrotoxicity. In toxicological studies, however, the transport of these compounds by the proximal tubule has often been oversimplified or misunderstood. Renal slices accumulated TEA and PAH to intracellular levels 5-fold greater than the extracellular media (Fig. 1A and B). Exposure of renal slices to the monovalent cation 1-BQ at a concentration of 1000 μM resulted in approximately a 90% reduction in the steady-state accumulation of TEA and PAH (Fig. 1A and B). Exposure to 100 μM 1-BQ reduced TEA accumulation by ~50%, but had no effect on the accumulation of PAH. Thus, the inhibition of PAH accumulation by 1000 μM 1-BQ may be the result of a toxic effect on cell function or viability.

Tubule suspensions accumulated TEA to intracellular levels 15-fold greater than the extracellular media and 3-fold greater than in renal slices (Fig. 1C and D). This difference in TEA accumulation between slices and tubules may be the result of a heterogeneous population of cells within the slice which do not contribute to TEA uptake. Preincubation with the cationic anticancer agent celiptium also caused a reduction in TEA accumulation in both *in vitro* systems (Fig. 1C and D). Preincubation of tubule suspensions with 100 μM celiptium for 15 min or more reduced steady-state TEA accumulation by ~88%. When the concentration of celiptium was reduced to 10 μM, inhibition of TEA accumulation was observed only after preincubation for more than 60 min (Fig. 1C). In renal slices preincubation with celiptium for 120 min reduced TEA accumulation by ~50% (Fig. 1D). TEA accumulation was further reduced after a 240-min preincubation. Celiptium produced a greater inhibition of TEA accumulation in tubule suspensions than in renal slices, possibly due to the presence of multiple cell types in a slice which will not transport TEA compared to the homogeneous proximal cell population in the tubule suspensions. Celiptium-induced inhibition of TEA accumulation may have been the result of a toxic effect on the cell function or viability or a direct effect on the organic cation carrier. However, the fact that PAH accumulation was unaffected by celiptium (data not shown) suggests that inhibition of TEA accumulation represented a direct inhibition of transport.

The observations noted above represent common examples of toxicological studies of transport. Although the data suggest that the tested compounds inter-

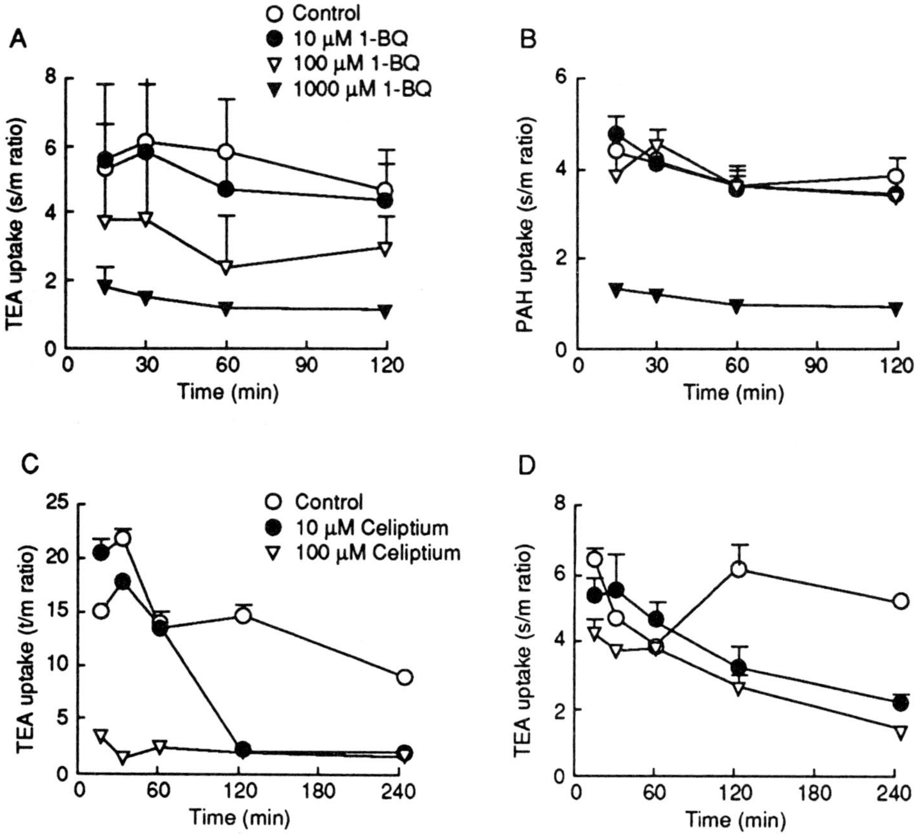

Figure 1 (A) Time-dependent effect of 1-benzylquinolinium (1-BQ) on [^{14}C]TEA accumulation in rabbit renal cortical slices. Each point represents the mean ± SEM of triplicate measurements from two experiments. (B) Time-dependent effect of 1-BQ on [^{14}C]PAH accumulation in rabbit renal cortical slices. Each point represents the mean ± SEM of triplicate measurements from two experiments. (C) Time-dependent effect of celiptium on [^{14}C]TEA accumulation in suspensions of rabbit renal proximal tubules. Each point represents the mean ± SEM of triplicate measurements from a representative experiment. (D) Time-dependent effect of celiptium on [^{14}C]TEA accumulation in rabbit renal slices. Each point represents the mean ± SEM of triplicate measurements from a representative experiment.

act with a specific transporter, neither the type of interaction (e.g., competitive or noncompetitive) nor evidence for transport of the agent in question is indicated. More detailed studies, such as those presented in subsequent paragraphs, are required to examine the transport characteristics of a particular chemical.

The uptake of TEA by tubule suspensions increased with time (Fig. 2A) and approached a steady-state level after 10 min (data not shown). Uptake through 60 sec was adequately described by a second-order polynomial, $U = a_0 + a_1 t + a_2 t^2$, where U is uptake at time t, and a_0, a_1, and a_2 are rate constants. The slope at time zero of this empirical relationship represents an estimate of the initial rate of TEA transport (15). Measurement of the initial rate of transport is a prerequisite to any subsequent effort to establish the kinetic characteristics of a transport phenomenon. Estimates of the rate of uptake at *time zero* suggested that 30-sec uptakes were within 3–5% of the initial rate of TEA transport. (Thus, 30-sec uptakes were used in subsequent kinetic experiments to estimate the initial unidirectional rate of TEA uptake into tubules.)

In the presence of 1 mM unlabeled TEA and TPeA, the uptake of $[^{14}C]$TEA was reduced by ~ 81% and ~ 95%, respectively. Since TPeA was such an effective inhibitor of TEA uptake, TPeA was added to the "stop" solution to prevent further loss of $[^{14}C]$TEA from tubules and decrease nonspecific binding. The efficacy of this procedure is evident in results presented below.

The kinetic characteristics of a transport system provide important information pertaining to the physiological role of the process. The kinetic parameters of transport J_{max} and K_t are defined, respectively, as the maximal capacity of a carrier for a substrate and the concentration of substrate at $1/2 J_{max}$ (16). The kinetic parameters of organic cation uptake were determined using the more traditional Michaelis–Menten plot of total TEA uptake in tubules (Fig. 2B, inset) and the isotope displacement procedure (the displacement of radioisotope by increasing concentrations of unlabeled substrate) (Fig. 2B) introduced by Malo and Berteloot (17). A Michaelis–Menten plot of the kinetics of TEA uptake resulted in a J_{max} and a K_t of 826 ± 47 pmol/30 sec/mg protein and 70 ± 8.3 μM, respectively. Using isotope displacement, the J_{max} and the K_t for TEA uptake for a representative experiment were 759 ± 108 pmol/30 sec/mg protein and 61 ± 8.9 μM, respectively. The isotope displacement procedure, like the Michaelis–Menten plot, can be used to determine the kinetics of transport of a radiolabeled substrate or to examine the kinetics of inhibition of substrate transport by different compounds. Either method also can be used to establish whether this inhibition is competitive or noncompetitive. For a more comprehensive overview and understanding of the kinetics of membrane transport, one can refer to any of a variety of works on the subject (16,18,19).

One fact that should be emphasized is that the ability of a compound to inhibit organic cation uptake is not synonymous with its transport by this system. To determine whether an inhibitor is actually a substrate for the organic cation tansporter, the effect of these *n*-tetraalkylammonium compounds on TEA efflux was examined (Fig. 2C). Both unlabeled TEA and TMA increased the efflux (i.e., transstimulated efflux) of $[^{14}C]$TEA from tubules, presumably as a consequence of an increase in turnover of the carrier, which is consistent with the hypothesis

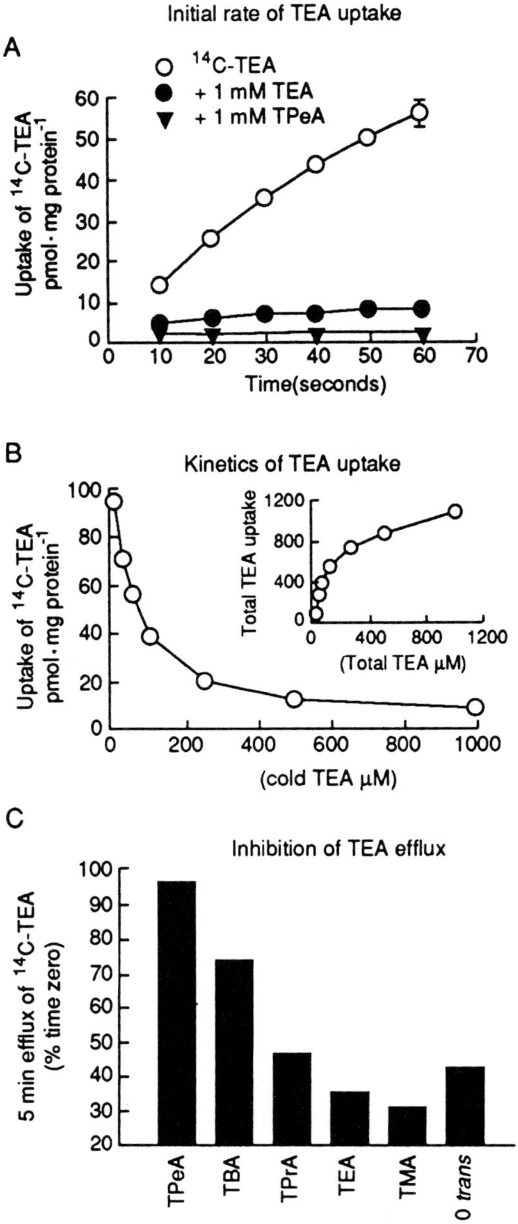

Figure 2 (A) Time-dependent uptake of [^{14}C]TEA in suspensions of rabbit renal proximal tubules in the presence and absence of unlabeled tetraethylammonium (TEA) and tetrapentylammonium (TPeA). Each point is the mean ± SEM of triplicate measurements from a representative experiment. (B) Kinetics of [^{14}C]TEA uptake in suspensions of rabbit renal proximal tubules. Initial rates for TEA uptake were estimated from 30-sec incubations. Kinetic parameters were determined using the isotope displacement method de-

that these agents are substrates for the organic cation transporter. Thus, this "transstimulation" strongly suggests that the transstimulating agent is itself a substrate for the carrier. In contrast, TPeA decreased the efflux of [^{14}C]TEA by 96%, which suggests that this compound binds to the organic cation transporter, but turnover of the carrier may occur slowly, if at all. The organic cations TBA and TPrA inhibited [^{14}C]TEA efflux by 74% and 46%, respectively, suggesting that carrier turnover in the presence of these agents is more rapid than with TPeA, but slower than that of an empty carrier or that in the presence of TEA or TMA. To summarize, the ability of a substrate to stimulate the efflux of a second substrate supports the contention that the two substrates share the same transporter, but failure to observe such a stimulation of efflux does not rule out the possibility of shared transport.

Cautionary Remarks

Renal cortical slices and isolated renal proximal tubule suspensions can easily be adapted to monitor organic ion uptake. However, several points should be considered when designing experiments for organic ion transport. A decrease in uptake and/or accumulation in the presence of a potential inhibitor does not always indicate a direct chemical or drug effect on the transporter, but may be an indirect or generalized response to toxicity. To differentiate an indirect toxic from a direct transport effect, similar experiments can be done with other transported substrates, such as glucose. Compounds that decrease only TEA or PAH uptake without any effect on glucose uptake are likely to be interacting only with the organic cation or anion transporters. On the other hand, a compound which affects glucose as well as TEA and PAH uptake is most likely producing a general toxic effect on the cell and its various metabolic processes, including transport. As shown for the inhibition of TEA and PAH accumulation by 1-BQ (Fig. 1A and B), reducing the dose of the test compound to nontoxic levels and/or the exposure time may help to clarify whether the changes observed are the result of toxicity or inhibition of uptake. Examination of the kinetics of organic ion transport in tubule suspensions using very acute exposures ($\leq$60 sec)

---

scribed in "Procedures." (Inset) A Michaelis–Menten plot of total TEA uptake. The lines were calculated using the kinetic parameters derived from the isotope displacement procedure. Each point is the mean ± SEM of triplicate measurements from a representative experiment. (C) Effect of long-chain *n*-tetraalkylammonium compounds on the efflux of [^{14}C]TEA from tubule suspensions. Each point is the mean ± SEM of triplicate measurements from a representative experiment. TBA, tetrabutylammonium; TPrA, tetrapropylammonium; TMA, tetramethylammonium; O trans, incubation buffer only.

provides a more definitive method to differentiate a direct interaction with a transporter from a toxic effect on cell function or viability.

A common error when interpreting transport data is the presumption that a compound which reduces TEA or PAH uptake is transported by the organic ion transport systems. Direct assessment of transport kinetics or inhibition of efflux (transstimulated efflux) experiments as described above can establish whether a chemical or a drug interacts directly with the transporter.

ACKNOWLEDGMENTS

We thank Dr. A. Jay Gandolfi and Dr. Stephen Wright for their helpful comments and suggestions. This work was supported by National Institutes Health award PO1 DK41006 and by National Science Foundation award DCB91-54416.

REFERENCES

1. P. S. Aronson, *in* "Annual Review of Physiology" (J. F. Hoffman and P. DeWeer, eds.), pp. 419–441. Annual Reviews, Palo Alto, California, 1989.
2. J. V. Moller and M. I. Sheikh, *Pharmacol. Rev.* **34**(4), 315 (1983).
3. B. M. Tune, M. B. Burg, and C. S. Patlak, *Am. J. Physiol.* **207,** 1057 (1969).
4. F. Roch-Ramel and I. M. Weiner, *Kidney Int.* **18,** 665 (1980).
5. B. Rennick, *Am. J. Physiol.* **240,** F83 (1981).
6. T. D. McKinney, *Am. J. Physiol.* **243,** F404 (1982).
7. D. Rodeheaver, M. Aleo, and R. Schnellmann, *In Vitro Cell Dev. Biol.* **26,** 898 (1990).
8. C. L. Krumdieck, J. E. dos Santos, and K. J. Ho, *Anal. Biochem.* **104,** 118 (1980).
9. A. J. Gandolfi and K. Brendel, *Toxicol. in Vitro* **4,** 337 (1990).
10. C. Ruegg, G. H. I. Wolfgang, A. J. Gandolfi and K. Brendel, *in* "In Vitro Toxicology: Model Systems and Methods" (C. A. McQueen, ed.), p. 201. Telford, New Jersey, 1989.
11. P. F. Smith, A. J. Gandolfi, C. L. Krumdieck, C. W. Putman, C. F. Zudoskli III, W. M. Davis, and K. Brendel, *Life Sci.* **36,** 1367 (1985).
12. P. Vinay, A. Gougoux, and G. Lemieux, *Am. J. Physiol.* **241,** F403 (1981).
13. K. Dickman and L. J. Mandel, *Am. J. Physiol.* **257,** C333 (1989).
14. C. E. Groves, E. A. Lock, and R. G. Schnellmann, *Toxicol. Appl. Pharmacol.* **107,** 54 (1991).
15. J. A. Jacquez, *in* "Physiology of Membrane Disorders" (T. E. Andreoli, J. F. Hoffman, and D. D. Fanestil, eds.), p. 147. Plenum, New York, 1978.
16. K. D. Neame and T. G. Richards, "Elementary Kinetics of Membrane Carrier Transport." Wiley, New York, 1972.
17. C. Malo and A. J. Berteloot, *J. Membr. Biol.* **122,** 127 (1991).
18. I. H. Segal, "Enzyme Kinetics: Behavior and Analysis of Rapid Equilibrium and Steady-State Enzyme Systems." Wiley, New York, 1975.
19. W. D. Stein, "Transport and Diffusion across Cell Membranes." Academic Press, Orlando, Florida, 1986.

11 Endoplasmic Reticulum Calcium Pump

Leon Moore

INTRODUCTION

Many toxicants significantly alter calcium in cells and tissues and alter intracellular Ca^{2+} homeostasis. When the cytosolic Ca^{2+} concentration is elevated to a supraphysiological level or for a prolonged period, activation of a variety of Ca^{2+}-dependent enzymes found at various locations within the cell can result in cellular necrosis. Ca^{2+}-responsive degradative enzymes activated in an uncontrolled manner may damage sites distant (e.g., the plasma membrane) from the original site within the cell at which the toxicant acts or the site at which the toxicant is activated. Potentially, a scheme of early redistribution of intracellular calcium, elevation of Ca^{2+} in cytosol, and overstimulation of Ca^{2+}-responsive enzymes may prove to be a mechanism for initiation of irreversible cellular injury common to a wide variety of toxic substances and target tissues.

Endoplasmic Reticulum Calcium Pump

The endoplasmic reticulum Ca^{2+} pump exhibits Ca^{2+} uptake catalyzed by a Ca^{2+} pump ATPase. The pump has an acyl-phosphoenzyme intermediate (M_r 116,000–118,000) (1) and is encoded as a family of structurally related enzymes, called the sarcoplasmic or endoplasmic reticulum Ca^{2+}-ATPases (2). Three separate genes encode this family of calcium pumps and these Ca^{2+}-ATPases have a distinct pattern of tissue-specific and developmentally regulated gene expression. A calcium pump activity in liver nuclear membranes is claimed to be identical to that found in the liver endoplasmic reticulum (3).

Toxicants and the Endoplasmic Reticulum Calcium Pump

The endoplasmic reticulum has a Ca^{2+} pump that uses Mg-ATP as the energy source for Ca^{2+} translocation (Fig. 1). This pump sequesters calcium from cytoplasm and stores it within the reticulum. Membrane preparations (microsomes) from cultured cells or from animal tissue are used to determine endoplasmic reticulum calcium pump activity. In rat liver or cultured hepatocytes, one of the earliest effects observed after halocarbon intoxication ($BrCCl_3$, CCl_4, $CHCl_3$,

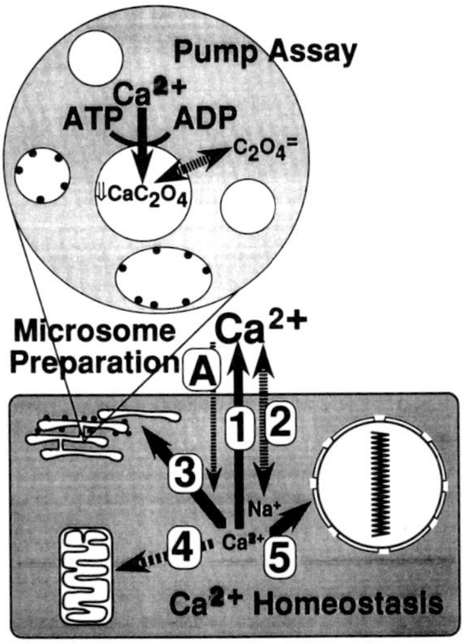

Figure 1 Ca^{2+} homeostasis and the endoplasmic reticulum calcium pump assay. Cellular Ca^{2+} homeostasis depends on a number of Ca^{2+} transport processes. Cytoplasmic Ca^{2+} is compartmentalized by Ca^{2+} pumps that depend on energy from ATP for the Ca^{2+} translocation process: (1) the plasma membrane Ca^{2+} pump, (3) the endoplasmic reticulum Ca^{2+} pump, and (5) an endoplasmic reticulum Ca^{2+} pump associated with the nuclear membrane. The endoplasmic reticulum Ca^{2+} pump not only regulates cytoplasmic Ca^{2+} levels; it also sequesters an intracellular store of calcium that can be released by physiological processes or by toxicants. A Na^{+}/Ca^{2+} exchanger (2) is able to move Ca^{2+} into or out of the cell. Ca^{2+} will move out of the cell via this mechanism when Na^{+} moves into the cell, down its concentration gradient. Passive Ca^{2+} entry (A) moves Ca^{2+} into the cell. The plasma membrane normally is very Ca^{2+} impermeable. The mitochondrial antiport (4) depends on electron flow as the energy source for Ca^{2+} translocation, but can utilize ATP as the energy source for Ca^{2+} accumulation. During homogenization and isolation of microsomes, the endoplasmic reticulum is ruptured and reseals as inverted (inside-out) vesicles. Transport activity of the endoplasmic reticulum calcium pump may be determined with an *in vitro* assay and the microsome preparation. Mg-ATP powers the transport process and is hydrolyzed to ADP. Oxalate salts ($C_2O_4^{=}$) are used to trap (by precipitation) Ca^{2+} transported into the microsomal vesicle. Trapping transported Ca^{2+} allows determination of the rate of the Ca^{2+} transport process uncomplicated by a passive diffusion of Ca^{2+} out of the vesicle.

1,1-dichloroethylene, and halothane) is inhibition of an ATP-dependent Ca^{2+} pump in the endoplasmic reticulum (4–8). Within 30 min after exposure to CCl_4, morphology of the endoplasmic reticulum changes as the cisternae become dilated, polyribosomes disaggregate, protein synthesis is inhibited, and some microsomal enzyme activities (endoplasmic reticulum Ca^{2+} pump and mixed function oxidase activities) are depressed (9). Inhibition of the pump depends on metabolism of the halocarbon to a reactive intermediate. Correlative studies have demonstrated that inhibition of the endoplasmic reticulum pump is related to hepatotoxicity temporally, by modulation of metabolism to reactive intermediates, and by potency of related halocarbons (5,10). Many hepatotoxicants that inhibit the endoplasmic reticulum pump are halocarbons, but there are at least two nonhalocarbons that also do so [carbon disulfide (7) and diquat (11)]. In contrast, hepatotoxic doses of acetaminophen, bromobenzene, or CCl_4 (in addition to its effect on the endoplasmic reticulum calcium pump) inhibit another liver calcium pump, the plasma membrane Ca^{2+} pump (12). While acetaminophen, diquat, and CCl_4 each produce liver injury by different chemical mechanisms (covalent binding and thiol depletion, oxidant stress, covalent binding, and lipid peroxidation), they share the ability to inhibit calcium pumps, and a rise in intracellular Ca^{2+} accompanies the hepatotoxic effect of each of these compounds.

MATERIALS AND REAGENTS

Reagent	Stock concentration	Final concentration
KCl	1 *M*	100 m*M*
Imidazole–histidine buffer (pH 6.8)	300 m*M*	30 m*M*
Ammonium oxalate	50 m*M*	5 m*M*
Sodium azide	50 m*M*	5 m*M*
$MgCl_2$	50 m*M*	5 m*M*
ATP (pH adjusted with 1 *M* imidazole)	50 m*M*	5 m*M*
$CaCl_2$	200 μ*M*	20 μ*M*
$^{45}CaCl_2$	0.1 μCi/ml	0.01 μCi/ml

All chemicals may be obtained from the usual suppliers of laboratory-grade reagents and are prepared at least once a month. The imidazole–histidine buffer is prepared by titration of a histidine solution (300 m*M*) with imidazole (300 m*M*) to pH 6.8. All reagents, with the exception of ATP, are stored at 4°C in polypropylene containers. ATP is prepared by titration of a solution of ATP (commonly the disodium salt) with imidazole (1 *M*) to pH 6.8. The final volume is adjusted to achieve an ATP concentration of 50 m*M*. The ATP solution is stored frozen (−20°C) in polystyrene tubes and thawed immediately (within 30 min) before beginning the endoplasmic reticulum calcium pump assay. The pH of the final mixture should be 6.8. Nitrocellulose membrane filters (0.45 μm), filter rinsing solution (250 m*M* sucrose), a vacuum-filtration manifold, a shaking water bath, and a liquid scintillation spectrophotometer are needed for the assay.

PROCEDURES

Microsome Preparation

Microsome preparations should be prepared in either salt [KCl (13)] or sucrose solutions (4). Tissue samples may be homogenized in isotonic solutions (150 m*M* KCl or 250 m*M* sucrose). Cultured cells often require a hypertonic solution (500 m*M* sucrose) for adequate homogenization. Typically, liver microsomes are isolated as follows: liver samples (1 g) are homogenized with six strokes of a motor-driven (1000 rpm) Teflon pestle in 10 vol of 250 m*M* sucrose with a Potter–Elvehjem homogenizer (Teflon–glass). Homogenization and all centrifugation steps are done at 0–4°C. The homogenate is filtered through a doubled layer of cheesecloth and centrifuged at 12,500 *g* for 20 min. Microsomal vesicles from this supernatant are sedimented at 105,000 *g* for 60 min. Microsome pellets are resuspended with a Potter–Elvehjem homogenizer in a sufficient volume of a solution containing 125 m*M* sucrose and 75 m*M* KCl to yield a protein concentration of 0.75–2 mg/ml. This solution may be rapidly frozen for storage (see "comments") or assayed within 30 min. Before the calcium pump assay and protein determination, the microsome suspension is diluted another 1:10 into a solution containing 125 m*M* sucrose and 75 m*M* KCl (to a protein concentration of 0.075–0.2 mg/ml).

Endoplasmic Reticulum Calcium Pump Assay

The eight assay medium components and water are combined in equal volumes (100 μl of each, or a total of 900 μl for a single time point) as an assay cocktail. Nine volumes (900 μl for a single time point or multiples of this volume for a time course) of the assay mixture are dispensed into polystyrene tubes (17 × 100 mm) and the mixture is brought to 37°C in a shaking water bath (60 oscillations per minute). One volume (100 μl for a single time point or multiples of this volume for a time course of transport) of the microsome preparation (0.075–0.2 mg protein/ml in a solution containing 125 m*M* sucrose and 75 m*M* KCl) is added to each tube to initiate the calcium pump assay. The final concentration of microsome protein in the calcium pump assay should range from 7.5 to 20 μg/ml. Assay tubes are kept shaking in the water bath at 37°C for the duration of the assay.

After an appropriate interval (usually 10–30 min) a 500-μl sample is removed for rapid filtration through a 0.45-μm nitrocellulose filter on vacuum-filtration manifold. Most vacuum-filtration manifolds accommodate multiple nitrocellulose filers, commonly 12 filters. It is not difficult to use these 12 manifold positions to process 12 samples at each time point. At times an investigator will need to do a time course of transport assay (e.g., to demonstrate linearity of the transport process). On most vacuum-filtration manifolds it is not difficult to process a set of 12 filters every 10 min during the analysis of a transport assay time course. Following filtration of all samples at a given time point, but before the nitrocellulose filters are removed from the manifold, each filter is washed with 2 ml of the filter rinsing solution (0.25 *M* sucrose) to remove assay medium (and ^{45}Ca) trapped on and in the nitrocellulose filter. The filters are removed from the vacuum-filtration manifold and placed in a liquid scintillation cocktail for counting. After all assay samples have been collected, duplicate 100-μl samples of the assay mixture containing microsomes are removed from any of the assay tubes and applied to two unused nitrocellulose filters for use as standards to determine $^{45}Ca^{2+}$-specific activity. These duplicate standard filters each contain a known amount of calcium (2 nmol) and ^{45}Ca ($\sim$1 nCi). They are used to calculate specific activity of the $^{45}Ca^{2+}$ in the endoplasmic reticulum calcium pump assay mixture on a daily basis ($^{45}Ca^{2+}$ half-life is 163 days). These standards are also prepared for liquid scintillation spectrophotometry. The nitrocellulose filters containing the radioactive samples are quantified in a liquid scintillation spectrophotometer as if they contained ^{14}C.

Calculation of Endoplasmic Calcium Pump Activity

To determine calcium pump activity, one must know the calcium and protein concentrations in the assay medium, the amount of ^{45}Ca precipitated as calcium oxalate in microsome vesicles trapped on the nitrocellulose filters, and a measure of the specific activity of $^{45}Ca^{2+}$ in the assay medium. Calcium pump activity is usually reported as the number of nanomoles of Ca^{2+} transported per milligram of microsome protein per minute at 37°C.

The calcium concentration of the assay medium is fixed at 20 μM. The protein concentration in the assay mixture is determined by measuring the protein concentration of the microsome suspension used to initiate the calcium pump assay (mg/ml). This solution is diluted 10-fold when it is pipetted into the calcium pump assay medium to begin the assay. Quantification of ^{45}Ca on the assay filters provides the amount of ^{45}Ca precipitated as calcium oxalate in the microsome vesicles (cpm). Quantification of ^{45}Ca on the standard filters provides a measure of the specific activity (MSA) of $^{45}Ca^{2+}$ on the day the assay is performed. These standard filters contain 2 nmol of $CaCl_2$ (100 μl of 20 μM $CaCl_2$). Calcium pump activity is calculated as:

$$\text{nmol Ca}^{2+}\text{/mg microsome protein/min} = \frac{(\text{cpm})(\text{MSA})}{(k)(\text{mg/ml})(\text{min})}$$

where cpm represents counts per minute of ^{45}Ca on each assay filters, MSA is 2 nmol of $CaCl_2$/cpm ^{45}Ca on the standard filters, k = 0.05 (a constant to account for the 1:10 dilution of the microsome suspension in the assay medium and sampling 500 μl of the assay medium for liquid scintillation spectrophotometry). If either of these factors is changed, the constant must be appropriately altered. Here mg/ml represents the protein concentration of the microsome suspension added to the calcium pump assay medium (10-fold the concentration in the assay), and min indicates the length of the assay.

COMMENTS

Homogenization of cells or tissue must be as gentle as possible. In general, a Dounce homogenizer (glass–glass) is adequate for cultured cells and a Potter–Elvehjem homogenizer (Teflon–glass) is appropriate for brain, liver, kidney, and most smooth muscle tissues. Care must be taken to rapidly cool tissue samples or cells and to keep all solutions as close to 4°C as possible during the entire isolation procedure. Endoplasmic reticulum calcium pump activity is very sensitive to temperature, until the microsomes are in the assay medium. Ideally, the microsome preparations are assayed for endoplasmic reticulum calcium pump activity immediately after preparation. If the resuspended microsomes are to be frozen, resuspend the microsomes in a sucrose (125 m*M*)–KCl (75 m*M*) solution to preserve endoplasmic reticulum calcium pump activity. The resuspended microsomes should then be quickly frozen (in a liquid nitrogen or dry ice/ethanol bath) in small ($\leq$0.5-ml) aliquots usually in 12 × 75-mm glass tubes. Frozen microsomes are stored at −70°C. The frozen samples should be rapidly thawed immediately before beginning the endoplasmic reticulum calcium pump assay ($\leq$5 min). When microsomes are prepared, frozen, and stored in this manner, approximately one-half of the liver endoplasmic reticulum calcium pump activity is lost during 90 days of storage.

Mg-ATP powers the transport process and is hydrolyzed to ADP by the calcium pump enzyme. Oxalate salts are used to trap (by precipitation) Ca^{2+} transported into the microsomal vesicle. Sodium azide inhibits the mitochondrial calcium antiporter. It is included in the assay mixture to prevent sequestration of calcium by any contaminating mitrochondria or mitochondrial vesicles.

Determination of endoplasmic reticulum calcium pump activity can provide an early measure of toxicant-induced damage to the endoplasmic reticulum (14). Studies of the calcium pump have also proven useful to study possible mechanisms of toxicant action (4–8,11–13). Althgough the procedure is presented as an endoplasmic reticulum calcium pump assay, with suitable modifications it is used for other subcellular fractions, including the plasma membrane (12,15,16) and nuclei (17,18). In addition, it may be used to determine endoplasmic reticulum calcium pump activity in crude membranes isolated from whole-cell homogenates isolated from cultured cells or animal tissue (13,14,19).

ACKNOWLEDGMENT

Work in this laboratory was supported by U.S. Public Health Service grant ES03437. The opinions or assertions contained herein are the private ones of the author and are not to be construed as official or reflecting the views of the Department of Defense or The Uniformed Services University of the Health Sciences. Experiments were conducted according to the principles set forth in the *Guide for Care and Use of Laboratory Animals,* Institute of Animal Resources, National Research Council, DHHS Publication No. (NIH) 78–23.

REFERENCES

1. C. Heilmann C. Spamer, and W. Geork, *Cell Calcium* **10,** 275 (1989).
2. J. Lytton, M. Westlin, S. E. Burk, *et al., J. Biol. Chem.* **267,** 14483 (1992).
3. L. Lanini, O. Bachs, and E. Carafoli, *J. Biol. Chem.* **267,** 11548 (1992).
4. L. Moore, T. Chen, H. R. Knapp, Jr., *et al., J. Biol. Chem.* **250,** 4562 (1975).
5. L. Moore, *Biochem. Pharmacol.* **29,** 2505 (1980).
6. K. P. Lowrey, E. A. Glende, Jr., and R. O. Rechnagel, *Biochem. Pharmacol.* **30,** 135 (1981).
7. L. Moore, *Biochem Pharmacol* **31,** 1465–1467 (1982).
8. G. C. Farrell, J. Mahoney, M. Bilous, *et al., J. Pharmacol. Exp. Ther.* **247,** 751 (1988).
9. R. O. Recknagel, *Pharmacol. Rev.* **19,** 145 (1967).
10. R. M. Long and L. Moore, *Biochem. Pharmacol.* **35,** 4131 (1986).
11. J. O. Tsokos-Kuhn, C. V. Smith, H. Hughes, *et al., Mol. Pharmacol.* **34,** 209 (1988).
12. J. O. Tsokos-Kuhn, E. L. Todd, J. B. McMillin-Wood, *et al., Mol. Pharmacol.* **28,** 56 (1985).
13. L. M. De Witt, T. W. Jones, and L. Moore, *Toxicol. Appl. Pharmacol.* **92,** 157 (1988).
14. R. M. Long and L. Moore, *Toxicol. Appl. Pharmacol.* **92,** 295 (1988).
15. L. Moore, D. F. Fitzpatrick, T. S. Chen, *et al., Biochim Biophys. Acta* **245,** 405 (1974).
16. F. A. X. Schanne and L. Moore, *J. Biol. Chem,* **261,** 9886 (1986).
17. P. Nicotera, D. J. McConkey, D. P. Jones, *et al., Proc. Natl. Acad Sci U.S.A.* **86,** 453 (1989).
18. P. Nicotera, S. Orrenius, T. Nilsson, *et al., Proc. Natl Acad Sci. U.S.A.* **87,** 6858 (1990).
19. L. Moore and I. Pastan, *Ann. N.Y. Acad. Sci.* **307,** 177 (1978).

12 Measurement of Oxygen Consumption

Rick G. Schnellmann

Measurements of cellular oxygen consumption and oxygen consumption of subcellular organelles have been used extensively to study cell metabolism. With increased emphasis on determination of the mechanisms of toxicity of drugs, environmental pollutants, and industrial chemicals, and the observation that mitochondrial dysfunction plays a critical role in the cell death produced by a variety of toxicants, the use of cellular oxygen consumption measurements is increasing in the field of toxicology. Numerous toxicants have been shown to produce mitochondrial dysfunction in a number of cell types. For example, the nephrotoxicants mercuric chloride, ochratoxin A, and the haloalkane and haloalkene cysteine conjugates, tetrafluoroethyl-L-cysteine and pentachlorobutadienyl-L-cysteine, produce mitochondrial dysfunction, which plays a critical role in the subsequent renal proximal tubule cell death (for a review see Ref. 1). Furthermore, different toxicants produce different types of mitochondrial dysfunction. For example, pentachlorobutadienyl-L-cysteine initially uncouples oxidative phosphorylation in renal proximal tubules by dissipating the proton gradient (2–5). Subsequently, there is an overall collapse of mitochondrial function. In contrast, the related compound tetrafluoroethyl-L-cysteine does not uncouple oxidative phosphorylation, but rather inhibits state 3 respiration by inhibiting sites I and II of the electron transport chain (5,6). Of particular interest is that the mitochondrial dysfunction produced by these compounds is extensive and occurs significantly before the onset of cell death.

It is difficult to develop cause-and-effect relationships between mitochondrial changes and subsequent cell death and organ failure following an *in vivo* exposure. The reason for this difficulty relates to the fact that the population of cells or mitochondria isolated from a treated animal is unknown. That is, cells (or multiple cell types) will be taken or mitochondria isolated from both affected and nonaffected areas. Furthermore, cellular and mitochondrial changes may have occurred during the isolation process. Treated cells or mitochondria may be more sensitive to the isolation techniques and thereby be further compromised or lost in the isolation process. In either case the investigator should be aware that false-negatives and false-positives are distinct possibilities. If an *in vivo* study is conducted, cells or mitochondria should be isolated prior to the

METHODS IN TOXICOLOGY, Volume 1B

onset of necrosis, since it is extremely difficult to draw conclusions once cell death has begun.

The most direct method to determine whether a given toxicant produces mitochondrial dysfunction and whether this mitochondrial dysfunction plays a role in cell death is through the use of an appropriate *in vitro* cellular model. Several important facts concerning the toxicant should be considered when planning these experiments. First, is the parent compound or a metabolite responsible for the toxicity? In addition, what is the relative concentration of the parent compound or metabolite in the target cell or organ following a toxic *in vivo* exposure? This information will greatly help the investigator by focusing the *in vitro* studies on the actual compound responsible for the cellular toxicity and the potential mitochondrial toxicity. Second, *in vivo* pathology studies should identify the cell type that is affected and this cell type should be used for the cellular studies.

The measurement of cellular oxygen consumption is one of the best ways to assess mitochondrial function. This method allows for direct and continual monitoring of mitochondrial function over time. Other chapters in this book discuss the use and measurement of adenine nucleotide levels, mitochondrial charge, and glycolysis in the determination of energy metabolism (7–9). Measurement of oxygen consumption is fast, relatively easy, and can be done using a variety of tissue models. For example, it is routinely used to measure the function of submitochondrial particles, mitochondria, isolated cells, and proximal tubules, and can be used with renal and hepatic slices.

It is important to note problems that may arise during the measurement of oxygen consumption in tissue slices. First, tissue slices thicker than 300 μm have been shown to be hypoxic in their centers and thus have limited oxygen and metabolic substrate diffusion (10,11). Limited information is available concerning the state of oxygen and metabolic substrate diffusion in 250- to 300-μm slices. However, slices of this size incubated in dynamic organ culture systems do maintain ATP and potassium contents (12). Second, slices contain numerous cell types. If a toxicant has an effect on one cell type, and depending on the number of these cells in the slice, it may be difficult to detect changes in oxygen consumption. Irrespective of the model used, it is important to measure oxygen consumption prior to the onset of cell death (cell lysis), since it is difficult to determine cause-and-effect relationships when cell death has started.

Mitochondrial function (thus, oxygen consumption) is dependent on the availability of oxygen and metabolic substrates. Consequently, it is imperative that the appropriate type and amount of metabolic substrates and oxygen are included in the incubation medium. This raises two interesting points concerning cultured cells. First, cultured cells maintained under standard culture conditions are in a state of hypoxia (13) and derive a large part of their metabolic energy from glycolysis (14–17). Thus, mitochondrial function may be diminished in cultured cells, and glycolysis may maintain cellular functions in the case of a mitochondrial deficit. Second, many of the media available from commercial vendors are designed to support the growth and function of cultured cells deriving their energy from glycolysis. Consequently, many of the media do not contain the required types and amounts of metabolic substrates required to support mitochondrial function.

Many of the techniques and conditions described below were developed originally to study cell metabolism and ion transport in renal proximal tubules (10,11,18) and have been modified to study the mechanism of toxicity of a number of nephrotoxicants (2,19–23).

EQUIPMENT

YSI Model 5300 biological monitor and YSI Model 5331 standard oxygen probe (Fisher, Pittsburgh, PA.)
Water-jacketed cell (1.5 ml;) Model 01271002, Gilson, Middleton, WI)
Lauda heating circulator (Model MS-3, Fisher)
Lab-Line magnetic stirrer (Model 1250, VWR, West Chester, PA)
Soltec flat-bed recorder (Model 1242, Soltec, Sun Valley, Fernando, CA)
Stir bars (2×7 mm; VWR)
Polyethylene tubing (PE-20 and PE-50, Clay Adams, Division of Becton Dickinson, Parsippany, NJ)
Fixed-needle beveled Hamilton syringes [10 μl (Model 701N) and 25 μl (Model 702N); VWR]
Latex tubing

The above items are routinely used in our laboratory and have withstood the test of time. However, numerous other companies make products that could easily be substituted. Instech Laboratories (Horsham, PA) has a small-volume (0.6-ml) oxygen measurement system that includes a water-jacketed chamber with a magnetic stirrer, oxygen electrode amplifier, and oxygen probe. One advantage of this system is the small oxygen probe and chamber. We have used this probe, which will also work with the YSI biological monitor, in a custom-designed glass water-jacketed chamber with a volume of 0.4 ml. The disadvantages of this small probe are stability and the routine coating of the probe tip.

The general setup of the equipment is illustrated in Fig. 1. The heating circulator should be started and the chamber allowed to reach the desired temperature (usually 37°C). Place a new membrane on the oxygen probe each day. Hold the oxygen probe vertically and place 1 drop of the KCl solution that comes with the membranes on the tip of the oxygen probe (see oxygen probe

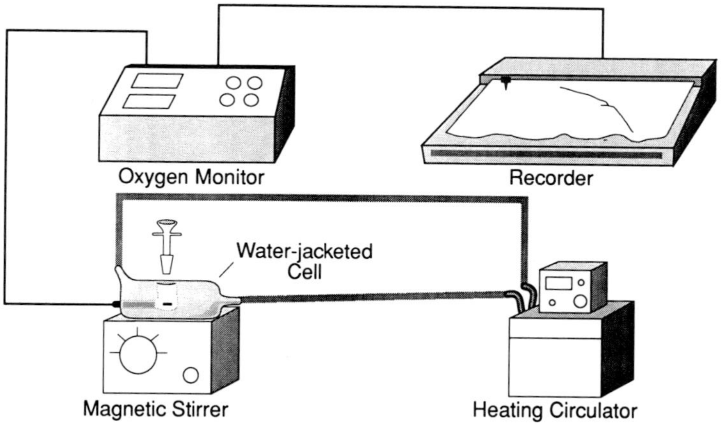

Figure 1 A schematic of the oxygen consumption apparatus.

instructions). Gently place a 1- to 1.5-cm^2 piece of membrane on the drop of half-saturated KCl solution. Spread the O-ring with the "golf tee" supplied with the membranes and in one motion set the tee on the oxygen probe and push the O-ring onto the oxygen probe. Make sure that there are no air bubbles between the membrane and the oxygen probe and trim away excess membrane around the O-ring. Lightly wet the slot in which the oxygen probe is placed into the chamber with water to facilitate oxygen probe entry without disturbing the membrane. Rinse the chamber several times with 150 m*M* NaCl (Fisher Scientific, Fairlawn, NJ). Leave 150 m*M* NaCl in the uncapped chamber following the last rinse. Once the membrane has been wetted, do not allow it to dry out. Turn on the biological monitor and the magnetic stirrer and allow them to equilibrate for 10–15 min. Adjust the speed of the stirrer such that there is good mixing without the formation of a vortex. With the biological monitor set on the O_2 setting, the percent O_2 reading should be ~21%. If the reading is significantly different from 21%, check or replace the membrane and rinse or wash the chamber. After the 21% reading has stabilized, add a few grains of sodium dithionite (Baker, Phillipsburg, NJ) to the chamber to remove the O_2. The reading on the biological monitor should go to zero within a few minutes. If it does not go to zero, you may add a few additional grains of sodium dithionite. The most common reason that the instrument will not "zero" is a bad membrane or a dirty oxygen probe. Clean the oxygen probe with a cotton-tipped swab dipped in 3% NH_4OH (see oxygen probe instructions). Zero the chart recorder while the biological monitor is reading zero. Rinse the chamber five or six times with 150 m*M* NaCl, leaving 150 m*M* NaCl in the chamber following the last rinse. Tune the biological monitor to the air setting and the reading should be ~ 100%. Allow the chamber to equilibrate for 20–30 min. Set the biological monitor to 100% and then the chart recorder to 100% full scale. Tune the biological monitor to the O_2 setting. The equipment is now ready for oxygen consumption experiments.

CHEMICALS

Digitonin and nystatin (Calbiochem, San Diego, CA)
Carbonyl cyanide *p*-trifluoromethoxyphenylhydrazone (FCCP), butyrate, heptanoate, and valerate (Aldrich, Milwaukee, WI)
Adenosine diphosphate, alanine, ascorbic acid, EGTA, glucose, glutamate, HEPES, lactate, malate, ouabain, rotenone, succinate, *N,N,N′,N′*-tetramethyl-*p*-phenylenediamine (TMPD), and various salts (Sigma, St. Louis, MO)

BUFFERS

Incubation buffer: 115 m*M* NaCl, 5 m*M* KCl, 25 m*M* $NaHCO_3$, 2 m*M* $NaHPO_4$, 1 m*M* $MgSO_2$, 1 m*M* $CaCl_2$, 1 m*M* alanine, 5 m*M* glucose, 4 m*M* lactate, 5 m*M* malate, and 2 m*M* butyrate (osmolality 296 mOsml, pH 7.4)
Intracellular buffer: (120 m*M*) KCl, 5 m*M* KH_2PO_4, 1 m*M* $MgSO_4$, 5 m*M* glutamate, 5 m*M* malate, 1 m*M* valerate, 10 m*M* HEPES, and 2 m*M* EGTA (pH 7.4)

The above buffers have been used extensively in measuring the oxygen consumption of renal proximal tubules. The type and amount of metabolic substrates may need to be altered for other cell types. The 5 m*M* glutamate and 5 m*M* malate (mitochondrial site I substrates) in the intracellular buffer may be replaced with 10 m*M* succinate and 0.1 μM rotenone to examine site II of the electron transport chain.

SOLUTIONS

40 mg/ml nystatin in dimethyl sulfoxide (make fresh daily)
10 m*M* ouabain in deionized water (store in small aliquots at 4°C for up to 1 month; use a fresh aliquot each day)
10 mg/ml digitonin in dimethyl sulfoxide (make fresh daily)
40 m*M* ADP in deionized water (store in small aliquots at −20°C for up to 1 month; use a fresh aliquot each day)

0.25 *M* ascorbate/0.25 *M* TMPD (pH 7.4) (store at −20°C)
300 μ*M* FCCP in ethanol (store in small aliquots at -20°C for up to 1 month, use a fresh aliquot each day)
30 μ*M* rotenone in dimethyl sulfoxide (make fresh daily)
30 μ*M* antimycin A in dimethyl sulfoxide (make fresh daily)

MEASUREMENT OF OXYGEN CONSUMPTION

Calibrate the oxygen consumption apparatus prior to the initiation of the experiment. Bring the cellular model to temperature (usually 37°C) in a gyratory shaker bath under an atmosphere of 95% air/5% CO_2 or 95% O_2/5% CO_2 for 15–30 min prior to the measurement of oxygen consumption or addition of the toxicant. At the appropriate times rinse the oxygen consumption chamber with incubation buffer, add an aliquot of the cellular model to the chamber, cap the chamber with the stopper, ensuring that there are no air bubbles in the chamber, and start the chart recorder. For optimal sensitivity adjust the chart recorder speed to achieve a slope between 30° and 45° for basal oxygen consumption. Record basal oxygen consumption until a linear response greater than 2 cm is obtained. Add nystatin (0.16 mg/ml final concentration) to determine nystatin-stimulated oxygen consumption (see Fig. 2 for a representative tracing) and record until a linear response greater than 2 cm is obtained. Make all additions to the chamber without removing the cap, using a Hamilton syringe with a piece of polyethylene tubing attached. Add the Na^+,K^+-ATPase inhibitor ouabain (0.1 m*M* final concentration) to determine the oxygen consumption not associ-

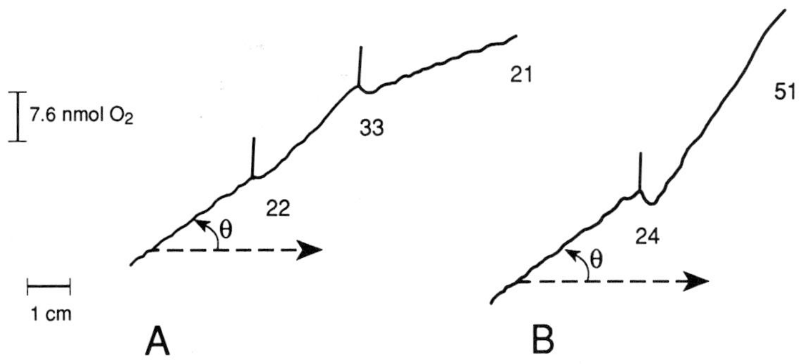

Figure 2 A representative oxygen consumption tracing obtained from rabbit renal proximal tubules. θ is the angle used to calculate the rate of oxygen consumption. The chart speed was 2 cm/min. Numbers represent the rate of oxygen consumption in nmol O_2/mg protein/min. (A) The first event marker indicates the addition of nystatin; the second indicates the addition of ouabain. (B) The event marker indicates the addition of FCCP.

ated with Na^+,K^+-ATPase activity and record until a linear response greater than 2 cm is obtined. Ouabain-sensitive oxygen consumption can be determined by substracting the ouabain-insensitive oxygen consumption rate from the basal oxygen consumption rate. Alternatively, add the uncoupler of oxidative phosphorylation, FCCP (1 μM final concentration), after measuring basal oxygen consumption to determine the uncoupled rate of oxygen consumption. The rate of oxygen consumption can be determined from the output of the chart recorder, using the following equation:

$$\frac{\text{tangent } \theta \times 38 \text{ nmol } O_2/\text{ml/cm} \times \text{chart speed (cm/min)}}{\text{cellular protein (mg/ml)}} = \text{nmol } O_2/\text{mg cellular protein/min}$$

where θ is the angle between the horizontal lines on the chart recorder paper and the linear portion of the oxygen consumption tracing (see Fig. 2). The constant, 38 nmol O_2/ml/cm, is based on the solubility of O_2 in physiological saline at 37°C (24) and a chart recorder calibrated from 0% to 100% over the width of 25 cm chart paper. By adjusting the range of the recorder, it is possible to expand the 0–20% range for clarity and accuracy. Altering the range of the recorder by a factor of 5 necessitates the changing of the constant 38 nmol O_2/ml/cm to 7.6 nmol O_2/ml/cm. Cellular oxygen consumption is commonly normalized to cellular protein (mg/ml) but may also be normalized to cell number or cellular DNA. We routinely measure renal proximal tubule oxygen consumption at a tubule concentration of 1–5 mg of tubular protein/ml. Depending on the cell type used and the concentration of the cells, the concentration of nystatin and ouabain may need to be adjusted. For example, renal proximal tubule cells from the rat are very insensitive to ouabain (25).

We have used nystatin-stimulated oxygen consumption as a stress test to uncover early mitochondrial dysfunction. Briefly, the pore-forming polyene antibiotic nystatin increases sodium influx (Fig. 3). The increase in intracellular sodium stimulates the Na^+,K^+-ATPase and results in the consumption of ATP and an increase in ADP. The increase in ADP produces maximal mitochondrial ATP formation. Under normal conditions the rate-limiting step in this process is

Figure 3 A schematic of the relationships between mitochondrial ATP production and Na^+,K^+-ATPase activity. (Upper right) The influx of sodium following the addition of nystatin, the activation of Na^+,K^+-ATPase, and the stimulation of mitochondrial ATP formation by ADP. (Lower left) The inhibition of Na^+,K^+-ATPase following the addition of ouabain and the consumption of mitochondrial ATP by other processes in the cell. (Lower right) The three points that may result in a decrease in nystatin-stimulated oxygen consumption: mitochondrial dysfunction, loss of adenine nucleotides, and direct inhibition of the Na^+,K^+-ATPase.

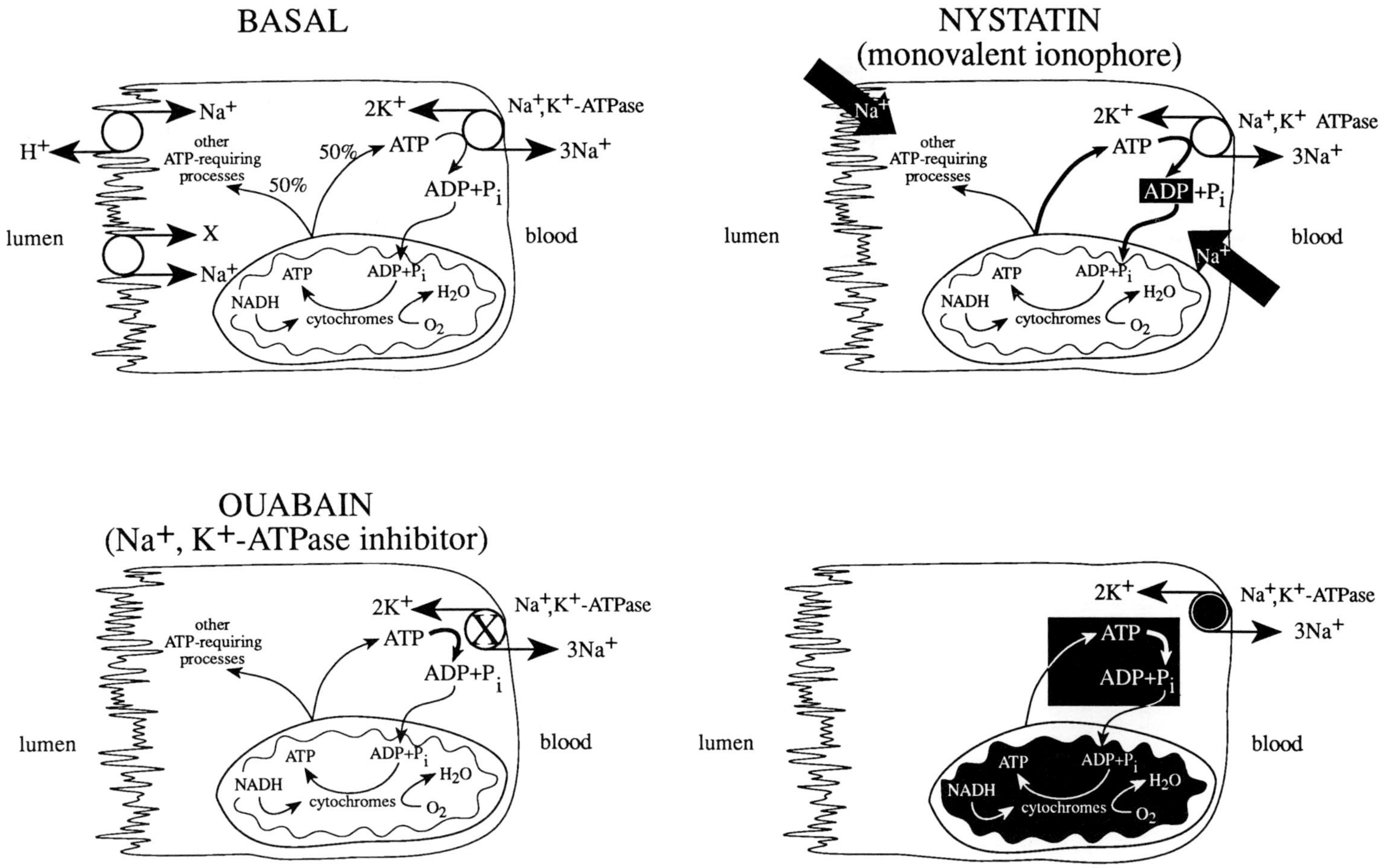
BASAL
H^+
Na^+
other ATP-requiring processes
50%
50%
$2K^+$
ATP
Na^+,K^+-ATPase
$3Na^+$
$ADP+P_i$
lumen
X
Na^+
blood
ATP
$ADP+P_i$
NADH
H_2O
cytochromes
O_2
NYSTATIN
(monovalent ionophore)
Na^+
other ATP-requiring processes
$2K^+$
ATP
Na^+,K^+ ATPase
$3Na^+$
ADP $+P_i$
lumen
blood
Na^+
ATP
$ADP+P_i$
NADH
H_2O
cytochromes
O_2
OUABAIN
(Na^+, K^+-ATPase inhibitor)
other ATP-requiring processes
$2K^+$
ATP
Na^+,K^+-ATPase
$3Na^+$
$ADP+P_i$
lumen
blood
ATP
$ADP+P_i$
NADH
H_2O
cytochromes
O_2
$2K^+$
Na^+,K^+-ATPase
ATP
$3Na^+$
$ADP+P_i$
lumen
blood
ATP
$ADP+P_i$
NADH
H_2O
cytochromes
O_2

the mitochondrial ATP formation (18). Since renal cells use only 50–60% of their mitochondrial capacity (18), significant mitochondrial dysfunction may occur prior to a decrease in basal oxygen consumption. Thus, the measurement of nystatin-stimulated oxygen consumption may uncover an early mitochondrial deficit prior to its appearance as a decrease in basal oxygen consumption. However, a decrease in nystatin-stimulated oxygen consumption does not necessarily indicate mitochondrial dysfunction. A decrease in nystatin-stimulated oxygen consumption may result also from the loss of adenine nucleotides (particularly ADP) or direct inhibition of the Na^+,K^+-ATPase (Fig. 3). Consequently, direct probing of mitochondrial function is required to confirm mitochondrial dysfunction (see below).

Using ouabain, it is possible to divide oxygen consumption into two components. The oxygen consumption that is ouabain sensitive is that which is associated with Na^+,K^+-ATPase activity and sodium transport. For example, if a toxicant increases sodium influx into the cell, then the rate of ouabain-sensitive oxygen consumption would increase. The oxygen consumption that is insensitive to ouabain is associated with the other oxygen-consuming reactions within the cell and has not been well characterized. However, if a toxicant uncouples oxidative phosphorylation, ouabain-insensitive oxygen consumption would increase.

DIRECT MEASUREMENT OF MITOCHONDRIAL FUNCTION IN CELLS

The direct measurement of mitochondrial function in cells complements studies using isolated mitochondria and decreases the potential of false-negatives and false-positives that may occur with isolated organelles. Following exposure to a given toxicant, pellet the cells by low-speed centrifugation and resuspend them in intracellular buffer (5 mg of cellular protein/ml). Place an aliquot of the cell suspension in the oxygen consumption chamber, cap the chamber, and start the chart recorder. Add digitonin (0.33 m*M* final concentration) to permeabilize the plasma membrane to ADP and other mitochondrial probes (Fig. 4). Digitonin can selectively permeabilize the plasma membrane without affecting mitochon-

Figure 4 A schematic of the probes used to determine mitochondrial dysfunction directly in the cell. Cells are suspended in intracellular buffer (high K^+) in the presence of digitonin to permeabilize the plasma membrane. (Upper left) The use of the site I substrates pyruvate/malate. (Upper right) The use of the site II substrate succinate and the site I inhibitor rotenone. (Lower left) The direct stimulation of cytochrome-*c*-cytochrome oxidase by ascorbate/TMPD. (Lower right) The uncoupling of electron transport from ATP formation using FCCP.

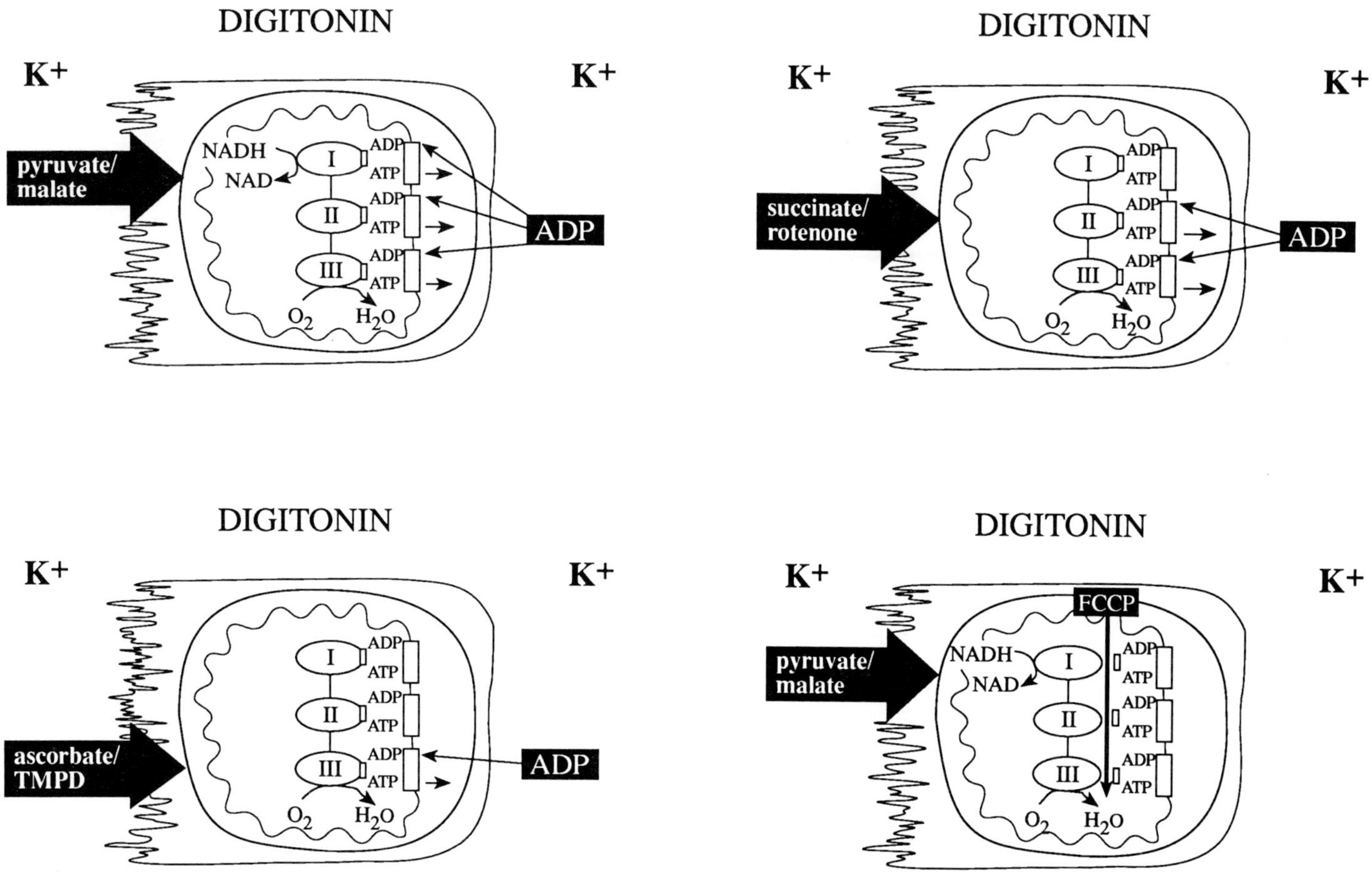
DIGITONIN
K+
K+
pyruvate/ malate
NADH
NAD
I
II
III
ADP
ATP
O2
H2O
ADP
DIGITONIN
K+
K+
succinate/ rotenone
I
II
III
ADP
ATP
O2
H2O
ADP
DIGITONIN
K+
K+
ascorbate/ TMPD
I
II
III
ADP
ATP
O2
H2O
ADP
DIGITONIN
K+
K+
pyruvate/ malate
FCCP
NADH
NAD
I
II
III
ADP
ATP
O2
H2O

drial function (18,26). However, this selective permeabilization is concentration dependent, and concentration–response curves should be run for different types of cells and at different protein concentrations. Immediately after digitonin addition, add excess ADP (0.4 m*M* final concentration) to determine mitochondrial-state 3 respiration. State 3 respiration is the maximal rate of mitochondrial respiration and occurs when there is sufficient substrate, ADP (and inorganic phosphate), and oxygen (27,28). The metabolic substrates in the intracellular buffer can be site I substrates [pyruvate/malate or glutamate/malate (5/5 m*M*)] or the site II substrate succinate (10 m*M*). When using the site II substrate succinate, rotenone (0.1 μM) is added to inhibit site I. Alternatively, ascorbate/TMPD (1/1 m*M*) can be added to examine cytochrome-c/cytochrome oxidase activity, FCCP (1 μM) can be added to examine uncoupled respiration, or a variety of other mitochondrial probes can be added to dissect the site of action of a mitochondrial toxicant.

ACKNOWLEDGMENTS

I thank Drs. M. D. Aleo and C. E. Ruegg and Mr. R. D. Griner for reviewing the manuscript. This work was supported by National Institutes of Health grant ES-04410.

REFERENCES

1. R. G. Schnellmann and R. D. Griner, Mitochondrial mechanisms of tubular injury. *In* "Mechanisms of Injury in Renal Disease and Toxicity" (R. S. Goldstein and M. E. Davis, eds.), in press. Telford Press, 1994.
2. R. G. Schnellmann, E. A. Lock, and L. J. Mandel, *Toxicol. Appl. Pharmacol.* **90,** 513 (1987).
3. A. Wallin, T. W. Jones, A. E. Vercesi, I. Cotgreave, K. Ormstad, and S. Orrenius, *Arch. Biochem. Biophys.* **285,** 365 (1987).
4. R. G. Schnellmann, T. J. Cross, and E. A. Lock, *Toxicol. Appl. Pharmacol.* **100,** (1989).
5. P. J. Hayden and J. L. Stevens, *Mol Pharmacol,* **37,** 468, (1990).
6. C. E. Groves, P. J. Hayden, E. A. Lock, and R. G. Schnellmann, *J. Biochem. Toxicol.* **8,** 75 (1993).
7. Y. Park, T. Y. Aw, and D. P. Jones, this volume, Chapter 13.
8. M. J. Olson, this volume, Chapter 14.
9. Deleted in press.
10. R. S. Balaban, S. P. Soltoff, J. M. Storey, and L. J. Mandel, *Am. J. Physiol.* **238,** F50 (1980).
11. L. J. Mandel, *Fed. Proc., Fed. Am. Soc. Exp. Biol.* **41,** 36 (1982).
12. I. G. Sipes, R. L. Fisher, P. F. Smith, E. R. Stine, A. J. Gandolfi, and K. Brendel, *Arch. Toxicol., Suppl.* **11,** 20 (1987).
13. R. J. Werrlein and A. D. Glinso, *Nature (London)* **251,** 317 (1974).
14. L. Levinton and H. Eagle, *Annu. Rev. Biochem.* **30,** 605 (1961).

15. J. Paul, "*Cells and Tissues in Culture*" (E. N. Willmer, ed.), Academic Press, New York, 1965.
16. L. M. Sakhrani, B. Badie-Dezfooly, W. Trizna, N. Mikhail, A. G. Lowe, M. Taub, and L. G. Fine, *Am. J. Physiol.* **246,** F757 (1984).
17. M. D. Aleo, and R. G. Schnellmann, *Am. J. Physiol.* **262,** F77 (1992).
18. S. I. Harris, R. S. Balaban, L. Barrett, and L. J. Mandel, *J. Biol. Chem.* **256,** 10319 (1981).
19. R. G. Schnellmann, E. A. Lock, and L. J. Mandel, *Toxicol. Appl. Pharmacol.* **90,** 420 (1987).
20. R. G. Schnellmann, *Am. J. Physiol.* **255,** C28 (1988).
21. M. D. Aleo, R. D. Wyatt, and R. G. Schnellmann, *Toxicol. Appl. Pharmacol.* **109,** 455 (1991).
22. M. D. Aleo, R. D. Wyatt, and R. G. Schnellmann, *Toxicol. Appl. Pharmacol.* **107,** 73 (1991).
23. R. K. Zalups, K. L. Knutson, and R. G. Schnellmann, *Toxicol. Appl. Pharmacol.* **119,** 221 (1993).
24. J. Sendroy Jr., R. T. Dillon, and D. D. Van Slyke, *J. Biol. Chem.* **105,** 597 (1934).
25. G. Gstraunthaler, W. Pfaller, and P. Kotanko, *Renal Physiol.* **8,** (1985).
26. P. F. Zuurendonk and J. M. Tager, *Biochim. Biophys. Acta* **333,** 393 (1974).
27. B. Chance and C. M. Williams, *Adv. Enzymol.* **17,** 65 (1956).
28. L. J. Mandel and R. S. Balaban *Am. J. Physiol.* **240,** F357 (1981).

13 ATP and Other Energetic Parameters as Indicators of Cell Injury

Youngja Park, Tak Yee Aw, and Dean P. Jones

INTRODUCTION

The ability to extract energy from the environment and utilize that energy to create and maintain order is one of the fundamental characteristics of living cells. It is therefore of little surprise that death is inexorably linked to disruption of the energy-extracting and -utilizing systems. Thus, measures of cellular energetics provide useful ways to assess cell injury and unravel the critical sequence of events involved in toxicity.

There are three commonly used indicators of cellular energetics (1,2), namely, the oxidation–reduction state of electron carriers such as NADH and NADPH (3), the energy available from movement of ions across membranes in response to an electrochemical ion gradient (2), and the amount of energy available from the hydrolysis of ATP to ADP and inorganic phosphate (4,5). Measurements of the availability of energy in the form of ATP are the most commonly used single parameter to describe cellular energetics because retention of high ATP usually means that the ATP-producing machinery is functionally intact and that toxicological processes have not drastically increased membrane permeability or excessively stimulated ATP utilization. However, there are limitations to the use of changes in ATP as a parameter of toxicity. These limitations must be recognized and use of additional criteria for toxicity is warranted.

First, reversible changes in ATP can occur without loss of viability. Such changes have been extensively studied in hypoxic and anoxic cells, and the results clearly establish that decreased ATP per se is not necessarily associated with irreversible injury. This conclusion is further supported by studies with potassium cyanide (KCN) in the presence of dicalciphor, the dimer of 16,16-dimethyl-15-dehydroprostaglandin B_1 (6). In each of these cases, cells can remain viable for 3 hr, even though ATP is depleted substantially within the first 30 min of incubation.

A second major limitation is that the ATP concentration always decreases in dead cells, regardless of the mechanism of cell death (7). However, in cells undergoing apoptosis, the ATP concentration can be preserved long after a cell program leading to death has been activated (8). Thus, depending on the mech-

METHODS IN TOXICOLOGY, Volume 1B

anism of toxicity, changes in ATP may be a relatively late event that poorly reflects the early irreversible steps of cell death.

Third, the measurement of ATP concentration alone is of limited utility in defining whether toxicant-induced failure of mitochondrial function is important in the mechanism of toxicity. A more accurate representation of cell energetics may be the measurement of the adenylate charge $[(ATP + \frac{1}{2}ADP)/(ATP + ADP + AMP)]$ and/or the ATP/ADP ratio (9), since the adenine nucleotide pool contributes to the overall ATP homeostasis. The importance of distinguishing between changes in ATP concentration per se and the ATP/ADP ratio can be seen from ethionine intoxication (10). Ethionine traps adenosyl residues in *S*-adenosylethionine and results in marked decreases in ATP concentration. In order for changes in ATP to be useful as a parameter of toxicity, the measurement of ATP should be done in conjunction with other indicators, including total adenylate level, cellular O_2 consumption, and mitochondrial membrane integrity. In studies of interrupted supply of oxidizable substrate or electron transport, the O_2 consumption rate can easily be measured. Changes in mitochondrial membrane permeability can be assessed by measures of the mitochondrial membrane potential ($\Delta\psi$) (11,12) and the transmembrane pH gradient (ΔpH) (13).

In this chapter we describe two high-performance liquid chromatography (HPLC) methods (14,15) that we use to measure mitochondrial and cytosolic ATP. The advantage of HPLC is that it provides simultaneous measures of ADP and AMP, which allow determinations of total adenylates, ATP/ADP ratio, and energy charge as indicators of cellular energetics. One method also allows measurement of NAD^+ and $NADP^+$, as well as NADH and NADPH with a minor modification (14). To estimate mitochondrial and cytosolic adenylates and the mitochondrial $\Delta\psi$ and ΔpH, we use a digitonin fractionation technique for separation of mitochondrial and cytosolic pools in isolated cells (16). Detection of major changes in mitochondrial membrane potential in cells can also be obtained with fluorescent lipophilic cations (17), and enzyme-based methods for measuring adenylates and pyridine nucleotides are available (18,19). Selective utilization of these measurements provides a general approach to assess whether disruption of energy metabolism is an early event in specific types of toxicant-induced injury. Here, results from studies with hepatocytes are given as examples of bioenergetic changes during toxic and nontoxic changes in mitochondrial function.

MATERIALS AND REAGENTS

AMP, ADP, ATP, KH_2PO_4, collagenase (type IV), digitonin, HEPES, bovine serum albumin, EGTA, EDTA, 2-(*N*-morpholino)ethanesulfonic acid (MES), and tetrabutylammonium hydrogen sulfate are obtained from Sigma (St. Louis, MO). Acetonitrile and perchloric acid ($HClO_4$) are from Fisher (Pittsburgh, PA). Silicone oil, density 1.05, and mineral oil (white, heavy), density 0.862, are obtained from Aldrich (Milwaukee, WI). Ultrahigh-purity argon ($< 0.001\%$ O_2) is purchased from Linde Specialty Gases (Birmingham, AL). The [*methyl*-^{3}H]TPMP (triphenylmethyl phosphonium iodide; specific activity, 46.1 Ci/mmol), ^3H_2O (specific activity, 10mCi/g), [2-^{14}C]DMO (dimethadione; specific activity, 60 mCi/mmol), and [carboxyl-^{14}C]inulin (specific activity, 2.3 mCi/g) are obtained from New England Nuclear (Boston, MA). Biodegradable counting scintillant is obtained from Amersham (Arlington Heights, IL). KCN is from Merck (Rathway, NJ). All other chemicals used are reagent grade or high purity and are obtained from commercial suppliers. Dicalciphor, synthesized and purified as previously described (20), is provided by the Office of Naval Research (Baltimore, MD). Dicalciphor is an oily solid and was frozen at −80°C until used. To solubize the dicalciphor, 3% $NaHCO_3$ in water is added and heated to 40–50°C. Once in solution, it is kept on ice until use.

PROCEDURES

Isolation and Incubation of Hepatocytes

Hepatocytes are isolated from male Sprague-Dawley rats (200–250 g, Sasco Animal Laboratories, Oregon, WI) by recirculating collagenase perfusion (21). Immediately upon isolation, cells are $> 90\%$ viable as measured by trypan blue (0.2%) exclusion. Cells can be maintained for 5–6 hr under air at room temperature in a gyratory shaker without significant loss of viability. For studies of anoxia, incubations (10^6 cells/ml) are performed in rotating round-bottomed flasks in Krebs–Henseleit buffer containing 25 m*M* HEPES (pH 7.2) at 37°C under argon. For KCN studies cells are incubated under air with or without 0.5 m*M* KCN. The buffer is preequilibrated for 30 min before addition of hepatocytes. The pH of the medium remains between 7.2 and 7.4 over the time course of the experiment. For toxicity studies, variation in pH can have an important influence on viability because low pH protects against cell injury from a variety of agents (22). Viability is ascertained by trypan blue exclusion, which corresponds well with viability as assessed by release of lactate dehydrogenase.

ATP Measurements

We typically measure ATP by HPLC using isocratic or gradient methods (14,15). The major disadvantage of this approach is that it is time consuming and cannot be readily applied to large numbers of samples. For large numbers of samples, we use either a luciferase assay (18) or a fluorometric method enzyme assay (19,23). As described below, simultaneous measures of ADP and AMP are usually advantageous, and the HPLC methods are much more reliable for these measurements.

After incubation, cell suspensions (10^6 cells/ml) are treated with ice-cold 3 *M* $HClO_4$ (0.5 ml/ml of cell incubation) and maintained on ice. At this stage samples can be stored for several days at −80°C without much hydrolysis of ATP; storage at −2°C is also possible, but should be empirically validated by analysis after addition of known amounts of ATP to tissue extracts and timed storage. Aliquots of the $HClO_4$ extracts (usually 300μl) are neutralized with 30 μl each of ice-cold 1 *M* KH_2PO_4 buffer (pH 8.0) and ice-cold 10 *M* KOH. The pH is checked with pH paper to ensure that neutralization is complete. Incomplete neutralization results in slow precipitation of $KClO_4$ and damage to the column. The neutralized aliquots are centrifuged at 13,000 *g* for 1 min at room temperature to remove $KClO_4$, and the supernatant is used for ATP determination. Values are expressed as nmol/10^6 cells.

Isocratic Method (14) (Fig. 1A)

This is an ion-pairing method using a reversed-phase C_{18} column (Beckman, Fullerton, CA) and ultraviolet detection that allows rapid separation and quantitation of the adenylates. The operating conditions are as follows: The running buffer contains 215 m*M* KH_2PO_4, 2.3 m*M* tetrabutylammonium hydrogen sulfate, 0.5% (v/v) methanol, and 3.5% (v/v) acetonitrile (pH 6.25). The flow rate is maintained at 0.8 ml/min. The ATP, ADP, and AMP peaks are detected at 254 nm on a fixed-wavelength absorbance detector or at 260 nm on a variable-wavelength detector (see Fig. 1). Detection limit for each adenylate is below 100 pmol. Quantitation relative to standards can be readily obtained by peak height, but is more conveniently and accurately performed by integration with a commercial integrator.

Gradient Method (15) (Fig. 1B)

ATP is also determined using a gradient system without ion pairing. This involves separation on a reversed-phase C_{18} column with a two-pump gradient system. For this separation we have used several columns made by different companies, most of which provided acceptable separation. Occasionally, we are unable to separate ATP and ADP due to either a very broad ADP peak or the coelution of ATP and ADP. Although we are unable to identify specifically the cause of this problem, we find that the Waters Radial Pak columns (Waters, Milford, MA) do not have this problem. We also find that dedication of a column to adenylate analysis is usually preferred, because the use of phosphate in the solvent alters the characteristics of the column for other assays. In using this method, it should be noted that washing an HPLC column with methanol will

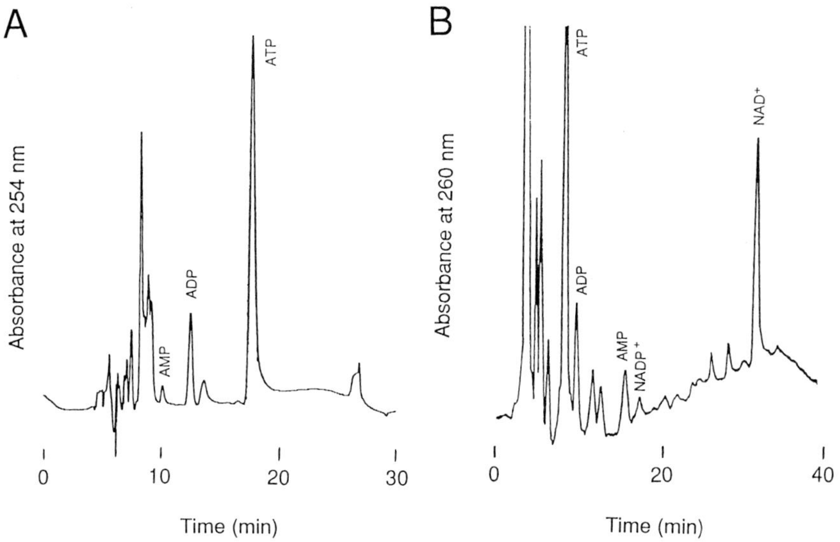

Figure 1 Chromatograms from high-performance liquid chromatography analysis of adenylates in isolated hepatocytes. (A) Isocratic method with a 20-μl extract of 10^6 cells/ml. (B) Gradient method with a 20-μl extract from 10^6 cells/ml.

precipitate phosphate on the column. This can be avoided by washing with water before washing with methanol for storage of the column.

Adenylates are eluted rapidly under isocratic conditions with buffer A (100 m*M* potassium phosphate, pH 6.0). However, we routinely use a gradient with an increasing concentration of methanol [buffer B: 100 m*M* potassium phosphate, pH 6.0, containing methanol (final concentration 5%, v/v)], which provides separation of $NADP^+$ and NAD^+ as well as ATP, ADP, and AMP. The program is run under the initial condition of 100% buffer A for 8.5 min and then changed to 80% buffer A and 20% buffer B over 0.5 min. This condition is maintained for 6 min and then the percentage of B is increased from 20% to 100% over 5 min. Flow is maintained at 100% B for 20 min before being returned to 100% A for at least 10 min for equilibration. For some columns, better resolution is obtained at a slightly lower pH (i.e., 5.93). We usually maintain flow rate at 1 ml/min, but the method works well with flow rates up to at least 4 ml/min.

For measurement of NADH and NADPH it is necessary to extract tissues with an alkaline medium to prevent hydrolysis of the nicotinamide group (19). For this we use ice-cold 0.5 *M* KOH in 50% ethanol containing 35% (w/v) cesium chloride, which is added at 0.1 ml/ml of cell incubation. Protein is removed by centrifugation at 13,000 *g* for 1 min, and HPLC is performed as above with spectrophotometric detection at 340 nm or fluorometric detection with excitation at 340 nm and emission detection at 450 nm.

Separation of Mitochondrial and Cytoplasmic Components

Separation of cytoplasmic and mitochondrial components is performed by digitonin fractionation (16). Separation of cytosolic and mitochondrial compartments is achieved by including 0.12 mg/ml digitonin in MES buffer (20 m*M* EDTA, 20 m*M* EGTA, 250 m*M* mannitol, and 20 m*M* MES, pH 7.4). Microcentrifuge tubes (1.5 ml) are layered from the bottom with 0.1 ml of 40% glycerol, 0.5 ml of a silicone oil (density 1.050)–mineral oil (density 0.862) mixture (ratio 6 : 1), and 0.1 ml of MES buffer. A 0.5-ml aliquot of a cell incubation is added to the top layer and centrifuged at room temperature for 30 sec at 13,000 *g* in a microcentrifuge. To identify the cytosolic and mitochondrial compartments, samples from the supernatant and glycerol layer are assayed spectrophotometrically for lactate dehydrogenase (24) and glutamate dehydrogenase activities (25), and compared to cells lysed with Triton *X*-100 for total enzyme activity.

$\Delta\psi$ and ΔpH

The mitochondrial membrane potential ($\Delta\psi$) or ΔpH is determined from the distribution ratio of [^{3}H]TPMP$^+$ or [^{14}C]DMO between the cytoplasmic and mitochondrial compartments, respectively (11–13). Cells are incubated with the radiotracer ([^{3}H]TPMP$^+$ or [^{14}C]DMO, 0.5 μCi/ml) at 37°C for 20 min to allow equilibration, and the mitochondrial and cytosolic compartments are separated by digitonin fractionation as described above (16), except that 0.1 ml of 15% trichloroacetic acid (TCA) is substituted for glycerol as the bottom layer in the centrifuge tubes. Aliquots from the supernatant and the TCA layer are taken for analysis of the total cellular (without digitonin) and mitochondrial (with digitonin) accumulation of [^{3}H]TPMP$^+$ or [^{14}C]DMO. Parallel incubations are performed using ^3H_2O (2 μCi/ml) and [^{14}C]inulin (0.3 μCi/ml) to determine the cell volume and the extracellular space (13). The accumulation of [^{3}H]TPMP$^+$ is determined in the mitochondrial compartments, and from the accumulation ratio (mitochondria to total) the $\Delta\psi$ is calculated using the Nernst equation: $\Delta\psi = (-RT/\mathrm{F}) \ln \mathrm{Cr}$, in which R is the gas constant, T is the absolute temperature, F is the Faraday constant, and Cr is the accumulation ratio (12). Nonspecific binding of [^{3}H]TPMP$^+$ or [^{14}C]DMO is determined by incubation of boiled cells. This binding is subtracted from the total cellular and mitochondrial accumulation of [^{3}H]TPMP$^+$ or [^{14}C]DMO. Parallel experiments are performed to determine the total water space and extracellular space of hepatocytes. ΔpH values are measured from the distribution of DMO using the same general approach using the equation $\mathrm{pH} = \log[\mathrm{Cr}(10^{\mathrm{pK}+\mathrm{pH}_{\mathrm{out}}}) - 10^{\mathrm{pK}}]$, where Cr is the accumulation ratio, $\mathrm{pH}_{\mathrm{out}}$ is for extracellular pH, and pK for DMO at 37°C is 6.13 (11,13).

A qualitative measure of altered mitochondrial $\Delta\psi$ can be obtained using the fluorescent lipophilic cation rhodamine-123. The method described by Johnson *et al.* (17) is recommended. The accumulation ratio of this compound into the cells is highly dependent on the mitochondrial $\Delta\psi$, and direct measurement of the change in fluorescence associated with cells following a treatment indicates whether the mitochondrial $\Delta\psi$ has changed.

Oxygen Consumption

For a detailed discussion of this topic, the reader is referred to the chapter by Schnellmann in Ch. 12 of this volume.

RESULTS AND INTERPRETATION

Time Course of Viability Changes

Most toxic processes have two critical variables that must be considered in studies of mechanism, namely, the intensity of the toxic challenge and the time course of toxic response. To define the mechanism of toxicity, both must be considered. Similarly, bioenergetic changes must also be considered from both perspectives, because profound decreases in ATP can be tolerated for brief durations, while modest decreases may be pathological over extended periods.

A comparison of two mechanisms to induce mitochondrial failure is given in Fig. 2. Addition of 0.5 m*M* KCN to aerobic hepatocytes causes nearly the same amount of ATP decrease as that detected when cells are made anoxic (26). In contrast, loss of viability, as measured by trypan blue exclusion, occurs within 1–2 hr with KCN, but not until after 2 hr with anoxia. In both cases ATP decrease precedes loss of membrane integrity; however, the results show either that the decrease in ATP is not causal in the sequence of viability loss or that other factors affect the time course of toxicity.

Mitochondrial Function and ATP Content in Anoxic and KCN-Treated Hepatocytes

In examination of the factors that can explain this difference between anoxia and KCN-induced cell death, we find that the maintenance of mitochondrial pH gradient and membrane potential more closely reflect loss of viability than do the decrease of ATP concentration (7,27). The differences in time courses suggest that anoxia elicits protective responses that allow preservation of mitochondrial $\Delta\psi$, ΔpH, and osmotic regulation that do not occur in the unprotected KCN-treated cells (Table I). Thus, although ATP measurements indicate that the cells are under severe bioenergetic limitations, the better indicators of loss of cell viability are the loss of mitochondrial and cellular membrane poten-

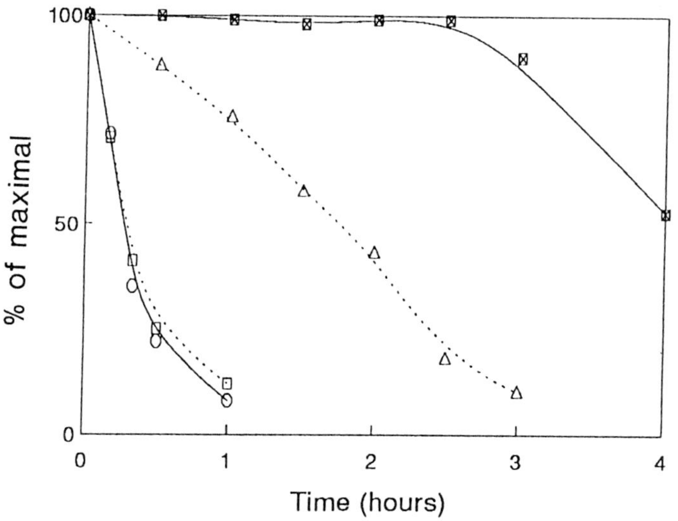

Figure 2 Time course of changes in ATP concentration and viability in hepatocytes exposed to anoxia (solid lines) and KCN (dotted lines). Hepatocytes (10^6 cells/ml) are incubated in modified Krebs–Henseleit buffer and cell viability is measured by exclusion of trypan blue. ATP values are given for KCN treatment as open squares and for anoxia as circles. Viability values are given for KCN treatment as open triangles and for anoxia as crossed-squares.

tials, loss of the pH gradient, and initiation of mitochondrial swelling. Further evidence for the critical role of mitochondrial membrane potential in cell survical is provided by studies of the mitochondrial protectant, dicalciphor, on ATP concentration and cellular energetics in KCN-treated cells (6). The results in Table II show that it is the maintenance of the mitochondrial proton motive force ($\Delta\psi$ and ΔpH) by dicalciphor, rather than cell ATP concentration per se, that preserves cell viability.

Table I Cell Viability, Mitochondrial Function, and ATP Content during Anoxia[a]

	Cell viability (%)	$\Delta\psi$	ΔpH	ATP (nmol/10^6 cells)
Control	90	−162	0.78	23.0
Argon	88	−133	0.76	3.6

[a] Cell viability was determined by exclusion of trypan blue (0.2%) at 30 min of incubation. Control, hepatocytes (10^6 cells / ml) were incubated under air; argon, hepatocytes (10^6 cells / ml) were incubated under argon. Mitochondrial membrane potential ($\Delta\psi$), ΔpH, and ATP were determined at 30 min of incubation. Data are expressed as means; n = 3–4 for all points.

Table II Effect of Dicalciphor on Cell Viability, Mitochondrial Function, and ATP in the Presence of KCN[a]

	Cell viability %	$\Delta\psi$	ΔpH	ATP (nmol/10^6 cells)
Control[b]	90	−156	0.78	26.8
0.5 m*M* KCN	83	−95	0.44	5.7
0.5 m*M* KCN + 10 μM dicalciphor	88	−143	0.70	8.1

[a] Conditions used in this experiment are the same as in Table I. All assays are performed at 30 min incubation so that the KCN-induced cell death had not occurred to an extent that would interfere with the analyses.
[b] Control, hepatocytes (10^6 cells/ml) are incubated under air; 0.5 m*M* KCN, hepatocytes are incubated in the presence of 0.5 m*M*KCN; 0.5 m*M* KCN + 10 μM dicalciphor; 10 μM dicalciphor is added to hepatocytes in the presence 0.5 m*M* KCN.

Effect of FCCP and Antimycin A on O_2 Consumption Rate and ATP/ADP Ratio

Insight into the utility of various types of bioenergetic measurements can be obtained by measuring the responses of O_2 consumption, ATP, or the ATP/ADP ratio to poisons that cause cell death due to mitochondrial failure. Although changes in cellular O_2 consumption per se do not necessarily indicate cell toxicity, O_2 consumption provides important information on mitochondrial function when taken into context with ATP, ATP/ADP, and $\Delta\psi$ measurements. In these determinations we normally make such analyses prior to significant loss of viability to eliminate ambiguities related to variations in the percentage of cell viability. Addition of the protonphore FCCP[1] causes a marked stimulation of O_2 consumption, with a decrease in ATP concentration and ATP/ADP (Fig. 3). Under these conditions a loss of mitochondrial $\Delta\psi$ occurs and cells go on to die. A different type of response occurs to the electron transport inhibitor antimycin A. This toxin causes a marked inhibition of O_2 consumption, with a decrease in ATP and ATP/ADP. Under these conditions the mitochondrial $\Delta\psi$ decreases dramatically and the cells die.

Oligomycin and carboxyatractyloside are also mitochondrial poisons that result in significant decreases in cell ATP and the ATP/ADP ratio (27). However, these agents have rather modest effects on O_2 consumption rate and mitochondrial $\Delta\psi$. In such instances interference with cytosolic ATP availability or the ATP/ADP ratio can result in toxicity despite preservation of the mitochondrial $\Delta\psi$. The above discussion suggests the limited utility of any single energetic parameter in defining toxicant-induced mitochondrial dysfunction in the mechanism of cell toxicity.

[1] FCCP, Carbonyl cyanide *p*-trifluoromethoxyphenylhydrazone.

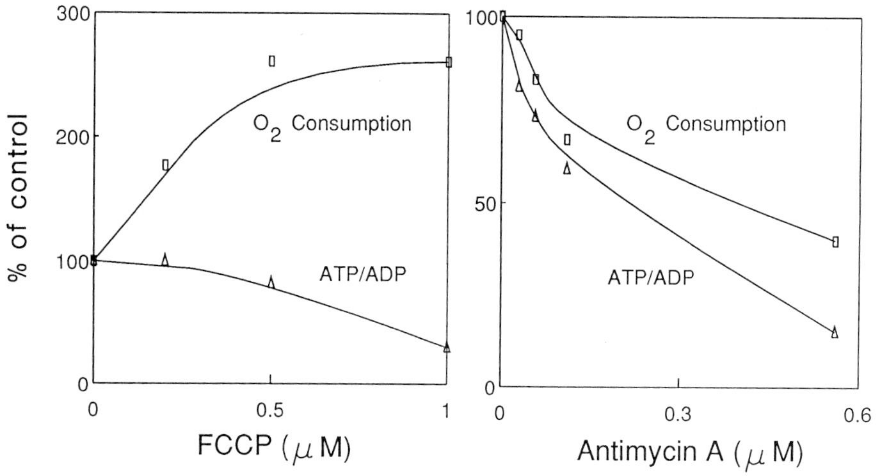

Figure 3 Comparison of the effects of carbonyl cyanide *p*-trifluoromethoxyphenylhydrazone (FCCP) and antimycin A on the O_2 consumption rate and ATP/ADP ratio in hepatocytes. O_2 consumption is measured polarigraphically with a Clark-type electrode standardized relative to air, and the experimental zero is obtained with sodium dithionite. O_2 consumption rates are measured at 37°C within the first 5 min following addition of either FCCP or antimycin A at the concentrations indicated. For ATP and ADP measurements cells (10^6 cells/ml) are incubated with FCCP or antimycin A at the concentrations indicated for 30 min and extracted and analyzed by the gradient method as described in the text. FCCP is added from a stock solution made up in ethanol, and antimycin A is added from a stock solution made up in dimethylformamide. Solvent additions do not affect either O_2 consumption or ATP/ADP ratio under the conditions of the experiments.

COMMENTS

The level of ATP has been considered one of the most important markers of irreversible injury to cells. However, in the past several years, studies on the mechanism of cell injury have been demonstrated that decreases in ATP level alone cannot account for cell death under many conditions (28,29).

ATP is mainly produced by mitochondrial oxidative phosphorylation using O_2 as a final electron acceptor. During mitochondrial oxidative phosphorylation electron transport from NADH to O_2 is coupled to the pumping of protons out of the mitochondrial matrix, which establishes an electrochemical proton gradient termed the protonmotive force (Δp). Δp functions as the intermediate in the coupling mechanism of mitochondrial substrate oxidation and ATP synthesis (30) and provides energy for ATP/ADP exchange (ATP out of mitochondria, ADP into mitochondria) and other ion movements. Interruption of function occurs due to deregulation of substrate oxidation, damage to electron transfer components, inhibition of ion flux, loss of mitochondrial membrane permeability barrier, or the destruction of ATP synthase (1). Thus, failure of cellular energy production can occur at numerous sites and by different mechanisms (1).

Determination of the role of energetic failure in toxicity therefore requires measurement using multiple indicators. In general, measurements of O_2 consumption rate, mitochondrial $\Delta\psi$, or cytoplasmic ATP/ADP provides a good overview of bioenergetic functions and provides the basis for concluding whether bioenergetic failure precedes or coincides with cell death. Such a determination requires that one recognize that cell death is a quantum property, while the above bioenergetic measures are continuous. Thus, an ATP measurement on a cell extract provides no distinction between a 50% change in 100% of the cells and a 100% change in 50% of the cells. To address this latter issue, efforts are under way to develop methods to measure energy status on a single-cell basis. The most promising available methods focus on the *in situ* measurement of the mitochondrial uptake and retention of fluorescent lipophilic cations (31). A variety of these compounds are commercially available and, in principle, can be used to assess mitochondrial integrity. In using such compounds, one must recognize that without simultaneous measures of O_2 consumption and cytoplasmic ATP/ADP, it is not possible to distinguish between regulated changes in response to functional load, toxicant-induced failure, and toxicant-induced protective responses. Thus, there remains an important need for improved indicators of bioenergetic functions that are suitable for analysis of single cells.

Finally, there is also an unresolved issue concerning the use of cultured cells for toxicological studies that involve mitochondrial dysfunction. Most primary cultures and cell lines have considerably reduced mitochondrial content compared to their counterparts in normal tissues (32,33). Even without qualitative changes in enzymes and transport systems, this quantitative difference reduces the reliance of the cell on mitochondrial energy production and increases the relative importance of glycolysis. In principle, this shift could result in susceptibility to failure at different sites and result in a different mechanism of toxicity. Consequently, conclusions based on *in vitro* cell culture studies must be verified with experiments *in vivo*.

ACKNOWLEDGMENTS

The research on which this manuscript was based was supported by National Institutes of Health grant HL39968 and by the Office of Naval Research grants N-00014-89-J-1738 and N-00014-89-J-1027.

REFERENCES

1. D. P. Jones, X. Shan, and Y. Park, *Annu. Rev. Nutr.* **12,** 327 (1992).
2. L. M. Mela-Riker, *Annu. Rev. Physiol.* **47,** 645 (1985).

3. F. W. Heineman and R. S. Balaban, *Annu. Rev. Physiol.* **52,** 523 (1990).
4. R. S. Balaban, *Am. J. Physiol.* **258,** C377 (1990).
5. M. Erecinska and D. F. Wilson, *J. Membr. Biol.* **70,** 1 (1982).
6. Y. Park, T. M. Devlin, and D. P. Jones, *Am. J. Physiol.* **263,** C405 (1992).
7. T. Y. Aw, B. Andersson, and D. P. Jones, *Am. J. Physiol.* **252,** C356 (1987).
8. L. B. Chen, *Methods Cell Biol.* **29,** 103 (1989).
9. D. E. Atkinson, *in* "The Enzymes" (P. D. Boyer, ed.), Vol. 1, p. 461. Academic Press, New York, 1970.
10. T. Y. Aw and D. P. Jones, *J. Biol. Chem.* **257,** 8997 (1982).
11. J. B. Hoek, D. G. Nicholls, and J. R. Williamson, *J. Biol. Chem.* **255,** 1458 (1980).
12. H. Rottenberg, *J. Membr. Biol.* **81,** 127 (1984).
13. W. J. Waddell and T. C. Butler, *J. Clin. Invest.* **38,** 720 (1959).
14. O. F. M. Sellevold, P. Jynge, and K. Aarstad, *J. Mol. Cell. Cardiol.* **18,** 517 (1986).
15. D. P. Jones, *J. Chromatogr.* **225,** 446 (1981).
16. B. Andersson and D. P. Jones, *Anal. Biochem.* **146,** 164 (1985).
17. L. V. Johnson, M. L. Walsh, B. J. Bockus, and C. B. Chen, *J. Cell Biol.* **88,** 526 (1981).
18. J. J. Lemasters and C. R. Hackenbrock, *in* "Methods in Enzymology" (S. Fleischer and L. Packer, eds.), Vol. 56, p. 530. Academic Press, New York, 1979.
19. J. R. Williamson and B. E. Corkey, *in* "Methods in Enzymology" (J. M. Lowenstein, ed.) Vol. 13, p. 434. Academic Press, New York, 1969.
20. G. L. Nelson and G. L. Verdine, *Tetrahedron Lett.* **24,** 991 (1983).
21. P. Moldeus, J. Hogberg, and S. Orrenius, *in* "Methods in Enzymology" (S. Fleischer and L. Packer, eds.), Vol. 52, p. 60. Academic Press, New York, 1978.
22. G. J. Gores, A. Nieminen, K. E. Fleishman, T. L. Dawson, B. Herman, and J. J. Lemasters, *Am. J. Physiol.* **255,** C315 (1988).
23. R. W. Estabrook, J. R. Williamson, R. Frenkel, and P. K. Maitra, *in* "Methods in Enzymology" (R. W. Estabrook and M. E. Pullman, eds.), Vol. 10, p. 474. Academic Press, New York, 1967.
24. H. U. Bergmeyer and E. Bernt, *in* "Methods of Enzymatic Analysis" (H. U. Bergmeyer, ed.), Vol. 2, p. 574. Academic Press, New York, 1974.
25. E. Schmidt, *in* "Methods of Enzymatic Analysis" (H. U. Bergmeyer, ed.), Vol. 2, p. 650. Academic Press, New York, 1974.
26. T. Y. Aw and D. P. Jones, *Am. J. Physiol.* **257,** C435 (1989).
27. B. S. Andersson, T. Y. Aw, and D. P. Jones, *Am. J. Physiol.* **252,** C349 (1987).
28. A. Gasbarrin, A. B. Borle, H. Farghali, C. Bender, A. Francavilla, and D. Van Thiel, *J. Biol. Chem.* **267,** 6654 (1992).
29. A. Gasbarrin, A. B. Borle, H. Farghali, A. Francavilla, and D. Van Thiel, *J. Biol. Chem.* **267,** 7545 (1992).
30. P. Mitchell, *Science* **206,** 1148 (1979).
31. S. T. Smiley, M. Reers, C. Mottola-Hartshorn, M. Lin, A. Chen, T. W. Smith, G. D. Steele, Jr., and L. B. Chen, *Proc. Natl. Acad. Sci. U.S.A.,* **88,** 3671 (1991).
32. M.-J. Tang, K. R. Suresh, and R. L. Tannen, *Am. J. Physiol.* **256,** C532 (1989).
33. T. Y. Aw and D. P. Jones, *in* "Microcompartmentation" (D. P. Jones, ed.), p. 191. CRC Press, Boca Raton, Florida, 1988.

14

Evaluation of Glucose Metabolism *in Vitro:* Altered Competence of Intermediary Metabolism as an Index of Hepatotoxicity

Michael J. Olson

INTRODUCTION

The history of modern biochemistry is intimately coupled to elucidation of the pathways of glucose synthesis, storage, and utilization. In mammals the liver is recognized as integral in the regulation of bodily carbohydrate stores, as well as maintaining circulating levels of glucose within the bounds required for normal function of glucose-dependent extrahepatic tissues. Furthermore, the liver serves as a key organ effecting metabolism of xenobiotic substances and, as such, is a common target tissue for chemical toxicants. The polyenzymatic process whereby glucose and glycogen are biosynthesized, degraded, and interconverted offers many points at which exogenous chemicals may interfere with intermediary metabolism. At the molecular level the overall flux of intermediates through the pathways of glucose metabolism may be altered by toxicants which directly impair the function of enzymes integral to glucose metabolism. In addition, alterations in the efficiency of oxygen uptake or mitochondrial electron transport, and thereby, the balance of cofactors (e.g., NADH) required by some glucose-metabolizing enzymes, may alter rates of glucose metabolism.

In the context of toxicology, evaluation of the functional competence of a highly regulated and elaborate cellular process such as glucose metabolism provides greater sensitivity of detection for toxic events than assessments of overt cytolethality, such as increased membrane permeability to dyes (1) or NADH (2), release of previously incorporated ^{51}Cr (3), or loss of 5′-[^{14}C]AMP from cells incubated with [^{14}C]adenosine (4). In addition, assessment of the ability of chemicals to alter functional competence may be useful in organizing the chronology of events in studies of toxic mechanisms, inasmuch as modulation of cellular intermediary metabolism is often an early-onset effect of exposure to chemicals associated with more severe latent toxicity (5). Thus, evaluation of the effect of xenobiotics on rates of hepatic functions such as glycolysis,

METHODS IN TOXICOLOGY, Volume 1B

glycogenolysis, and gluconeogenesis is of great potential utility, whether one is seeking to define mechanisms of toxicity, screen pharmaceuticals for potential toxicity, or rank the toxic potential of candidate chemicals for nontherapeutic applications.

This chapter describes methods for determining the functional competence of glucose metabolism in suspension cultures of freshly isolated rat hepatocytes and illustrates the effect of one hepatotoxicant, halothane, on rates of glycolysis and gluconeogenesis. Similar methods have been successfully applied to the study of modulation of intermediary metabolism by hormones and therapeutic or toxic chemicals in other liver-derived preparations, for example, primary cultures of rat hepatocytes (6), suspension cultures of rat hepatocytes adhered to microcarrier beads (7), and the isolated perfused rat liver (8–10). Finally, *in vitro* analyses of glucose metabolism as a parameter modulated by toxicant exposure are, in principle, possible with a wide variety of preparations from other tissues (e.g., kidney).

MATERIALS AND REAGENTS

Hepatocyte Preparation

The perfusion system and reagents necessary for preparation of isolated rat hepatocytes by liver perfusion have been well described in earlier publications (2,11,12). We use only a few deviations from the chemical materials described in the earliest of these publications (2,11). Briefly, the first perfusate is prepared with commercially available Hanks' balanced salt solution without Ca^{2+} (HBSS) (GIBCO, Grand Island, NY) containing 0.25 m*M* EGTA (Sigma, St. Louis, MO) but omitting albumin. The second (collagenase-containing) perfusion solution consists of Leibovitz' L-15 medium (Sigma) with 2 m*M* L-glutamine and 50 U /ml collagenase type IV (Sigma). When it is necessary to purchase collagenase, several lots of the enzyme are screened to determine which particular lot gives hepatocyte preparations with the highest viability. Both perfusion solutions are buffered with 10 m*M* HEPES, and immediately prior to use the pH is adjusted to 7. 2 (at 37°C).

Determination of Products of Intermediary Metabolism

For determination of the glycolytic products lactate and pyruvate, the gluconeogenic product glucose, and glycogen, enzymatic techniques linked to spectrophotometric determination of reduced pyridine nucleotide cofactors are used (13–16). A central advantage of the use of isolated hepatocytes is the availability of large numbers of cells from a single rat liver such that more sensitive, but also more costly or time-consuming, methods for assessment of glucose metabolism (e.g., the use of radiolabeled substrates) are unnecessary. We have relied on materials ordered from a single supplier (Sigma) for convenience. However, numerous commercial sources are available for the enzymes, cofactors, and buffer components specified below, although the reader is advised to consult Refs. 13–16 for cautionary notes regarding the quality of enzyme preparations selected.

The assays described below were validated in my laboratory to ensure that all cofactors and enzymes are present in sufficient excess to allow complete enzyme-catalyzed destruction of the substrate of interest. The following solutions are necessary for determination of lactate in hepatocyte culture media:

Glycine/hydrazine buffer: Dissolve 750 mg of L-glycine and 59 mg of NaOH in 200 ml of deionized water, and adjust the pH to 9.5 with dilute (~2 N) NaOH or HCl if necessary. Add 4 ml of hydrazine hydrate just prior to use

NAD solution: Dissolve 66.3 mg of NAD (monosodium salt) in 5 ml of deionized water

L-Lactate dehydrogenase (LDH; EC 1.1.1.27) solution: Dilute a sufficient amount of $(NH_4)_2SO_4$ suspension of LDH (~250 U/ml) in 1 ml of deionized water to yield a solution of 12.5 U of enzyme/ml

For determination of pyruvate, prepare the following solutions:

Triethanolamine/EDTA buffer: Dissolve 18.63 g of triethanolamine and 0.47 g of EDTA (disodium salt) in 250 ml of deionized water, and adjust the pH to 7.0 as above

NADH solution: Dissolve 5 mg of NADH (disodium salt) in 1 ml of 5% $NaHCO_3$ solution

LDH solution: Dilute sufficient LDH, as an $(NH_4)_2SO_4$ suspension (~250 U/ml), to yield a solution of 12.5 U of enzyme/ml in 1 ml of deionized water

Assessment of glucose in cell culture media requires these solutions:

Buffer: Add 49.3 mg of magnesium sulfate heptahydrate ($MgSO_4 \cdot 7H_2O$), 48.4 mg of ATP (disodium salt), and 63 mg of NADP (disodium salt) to 50 ml of triethanolamine/EDTA buffer (see above), and adjust the pH to 7.7 with dilute (~2 N) NaOH or HCl if necessary

Glucose-6-phosphate dehydrogenase (EC 1.1.1.49) solution: Add sufficient enzyme suspension (~250 U/ml in $(NH_4)_2SO_4$) to 50 ml of buffer to yield 2 U of enzyme/ml

Hexokinase (EC 2.7.1.1) solution: Add sufficient enzyme suspension in $(NH_4)_2SO_4$ to 50 ml of the glucose-6-phosphate dehydrogenase buffer to produce a final dilution of 0.15 U of enzyme/ml

Determination of glycogen in hepatocytes requires the reagents just described for glucose determination in addition to the following solutions:

Buffer: Combine 230 μl of glacial acetic acid and 816 mg of sodium acetate trihydrate ($C_2H_3O_2Na \cdot 3H_2O$) in 100 ml of deionized water, and adjust the pH to 4.8 as above

Amyloglucosidase (EC 3.2.1.3; exo-1,4-α-D-glucosidase) solution: Add sufficient enzyme suspension [~50 U/mg of protein in $(NH_4)_2SO_4$] to yield 20 U of enzyme/ml in 20 ml of the buffer prepared in step 1

PROCEDURES

Hepatocyte Preparation

Isolated hepatocytes are prepared from the livers of adult (200- to 250-g) male Fischer 344 rats [CDF^R(F-344)Crl BR, VAF/Plus, Charles River Laboratories, Kingston, NY] by a two-step *in situ* perfusion of the liver via the portal vein as described in Refs. 11 and 12. For evaluation of rates of gluconeogenesis only, rats are fasted for 18 hr (3 PM to 9 AM) immediately prior to hepatocyte preparation.

Immediately after isolation, the cells are collected by 3-min centrifugation at 50 *g* with refrigeration (4°C). The sedimented cells are suspended in cold L-15 medium supplemented with 0.2% bovine serum albumin and 10 m*M* HEPES (pH 7.2), and a small amount of the suspension is made 0.04% (v/v) in trypan blue for microscopic determination of dye exclusion as an index of initial cell viability (1). Cells are enumerated using a Neubauer-type hemocytometer, and the volume of the cell suspension is adjusted to achieve 5–12 $\times$ 10^6 cells/ml. Hepatocytes are further processed by an isodensity centrifugation method with Percoll (Pharmacia LKB Biotechnology, Piscataway, NJ) (17). The postcentrifugation cell pellet is washed twice in cold Krebs–Henseleit (KH) buffer (18) with 10 m*M* HEPES (pH 7.2), resuspended in the same buffer, and analyzed for trypan blue exclusion as before. The Percoll step may be omitted if cells are of very high initial viability (~90%). However, we routinely use cell processing with Percoll to both improve and normalize initial viability from hepatocyte preparation to preparation.

For assessment of chemical effects on glycolysis and glycogenolysis, hepatocytes from fed rats are suspended in KH buffer plus 10 m*M* HEPES (pH 7.2) and adjusted to a concentration of 2 $\times$ 10^6 cells/ml. In experiments evaluating the rate of gluconeogenesis, hepatocyte preparations from fasted rats are used and the suspension medium contains lactate (5 m*M*) and pyruvate (1 m*M*) to support gluconeogenesis. Portions (3 ml) of the cell suspensions are transferred to 25-ml screw-top Erlenmeyer flasks. At this point the test chemical, dissolved in KH buffer or a minimal volume of solvent (e.g., dimethyl sulfoxide, acetone, or methanol), may be added. The final solvent concentration should be kept at or below 1% (v/v), and appropriate solvent controls should be included.

If gaseous or volatile toxicants are to be evaluated, the hepatocyte-containing flasks are capped with Teflon-faced septa and screw caps. Immediately after closure, flasks are flushed with hydrocarbon-free air containing the appropriate dilution(s) of gaseous toxicant via a syringe needle passed through the rubber stopper while a separate needle provides pressure relief. Gas mixtures for introduction into cell culture flasks are conveniently prepared by simultaneously mixing the pure toxicant gas and hydrocarbon-free air, or a $O_2/CO_2/N_2$ mixture, with multiple gas-flow controllers (Dwyer, Michigan City, IN). Care should be taken to ensure that the oxygen content of the flask head space is at or very near 21%, especially if hepatocyte incubation is to exceed 1 hr. Volatile liquid toxicants may be added in liquid form and allowed to evaporate from a small plastic shelf suspended inside the flask. Alternatively, sufficient volatile liquid to yield a 100% atmosphere may be allowed to evaporate in a 1-liter (or other size, as appropriate) gas sampling bag (SKC, Eighty Four, PA) which was initially evacuated. Aliquots of the atmosphere in the gas-filled bag may then be transferred to the flasks with a gastight syringe to give the final gas phase toxicant concentrations desired.

After adding the test agents, cell cultures are placed immediately in a gyratory water bath and maintained at 37°C and 80–100 oscillations/min for the desired incubation period.

Determination of Rates of Glycolysis and Gluconeogenesis

After incubation for an interval deemed appropriate by the investigator,[1] the contents of each culture flask are emptied into conical-bottomed centrifuge tubes and the hepatocytes are separated from the culture medium by centrifugation at room temperature for 5 min at 50 *g*. The supernatant medium is deproteinized with 0.6 *M* perchloric acid ($HClO_4$; final concentration 0.1 *M*), neutralized with potassium carbonate (K_2CO_3), centrifuged at 1750 *g* for 10 min, and assayed in duplicate for the products of glycolysis (lactate + pyruvate),

[1] When initiating experiments, care should be taken to determine the time course of hepatocyte incubation over which rates of glucose metabolism remain linear in the presence and absence of toxicant. While kinetic data of this type are themseleves of interest, such knowledge is of critical importance in the design of experiments in which the effect of a toxicant on glucose metabolism is to be determined by comparison to an untreated control at only a single time point.

glycogenolysis (glucose), or gluconeogenesis (glucose) (see below). The cell pellet (formed from 3 ml of a suspension of 2×10^6 cells/ml, ~200 mg of wet weight) is resuspended in 500 μl of 0.6 *M* $HClO_4$ and disrupted with a probe sonicator (Sonifier Cell Disruptor, Model W140, Heat Systems Ultrasonics, Plainview, NY). The resulting homogenate is neutralized with K_2CO_3 and used for assessment of glycogen synthesis (see below).

Although the methods described here are designed for end-point analysis of batch samples, very similar analyses by kinetic methods may also be used as described in Refs. 13–16. Determination of lactate content of hepatocyte culture media is as follows:

> Combine 670 μl of glycine/hydrazine buffer, 100 μl of NAD solution, 200 μl of deproteinized neutralized cell culture medium, and 1 ml of deionized water. Mix well, and determine absorbance at 340 nm (A_{340}). Then add 20 μl of LDH solution per sample, mix, incubate at room temperature for at least 1 hr, and determine A_{340}. Calculate ΔA_{340} (the difference in A_{340}) by subtracting the initial absorbance value from the final value.

The pyruvate concentration of hepatocyte culture media is determined by this method:

> Combine 250 μl of triethanolamine/EDTA buffer, 20 μl of NADH solution, and 500 μl of deproteinized neutralized cell culture medium. Mix well, and determine A_{340}. Then add 10 μl of LDH solution per sample, mix, incubate at room temperature for at least 30 min, and determine A_{340}. Calculate ΔA_{340} (subtract the final absorbance value from the initial value).

Glucose in the liquid media used to suspend hepatocytes is determined by this method:

> Prepare complete assay buffer with $MgSO_4 \cdot 7H_2O$, ATP (disodium salt), NADP (disodium salt), glucose-6-phosphate dehydrogenase, and hexokinase. Determine A_{340}. Then add 50 μl of deproteinized neutralized cell culture medium to 1 ml assay buffer, mix, incubate at room temperature for 2 hr, and determine ΔA_{340}. Calculate ΔA_{340}.

The glycogen content of the cell pellet may be evaluated as follows:

> Combine 300 μl of neutralized hepatocyte homogenate and 500 μl of amyloglucosidase in acetate buffer. Incubate at 37°C for 2 hr with continuous vigorous shaking using a wrist-action shaker. Add 500 μl of 0.6 N $HClO_4$,

mix, and centrifuge at room temperature at 1750 *g* for 10 min. Transfer the clear supernatant to a clean tube and neutralize with K_2CO_3. Assay 50 μl of neutralized sample for glucose as described above. The resulting value must be corrected for the glucose content of the hepatocyte homogenate prior to amyloglucosidase treatment.

Calculation of intermediary metabolite concentrations:

For all metabolites the molar extinction coefficient (ϵ) for NADH or NADPH at 340 nm, 6.3×10^2 liter $\times$ mol^{-1} $\times$ mm^{-1}, is used (19). If absorption measurements are made in a standard 10-mm path-length cuvette and the metabolite concentration is expressed as μmol/ml (m*M*), ϵ becomes 6.3 liter $\times$ $mmol^{-1}$. The concentration (c) of analyte (e.g., lactate) in a sample of incubation medium may be calculated as:

$$c = (\Delta A_{340} \times V)/(6.3 \times v)$$

Here, V is the total volume of the assay mixture (in ml) and v is the volume of sample (also in ml) used in the assay. c is expressed as a m*M* concentration in the sample, but must be corrected for dilution (e.g., with $HClO_4$ and K_2CO_3) and for the initial volume of the hepatocyte suspension medium to reflect the true yield of metabolite. Results are conveniently expressed as molar quantity of metabolite (μmol) formed/unit of time/1×10^6 cells, or may be normalized to cell protein or another appropriate parameter.

In some cases when data from multiple experiments are combined, it may be found that significant differences exist from experiment to experiment in the basal rates of intermediary metabolic processes. Provided that adequate care has been taken to account for the nutritional status of the rats prior to hepatocyte preparation (e.g., use of rats of same age/body weight and hepatocyte preparation at same time of day in each experiment), the basal rate of metabolite formation in untreated control incubations may be set to 100% and toxicant-induced alterations may be expressed with reference to this normalized rate.

Assessment of Cytolethality

At intervals during hepatocyte incubation and at the conclusion of incubation, it is desirable to assess cell viability in order to determine whether alterations in rates of glucose metabolism are due to overt cytolethality or to more subtle perturbations of cell function. For this purpose quantitation of LDH activity released into the cell suspension medium and trypan blue penetration into hepatocytes are commonly used, and easily measured, parameters. The methods described by Jauregui *et al.* (1), Moldeus *et al.* (2), or Acosta (20) are of utility in that they allow for expression of LDH release as a percentage of total LDH in individual culture samples, thereby normalizing for slight differences in cell number from culture to culture.

COMMENTS

In this laboratory accumulation of the products of glycolysis and gluconeogenesis in the suspension media of hepatocytes is linear for at least 4 hr (data not shown). Under the conditions described, basal rates of synthesis of lactate, pyruvate, and glucose in a representative set of hepatocyte suspensions isolated from fed rats averaged about 190, 40, and 380 μmol/hr/1 $\times$ 10^6 cells, respectively, in the absence of exogenous substrates (21). Dependent on factors such as nutritional status, age, and genetic background, a range of values is possible. Comparison of absolute rates of metabolite production with these or historical values in the literature is probably less useful for judging the metabolic performance of a specific hepatocyte preparation than comparison to the average of values accumulated under similar circumstances in the same laboratory. The lactate/pyruvate ratio (L/P) calculated for this set of hepatocyte suspensions in our laboratory is 4.8 ± 0.7 (mean ± SD, $n = 4$), which compares favorably to values of 3.5–4 reported for the effluent perfusate from the isolated perfused rat liver (10). Determination of L/P from concentrations of glycolytic products provides a sensitive index of the cytosolic redox state, since this metabolite pair is in equilibrium with cytoplasmic NAD/NADH in liver (22,23).

The relatively low L/P in the medium suspending hepatocytes under the conditions described here suggests that oxygenation is adequate. We have, furthermore, verified that L/P is quite sensitive to hypoxia in this primary cell culture system (Fig. 1). Elevated lactate production reflects a hypoxia-induced increase in cytoplasmic NADH which shifts the equilibrium of the pyruvate–lactate couple. In addition, as the degree of hypoxia is increased, glucose output decreases, perhaps due to increased glycolytic flux (Fig. 1). As described below, modulation of glycolytic activity, and thus L/P, occurs upon exposure to toxicants as well as during hypoxia.

Cells derived from 18-hr-fasted rats produced glucose at an average rate of ~220 μmol/hr/1 $\times$ 10^6 cells in the presence of saturating concentrations of exogenous lactate and pyruvate (21). As with glycolysis, rates of gluconeogenesis are also subject to modulation by the availability of O_2; anoxia depresses rates of gluconeogenesis by decreasing cellular ATP levels (21,24).

To model some toxicant-induced perturbations which may be observed in rates of glucose metabolism in isolated hepatocytes, we investigated the effects of the anesthetic halocarbon halothane, which is hepatotoxic under some cir-

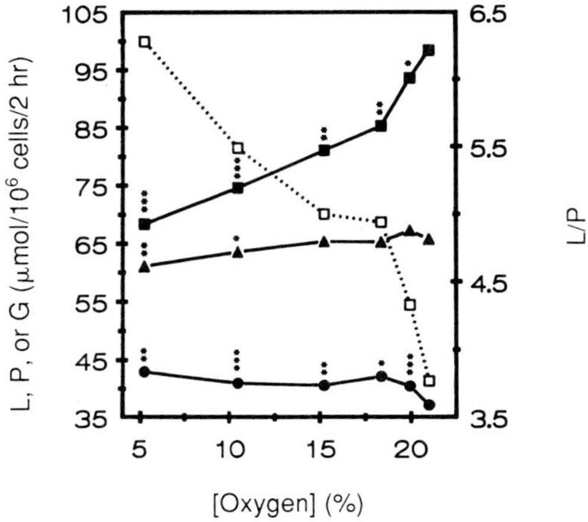

Figure 1 Stimulation of glycolysis by hypoxia in hepatocytes isolated from a fed rat. Hepatocytes suspended in Krebs–Henseleit buffer (6×10^6 cells in 3 ml of buffer) were incubated at 37°C in sealed 25-ml flasks. Head space O_2 concentrations at the initiation of incubation are shown on the abscissa. After 2 hr, culture media were assayed for lactate (L; ●), pyruvate (P; ■), and glucose (G; ▲) as described in "Procedures" and L/P (□) was calculated. Values for L and G have been multiplied by 10^{-1} for convenience in scaling the figure. All values are reported as the mean of duplicate determinations on two like-treated cell cultures; the standard deviation was less than 5% of the mean at all points. Comparison to 21% O_2 (one-way analysis of variance and t test): * $P \leq 0.05$, ** $P \leq 0.02$, *** $P \leq 0.01$.

cumstances *in vivo* (25,26). In both intact rats and the isolated perfused rat liver, halothane has pronounced effects on glycolysis and gluconeogenesis at concentrations less than those associated with induction of overt cytotoxicity (8,27). At concentrations as low as 312 ppm, halothane caused a substantial increase in L/P in the media sustaining hepatocytes isolated from fed rats (Fig. 2A). This was due to stimulation of the production of both glycolytic metabolites; a large increase in lactate output was accompanied by a relatively smaller, but significant, increase in pyruvate production (Fig. 2A). In addition, halothane decreased the production of glucose in cells of fed rats in concert with increased lactate and pyruvate production (Fig. 2A). As opposed to the stimulation of glycolysis in hepatocytes isolated from fed rats, inclusion of halothane at subcytotoxic concentrations decreased rates of gluconeogenesis in the cells of fasted rats (Fig. 2B). Perturbation of hepatocellular glucose metabolism in preparations from fed rats was less severe with 1250 ppm halothane, probably because of overt cytotoxicity, than with lower halothane concentrations. In fact, inclusion of 1250 ppm halothane resulted in a release of 37% (±1%) of total LDH during 2-hr incubations as opposed to a loss of only 24% (±3%) of total

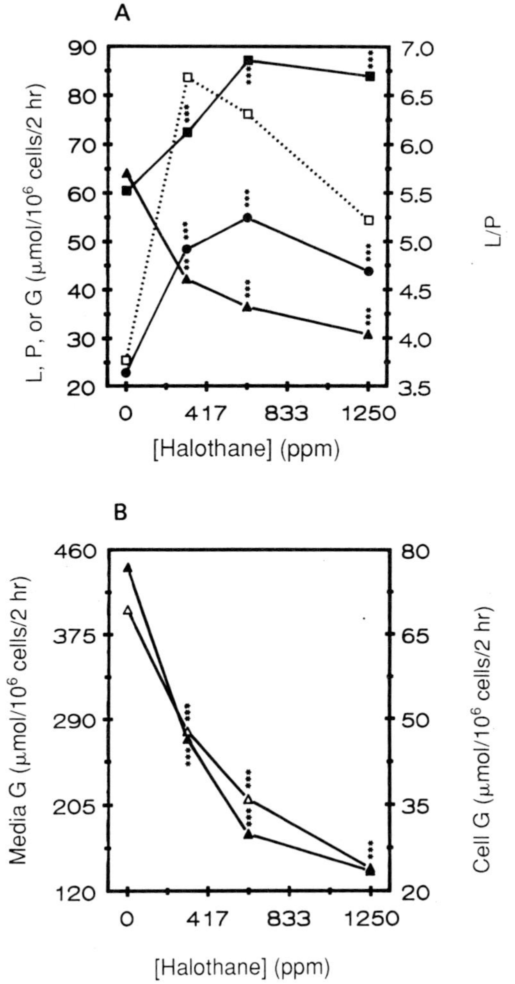

Figure 2 The effect of halothane on glycolysis in hepatocyte suspensions from a fed rat (A) or gluconeogenesis in hepatocytes of a fasted rat (B). (A) Hepatocytes suspended in Krebs–Henseleit (KH) buffer (6×10^6 cells in 3 ml of buffer) were incubated in sealed 25-ml flasks for 2 hr after adding sufficient liquid halothane to yield calculated gas phase concentrations of 312.5, 625, and 1250 ppm. Culture media samples were assayed for lactate (L; ●), pyruvate (P; ■), and glucose (G; ▲); L/P (□) was calculated. Values for L and G have been multiplied by 10^{-1} for convenience in scaling the figure. (B) For determination of gluconeogenesis only, the KH buffer was supplemented with lactate (5 m*M*) and pyruvate (1 m*M*) and G was determined in suspension media (▲) and hepatocytes (△). Results are reported as the mean of two assays on each of two like-treated cell cultures; the standard deviation was less than 5% of the mean in all cases. Comparison to control: ** $P < 0.02$, *** $P \leq 0.01$.

cellular LDH in untreated control cultures ($P \leq 0.02$); concentrations of halothane lower than 1250 ppm had no effect on LDH release compared to controls.

Interpretation of alterations in rates of glucose-utilizing or glucose-producing metabolic pathways by toxicants requires consideration of possible toxicant action in the cytosolic as well as the mitochondrial compartments. Although the enzymes effecting glucose metabolism are exclusively cytosolic, it has been amply demonstrated that toxicants which affect the tricarboxylic acid cycle or mitochondrial electron transport also alter rates of glycolysis. Thus, for an agent such as halothane, effects on glycolysis and gluconeogenesis may be potentially attributed to chemically induced decreases in the efficiency of aerobic ATP generation. Indeed, halothane has been shown to inhibit oxygen consumption in isolated mitochondria, presumably by imposing a blockade of the mitochondrial electron transport chain (28). Halothane apparently alters lipid–protein interactions directly by solvent activity, rather than through interactions of halothane-derived metabolites with membrane constituents, since hepatocytes from phenobarbital-treated rats exhibit impaired oxygen consumption and gluconeogenesis only to the same degree as cells from uninduced rats (29). Consequently, determination of the target site of action of a toxicant within the cell will invariably require further investigation, including analyses of factors such as ATP levels and rates of respiration.

In summary, determination of rates of glucose metabolism, as described, provides a simple and rapid metric for determination of the functional viability of isolated cells during exposure to known or suspected toxicants. Without reiterating the many advantages of the use of isolated rat hepatocytes, it should be pointed out that this cell type, because of inherently high rates of glycolysis, gluconeogenesis, and xenobiotic metabolism, is especially well suited for use as an indicator cell type in the study of chemically induced alterations in intermediary metabolism.

ACKNOWLEDGMENT

I am grateful to Charles A. Reidy, now at Eli Lilly & Co., Indianapolis, IN, for assistance during development and validation of the techniques described.

REFERENCES

1. H. O. Jauregui, N. T. Hayner, J. L. Driscoll, R. Williams-Holland, M. H. Lipsky, and P. M. Galletti, *In Vitro* **17**, 1100 (1981).
2. P. Moldeus, J. Hogberg, and S. Orrenius, in "Methods in Enzymology" (S. Fleischer and L. Packer, eds.), Vol. 52, p. 60. Academic Press, New York, 1978.
3. R. Zawydiwski and G. R. Duncan, *In Vitro* **8**, 707 (1978).
4. V. Shirhatti and G. Krishna, *Anal. Biochem.* **147**, 410 (1985).

5. F. Goethals, G. Krack, D. Deboyser, P. Vossen, and M. Roberfroid, *Fundam. Appl. Toxicol.* **4**, 441 (1984).
6. D. M. Bissell, L. Hammaker, and U. A. Meyer, *J. Cell Biol.* **59**, 722 (1973).
7. A. Athari, K. Unthan-Fechner, P. Schwartz, and I. Probst, *In Vitro* **24**, 1085 (1988).
8. J. F. Biebuyck, P. Lund, and H. A. Krebs, *Biochem. J.* **128**, 711 (1972).
9. R. Scholz, W. Hansen, and R. G. Thurman, *Eur. J. Biochem.* **38**, 64 (1973).
10. R. G. Thurman and R. Scholz, *Eur. J. Biochem.* **75**, 13 (1977).
11. G. M. Williams, E. Bermudez, and D. Scaramuzzino, *In Vitro* **13**, 809 (1977).
12. C. A. McQueen, this series, Vol. 1, Part A, p. 255.
13. F. Noll, *in* "Methods of Enzymatic Analysis" (H. U. Bergmeyer, ed.), Vol. VI, p. 582. Verlag Chemie, Deerfield Beach, Florida, 1984.
14. W. Lamprecht and F. Heinz, *in* "Methods of Enzymatic Analysis" (H. U. Bergmeyer, ed.), Vol. VI, p. 570. Verlag Chemie, Deerfield Beach, Florida, 1984.
15. A. Kunst, B. Draeger, and J. Ziegenhorn, *in* "Methods of Enzymatic Analysis" (H. U. Bergmeyer, ed.), Vol. VI, p. 163. Verlag Chemie, Deerfield Beach, Florida, 1984.
16. D. Keppler and K. Decker, *in* "Methods of Enzymatic Analysis" (H. U. Bergmeyer, ed.), Vol. VI, p. 11. Verlag Chemie, Deerfield Beach, Florida, 1984.
17. B. L. Kreamer, J. L. Staecker, N. Sawada, G. L. Sattler, M. T. S. Hsia, and H. C. Pitot, *In Vitro* **22**, 201 (1986).
18. H. A. Krebs and K. Henseleit, *Hoppe-Seyler's Z. Physiol. Chem.* **210**, 33 (1932).
19. H. U. Bergmeyer, *in* "Methods of Enzymatic Analysis" (H. U. Bergmeyer, ed.), Vol. VI, p. 694. Verlag Chemie, Deerfield Beach, Florida, 1984.
20. A. A. Welder and D. Acosta, this volume, Chapter 4.
21. M. J. Olson, C. A. Reidy, and J. T. Johnson, *Fundam. Appl. Toxicol.* **15**, 270 (1990).
22. T. Bucher, B. Brauser, A. Conze, F. Klein, O. Langguth, and H. Sies, *Eur. J. Biochem.* **27**, 301 (1972).
23. D. P. Jones and H. S. Mason, *J. Biol. Chem.* **253**, 4874 (1978).
24. P. O. Seglen, *Biochim. Biophys. Acta* **338**, 317 (1974).
25. B. R. Brown and I. G. Sipes, *Biochem. Pharmacol.* **26**, 2091 (1977).
26. S. A. Rice, M. Maze, C. M. Smith, J. C. Kosek, and R. I. Mazze, *Toxicol. Appl. Pharmacol.* **87**, 411 (1987).
27. J. F. Biebuyck and P. Lund, *Mol. Pharmacol.* **10**, 474 (1974).
28. B. A. Britt, W. Kalow, and L. Endrenyi, *Biochem. Pharmacol.* **21**, 1159 (1972).
29. A. A. J. Van Iersel, A. J. De Boer, C. W. M. Van Holsteijn, and B. J. Blaauboer, *Toxicol. in Vitro* **2**, 75 (1988).

15 Quantitation of DNA by Fluorometry

Sean R. Gallagher and Zbigniew Rymaszewski

INTRODUCTION

Quantitation of DNA by fluorometry with the fluorochrome Hoechst 33258 has many advantages over the more traditional absorption spectroscopy (1–4). These include greatly increased sensitivity, specificity, and dynamic range. Furthermore, contaminants such as protein and RNA do not normally interfere.

This chapter presents four DNA assays, all of which are based on the increased fluorescence of H33258 upon binding to DNA. Although other fluorochromes (e.g., ethidium bromide; Table I) have also been used for DNA quantitation, they generally also bind RNA and thus are not specific for DNA (4). However, for relatively pure samples, RNA-binding fluorochromes can be quite useful for RNA quantitation. Recently, several new DNA- and RNA-binding fluorochromes have been developed by Molecular Probes (Table I) (5). Because of their low intrinsic fluorescence and wide range of excitation and emission wavelengths, these fluorochromes show promise for a variety of applications and should readily adapt to the procedures presented below.

The first protocol is the standard assay. The second is a modification that permits isolating both intact DNA and mRNA during the same extraction. The last two procedures deal with small-volume measurements, one in a 9-μl capillary cuvette and other in 96-well microwell plates.

To perform the assay, a small amount of DNA (generally 1–1000 ng total) is mixed with the fluorochrome H33258 (365-nm excitation and 455-nm emission) in a high-salt neutral-pH buffer. A reading of this standard is taken in relative fluorescence units. Because the assay is linear over a wide range of DNA concentration, a one-point calibration is generally all that is required (see step 5 under the standard assay protocol). However, a multipoint calibration curve is useful to verify linearity over the range of DNA concentrations to be measured (see step 6 under the standard assay protocol). Once standardized, the concentration of DNA in the unknown is directly read from the instrument or determined with a calibration curve (see "Linear Regression," below).

METHODS IN TOXICOLOGY, Volume 1B

Table I Characteristics of Nucleic Acid Stains Used for DNA Quantitation[a]

Dye	EX_{max}/EM_{max} (nm)	Molecular weight	Specificity
H33258	346/460	533.89	DNA
DAPI (HCL)	359/461	350.25	DNA
Ethidium bromide	302, 510/595	394.31	DNA/RNA
Ethidium homodimer 1	528/617	856.77	DNA/RNA
YO-PRO-1	485/530	629.32	DNA/RNA

[a] EX, Excitation; EM, emission.

STANDARD ASSAY

The standard assay is based on the procedure of Labarca and Paigen (1). Designed for 2-ml assay volume in standard fluorometry cuvettes, typical sample volumes are 2 μl containing a minimum of 20 ng of DNA total. This is equivalent to a sample representing a total of 1000–2000 cells. The low-salt assay is suitable for reasonably purified DNA, while the high-salt assay is required for maximum fluorescence from samples of crude cell homogenates (1).

Equipment and Solution

Fluorometer, either fixed wavelength (TKO 100, Hoefer, San Francisco, CA) or variable wavelength (RF 5000, Shimadzu, Columbia, MD)

Fluorometry cuvette (because fluorometers detect at 90° relative to the excitation beam, fluorometry cuvettes are optically polished on all four sides. Spectrophotometer cuvettes are not recommended)

Pipette (0–2 or 0–10 μl)

10× TNE buffer [2.0 *M* NaCl, 100 m*M* Tris (free base), pH 7.4, and 10 m*M* Na_2EDTA; adjust the pH to 7.4 with concentrated HCL]

1× TNE buffer, low salt: Dilute 10× TNE buffer 1 : 10 with distilled water and filter (0.45 μm, MSI Dublin, CA, or equivalent) before use

1× TNE buffer, high salt (2.0 *M* NaCl, 10 m*M* Tris, pH 7.4, and 1 m*M* Na_2EDTA; adjust the pH to 7.4 with concentrated HCL). Filter (0.45 μM) before use

H33258 stock solution. Dilute to 1 mg/ml in distilled water. The stock is stable for at least 6 months at 4°C. Store away from light in an amber bottle. H33258 is a possible carcinogen and should be treated with caution. Wear gloves, goggles, and dust mask when weighing. Wash hands thoroughly after use

H33258 assay solution (0.1 μg/ml H33258), standard DNA concentration range. This will give a linear response over the range 10–500 ng DNA/ml (final assay concentration):
10 μl of H33258 stock mixed into 100 ml of 1× TNE buffer (low salt for purified or partially purified DNA or high salt for crude cell lysates)
H33258 assay solution (1 μg/ml H33258), extended DNA concentration range. This will give a linear response over the range 100–10,000 ng DNA/ml (final assay concentration):
100 μl H33258 stock mixed into 100 ml of 1× TNE buffer (low salt for purified or partially purified DNA or high salt for crude cell lysates)
DNA reference standard (must be high purity and intact double stranded; calf thymus, highly polymerized; Hoefer Cat. No. TKO 102; Sigma (St. Louis, MO) Cat. No. D-4764):
100 μg/ml in 1× TNE buffer (standard assay)
1000 μg/ml in 1× TNE buffer (extended-range assay)

Verify both concentration and purity of the DNA stock with absorption spectroscopy (A_{260} = 1.0 for 50 μg/ml; 0.2 for 10 μg/ml). High-purity DNA should have an optical density OD_{260}/OD_{280} ratio of 1.8 or better. Lower ratios indicate protein contamination (4).

Experimental Protocol

1. Set the excitation wavelength of the fluorometer to 365 nm and emission to 460 nm.
2. Pipette 2 ml of the assay solution into a fluorometer cuvette and place the cuvette into the fluorometer sample chamber. Make sure that the cuvette is in the same orientation for every reading.
3. Determine the relative fluorescence of the blank. Some instruments (e.g., TKO 100) permit adjusting of the blank to read zero at this point.
4. With the cuvette still in the sample chamber, pipette 2 μl of the DNA reference standard (100 μg/ml DNA for the standard concentration range assay and 1000 μg/ml for the extended-range assay) into the cuvette and mix by drawing solution in and out with a disposable pipette. Errors are common during small-volume pipetting. Use high-accuracy pipettes and minimize carryover by wiping the disposable tips after withdrawing the sample into the pipette.
5. Determine the relative fluorescence of the standard. Some instruments (e.g., TKO 100) permit setting the sensitivity so that the readout is in concentration units. For example, if 2 μl of the 100 μg/ml DNA standard is mixed with 2 ml of the assay solution, the final concentration of DNA is 100 ng/ml. By adjusting the fluorometer to read 100, all subsequent measurements are in units of DNA concentration.

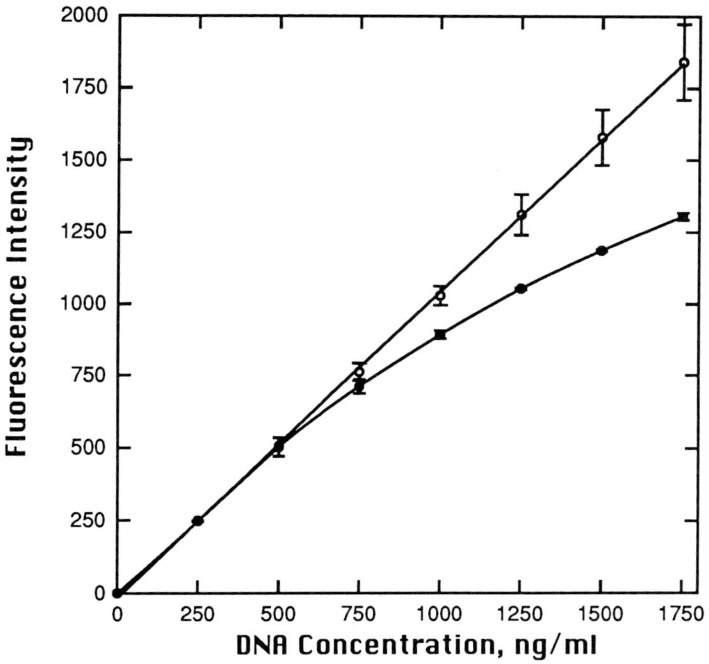

Figure 1 DNA standard curve. A 2-μl aliquot of calf thymus DNA was added to 2 ml of either 0.1 μg (●) or 1 μg (○) H33258 per milliliter of solution containing 0.2 *M* NaCl, 10 m*M* Tris-Cl, and 1.0 m*M* EDTA (pH 7.4). The higher dye concentration is required to extend the range of the assay above 500 ng DNA/ml.

6. Prepare a standard curve using 2, 4, 6, 8, and 10 μl of 100 (standard range; Fig. 1) or 1000 (extended range) μg/ml DNA. Two-microliter increments of the standard can also be added sequentially to the same assay solution to produce a standard curve. Verify the linearity by performing linear regression on the results (see "Linear Regression," below).

7. Repeat steps 3 and 4 for the unknown and determine the amount either from direct concentration readout or a standard curve.

mRNA EXTRACTION AND DNA QUANTITATION

The following protocol is designed to quantitate DNA under conditions that also allow isolation intact mRNA (6). Based on an acid guanidinium thiocyanate-phenol (AGTP) lysis procedure, the lysates can be stored for several weeks due to the stability of the DNA in AGTP. Prior to reading the sample, the lysate is treated with pH 13.3 EDTA followed by neutralization to pH 7.0 with KH_2PO_4.

Additional Equipment and Supplies

RNAzol B (AGTP; Biotecx, Houston, TX)
10 m*M* EDTA (pH 13.3)
1 *M* KH_2PO_4
Phosphate-buffered saline (PBS; 0.01 *M* NaH_2PO_4–Na_2HPO_4, 0.15 *M* NaCl, pH 7.4)
DNA standard (must be high purity and intact double-stranded DNA) (see under "Standard Assay"). Dilute 20 μl of 1 mg/ml calf thymus reference standard DNA in 0.98 ml of RNAzol to get 20 μg/ml and then, by serial dilution, to get 10, 5, 2.5, and 1.25 μg/ml in RNAzol. This is equivalent to DNA concentrations of 400, 200, 100, 50, and 25 ng per 20-μl sample

Experimental Protocol

Preparation of the Sample

1. Discard media from cultured cells. Wash cells gently with one volume of PBS.

2. Dissolve cells in no less than 0.2 ml of RNAzol/1 million cells (5 million cells/ml). Flux the cells with a wide-bore pipette 10 times to ensure that the cells are well dissolved.

3. Remove a portion of the lysate for DNA measurement and dilute it with RNAzol to a concentration in the range of 5000–100,000 cells/20 μl (i.e., 250,000 to 5 million cells/ml) (Fig. 2). For example, if step 2 gives a concentra-

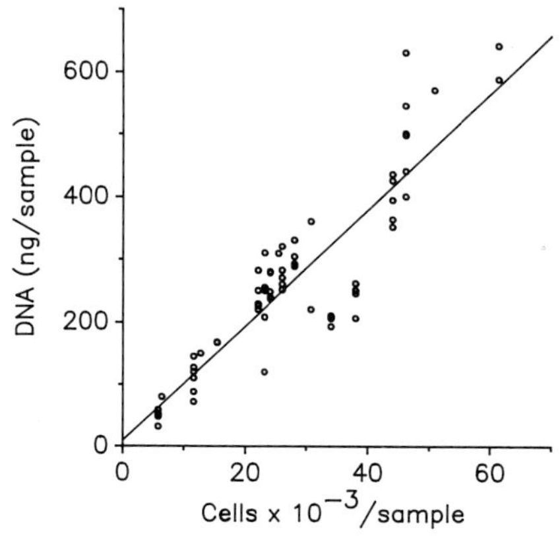

Figure 2 DNA content as a function of cell number in 69 separate determinations ("mRNA Extraction and DNA Quantitation") performed on human umbilical vein endothelial cells (hUVEC). Correlation coefficient r = 0.89, intercept 9.1 ± 17.9 ng, slope 9.2 ± 0.6 ng/10^3 cells (6).

tion of 10 million cells/ml (2 million cells/0.2 ml of RNAzol), then 100,000 cells = 10 μl. To get 100,000 cells/20 μl, simply add 10 μl of RNAzol to 10 μl of the original lysate.

4. Leave the sample from step 3 at room temperature for 2 hr. Samples may be stored for several weeks at 0–4°C before measurement.

Measurement

1. Add 20 μl of the standard DNA and 20 μl of the sample to separate 13 × 100-mm glass tubes.
2. Add 165 μl of 10 m*M* EDTA (pH 13.3) to each tube and vortex briefly. (Note: After addition of EDTA, the pH of the solution should be ≈12.3. Because the amount of water bound to the dry reagent varies, each time EDTA and KH_2PO_4 solutions are made up, the volume added must be checked to ensure that the correct pH is achieved.)
3. Place the tubes in a test tube rack and incubate in a water bath or oven at 36°C for 30 min. Allow them to cool to room temperature.
4. Add 120 μl of 1 *M* KH_2PO_4 and briefly shake the rack by hand. (Note: After addition of KH_2PO_4, the pH of the solution should be ≈7.3.)
5. To each tube add 2 ml of a 0.2 μg/ml H33258 dye solution made fresh from H33258 stock [diluted 1 mg/ml in distilled water; dilute 20 μl of stock per 100 ml of TNE (low-salt) buffer]. Briefly vortex.
6. Flux the solution a few times with a plastic pipette to mix. Let the samples stand in the dark for 5 min at room temperature.
7. The TKO 100 fluorometer should be on 15 min before taking measurements. Keep the samples in a covered box while not measuring.
8. Add blank solution to a clear cuvette to obtain a background reading. Remove the cuvette and measure standards and samples in separate cuvettes. Check the blank occasionally.

CAPILLARY ASSAY

Small-volume (3- to 9-μl) quantitation of DNA is possible in capillary tubes. To use the capillary system, the simplest approach is to mix 1 part of a 2× capillary assay solution (CAS) with 1 part DNA solution. To ensure accurate results, make sure that the blank solution used to zero the TKO 100 has the same final dye concentration as the samples containing DNA. For the Hoefer TKO 130 capillary holder (Fig. 3), the minimum volume of the sample solution needed in the 9-μl capillary tube is 3 μl. It may be necessary to mix up a little more than 3 μl of the sample solution to ensure that at least 3 μl gets into the capillary tube.

Although the total amount of DNA in the 9-μl capillary is small (detection limit, <1 ng total), the concentration is relatively high (e.g., 1 ng in 3 μl = 0.33 μg/ml). As the amount of DNA increases, so must the amount of H33258 in

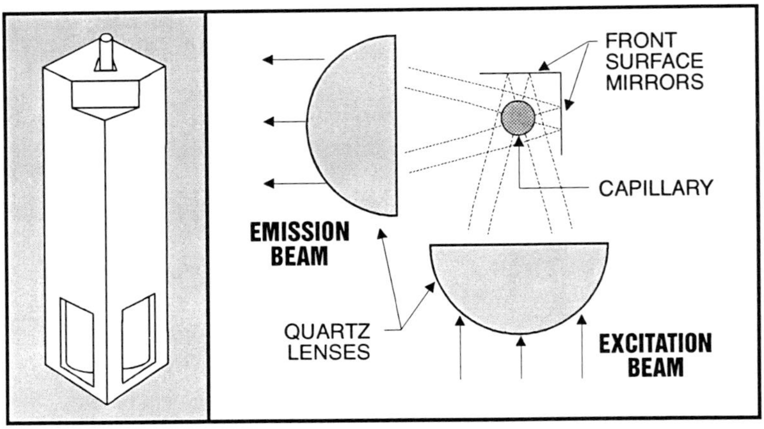

Figure 3 Capillary cuvette for fluorometers (Hoefer) is shown on the left. A 9-μl capillary containing the sample is inserted into the cuvette. Focusing lenses and mirrored surfaces provide increased sensitivity.

order to maintain assay linearity. Thus, two assay solutions for two ranges are presented below. (Note: It is important to avoid all sources of contamination. Use sterile pipette tips and sample tubes. Sterile gloves are also recommended. The TNE buffer should be made with double-distilled sterile water and highly pure chemicals.)

Equipment and Solutions

TKO 130 capillary cuvette kit (Fig. 3; from Hoefer) containing the cuvette that holds and positions the capillary tube, a vial of 9.33-μl capillary tubes, Critoseal (VWR Scientific) sealant for the ends of the tubes, and a hex wrench for cuvette disassembly and cleaning

2× CAS: For 1–100 ng total DNA (~0.11–11 μg/ml in 9-μl volume), use a concentration of H33258 of 2 μg/ml for the 2× CAS (see recipe 1 below). For 100–1000 ng total DNA in the capillary (~11–111 μg/ml in the 9-μl volume), use the 2× CAS containing 20 μg/ml H33258 (see recipe 2 below)

1. For 1–100 ng DNA (total): To make a 2 μg/ml H33258 solution in 1× TNE buffer, mix 100 μl of 10× TNE buffer (pH 7.4), 2 μl of H33258 stock solution, and 898 μl of water
2. For 100–1000 μg DNA (total): To make 20 μg/ml H33258 in 1× TNE buffer, mix 100 μl of 10× TNE buffer (pH 7.4), 20 μl of H33258 stock solution, and 880 μl of water

Experimental Protocol

1. Set the excitation wavelength to 365 nm and emission to 460 nm. Follow the manufacturer's instructions for the setup and calibration of the fluorometer. In general, set the instrument for maximum sensitivity.

2. Place the capillary cuvette into the cuvette well in the fluorometer.

3. Align the cuvette with the excitation light and emission detection window of the sample chamber, with the TKO 100 filter fluorometer, place the cuvette in the sample chamber with the beveled index corner oriented to the top right.

4. The vial containing the capillary tubes has a small hole in the lid. To remove one capillary tube at a time, invert the bottle and give it a gentle shake.

5. Prepare the sample blank and DNA standards (use Table II for low range standards):

a. For the blank, combine an equal volume of 1× TNE buffer and 2× CAS. (For example, use 5 μl of 1× TNE buffer and 5 μl of 2× CAS.)

b. Dissolve the DNA sample or standard in distilled water, TE (10m*M* Tris, 1m*M* Na_2 EDTA, pH 7.4), or 1× TNE buffer and add an equal volume of the 2× CAS. (For example, use 5 μl of DNA/TNE solution and 5 μl of 2× CAS.)

6. Place an end of the capillary tube into the blank or the DNA sample solution and allow it to flow into the capillary. If the fluid does not easily flow up the capillary tube, tilt the tube so that it is horizontal. Capillary action should be able to pull nonviscous fluids into the capillary in 1–2 sec. Wipe the bottom outside of the capillary tube with a tissue to remove any excess liquid, taking care that the tissue does not touch the bottom opening in the tube.

7. Gently insert the capillary tube containing the blank solution down the small square hole at the top center of the capillary cuvette. It should slide smoothly until it touches the bottom of the cell. If the tube does not fully insert, gently twist until it falls into place. At this point about 4 mm of the capillary will be sticking out the top of the cell. [Note: The capillary tube sits in a conical hole in the bottom of the cuvette so that the sample fluid does not touch the plastic walls of the cuvette. Thus, if the tube is inserted gently into the cuvette, the sample fluid should not leak out. You can use a very small plug of Critoseal sealant (no more than 0.25 mm) to prevent accidental leakage. Take care that the sealant does not protude into the optical path. Most sealants, including Critoseal, fluoresce strongly and can interfere with DNA measurements.]

8. Determine the relative fluorescence of the blank. Some instruments such as the TKO 100 fluorometer permit subtracting the blank at this point.

9. Remove the blank capillary tube and insert one containing a known DNA standard (Table II).

10. Construct a calibration curve as described under "Linear Regression."

11. Insert the capillary containing the sample DNA and record the fluorescence. Compare to the calibration curve to calculate sample DNA concentration.

Table II Preparation of DNA Standards for the Microwell Assay

μl of 10 μg/ml DNA	μl of 1 μg/ml DNA	μl of TE buffer	DNA (ng/100 μl)
100	0	0	1000
75	0	25	750
50	0	50	500
25	0	75	250
10	0	90	100
0	75	25	75
0	50	50	50
0	25	75	25
0	10	90	10
0	0	100	0

MICROWELL ASSAY

Based on the procedure of Rago *et al.* (7), the following protocol can be used with any microwell-measuring fluorometer. An important variation of this procedure that is useful for cells which are difficult to dissolve (e.g., keratinocytes and mucus-secreting cells) was developed by Rao and Otto (8) and is presented as an alternative. These procedures also adapt well to the capillary procedure outlined above. In addition, the reagents are available as a kit from Molecular Probes (Eugene, OR).

Additional Equipment and Solutions

Microwell-reading fluorometer (Millipore CytoFluor 2350, Bedford, MA; Fluoroskan II, ICN Biomedical, Costa Mesa, CA)

FluoReporter Blue Fluorometric Assay Kit (Molecular Probes Cat. No. F-2962). The kit comes complete with 1× TNE (high-salt) assay buffer and H33258 in dimethyl sulfoxide (DMSO) (2.5 mg/ml)

Assay solution: 6.2 μg/ml H33258 in TNE (1×, high salt). Mix either 25 μl of H33258 in DMSO (FluoReporter Blue Fluorometric Assay Kit) or 62 μl of 1 mg/ml H33258 stock with 10 ml of TNE buffer. This is enough for 100 assays in the 96-microwell format

DNA Standard Curve

Prepare 1 ml of a 1 μg/ml and 10 μg/ml stock DNA standard (calf thymus; Sigma Cat. No. D-4764 or Hoefer Cat. No. TKO 102) in 1× TNE buffer

Experimental Protocol

Preparation of the Calibration Curve

1. Using Table II, prepare DNA standards for the calibration curve and transfer the 100-μl aliquots to the microwells. Samples should be tested in duplicate.
2. Add 100 μl of the H33258 assay solution to the 100-μl standard solutions in the microwells.
3. Measure the fluorescence using excitation and emission filters at 360 and 460 nm, respectively. Alternate filters compatible with the excitation and emission of H33258 bound to DNA may also be used. On the Millipore CytoFluor 2350 set the sensitivity to 5 or 6.
4. Subtract reagent blank fluorescence from standard readings prior to further analysis.
5. Plot the fluorescence versus DNA amount per well. Calculate the slope of the curve to give the fluorescence intensity per nanogram of DNA (see "Linear Regression"). Steps 1–5 above should be repeated at the same time the cell lysate assay is performed below. The calibration curve from each individual experiment will be used to calculate the amount of DNA per cell.

Determination of the DNA Amount per Cell

1. Transfer adherent cells of interest into a concentrated cell stock (10^6 cells/ml) in normal medium.
2. Prepare serial dilutions of cells in microwells. Use 1000–100,000 cells per well in a volume of 100 μl. (Note: When first performing the assay, prepare a standard curve of known cell number using a hemocytometer.)
3. Incubate the plate at 37°C for the time required for the cells to attach (4–16 hr) or proliferate.
4. Empty wells at a desired end point by overturning them onto paper towels. Store the plate at −80°C. (Note: To increase the number of replicates so standard error is minimized, plates may be stored for several weeks at −80°C.)
5. Thaw the plates to room temperature and add 100 μl of distilled water per well.
6. Incubate at 37°C for 1 hr.
7. Freeze the plates to −80°C and then thaw to room temperature. [Note: This will cause rapid cell lysis and results in the release of DNA to form a relatively homogeneous solution. An alternative lysis solution consisting of sodium dodecyl sulfate in saline sodium citrate buffer (SDS–SSC; see below) for cells which are difficult to dissolve was developed by Rao and Otto (8). Furthermore, the SDS–SSC lysis solution makes the assay resistant to the loss of fluorescence caused by DNase activity. Briefly, after rinsing the wells containing the plated

cells twice with PBS, the wells are drained and either analyzed immediately or stored frozen. To each well (fresh or frozen), 100 μl of 0.02% SDS in 1× SSC (0.154 *M* NaCl, 0.015 *M* Na_3 citrate, pH 7.0) is added to lyse the cells; 8 *M* urea is added to the SDS–SSC lysis solution when analyzing keratinocytes. The plate is then incubated at 37°C for 1 hr with occasional agitation. One hundred microliters of 1.0 μg/ml H33258 in 1× SSC is then added to each well. Finally, the plate is read in a microwell-reading fluorometer. Standard DNA, dissolved in 100-μl aliquots of SDS–SSC, should be run in parallel with the cell samples.]

8. Add 100 μl of H33258 assay solution. (Note: Increase the final concentration of H33258 in solution (50 μl of DMSO stock [FluoReporter Blue Fluorometric Assay Kit] or 124 μl of the 1 mg/ml stock in 10 ml of TNE buffer) when measuring more than 100,000 cells per well. The higher dye concentration is required to maintain the linearity of the assay.)
9. Measure the fluorescence using excitation and emission filters at 360 and 460 nm, respectively. Alternate filters compatible with the excitation and emission of H33258 bound to DNA may also be used. On the Millipore CytoFluor 2350 set the sensitivity to 5 or 6.
10. Subtract the reagent blank fluorescence from sample and DNA standard readings prior to further analysis.
11. Calculate the amount of DNA per cell:

a. Determine the fluorescence per nanogram of standard DNA from the calibration curve (see above).
b. Determine the fluorescence per cell (see above).
c. ng of DNA/cell = fluorescence intensity per cell/fluorescence intensity per ng of DNA.

Using a calibration range of 5–500 ng of calf thymus DNA, a value of 13.3 pg of DNA per 3T3 cell was obtained (Molecular Probes).

LINEAR REGRESSION

Frequently, the fluorometer will give arbitrary fluorescence units and a calibration curve will be needed to determine the concentration of DNA.

Most scientific calculators or plotting programs will determine a calibration curve in the form of a linear regression through the data points. Consult your calculator manual or introductory statistics book for instructions. Thus:

For a line: $y = mx + b$, m = slope and $b = y$ intercept, or
Fluorescence = (slope)(DNA amount) + y intercept

To determine the amount of DNA, simply take the fluorescence value (preferably an average of three readings), subtract the averaged reagent blank fluorescence if necessary, and solve for x, the DNA amount, using the following formula:

$$x = (y - b)/m$$

Thus, DNA amount = (Fluorescence reading − y intercept)/slope.

COMMENTS

The fluorescence measured in this assay is due to the interaction between H33258 and DNA. Typically, the DNA is mixed with H33258 suspended in pH 7.4 TNE assay solution and the fluorescence per microgram of DNA is determined. A neutral pH is required to minimize background fluorescence (1), while the high ionic strength (>200 m*M* NaCl) is recommended to maximize fluorescence of the H33258–DNA complex (see also below). A combination of low ionic strength (<100 m*M* NaCl) and high concentration of H33258 (e.g., 1 μg/ml) can result in no fluorescence increase when DNA is added.

The amount of fluorescence and the linearity of the assay are a function of both the concentration of the DNA and the H33258 dye in the assay solution. However, because unbound dye fluorescences, excess H33258 can be a major cause of poor sensitivity. New dyes such as YO-PRO-1 (5) exhibit a much larger fluorescence increase upon DNA binding than H33258, and consequently produce lower unbound fluorescence background signals. However, these dyes, unlike H33258, are sensitive to RNA (see Table I). In contrast, too little dye relative to the amount of DNA will cause a nonlinear tailing downward and eventual flattening of the standard curve (Fig. 1). Thus, depending on the final volume of the assay and the amount of DNA to be measured, the concentration of H33258 ranges from 0.1 to 20 μg/ml. In general, to maintain linearity, the ratio of DNA to H33258 (w/w) should be no higher than 5–10.

The fluorescence per microgram of DNA is also dependent on the DNA composition (1–3,9). H33258 preferentially binds to double-stranded AT sequences of DNA. Loontiens *et al.* (10) has provided a detailed description of the binding properties of H33258. Like the DNA binding fluorochrome 4′,6-diamidino-2-phenylinode (DAPI), H33258 also shows a relationship between log fluorescence units and GC mol% (9). In practice, this is not usually a problem with animal DNA, in which the composition is ≈42% GC (11) and calf thymus DNA is a suitable standard. However, with prokaryotic DNA the composition can vary tremendously depending on the organism and the standard DNA should be close in composition to the DNA to be measured. High-purity DNA of varied GC% can be purchased from Sigma. 5-Bromouridine incorporated into the DNA will also reduce fluorescence (10).

In addition to the GC%, DNA strandedness also affects fluorescence. Single-stranded genomic DNA gives about one-half the fluorescence of the double-stranded DNA (1). Although small double-stranded DNA fragments (e.g., polymerase chain reaction products) also work well with this assay, small single-stranded pieces of DNA (e.g., oligonucleotides) yield little or no fluorescence and cannot be accurately quantitated with H33258.

Very few compounds interfere with the DNA assay. RNA and protein, in particular, do not significantly affect the readings when the assay is performed under optimal conditions (1,3). SDS will, however, interfere and cause both higher readings and nonlinearity when above a final assay concentration of 0.01% (3) to 0.04% (8). It is likely that any detergent present in a concentration above its critical micelle concentration will cause a similar interference.

Caution must also be used when either quenching agents or other fluorescent compounds are present in the sample, and a standard curve using known quantities of purified DNA should be used in the presence of the sample to verify the accuracy of the assay (1,2).

Proteins that interact with DNA will reduce fluorescence, presumably by preventing the H33258 from fully binding (1). Under these conditions (e.g., crude homogenates) several methods of solubilization have been developed. NaCl(2 *M*) was originally recommended by Labarca and Paigen (1) to enhance fluorescence by minimizing protein binding to the DNA, and Rago *et al.* (7) used freeze–thaw lysis in combination with 2 *M* NaCl to develop the microwell plate assay described above. The freeze–thaw microwell lysis procedure may result in reduced assay sensitivity with cells that produce excessively particulate suspensions, such as mucus-secreting gastrointestinal tumor cells or fibrous protein-containing keratinocytes (8). In place of distilled water, a lysis solution of 0.02% SDS in 1× SSC is recommended in order to maximize the assay sensitivity and minimize nuclease degradation. An additional 8 *M* urea is required to efficiently lyse and disperse keratinocytes.

Downs and Wilfinger (12) found that, during cell lysis or whole-tissue homogenization, intact DNA was most efficiently solubilized with an ammonium hydroxide–Triton X-100 solution. A commercial kit for the Downs and Wilfinger (12) procedure is available from Pierce (Rockford, IL). An alternative for tissue-cultured mammalian cells was developed by West *et al.* (13) in which DNA is extracted with pH 12.5 EDTA. After neutralization to pH 7.0, the DNA is quantitated with the standard H33258 assay. In the second protocol above, Rymaszewski *et al.* (6) modified this EDTA extraction procedure to permit both mRNA and DNA quantitation.

CONCLUSION

Fluorometric detection and quantitation of DNA with H33258 combines specificity, speed, and high sensitivity into one simple assay. Accurately detecting DNA in cell lysates without interference from RNA and protein makes this procedure unique. Lower detection limits range from 1 to 10 ng of DNA total in assay volumes extending from 3 μl to 2 ml. Furthermore, the assay can be automated through the use of microwell-reading fluorometers. With the development of new fluorochromes, it is likely that the applications for fluorometric DNA quantitation will continue to expand.

ACKNOWLEDGMENTS

We thank Iain Johnson and Liz Marcus (Molecular Probes) for their help in preparing the section titled "Microwell Assay" and for reviewing the final manuscript.

REFERENCES

1. C. Labarca and K. Paigen, *Anal. Biochem.* **102,** 344 (1980).
2. C. F. Brunk, K. C. Jones, and T. W. James, *Anal. Biochem.* **92,** 497 (1979).
3. C. F. Cesarone, C. Bolognesi, and L. Santi, *Anal. Biochem.* **100,** 188 (1979).
4. S. R. Gallagher, *in* "Current Protocols in Molecular Biology" (F. A. Ausubel, R. Brent, R. E. Kingston, D. D. Moore, J. G. Seidman, J. A. Smith, and K. Struhl, eds.), pp. A.3.9–A.3.15. Greene and Wiley (Interscience), New York, 1989.
5. R. P. Haugland, "Molecular Probes Handbook of Fluorescent Probes and Research Chemicals." Molecular Probes, Eugene, Oregon, 1992.
6. Z. Rymaszewski, W. A. Abplanalp, R. M. Cohen, and P. Chomczynski, *Anal. Biochem.* **188,** 91 (1990).
7. R. Rago, J. Mitchen, and G. Wilding, *Anal. Biochem.* **191,** 31 (1990).
8. J. Rao and W. R. Otto, *Anal. Biochem.* **207,** 186 (1992).
9. G. A. Daxhelet, M. M. Coene, P. P. Hoet, and C. G. Cocito, *Anal. Biochem.* **179,** 401 (1989).
10. F. G. Loontiens, P. Regenfuss, A. Zechel, L. Dumortier, and R. M. Clegg, *Biochemistry* **29,** 9029 (1990).
11. J. Marmur and P. Doty, *J. Mol. Biol.* **5,** 109 (1962).
12. T. R. Downs and W. W. Wilfinger, *Anal. Biochem.* **131,** 538 (1983).
13. D. C. West, A. Sattar, and S. Kumar, *Anal. Biochem.* **147,** 289 (1985).

16 Techniques for Measuring Cell Proliferation

Frank Dolbeare and Martin Vanderlaan

INTRODUCTION

Exposure to chemicals and radiation in the environment can inhibit cell growth by blocking mitosis, delaying entry into the DNA synthesis phase (S phase) of the cell cycle, and/or slowing progression through the S phase. In addition, increased cell proliferation is also sometimes observed following chemical or radiation exposure as a consequence of wounding or inflammation. Several methods are available for determining the level of cell proliferation in toxicology studies. These methods are based on the incorporation into newly synthesized DNA of either radiolabeled nucleosides or halogen-containing analogs of thymidine. Cells are exposed to a nucleoside analog (either radiolabeled or halogen labeled), which is transported into the cell, phosphorylated with appropriate kinases, and incorporated into DNA. Incorporated radioactive analogs are detected using radiographic film or scintillation counting, while incorporated halogen analogs are detected immunocytochemically with antibodies.

The incorporation of tritiated thymidine ([^{3}H]dThd) was originally used to study cell proliferation in plant root cells (1). This study led to the formulation of a specific equation for the progress of cells through the cell cycle. The addition of a second label, ^{14}C-labeled thymidine or cytosine, permitted a more complex interpretation of cell cycle events (2–4).

Radiolabel incorporation may be quantified either in batches of cells by liquid scintillation counting or by scoring individual cells with the radiolabel, as visualized by autoradiography. In the former case only the overall DNA synthesis rate of a population of cells can be determined. This average statistic for the population is occasionally sufficient. For example, in the case of mixed lymphocyte cultures, cells do not synthesize DNA unless they are stimulated by foreign major histocompatibility antigens. The alternative quantification method, that of counting the fraction of cells with silver grains formed in autoradiography film, results in more precise definition of cell cycle parameters (see Fig. 1). Following a pulse exposure to [^{3}H]dThd, for example, the fraction of cells with radiolabel is the fraction of cells in S phase at the time of the pulse. Continuous exposure to [^{3}H]dThd causes all cells that pass through S phase during the exposure period

METHODS IN TOXICOLOGY, Volume 1B

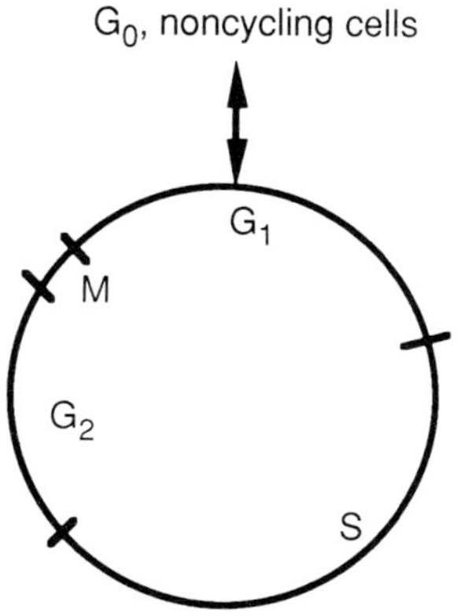

Figure 1 The cell cycle may be divided into four periods: G_1, prior to DNA replication; S, when DNA is replicated and nucleoside analogs are incorporated into nascent DNA; G_2, following DNA synthesis; and M, mitosis.

to become labeled. If the exposure to [^{3}H]dThd is long relative to the cycle time, then any cells remaining unlabeled must be from a noncycling (G_0) subpopulation. A variable time delay between a pulse of [^{3}H]dThd and sampling allows some of the labeled S phase cells to progress to mitosis, and the fraction of labeled mitosis may then be scored. By varying the time interval between [^{3}H]-dThd pulse and sample collection, one can estimate the rate of progression of the cells through the cycle and the total cell cycle time. Alternatively, cell progression can be measured using two-pulse exposures with distinguishable radiolabels (e.g., double labeling with [^{3}H]dThd and [^{14}C]dThd given at different times).

The introduction of antibodies developed against bromodeoxyuridine (BrdUrd) (5–7) permitted the immunochemical quantification of BrdUrd incorporated into DNA. In this case antibodies are used as immunological reagents to quantitate halogenated thymidine analogs incorporated into DNA. Depending on specificity, antibodies will detect either BrdUrd or iododeoxyuridine (IdUrd) or both when associated with DNA. With fluorescently tagged antibodies and the appropriate staining technique, the florescence intensity is proportional to the amount of BrdUrd incorporated and may be quantified by flow or image cytometry. The BrdUrd method also avoids the necessity of having to use radiolabeled chemicals and possible contamination or disposal problems. The use of flow cytometers to quantify the fraction of labeled cells eliminates the tedium associated with microscopically scoring labeled cells based on autoradiography. Alternatively, antibodies may be tagged with enzymes or colloidal gold and used to stain histological sections for the presence of BrdUrd-containing cells.

DNA-intercalating fluorophores (e.g., propidium iodide [PI], Hoechst 33342, and ethidium bromide) allow quantification of the DNA content of individual cells. G_1 and G_2 cells differ by a factor of 2 in DNA content. Intermediate DNA values are found in S phase cells, with the amount of DNA increasing as the cells traverse the S phase. While measurement of DNA content alone can provide a reasonable estimation of the fraction of cells in the G_1, S, and G_2 phases, the measurement is often compromised. Coefficients of variation in the DNA measurements greater than a few percent lead to significant spillover of the G_1 and G_2 cells into the region of intermediate DNA content occupied by the S phase cells. Single-parameter DNA analysis also fails when used with perturbed cell populations, in which the majority of cells are in the S or G_2 phase, as may occur in toxic exposure studies (8).

The incorporation of BrdUrd into cells offers a more accurate estimation of the fraction of cells in S phase than does DNA measurement alone, and the optimal method is the simultaneous measurement of both DNA content and incorporated BrdUrd in each cell (9). Two-parameter histograms of cell populations, as illustrated in Fig. 2, resolve all cell populations. In this figure fluorescein-conjugated anti-BrdUrd antibodies provide a green fluorescent signal that is proportional to incorporated BrdUrd and plotted on a logarithmic y axis. PI intercalation provides a red fluorescent signal that is proportional to DNA content and is plotted on a linear x axis. G_1 and G_2 cells are low in green fluorescence, but are well resolved on the basis of red fluorescence. S phase cells have intermediate DNA contents, but are readily distinguished by their green fluorescence staining.

BrdUrd label can be used in a fashion analogous to those developed for $[^3H]$dThd to provide detailed cell kinetics measurements. Continuous exposure to BrdUrd provides an estimate of the fraction of noncycling cells, and pulse–chase experiments provide quantitative measures of cell cycle progression. For use with human material, in which only limited sampling may be practical, the pulse–chase approach has been refined to a single time point method (10). The introduction of halogen-selective antibodies (e.g., anti-BrdUrd selective and anti-IdUrd selective) (11,12) allows double-labeling experiments such as those using ^3H and ^{14}C.

A third method of estimating cell proliferation depends on the appearance of specific antigens as the result of cell cycle phase-dependent protein synthesis during progression through the cell cycle. Proteins such as proliferating cell nuclear antigen (PCNA, or cyclin) (13,14) and Ki67 (15) are produced in G_1 in advance of DNA replication, remain high during active synthesis, and are degraded to almost zero by mitosis. The fraction of antigen-positive cells is therefore generally larger than the fraction of S phase cells, and the antigen cannot be followed during cell progression as in pulse–chase methods. The advantage of staining for these antigens over the other methods lies primarily with clinical studies, in which one does not have to expose a patient to $[^3H]$dThd or BrdUrd.

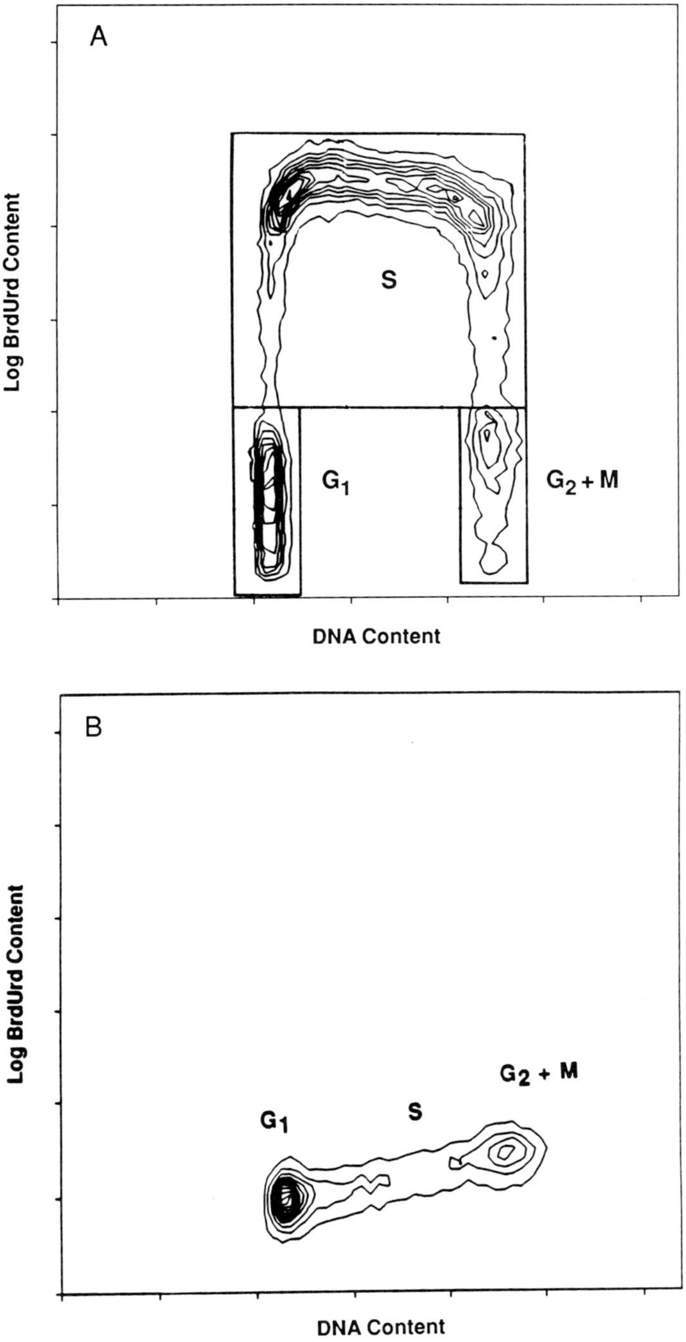

Figure 2 (A) Bivariate histogram showing DNA content (linear *x* axis, propidium iodide fluorescence) and bromodeoxyuridine (BrdUrd) content (logarithmic *y* axis, fluorescein fluorescence) of Chinese hamster ovany (CHO) cells following a 30-min pulse of 1 m*M* BrdUrd. (B) Bivariate histogram showing DNA content and BrdUrd content of CHO cells not receiving BrdUrd pulse.

A disadvantage is that these antigens are often fixation sensitive, and may not be detectable after routine tissue-processing methods.

A review of the flow-cytometric analysis of cell cycle-related antigens has recently been published (16). Some of these proteins are involved with the mechanisms of DNA replication and cell cycle regulation (e.g., DNA polymerase α, which is maximally expressed during the S phase). In addition to the S phase-associated nuclear antigens PCNA and Ki67, another nuclear antigen, p105 is expressed maximally in G_2, and a membrane antigen, transferrin, is expressed maximally at the G_1/S boundary. Statin, a nuclear envelope antigen, has the reverse expression pattern, being expressed maximally in quiescent G_0 cells. Some oncogene products also show variation in expression during the cell cycle.

This chapter presents laboratory procedures for quantifying [^{3}H]dThd and halogenated pyrimidine incorporation into DNA and immunochemical procedures for the quantification of PCNA and Ki67. We also present alternative methods with a discussion of some of the applications, technical problems associated with the methods, and possible advantages and disadvantages of each method.

APPLICATIONS

General Comments on the Measurement of Cell Proliferation

Incorporation of labeled nucleosides can be used for the *in vitro* and *in vivo* assay of cell proliferation and cell cycle kinetic measurements. Specific effects of agents which stimulate cell proliferation, block specific phases of the cell cycle, or slow the progression through the cell cycle can be quantified. The combination of one or more nucleoside analogs with varying amounts of time between cell exposure and sample collection can be used to determine the total cell cycle time and the duration of the various cell cycle compartments.

One application is determination of the fraction of cells in the S phase. Typical S phase durations in mammalian cells are 5–15 hr, so a pulse exposure of 0.5 hr to labeled nucleosides will label only those cells actively in the S phase. Lighter-than-average incorporation of label will occur for those cells entering and leaving the S phase during the time of the pulse. For *in vivo* exposures an exogenously administered analog is rapidly cleared from the blood, effectively limiting the pulse of exposure to about 30 min.

Pulse–chase experiments provide more detailed data on cell kinetics. After a brief exposure to labeled nucleoside, cells are allowed to progress thorough the cell cycle before sampling. The quantitative equations for determining phase durations (e.g., time duration of G_1, time duration of S phase, and cell cycle time), were derived by Takahashi (2). The mathematics provided by these models are beyond the scope of this methods chapter; however, a simplified mathematical equation can describe the movement of cells from compartment to compartment (17). For example, the rate of change in the number of cells in compartment i at time t, $N_i(t)$, might be described as:

$$dN_i(t)/dt = \lambda_{i-1}N_{i-1}(t) - \lambda_i N_i(t)$$

where λ_i defines the rate at which cells leave compartment i + 1. For compartment 1, the equation becomes

$$dN_1(t)/dt = 2\lambda_k N_k(t) - \lambda_1 N_1(t)$$

where k is the number of the last compartment in the cycle and the factor 2 takes account of the fact that the cell number doubles as cells move from the G_2/M phase to the G_1 phase.

Other applications of labeled nucleoside analog techniques include (1) analogs incorporated into DNA during the repair of DNA damage (unscheduled DNA synthesis) (18,19), (2) incorporation of BrdUrd into DNA for demonstrating sister chromatid exchanges by fluorescent antibody labeling (20), and (3) isolation of nascently replicated DNA using immunoaffinity columns directed against incorporated BrdUrd (21).

Comments on Tritiated Thymidine Labeling

The method is suitable for autoradiographic analysis of cells mounted on slides (e.g., cells grown on slides or centrifuged onto slides, or slide-mounted histological sections) and the scintillation quantification of radioactivity in batches of cells treated with dThd. Cell cycle analysis may also be performed by incorporating pulse-labeled analog into growing cells, staining the cells with an appropriate DNA stain, and then sorting a fixed number of cells from cell cycle phase fractions onto glass fiber filters for quantification by scintillation counting (22).

Comments on BrdUrd Labeling

The primary applications of the technique are the quantification of cell cycle phase fractions, phase durations, doubling time, labeling index, and growth fractions. The method has been applied to the analysis of cells from dispersed solid tumors, various leukemias, bone, spleen, liver, bladder epithelia, neural, dermal, and cultured mammalian cells. One may use multiple (9) or single sample points (10,23) to obtain labeling index and potential doubling times. The method can also be used to measure DNA repair synthesis (18,19). A modification of the method has been used to determine the fraction of cells in mitosis as well as in G_1, S, and G_2 (24). More recently, simplified methods have permitted the detection not only of BrdUrd and DNA but also surface antigens for lymphoid subset typing (25). Clinical studies have been conducted to determine the proliferation rate of tumor and normal cells, and to monitor the efficacy of cell cycle phase-selective chemotherapeutic agents and radiation. For these, either the patient is infused with BrdUrd or tissue samples are incubated in media containing the analog (26). For example, in the study by Shibuya *et al.*, cited in detail in the following methods sections, human subjects with brain tumors were infused with BrdUrd (30 min, 200 mg/m^2), and tissue samples were removed during surgery and then incubated in culture medium containing 100 μM IdUrd for 1 hr at 37°C.

Comments Specific to Proliferation Antigens

PCNA (also called cyclin), Ki67, p105, DNA polymerase α, and transferrin are endogenous protein antigens whose expression level are often linked to the cell cycle. Their detection implies that cells are proliferating, since they are found only at reduced levels, if at all, in nonproliferating cells. Several studies have attempted to link the expression level of these antigens to tumor grade and prognosis with varying levels of success. The significance of staining results must be established in the context of each tissue and experimental system studied.

MATERIALS

Materials Common to All Protocols

A cell source, typically logarithmically growing cultured cells with appropriate culture medium, or animal tissue

Phosphate-buffered saline (PBS), containing 0.15 *M* NaCl and 0.05 *M* sodium phosphate, pH 7.2

Materials for Tritiated Thymidine Labeling

5′-Methyl-[^{3}H]thymidine with a specific activity of ~40 Ci/mmol: Diluted [^{3}H]dThd to 0.1–0.2 mCi/ml final concentration in culture media

Ice-cold methanol/acetic acid (3/1, v/v) or cold 70% ethanol

Autoradiographic emulsion (Kodak Track Emulsion, Type ANTB2, Kodak, Rochester, NY)

Photographic developer (Model D19, Kodak)

Photographic fixative (Kodafix Kodak)

Counter stains, such as dilute Giemsa in water or hematoxylin and eosin

10% Cold trichloroacetic acid in water

70% Ethanol in water

Glass fiber filters, 1 μm (Millipore, Bedford, MA)

Scintillation vials (Packard, Downers Grove, IL)
Liquid scintillation fluid (e.g., Universol, ICN Biomedicals, Irvine, CA)
Scintillation counter (e.g., Model LS8100, Beckman, Fullerton, CA)

Materials for the Detection of Incorporated BrdUrd for Flow Cytometry

Pyrimidines: 5-BrdUrd, 5-IdUrd, 5-FdUrd, and dCytd, reagent grade (Sigma, St. Louis, MO)

Anti-halopyrimidine antibody: We describe below procedures using monoclonal antibodies against either BrdUrd or IdUrd. Animal antisera derived against one of the halopyrimidines may also be used, but historically these have lacked the needed selectivity. Table I lists commercially available anti-BrdUrd antibodies. The final sensitivity of the measurement depends on the purity, affinity, and specificity of the particular antibody. High-affinity antibodies permit quantification of low levels of BrdUrd incorporation (e.g., <0.1% substitution) (27). Antibodies directly conjugated to fluorophores may be used, or the anti-BrdUrd antibodies may be detected using indirect immunochemical methods. For methods involving the simultaneous detection of cell surface antigens and BrdUrd, direct conjugates are required. The monoclonal antibody pair of IU-4 and Br-3 (Caltag, South San Francisco, CA) allows double labeling with IdUrd and BrdUrd, since Br-3 shows halogen selectivity in binding, preferring BrdUrd to IdUrd (11,12)

Antibody diluting buffer: PBS as described above containing 2× salt sodium citrate (SSC = 0.15 *M* NaCl + 0.015 *M* sodium citrate) and 0.5% Tween-20 (Sigma) with a blocking protein to limit nonspecific sticking of the antibody. The blocking protein may be 1% bovine serum albumin (BSA), 1% gelatin, or 2% dry nonfat milk protein

RNase A stock solution: RNase A (Sigma Cat. No. R-5503) at 0.5 mg/ml in PBS. This solution may be stored for up to 6 months, refrigerated with 0.1 mg/ml sodium azide

Paraformaldehyde solution, electron microscopy grade (Polyscience, Warrington, PA): Prepare stock solution of 0.25% or 1% paraformaldehyde in PBS, pH 7.2

0.1 *M* HCl plus 0.5% Triton X-100: 5 g of Triton X-100 (Sigma) in 1 liter of 0.1 *M* HCl

Wash buffer: 5g of Tween-20 in 1 liter of PBS

Goat anti-mouse immunoglobulin G(IgG)–fluorescein conjugate: This antibody may be obtained from a number of sources (see *Linscott's Directory of Immunological and Biological Reagents,* published by Linscott's Directory). Depending on the particular needs of the experiment (e.g., membrane antigen labeling in addition to BrdUrd/DNA analysis), one

Table I Commerical Sources of Anti-Bromodeoxyuridine Antibodies[a]

Clone	Ig Type	State	Source
>1	IgG_1	Purified	Bioclone Australia
3D9	IgG_1	Purified	Oncogen Science
3D9	IgG_1	Purified–FITC	Oncogene Science
76-7	IgG_1	Purified	Amac, Biodesign, Serotec, and Sigma
B44	IgG_1	Purified	Becton Dickinson
B44	IgG_1	Purified–FITC	Becton Dickinson
BMC9318	IgG_1	Purified	Boehringer Mannheim
		Purified–FITC	Boehringer Mannheim
Br3	IgG_1	Purified	Caltag
Br3	IgG_1	Purified–biotin	Caltag
Br3		Purified–FITC	Caltag
BU5.1	IgG_{2a}	Purified/purified–FITC	Cymbus Bioscience, IBL Research Products, Paesel & Lorei, and Progen Biotechnik
BU1-75	Rat IgG	Ascites	Sera-Labs
		Purified	Accurate Chemical
		Supernatant	—
BU6-4	IgG_1	Purified	Pierce
Bu20a	IgG_1	Supernatant	Dako
BU-33	IgG_1	Purified	Sigma
MBU	IgG_1	Ascites	Medscand
IU4	IgG_1	Purified	Caltag
SB18	IgG_1	Ascites	Accurate Chemical
			Medica
			Sanbio
ZBU30	IgG_1	Purified	Zymed
		Purified–alkaline phosphatase	Zymed
		Purified–biotin	Zymed
		Purified–FITC	Zymed
		Purified–peroxidase	Zymed
		Purified–phycoerythrin	Zymed
Anti-BrdUrd	IgG_1	Ascites	Chemicon
Anti-BrdUrd	?		Janssen Biochimica and Accurate Chemical

[a] Most of the sources are listed in *Linscott's Directory of Immunological and Biological Reagents,* 7th ed., obtainable from Linscott's Directory, (Santa Rosa, CA). Complete addresses of all of the above sources and their international distributors are given in the directory. FITC, Fluorescein isothiocyanate.

may require an alternative fluorophore as a conjugate, such as the blue-emitting fluorophore aminomethylcoumarin acetic acid (AMCA) or a red-emitting fluorophore, such as Texas red, Princeton red, or phycoerythrin (Molecular Probes, Eugene, OR)

PI (Sigma): The working solution is 10 μg/ml in PBS, pH 7.2. A stock solution of 1 mg/ml PI in 70% ethanol stored in the refrigerator is stable for at least 1 year. PI is a suspected carcinogen and should be handled with proper caution

Exonuclease III and EcoRI: 10 Units of each enzyme per 1 ml of cell suspension (Bethesda Research Laboratories, Gaithersburg, MD)

0.1 *M* citric acid/0.5% Triton X-100

EcoRI buffer (see recommendations of the manufacturer for specific endonucleases): 0.1 *M* Tris-HCl (pH 7.5) containing 50 m*M* NaCl and 10 m*M* $MgCl_2$

Exonuclease III buffer: 50 m*M* Tris-HCl, (pH 8.0), 10 m*M* 2-mercaptoethanol, and 5 m*M* $MgCl_2$

100-μm nylon mesh (Small Parts, Miami Lakes, FL)

Labeling of Surface Antigens in Combination with BrdUrd Labeling

A biotin-conjugated antibody to cell surface antigen, such as biotin coupled with anti-CD4 (Becton Dickinson, San Jose, CA)

Streptavidin–phycoerythrin (Becton Dickinson)

1% Paraformaldehyde with 0.01% Tween-20 (Sigma)

DNase I (Sigma Cat. NO. D-4527): 50 Kunitz U/ml in PBS containing 1 m*M* Ca^{2+} and 4 m*M* Mg^{2+}

Reagents for Staining of BrdUrd in Tissue Sections on Slides

While there are many suitable techniques for immunohistochemical staining of paraffin-embedded histological sections, we have chosen the method of Shibuya *et al.* (26) as a particularly elegant illustration of the methods. This study reports methods for dual labeling of both incorporated BrdUrd and IdUrd, using the halogen-selective monoclonal antibody pair Br-3 and IU-4 and a combination of alkaline phosphatase enzyme immunohistochemistry and immunogold staining. Simpler methods can be developed by the reader, using parts of this comprehensive method.

6-μm histological sections mounted on glass slides from tissues exposed to BrdUrd and/or IdUrd, fixed in 70% ethanol, paraffin embedded, and sectioned.

4 N HCl

2.5% Glutaraldehyde

Gold-conjugated goat anti-mouse IgG and the silver enhancement kit (IntenSE M, Amersham, Arlington Heights, IL)

5% Acetic acid in water

Tris-buffered saline (TBS): 50 m*M* Tris (pH 7.6) and 0.15 *M* NaCl

Alkaline phosphate-conjugated rabbit anti-mouse Igs (Dako, Carpinteria, CA)
Alkaline phosphatase substrate kit I (Vector Immunochemicals, Burlingame, CA)
5% Gills No. 1 hematoxylin (Sigma)
Histo-Clear (National Diagnostics, Manville, NJ)
Permount (Fisher, Fairlawn, NJ)

Materials for Staining Proliferation Antigens

Antibodies: Fluorescein isothiocyanate (FITC) conjugated monoclonal Ki67 antibody (Accurate Chemical and Scientific, Westbury, NY) or PCNA antibody (Coulter, Hialeah, FL)
PI as a stock solution 1 mg/ml in 70% ethanol as noted above
Lysing solution: 0.5% Triton X-100, 1% BSA, 0.2 mg/ml EDTA in PBS
Fixatives: 70% ethanol at −20°C or 0.5% paraformaldehyde chilled on ice

INSTRUMENTS

General

Tissue culture facility or animal colony

Thymidine Labeling

Standard bright-field microscope with a 60× or 100× objective
Manual counter
Scintillation counter (optional, depending on the method)
Automated grain-counting image acquisition and processing software for the microscope (e.g., Quantimet 720 Image-Analysis System 20, Cambridge Instruments, Monsey, NY) (28).

BrdUrd Labeling

Any flow cytometer equipped with a single argon ion laser with two photomultiplier tubes is adequate. The instrument should also be equipped with a log amplifier to accommodate the large range of fluorescence signal generated by the anti-BrdUrd fluorescence. Both fluorescein and PI can be excited at 488 nm. Use a 514-nm band-pass filter for the fluorescein fluorescence (BrdUrd content) and a 600-nm long-pass filter for the PI fluorescence (DNA content). If AMCA is used as the fluorophore for antibodies, then excitation is at 363 nm and a 450-nm band-pass filter is used. The incorporation of a doublet eliminator will prevent accumulation of doublet G_1 and early S phase cells in windows that should contain either G_2 or late S phase cells

A phase or fluorescent microscope, depending on whether a fluorescent or enzyme-conjugated anti-BrdUrd is employed, can be used to determine labeling indices of cells stained on slides

Proliferation Antigens

Fluorescent microscope with filter combinations to view two-color fluorescence

Flow cytometer equipped with argon ion laser with 488-nm excitation and optical filters to allow discrimination between green and red fluorescence as described above

PROCEDURES

General Procedure for Incorporation of Nucleotide Analogs

Cells grown exponentially at a concentration of 10^5/ml under normal culture conditions used by investigators. [^{3}H]dThd or BrdUrd should be added to the culture in conditioned media at 37°C to prevent shock to the cells that might temporarily modify their proliferation. Final concentration of [^{3}H]dThd should be ~0.1 μCi/ml, and that or BrdUrd, ~2 μM

Detection of Tritium by Scintillation Counting

Pulse-label cells with 0.1 μCi/ml tritium [^{3}H]dThd for 30 min. Longer pulse-label times (up to 2 hr) may be desirable where a heavy label is wanted. Remove culture medium containing [^{3}H]dThd. Wash the cells with 10 ml of cold PBS (if further growth is not required). PBS will wash unincorporated [^{3}H]dThd out of the cells. The cells may then be trypsinized from monolayers with 2 ml of 0.025% trypsin in Ca^{2+}- and Mg^{2+}-free PBS for 2 min for batch analysis by scintillation counting

To prepare cells for scintillation counting, add 5 ml of cold 10% trichloroacetic acid (TCA). Allow the cells to remain on ice for 5 min. Add suspension to a vacuum filter funnel containing a 25-mm glass fiber filter. Apply a vacuum to collect the cells on the filter. Wash the filter with an additional 5 ml of cold 5% TCA and 5 ml of cold 70% ethanol

The glass filters are placed in a scintillation vial with 1 ml of tissue emulsifier at 37°C overnight. Add scintillation fluid and place vials in a scintillation counter for quantification of incorporated [^{3}H]dThd

Note: The procedure described above for monolayer cultures may also be applied to suspension cultures. The washing procedures require that cells be sedimented from the suspension at 500 *g* for 2 min. The wash buffer is aspirated and the cell pellet is gently resuspended. The trypsin step is not needed.

Detection of Tritium by Autoradiography

Cells growing on slides may be further prepared for autoradiography by washing the slides with cold methanol/acetic acid

The slides are dried and dipped in a photographic emulsion. Photographic emulsion NTB2 is melted at 40°C in a beaker in a water bath in the darkroom. Place the slides in the emulsion for 30 min.

Drain the slides, and place them horizontally to dry in air.

Place the slides in a black slide box for exposure at 4°C for several days to several weeks, depending on the levels of [^{3}H]dThd incorporation. Cells with cell cycle times of less than 20 hr incubated in 0.1 mCi of [^{3}H]dThd requires ~1 week. Cells with long (100-hr) cell cycle time will require ~3 weeks' exposure. After exposure the slides are washed for 2 min in distilled water and placed in a photographic developer (e.g., Kodak D19) and fixative (Kodafix) prescribed by specific manufacturers

Cells may be washed with 10 ml of distilled water and stained with a dilute Giemsa in 0.05 *M* phosphate buffer (pH 6.5). The slides are then evaluated for [^{3}H]dThd incorporation by counting silver grains microscopically using a bright-field microscope. Evaluate 500 cells per slide. Positive grain count can be determined by first evaluating background counts, that is, cytoplasmic grains in positive samples, or general grain count in cells not exposed to [^{3}H]TdR. Generally positive cells (i.e., cells incorporating [^{3}H]dThd) will have more than 20 grains per nucleus

BrdUrd Labeling for Flow-Cytometric Measurement

Thermal Denaturation Method (27, 29)

This basic method is widely used.

1. Use an aliquot of cells previously labeled with BrdUrd or IdUrd and fixed in cold 50% ethanol or methanol/acetic acid (3/1 v/v). Centrifuge at 500 *g* for 1 min. (Note: Avoid overcentrifugation, which can lead to serious cell clumping.) Pour off the supernatant. Loosen the cell pellet by gentle vortexing.
2. Add 1.5 ml of RNase stock solution and incubate for 10 min at 37°C.
3. Centrifuge at 500 *g* for 1 min, pour off, vortex the pellet, and suspend the cells in 3 ml of 0.25–1.0% paraformaldehyde solution for 30 min at room temperature.

4. Centrifuge as in step 1, decant the supernatant, and vortex to loosen the pellet. Wash with 3 ml of PBS. Centrifuge, decant the supernatant, and vortex the pellet.

5. Suspend the cells in 1.5 ml of 0.1 *M* HCl/Triton X-100 for 10 min on ice.

6. Add 5 ml of PBS and centrifuge for 2 min at 500 *g*. Drain the pellets well before vortexing.

7. Suspend the cells in 1.5 ml of distilled water and place in a water bath at 95°C for 10 min. This is the DNA denaturing step and often must be adjusted, depending on the cell type, to maximize denaturation while avoiding extensive cell loss. Cell loss will be evident both by visual observation and by the number of events recorded per unit of time with the flow cytometer.

8. Remove the samples from the hot water bath and place the tubes in an ice/water mixture until the suspensions are cold. Then add 3 ml of PBS, mix gently by vortexing, and centrifuge at 500 *g* for 2 min. Drain, and vortex the pellet. At this point some clumping may be observed. Disperse any clumps by pipetting or syringing through a 25-gauge needle. Failure to completely disperse the clumps may prevent antibody access to BrdUrd-labeled cells. These cells may appear later as apparently unlabeled, resulting in a measurement error. [Note: Steps 2–8 may be deleted if HCl denaturation is used (5,9). Cells are incubated at room temperature with 1.5–4 *M* HCl for 20 min and then washed twice with PBS buffer to restore the pH to neutral before antibody treatment.]

9. Suspend the cells in 100 μl of diluted anti-BrdUrd antibody for 30 min at room temperature. Antibody should be diluted in antibody buffer to 0.2–0.5 μg/ml. We have observed that staining is better at 25°C than at 4°C for the short incubation time.

10. Add 5 ml of wash buffer, and centrifuge at 500 *g* for 2 min. Drain well, and vortex pellet.

11. Add 100 μl of diluted second antibody (goat anti-mouse IgG–FITC conjugate, typically diluted 1 : 50 to 1 : 500 in antibody buffer) for 20 min at room temperature. This step may be omitted if a direct conjugate anti-BrdUrd is used.

12. Add 5 ml of wash buffer, centrifuge, drain well, and vortex the pellet.

13. Suspend the cells in 1.5 ml of PI working solution.

14. Filter by running the sample through nylon mesh and analyze with a flow cytometer. (Optical filters for the flow cytometer were described under "Instruments.")

Restriction Enzyme/Exonuclease III Method (30)

This method avoids the use of heat for denaturation, thus preserving many other antigens and minimizing cell loss.

1. Following treatment with RNase, wash the cells with 1 ml of PBS and incubate for 30 min in 1% paraformaldehyde at room temperature.

2. Wash the cells with 1 ml of PBS and incubate with 1 ml of cold 0.1 *M* citric acid containing 0.5% Triton X-100 for 10 min.

3. Wash the cells with 1 ml of 0.1 *M* Tris-HCl (pH 7.5) and incubate in 100 ml of 0.1 *M* Tris-HCl containing 50 m*M* NaCl and 10 m*M* $MgCl_2$ and 10 U of *Eco*RI for 30 min at 37°C.

4. Wash the cells with 1 ml of 0.1 *M* Tris-HCl (pH 7.5) and resuspend in 100 μl of exonuclease III buffer containing 30 U of exonuclease III.

5. Wash the cells with PBS and continue with the thermal denaturation protocol at step 9 above (incubation with anti-BrdUrd antibodies).

Double Pyrimidine Label Method (11,12,31)

This method permits a combination of pulse label (e.g., with BrdUrd) and extended labeling with IdUrd, making possible calculation of growth fraction in addition to cell kinetic parameters (phase duration, labeling index, and cell cycle time).

1. Following the denaturation step incubate the cells in the presence of 100 μl of Br-3 diluted 1 : 300 in antibody diluting buffer for 20 min at 25°C.

2. Without removing the Br-3, add 100 μl of a second antibody (with affinity IdUrd > BrdUrd; e.g., IU-4) at low concentration, such as 1 : 5000 dilution in antibody diluting buffer. Direct conjugate antibodies simplify the technique, since both Br-3 and IU-4 are mouse monoclonal IgG_1 subtypes. Simultaneous double-indirect antibody staining can be done if one of the antibodies is a mouse monoclonal antibody and the second is a rabbit polyclonal antibody.

3. Add 1 ml of wash buffer, centrifuge the cells at 500 *g* for 2 min, decant the supernatant, and gently loosen the pellet by vortexing. Add 1 ml of PBS containing 10 μg/ml PI.

Note: For single laser flow-cytometric analysis of the double-label, FITC–phycoerythrin antibody conjugates, 7-aminoactinomycin D can be used as the DNA stain.

Combined BrdUrd/DNA/Cell Surface Antigen [Method of Carayon and Bord (25)]

This method permits detection of cell surface antigens along with proliferation status, allowing determination of proliferation in each population in a mixture of cells.

1. Following BrdUrd incorporation wash the cells with 1 ml of PBS.

2. Resuspend the cells in 1 ml of PBS containing phycoerythrin-labeled anti-CD4 and incubate them for 30 min at 4°C.

3. Wash the cells once with 1 ml of PBS and resuspend in 1 ml of 1% paraformaldehyde/0.01% Tween-20 overnight at 4°C. This fixes the first antibody onto its antigen.

4. Wash the cells in 1 ml of PBS to remove paraformaldehyde. Incubate in 1 ml of PBS containing Mg^{2+} and Ca^{2+} and 50 Kunitz U of DNase I, 30 min at 37°C.

5. Wash with 1 ml of PBS and resuspend in 150 μl of PBS containing 10% BSA, 0.5% Tween-20, and 20 ml of FITC-coupled anti-BrdUrd for 45 min at room temperature.

6. Cells are then washed in 1 ml of wash buffer, resuspended in 1 ml of PBS containing PI (10 μg/ml), and analyzed on a flow cytometer using three-color fluorescence detection.

BrdUrd Labeling for Microscopic Detection

Many methods exist for the conjugation of enzymes, fluorophores, and colloidal gold to antibodies. A review of these immunological techniques is beyond the scope of this chapter, and readers are referred to the comprehensive methods book by Tijssen (32) for guidance in these techniques.

Fluorescent Staining Method

1. Cells centrifuged on slides by cytospin techniques or grown on slides may be stained by the above protocols, with times being reduced by 50% for washing, denaturation, and incubation with antibodies.

2. After fluorescent or colorimetric staining with anti-BrdUrd, slides may be washed with 5 ml of PBS, then 5 ml of distilled water. Fluorescence or phase microscopy may be used directly for determining labeling index. Labeling index is defined as BrdUrd labeled cells per total cells observed in the field. For brightfield microscopy after color staining, counterstain cells with 0.05% Giemsa in 0.05 *M* phosphate buffer (pH 6.5).

Histochemical Staining Method (26)

This method uses a combination of colloidal gold and alkaline phosphatase enzyme immunohistochemical methods to detect both BrdUrd and IdUrd incorporated into DNA in histological sections. Nuclei are counterstained with hematoxylin and mounted for microscopy.

1. Sections are deparaffinized by immersing for 5 min in xylene, followed by 1-min immersion in 90%, and then 50%, ethanol. DNA is denatured with 4 N HCl for 10 min at room temperature.

2. Incubate for 30 min with 100 μl of Br-3 diluted 1:20,000 in PBS with 5% normal goat serum as a blocking protein.

3. Rinse the slides with 5 ml of PBS.

4. Incubate for 30 min goat-conjugated goat anti-mouse IgG diluted 1 : 50 in PBS.

5. Fix with 100 μl of 2.5% glutaraldehyde for 10 min and rinse with 10 ml of deionized water.

6. Silver precipitate for 20–30 min with a silver enhancement kit as described by the protocol provided by the manufacturer. The result is a black staining of the nuclei containing BrdUrd.

7. Immerse the slides in 5% acetic acid for at least 1 hr. Shibuya *et al.* (26) noted that slides may be left overnight in this solution. Rinse the slides by immersion in TBS for 1 min following incubation.

8. Incubate for 30 min with IU-4 diluted 1 : 800 in TBS with 1% normal rabbit serum as a blocking protein. Rinse the slides with 5 ml of TBS following incubation.

9. Incubate for 30 min with 100 μl of alkaline phosphatase-conjugated rabbit anti-mouse Igs diluted 1 : 50 in TBS. Rinse the slides by a 1-min immersion in TBS following incubation.

10. Incubate with 100 μl of suitable alkaline phosphatase substrate (e.g., 0.2 m*M* naphthol ASMX phosphate plus 0.2 m*M* Fast red salt dissolved in 0.05 *M* Tris buffer, pH 8.5). The result is a red staining of the nuclei containing IdUrd. BrdUrd-containing nuclei also stain, but this is marginal against their previous black staining by Br-3. Rinse with 5 ml of TBS.

11. Counterstain the nuclei with 100 μl of 5% Gills No. 1 hematoxylin, giving a light blue color to nuclei not containing either BrdUrd or IdUrd.

12. Dehydrate the sections though graded alcohols, 50%, 80%, the 100%. Clear with Histo-Clear, and mount on a glass coverslip with Permount.

Proliferation Antigens (33–36)

1. Cells are fixed at −20°C in 1 ml of 45–70% ethanol or in ice-cold 0.5% paraformaldehyde for 15 min.

2. Permeabilize the cells by incubation in 1 ml of 0.1% triton X-100 for 5 min. Wash the cells in 1 ml of PBS.

3. The washed cells are suspended at 2×10^5 cells/ml in 100 μl of antibody diluting buffer containing specific antibody (anti-Ki67 or anti-PCNA) for 30 min at room temperature. Wash the cells in 1 ml of PBS.

4. Incubate with 100 μl of secondary antibody (anti-mouse IgG or anti-human IgG–FITC or other conjugate) diluted in PBS with 1% BSA blocking protein. Wash the cells in 1 ml of PBS.

5. One milliliter of DNA staining solution (10 μg/ml PI and 200 μg/ml RNase) is added then for 30 min at room temperature. During the staining procedure the cell samples should be gently agitated occasionally.

6. Samples may be analyzed by flow cytometry and are run in the PI-containing buffer after filtration, as described under "Instruments."

Variations on this method suitable for cryostat sections or flow-cytometric analysis of enzymatically dispersed solid tumors have been described in detail by Baisch and Gerdes (37) for Ki67.

CONTROLS AND STANDARDS

Thymidine Labeling

A negative control slide with no added [^{3}H]dThd should allow evaluation of the counting background. This should be incubated with photographic emulsion, as are the rest of the samples. Alternatively, cytoplasm approximately equal in area and adjacent to the nuclei can be counted as a measure of background in the immediate vicinity of the labeled nuclei. A positive control should include a standard cell line preparation with known cell cycle time and levels of uptake known from scintillation counting and slides for grain counting.

BrdUrd Labeling

1. To some extent, G_1 cells in the cell population serve as a negative control cell population. G_1 cells should have minimal green fluorescence from antibodies to BrdUrd, since they do not contain BrdUrd. Elevated G_1 staining indicates nonspecific antibody binding or autofluorescence. The latter may result from inappropriate fixation techniques, particularly those using aldehyde fixatives. The ratio of green fluorescence intensity of the mid-S phase to G_1 cells should be at least 10, and under ideal staining conditions may be several hundred. If the protocol used continuous BrdUrd labeling so unlabeled cells are not part of the sample, then a specific negative control sample in which BrdUrd has been omitted should be used.
2. To determine whether cross-talk is occurring between fluorescence channels (i.e., whether PI fluorescence is being detected by the fluorescein detector), add PI but no antibodies after the thermal denaturation step. If the green fluorescence is above background, then cross-talk is present. Correct this either by reducing the concentration of PI used or by selecting more appropriate filters for the light. We recommend a final PI concentration of ~10 μg/ml.

Proliferation Antigens

A supply of fixed cells with known levels of nuclear antigen (known from a previous experiment) is the best standard. Follow the same staining protocol as was done to achieve earlier results. Negative controls should include cells fixed, but with no antinuclear antibody added. If the method is an indirect one (i.e., requiring the addition of conjugated antibodies), then add only the secondary antibodies without the antinuclear antibodies.

CRITICAL ASPECTS OF THE PROCEDURES

General Comments on the Use of Nucleoside Analogs

Incorporation of labeled nucleoside into DNA at useful levels requires that several conditions have been met. The nucleoside analog must reach the cells in sufficient concentration to be incorporated into the cells at a detectable level. While this is seldom a problem with cultured cells exposed *in vitro*, it may be a problem with *in vivo* exposures, especially in tumor tissue, where vascularization may be poor. Failure to reach sufficient extracellular concentrations will result in little DNA incorporation. In the case of limited [^{3}H]dThd incorporation, longer exposure times for autoradiography may overcome this limitation if background radiation is not excessive. In the case of halogen-labeled analog, high-affinity antibodies are required if low-density labeling is to be detected. Most available antibodies will detect BrdUrd incorporated in place of 10% or greater of the DNA thymidines. High-affinity antibodies have been reported that will detect BrdUrd substitution down to 0.1% (38).

Also implicit in these methods is that exogenous nucleoside will be taken up by the cells, be phosphorylated with appropriate kinases, and successfully compete with endogenously synthesized nucleosides. Thymidine kinase-deficient cells lines may not be studied using thymidine nucleoside analogs. In addition, the endogenous pool of thymidine may effectively dilute the exogenously added label, particularly if the latter is present at only low levels. Endogenous thymidine synthesis may be blocked by addition of 5-fluorouracil to the media, which inhibits thymidylate synthetase in mammalian cells. For measurement of proliferation in bacterial cells, it may be necessary to use *thy*$^{-}$ mutant *Escherichia coli,* which require exogenous thymidine.

The incorporation of halogenated nucleosides is limited in part by their toxicity. IdUrd and BrdUrd are the least toxic analogs and only influence cell progression when given as continuous labels for several rounds of cell division. Damage to DNA caused by incorporation of these compounds is enhanced by concomitant exposure to ultraviolet light. Multiple rounds of BrdUrd incorporation lead to an elevation of sister chromatid exchanges, for example, and there should be minimal exposure to room lights while the cells are growing. Fluorodeoxyuridine, and chlorodeoxyuridine (CldUrd) are cytotoxic, poorly incorporated into DNA, and not suitable as labels.

Thymidine Labeling and Autoradiography

1. It is important to keep the level of [^{3}H]dThd in the range of 0.1–0.2 μC/ml to avoid inhibition of cell growth. Levels as high as 1 μCi/ml can severely delay progress of the cells through the cell cycle.

2. Autoradiography is useful for determining distribution of incorporation within a section, but does not permit simple quantitation of the amount of radiolabel incorporated. For this, batch counting by scintillation can be used for quantitation.

3. Avoid the use of contaminated glassware and avoid glass coverslips, since they contain varying levels of natural radioactivity.

BrdUrd Labeling with Antibodies

1. All antibodies to halogenated nucleosides suitable for cell kinetics studies reported to date recognize the incorporated analog only in the context of single-stranded DNA. As such, denaturation of the DNA is required before antibody staining. Extensive denaturation is neither required nor desirable, however, since denaturation leads to a loss of the ability to stain with DNA-intercalating dyes, causes unacceptably broad coefficient of variation in DNA staining, and increases cell loss. As such, there must be a balance between the need to denature the DNA for antibody recognition of the BrdUrd and the need to retain intact double-stranded DNA for PI binding. Limited denaturation either by heating or with HCl or partial DNA digestion by nucleases is the preferred method. Carefully controlled minimal denaturation may also allow resolution of tetraploid G_2 and M cells into distinct G_2 and M peaks in the bivariate histogram by exploiting the differences in denaturation of DNA in M and G_2 phase cells (24).

2. Paraformaldehyde fixation will lower the sensitivity of the staining reaction, probably by reducing the denaturability of the DNA. Even with 1% paraformaldehyde fixation, however, quantification of a 10 n*M* BrdUrd 30-min pulse is attainable. The paraformaldehyde treatment also helps to prevent cell loss, especially of lymphoid cells, during the staining procedure. We have also found that the fixation step improves the quality of the DNA histogram, with lower coefficients of variation for the G_1 peak.

3. Nonspecific fluorescence is due primarily to nonspecifically bound antibody (anti-BrdUrd or fluorescein-conjugated second antibody). Additional washes after antibody treatment or incorporation of 1–5% blocking protein in the wash buffer can reduce nonspecific binding of antibody. Since most nonspecific antibody binding is in the cytoplasm and on the cytoplasmic membrane, using nuclei rather than whole cells can also greatly reduce nonspecific fluorescence (35).

4. Cell loss generally results from clumping and cell adherence to the walls of the test tube being used to process the cells. Lymphoid cell loss is generally greater from this procedure, but may be greatly reduced by using lower centrifuge speeds during the pelleting of cells. Limit centrifugation to between 400 and 800 *g* for no more than 4 min. Clumping is also higher when cells have been fixed in methanol/acetic acid than when they are fixed in 50–70% ethanol. Frequently, large clumps appear after the thermal denaturation step. Clumps may be disaggregated by a combination of mild vortexing and syringing the suspension gently through a 25-gauge needle. Cell adherence to the centrifuge tube can be decreased either by siliconizing the tubes or by using microfuge the tubes to reduce the tube surface area.

5. When staining cells that have double halopyrimidine labels (e.g., with BrdUrd pulse and continuous IdUrd label), one should be concerned with the differences in specificities and affinities of the specific antibodies. If very specific antibodies are used, there may not be a problem. As an example of halogen specificity, IU-4 has affinity for the halopyrimidines in the order IdUrd > BrdUrd > CldUrd, whereas Br-3 has the following specificity: BrdUrd = CldUrd ≫ IdUrd. If some cross-reactivity occurs with one of the antibodies (e.g., IU-4 will react with both IdUrd and at lower affinity with BrdUrd), then add that antibody at a much lower concentration after the specific antibody Br-3 has incubated with the cells for 20–30 min Then continue the incubation for an additional 30 min. In this way the Br-3 will saturate BrdUrd sites but not react with the IdUrd sites. Adding the IU-4, then, will preferentially bind only to the exposed IdUrd sites. Using a lower concentration of this antibody will prevent displacement of the Br-3 from the BrdUrd sites.

6. Using correct optical filters during the flow-cytometric analysis will prevent the cross-talk between the photomultipliers detecting the fluorescein and PI signals. PI exhibits a broad band of fluorescence, ranging from 530 to 700 nm. If a 550-nm short-pass filter coupled with a 500-nm long-pass filter is used for the green fluorescence, then some PI fluorescence will be observed in the green fluorescence channels causing a skewing of the BrdUrd histogram. While commercial instruments have capabilities of, compensating for some excess cross-talk, they cannot correct for a large excess of one or the other fluorophore in the sample. As such, the absolute fluorescence intensity of the separate staining dyes should be approximately equal.

Proliferation Antigens

Fixation procedures may denature nuclear antigen, leading to a failure of antibody recognition during the staining procedure. Negative results must be interpreted with caution.

SUMMARY

We have described a number of laboratory procedures for the measurement of cell proliferation. These have included quantitation of radiolabeled and halogen-labeled thymidine incorporation into DNA and a method for measuring PCNAs. Quantitation of tritiated thymidine by autoradiography is time consuming and labor intensive compared to the other methods described. Immunohistochemical methods for halogenated pyrimidine incorporation and nuclear antigens also offer greater versatility in that both flow cytometry and image analysis may be used for quantitation. Halogenated pyrimidine quantitation offers the additional advantage over measurement of nuclear antigens in that cell cycle parameters, including total cell cycle time, phase durations, and growth fraction may be determined. Cell cycle-specific antigen staining does permit evaluation of relative proliferation status, but not cell cycle time or phase duration. The washless techniques described for several of the methods reduce the overall staining time so that the total procedure time is less than two 2 hr.

ACKNOWLEDGMENT

Part of this work was performed under the auspices of the U.S. Department of Energy at Lawrence Livermore National Laboratory under contract W-7405-Eng-48.

REFERENCES

1. H. Quastler and F. G. Sherman, *Exp. Cell Res.* **17,** 420 (1959).
2. M. Takahashi, *J. Theor. Biol.* **13,** 202 (1966).
3. R. Young, V. DeVita, and S. Perry, *Cancer Res.* **29,** 1581 (1969).
4. D. Wimbler and H. Quastler, *Exp. Cell Res.* **30,** 8 (1963).
5. H. Gratzner, *Science* **218,** 474 (1982).
6. A. Raza, H. Preisler, H. Mayers, and R. Bankert, *N. Engl. J. Med.* **310,** 991 (1984).
7. M. Vanderlaan and C. Thomas, *Cytometry* **6,** 501 (1985).
8. P. N. Dean, J. W. Gray, and F. A. Dolbeare, *Cytometry* **3,** 188, (1982).
9. F. Dolbeare, H. Gratzner, M. Pallavicini, and J. Gray, *Proc. Natl. Acad. Sci. U.S.A.* **80,** 5573 (1983).
10. A. C. Begg, N. McNally, D. C. Shrieve, and H. A. Karcher, *Cytometry* **6,** 620 (1985).
11. F. Dolbeare, W. L. Kuo, M. Vanderlaan, and J. Gray, *Proc. Am. Assoc. Cancer Res.* **29,** 1896 (1988).
12. S. Shibui, T. Hoshino, M. Vanderlaan, and J. Gray, *J. Histochem. Cytochem.* **37,** 1007 (1989).
13. K. Miyachi, J. Fritzler, and E. Tan, *J. Immunol.* **121,** 2228 (1978).
14. J. Celis, R. Bravo, P. Larsen, and S. Fey, *Leuk. Res.* **8,** 143 (1984).
15. J. Gerdes, U. Schwab, J. Lemke, and H. Stein, *Int. J. Cancer* **31,** 13 (1983).
16. M. Danova, A. Riccardi, and G. Mazzini, *Haematologica* **75,** 252 (1990).

17. J. W. Gray, F. Dolbeare, and M. Pallavicini, in "Flow Cytometry and Sorting" (M. R. Melamed, T. Lindmo, and M. L. Mendelsohn, eds.), 2nd Ed. Wiley–Liss, New York, 1990.
18. W. Beisker and W. Hittleman, *Exp. Cell Res.* **174,** 156 (1988).
19. J. Selden, F. Dolbeare, J. Clair, W. Nichols, J. Miller, K. Kleemeyer, R. Hyland, and J. DeLuca, *Cytometry* **14,** 154 (1993).
20. D. Pinkel, L. Thompson, J. Gray, and M. Vanderlaan, *Cancer Res.* **45,** 5795 (1985).
21. S. A. Leadon, *Nucleic Acids Res.* **14,** 8979 (1986).
22. J. Gray, J. Carver, Y. George, and M. Mendelsohn, *Cell Tissue Kinet.* **10,** 97 (1977).
23. R. White and M. Meistrich, *Cytometry* **7,** 486 (1986).
24. M. Nusse, M. Julch, E. Geido, S. Bruno, A. DiVinci, W. Giaretti, and K. Russo, *Cytometry* **10,** 312 (1989).
25. P. Carayon and A. Bord, *J. Immunol. Methods* **147,** 225 (1992).
26. M. Shibuya, S. Ito, R. L. Davis, and T. Hoshino, *Biotech. Histochem.* **67,** in press (1992).
27. W. Beisker, F. Dolbeare, and J. Gray, *Cytometry* **8,** 235 (1987).
28. R. J. Sklarew, *J. Histochem. Cytochem.* **30,** 35 (1982).
29. F. Dolbeare, W. L. Kuo, W. Beisker, M. Vanderlaan, and J. W. Gray, *Methods Cell Biol.* **33,** 207 (1990).
30. F. Dolbeare and J. Gray, *Cytometry* **9,** 631 (1988).
31. P. J. M. Bakker, J. Stap, C. J. Tucker, C. H. van Oven, C. H. N. Evenhof, and J. Aten, *Cytometry* **12,** 366 (1991).
32. P. Tijssen, "Practice and Theory of Enzyme Immunoassays". Elsevier, New York, 1985.
33. P. Kurki, M. Vanderlaan, F. Dolbeare, J. Gray, and E. M. Tan, *Exp. Cell Res.* **166,** 209 (1986).
34. J. Larsen, *Methods Cell Biol.* **33,** 227 (1990).
35. G. Landberg and G. Roos, *Cytometry* **13,** 230 (1992).
36. S. Bruno, H. A. Crissman, K. D. Bauer, and Z. Darzynkiewicz, *Exp. Cell Res.* **196,** 99 (1991).
37. H. Baisch, and J. Gerdes, *Methods Cell Biol.* **33,** 217, 1990.
38. M. Vanderlaan, B. Watkins, C. Thomas, F. Dolbeare, and L. Stanker, *Cytometry* **7,** 499 (1986).

17

Nuclease P1-Enhanced ^{32}P-Postlabeling Assay for Aromatic Carcinogen–DNA Adducts

M. Vijayaraj Reddy and Kurt Randerath

INTRODUCTION

The covalent binding of chemical carcinogens or their metabolites to DNA, forming DNA adducts, is an initial event in the multistage process by which many carcinogens induce cancer (1). Radiolabeled compounds are commonly used to detect and quantitate carcinogen–DNA adducts (2). However, to extend studies to compounds or complex mixtures that are not readily obtainable in radiolabeled forms and to measure DNA adducts in humans, alternative methods have been developed, which include fluorometric techniques (3,4), immunoassays (5–7), gas chromatography/mass spectrophotometry (8,9), and biochemical postlabeling methods (10–15). In addition to higher sensitivity and versatility, the latter method is unlike the others in that it does not require prior knowledge of the structure and origin of adducts in order to detect them.

The ^{32}P-postlabeling method, coupled with thin–layer chromatography (TLC), was first developed and validated for the measurement of normal bases and the modified base, m^{5}C, in DNA (10), and was then extended to DNA bases modified with structurally diverse mutagens/carcinogens (11–13). In the standard version of this assay (10–12), DNA is first digested to 3′-monophosphates of normal and adducted nucleotides, which are then ^{32}P-labeled using polynucleotide kinase and [γ-^{32}P]ATP, resolved by TLC, detected by autoradiography, and quantitated by Cerenkov counting (Fig. 1A, excluding step II).

Enhancement of the assay's sensitivity includes an additional step involving the removal of normal nucleotides prior to ^{32}P-labeling. Two commonly used approaches for this purpose in the case of aromatic adducts are extraction of adducts with butanol (14) and pretreatment of DNA digests with nuclease P1 (15) (Fig. 1A). The latter approach is simpler, more convenient, and faster than the former and is based on the discovery (15) that nuclease P1 preferentially removes the 3′-phosphates from normal nucleotides, thereby forming nucleosides, but not from most bulky or aromatic carcinogen-adducted nucleotides (Fig. 1A). Since nucleosides are not substrates for kinase, only adducted nucleotides are

METHODS IN TOXICOLOGY, Volume 1B

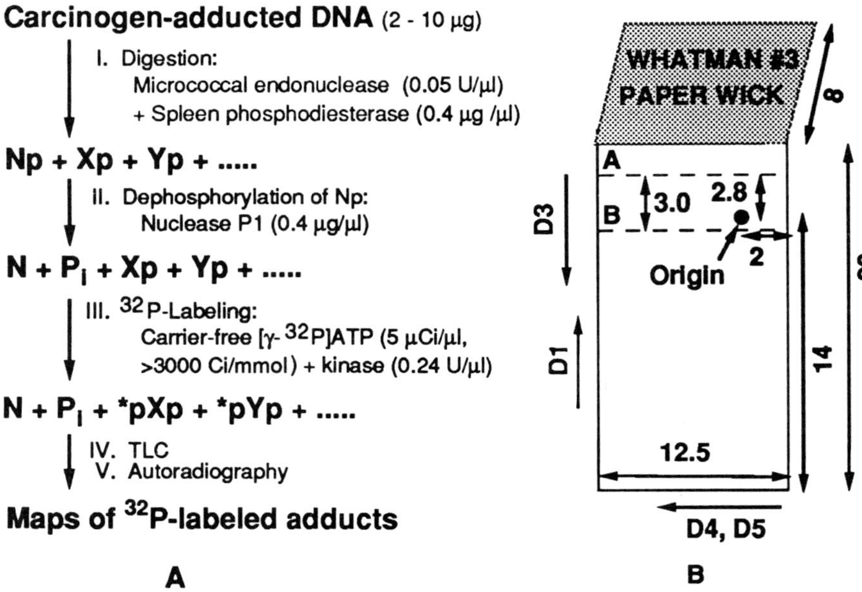

Figure 1 (A) Experimental strategy used in the analysis of aromatic carcinogen–DNA adducts by the nuclease P1-enhanced ^{32}P-postlabeling assay. Carcinogen-adducted DNA is digested to 3′-monophosphates of normal (Np) and adducted (Xp, Yp) deoxyribonucleosides (step I). The former are dephosphorylated to deoxyribonucleosides (N) by nuclease P1, while most aromatic and bulky adducts are not. The latter are labeled with ^{32}P, resolved by thin-layer chromatography (TLC), and detected by autoradiography. (B) Scheme of multidirectional TLC for purification and separation of adducted ^{32}P-labeled nucleotides. The scheme is a modification of a previous procedure (12). ^{32}P-Labeled DNA digest is applied at the origin of a polyethyleneimine (PEI)–cellulose sheet that had been attached to a Whatman No. 3 paper wick by stapling. The sheet is then developed in direction D1 in a nonurea solvent, which elutes leftover [γ-^{32}P]ATP and other unadducted ^{32}P-labeled material onto the wick, while most aromatic adducts are retained at the origin. After cutting at dashed line A and discarding the wick portion, the sheet is developed in directions D3 and D4 in solvents containing urea to resolve adducts. A final development in direction D5 in nonurea solvent may be performed to further remove adduct-unrelated radioactivity.

subsequently ^{32}P-labeled (Fig. 1A, step III). This chapter provides a detailed description of this procedure, as well as an abbreviated DNA isolation method.

MATERIALS AND REAGENTS

Reagents are dissolved and diluted in distilled water unless otherwise indicated. Enzyme solutions and buffers for enzyme reactions are stored in small aliquots at −20°C, except polynucleotide kinase, which is not aliquoted. TLC solvents are stored at room temperature (25°C).

Reagents for DNA Isolation

1% Sodium dodecyl sulfate (SDS), 1 m*M* EDTA: 100 ml. SDS and EDTA are from Sigma (St. Louis, MO)
0.1 *M* EDTA: 100 ml
1 *M* Tris-HCl (pH 7.4): 1 liter. Tris base [tris(hydroxymethyl) aminomethane] is from Sigma
1 *M* sodium acetate (pH 5.0): 100 ml. Prepared by titration of diluted acetic acid (Fisher, Pittsburgh, PA) with 50% NaOH solution (Fisher)
RNase A (10 μg/μl): 100 mg (Sigma). Dissolve in 10 ml of 0.05 *M* sodium acetate (pH 5.0). Incubate at 90°C for 10 min to inactivate DNases
RNase T1 (5 U/μl): 5000 U. (Calbiochem, San Diego, CA)
Proteinase K (10 μg/μl): 10 mg (Cat. No. 24568, EM Science, Gibbstown, NJ, an associate of Merck)
Saturated phenol: 500 g. To prepare buffer saturated phenol, add an excess of 50 m*M* Tris-HCl (pH 7.4) containing 1 m*M* EDTA to phenol (double distilled and packed under argon) from Boehringer-Mannheim (Indianapolis, IN), and mix the two layers. Store at −20°C in aliquots of 100 ml. Ensure that the solution is clear and colorless before use
Chloroform: 1 liter (Fisher)
Isoamyl alcohol: 500 ml (Fisher)
Saturated ether: 800 ml, spectrophotometric grade (Aldrich, Milwaukee, WI). Add 10 m*M* Tris-HCl (pH 7.4) containing 1 m*M* EDTA until present in excess
5 *M* NaCl: 500 ml (Fisher)
Absolute ethanol: 1 liter (Pharmaco, Bayonne, NJ)
70% Ethanol: 100 ml

Reagents for the ^{32}P-Postlabeling Assay

Micrococcal nuclease (0.5 U/μl): 500 U (Sigma)
Spleen phosphodiesterase (2 μg/μl): 1 ml, activity 2 U/mg (Boehringer-Mannheim). Dialyze the solution at 4°C for at least 3 hr against 1–2 liters of water, with three or four changes. Tie the dialysis bag tightly to avoid or minimize volume increase
400 m*M* sodium succinate (pH 6.0, 20×): 20 ml. Prepared by titration of a solution of succinic acid (Aldrich) with 50% NaOH solution (Fisher)
200 m*M* $CaCl_2$(20×): 20 ml
10× sodium succinate/$CaCl_2$ (pH 6.0): 10 ml. Mix 400 m*M* sodium succinate (pH 6.0) and 200 m*M* $CaCl_2$ in a 1 : 1 ratio

1 mM $ZnCl_2$: 10 ml (Cat. No. 22,999-7, Aldrich)
Nuclease P1 (4 μg/μl): 4 mg (Sigma)
400 mM sodium acetate (pH 5.0): 20 ml. Prepared by dilution of the above 1 M solution
1 M bicine–NaOH or CHES–NaOH (pH 9.6): 100 ml. Bicine [(bis-2-hydroxyethyl)glycine] or CHES [(N-cyclohexylamino)ethanesulfonic acid] is from Sigma. Adjust the pH with NaOH solution
T4 polynucleotide kinase (30 U/μl): 500 U (U.S. Biochemical, Cleveland, OH)
[γ-^{32}P]ATP: 5–10 mCi, concentration > 100 mCi/ml, specific activity > 3000 Ci/mmol. It is obtained commercially from either ICN Biomedicals (Cat. No. 35020, Costa Mesa, CA) or Amersham (Cat. No. PB 15068, Arlington Heights, IL) or prepared in the laboratory from carrier-free $^{32}P_i$ (ICN Biomedicals) by modifications (12,15) of the procedure of Johnson and Walseth (16). In our experience these different preparations give comparable results, although it is less expensive to prepare the reagent in the laboratory
10× kinase buffer: 20 ml. Contains 200 mM bicine, 100 mM $MgCl_2$, 100 mM dithiothreitol, and 10 mM spermidine (pH 9.6). Adjust the pH with NaOH solution
10 mM Bicine–NaOH or CHES–NaOH (pH 9.6): 100 ml. Prepared by dilution of the above 1 M bicine–NaOH or CHES–NaOH (pH 9.6)
Potato apyrase (50 mU/μl): 1000 U, grade I (Sigma)
Deoxyadenosine 3′-monophosphate (dAp) (2.5 pmol/μl): 1 ml (Sigma). Dissolve 10 mg in 1 ml of water and measure its concentration spectrophotometrically using $\epsilon = 15.2 \times 10^3 M^{-1}\ cm^{-1}$ at 260 nm. Dilute the solution to obtain 1 ml of 2.5 pmol/μl

TLC Solvents and Materials

1.1 M ammonium formate (pH 3.5): 1 liter. Prepared by titration of formic acid (Fisher) with concentrated ammonium hydroxide solution (Fisher)
0.1 M ammonium formate (pH 3.5): 1 liter. Prepared by dilution of the above 1.1 M solution
1.7 M sodium phosphate (pH 6.0) (D1 and D5 solvents): 2 liters. Prepared by titration of sodium phosphate (monobasic, Fisher), with concentrated. NaOH solution
1.0 M sodium phosphate (pH 6.0) (D1 and D5 solvents): 2 liters. Prepared by dilution of the above 1.7 M solution
0.12 M sodium phosphate (pH 6.0); 2 liters. Prepared by dilution of the above 1.7 M solution
4.5 M lithium formate and 8.5 M urea (pH 3.5) (D3 solvent): 2 liters. Prepared by titration of formic acid (Fisher) and urea (Aldrich Cat. No. U270-9) with lithium hydroxide (Fisher)

0.8 *M* sodium phosphate, 0.5 *M* Tris-HCl, and 8.5 *M* urea (pH 8.0) (D4 solvent): 2 liters. Prepared by titration of sodium phosphate (monobasic), tris, and urea with concentrated HCl

0.8 *M* lithium chloride, 0.5 *M* Tris-HCl, and 8.5 *M* urea (pH 8.0) (D4 solvent): 2 liters. Prepared by titration of lithium chloride (Fisher), tris, and urea with concentrated HCl

Polyethyleneimine(PEI)–cellulose plates: These are either purchased (20 × 40 cm) from Macherey-Nagel through Brinkmann (Westbury, NY) or prepared in the laboratory (12,17). Commercial plates are cut into 13.3 × 20 cm and the laboratory-made plates are cut into 12.5 × ~20 cm. The sheets are developed ascendingly in water for 15–20 hr with tank covers partially opened after the solvent reaches the top, to allow continuous development, and air-dried prior to use (12). In our experience laboratory-made sheets generally give sharper resolutions; however, commercial plates are adequate for most purposes. Since the latter usually retain adducts more strongly, we recommend that the concentra-

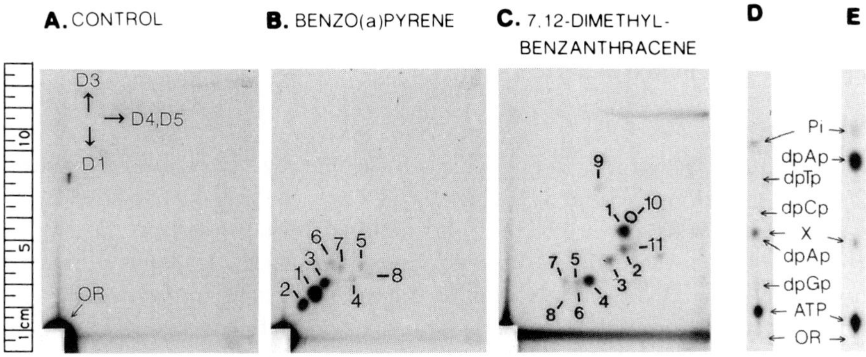

Figure 2 (A–C) Representative autoradiograms of PEI–cellulose maps of adducted nucleotides. DNA samples were isolated from cultured rat Zymbal glands exposed to solvent control or the indicated carcinogens (31). Samples were digested, labeled, and subjected to multidirectional thin-layer chromatography (TLC) as illustrated in Fig. 1A and B. The origin (OR) at the lower left–hand corner was removed before autoradiography. Orientation's of D1, D3, D4, and D5 developments are indicated. Adduct spots are identified by numbering. (D) A typical autoradiogram of one-dimensional polyethyleneimine (PEI)–cellulose TLC of ^{32}P-labeled DNA digest. DNA was digested with micrococcal nuclease, spleen phosphodiesterase, and nuclease P1, labeled, and resolved by one-dimensional TLC as described in the text. X, Unidentified material present in commercially obtained [γ-^{32}P]ATP. (E) A typical autoradiogram of one-dimensional PEI–cellulose TLC of ^{32}P-labeled dpAp. See the text for labeling and TLC conditions. X, Unidentified material; dpAp, Deoxyadenosine 3′, 5′-bisphosphate; dpTp, Thymidine 3′, 5′-bisphosphate; dpCp, Deoxycytidine 3′, 5′-bisphosphate; dpGp, Deoxyguanosine 3′, 5′-bisphosphate.

tions of salts other than urea in D3 and D4 solvents and in solvents for mapping normal nucleotides and deoxyadenosine 3′,5′-bisphosphate (dpAp) (Fig. 2) be increased by 15–25% over those indicated here, which are for laboratory-made plates

Stainless steel utility trays: 15 (Fisher Cat. No. 13-361C)

Heavy-duty warm air dryers: 4 (Fisher Cat. No. 09-210-5)

^{99}Tc ink: 1 mCi ([^{99}Tc]NH_4TcO_4 from Du Pont Cat. No. NEZ-085, New England Nuclear, Boston, MA.) Dilute ^{99}Tc ink 4-fold with black India ink

^{14}C ink (red): 1 mCi (ICN Biomedicals)

Du Pont Cronex-4 X-ray films and Kodak XAR-5 films: 100 films each, 8 × 10 inches (from a local supplier)

Cassettes (Wolf Deluxe or Kodak X-Omatic) and Du Pont Lightning Plus intensifying screens: 20–30, 8 × 10 inches (from a local supplier)

Polypropylene tubes: 500, natural, 0.5 and 1.5 ml (Eppendorf, Brinkmann). The tubes are prewashed by soaking in deionized water overnight

Poly-Q vials: 500, 18-ml size (Beckman, Fullerton, CA)

Micropipettes with built-in ejectors: Pipetman P2, P10, P20, P100, P200, P1000, and P5000 (Rainin, Emeryville, CA)

Handling of ^{32}P-Labeled Materials

General

The following safety practices are followed to minimize personnel exposure to ^{32}P (12,13): working behind $\frac{3}{8}$- to $\frac{1}{2}$-inch-thick transparent acrylic shields (custom made or from Research Product International, Mount Prospect, IL); wearing safety glasses, disposable gloves (two or three pairs), and a lead apron; reserving some pipettes for ^{32}P; frequently monitoring the work area and protective clothing for contamination with a Geiger counter; storing labeled materials and chromatograms in acrylic boxes; and frequently removing radioactive waste from the work area. Exposure (whole body and hand) is monitored by the required film badges.

Use of Special Devices

During labeling, microcentrifuge tubes are kept in transparent acrylic Beta-Bloks (Research Product International), a rectangular box (14), or a carousel rack (18), the latter being the most effective, as it eliminates the need for capping the radioactive tubes. A rectangular acrylic shield snugged onto the adjustable pipettes can provide shielding to hands (18,19). Labeled solution is applied to the TLC plate through a hole in a $\frac{1}{2}$-inch-thick acrylic sheet (18) or by an automatic spotting device for greater protection (18). Use of a multiplate holder and a mechanical device for washing plates (18) will also help to reduce exposures.

PROCEDURES

Isolation of DNA

DNA is isolated from cells or tissue by sequential treatments with RNases and proteinase K, followed by a series of solvent extractions (20). This procedure is a modification of published methods (21,22). It is significantly more rapid than a previous method (22), yet it provides the same quality protein- and RNA-free DNA. The other advantage is that it is adaptable for automated extraction of DNA using the 341 Purification System from Applied Biosystems (Foster City, CA).

Weigh out 0.25–0.5 g of a frozen tissue and suspend it in 2.94 ml of 1% SDS and 1 m*M* EDTA in a 8-ml polypropylene tube (Cat. No. 55.516, Sarstedt, Pennsauken, NJ). However, skin (up to 1 g) is cut into small pieces and suspended in the SDS solution with the EDTA concentration increased to 10 m*M*, which is necessary to inhibit excess DNase activity in this tissue. For tissues weighing < 0.1 g, reduce the volumes of SDS solution and all subsequent reagents to one-third. Add 60 μl of 1 *M* Tris-HCl (pH 7.4) and homogenize with a Tekmar Tissuemizer (Model STD-1810, Tekmar, Cincinnati, OH) at setting 70 for 15–30 sec. Skin is homogenized twice as long. Add 60 μl of RNase A (10 μg/μl) and 20 μl of RNase T1 (5 U/μl) to each tube. Vortex and incubate the mixture at 37°C for 45 min. Add 150 μl of proteinase K (10μg/μl) and further incubate at 37°C for 30–45 min. Add 3 ml of saturated phenol to the aqueous samples and mix by inverting the tubes for 1.5–2 min manually or on a tube rocker (American Dade, Division of American Hospital Supply, Miami, FL). Centrifuge the samples at 2000 *g* at 25°C for 5 min to separate the layers. Transfer the aqueous layer (top) to a new 8-ml polypropylene tube and discard the organic layer. Add 3 ml of a 1:1 mixture of saturated phenol and Sevag (chloroform:isoamyl alcohol, 24:1) to the aqueous layer and mix. Separate the layers as above. The aqueous layer may be extracted with 3 ml of saturated ether to remove traces of phenol that may contaminate DNA. Transfer the aqueous layer to a 13 × 100-mm Pyrex glass tube (Fisher Cat. No. 14-957C). Add 0.3 ml of 5 *M* NaCl and 3 ml of ice-cold absolute ethanol to the aqueous layer to precipitate DNA. Sediment the precipitate by centrifuging the samples at 2000 *g* at 25°C for 5 min. Carefully rinse the pellets adhering to the glass wall twice with 3 ml of 70% ethanol. Dissolve the DNA in 0.1–0.3 ml of water to give a final concentration of ~2μg/μl. Determine the DNA concentration spectrophotometrically using 20 A_{260} units = 1 mg of DNA. Store the DNA solution in 1.5 ml of prewashed (see above) Eppendorf polypropylene tubes (Brinkmann) at −80°C.

If the 341 DNA extractor is used, the homogenate is centrifuged at ~3000 *g* at 4°C for 10 min to remove unhomogenizable tissue and transferred to the vessels after addition of RNases. The machine performs automated digestions, extractions, and DNA precipitation as above. DNA retained on the filter is eluted in

0.2–0.3 ml of water into a 1.5-ml microcentrifuge tube placed on a continuous mixer (Model G-560, Scientific Industries, Bohemia, NY) for 15–20 min.

Analysis of DNA Adducts

DNA Digestion (10,15)

Pipette the DNA solution (2–10 μg) into 0.5- or 1.5-ml prewashed polypropylene Eppendorf microcentrifuge tubes, 0.5 ml if a carousel rack (18) is available and 1.5 ml if BetaBloks or a acrylic box (12) is used (see "Use of Special Devices," above). Add distilled water to bring the volume to 5 μl. If the volume exceeds 5 μl for the desired amount of DNA, it is reduced in a Savant Speed Vac Concentrator (Savant, Farmingdale, NY). Make a master mix of the following solutions: 1 μl of micrococcal nuclease (0.5 U/μl), 2 μl of spleen phosphodiesterase (2 μg/μl), 1 μl of 10× sodium succinate/$CaCl_2$ (pH 6.0), and 1 μl of water. The volume of the master mix should be 10–15% greater than that required for the desired number of samples. Add 5 μl of the master mix to each tube containing DNA and vortex. Centrifuge in a tabletop microcentrifuge (Brinkmann) at ~5000 *g* at 25°C for 3–5 sec to mix and make the solution homogeneous. Incubate at 37°C for 2–3.5 hr.

Dephosphorylation of dNp with Nuclease P1 (15)

Make a required volume of a master mix from the following solutions: 1.4 μl of nuclease P1 (4 μg/μl), 0.7 μl of 1 m*M* $ZnCl_2$, 0.7 μl of 400 m*M* sodium acetate (pH 5.0), and 1.2 μl of water. Add 4 μl of master mix to each tube. Mix and centrifuge in a microcentrifuge at ~8000 *g* at 25°C for 3–5 sec. Incubate at 37°C for 40 min. Add 2 μl of 1 *M* bicine–NaOH or CHES–NaOH (pH 9.6) to each tube.

Labeling of Adducts (10,15)

Before labeling, set up two additional tubes for measurement of specific activity of [γ-^{32}P]ATP by adding 4 μl of dAp (2.5 pmol/μl) and 2 μl of water to each tube. To shield radiation, place tubes in acrylic racks (see "Use of Special Devices," above).

Make a sufficient volume of a master mix from the following solutions: 2 μl of 10× kinase buffer, 0.16 μl of T4 polynucleotide kinase (30 U/μl), carrier-free [γ-^{32}P]ATP equivalent to 100 μCi, and 10 m*M* bicine–NaOH (pH 9.6) to bring the total volume to 4 μl. Add 4 μl of master mix to the sample and dAp tubes and mix. Incubate at 37°C for 30 min. DNA samples may be treated with apyrase to hydrolyze unreacted [γ-^{32}P]ATP to $^{32}P_i$ by adding 1 μl of apyrase solution (50 mU) to each tube, but this step is generally omitted in most experiments involving aromatic adducts. The labeled solution is ready for TLC.

TLC (12,15)

Dilution of Labeled Digests for Normal Nucleotide Mapping

After labeling, transfer a 2-μl aliquot from each labeled sample into a 5-ml polypropylene tube containing 373 μl of 10 m*M* bicine–NaOH (pH 9.6) and mix well. Store diluted solutions at −20°C if required, as they are further processed only after starting overnight TLC of adducts as below.

Mapping of Adducted Nucleotides

Two TLC procedures are used for purification and separation of adducts: (1) PEI–cellulose TLC for adducts derived from carcinogens with two or more aromatic rings (12) and (2) a combination of reversed–phase TLC and PEI–cellulose TLC for adducts derived from compounds containing one aromatic ring (23) or bulky nonaromatic rings (20). We describe the former method here, and the reader should consult Ref. 23 for reversed-phase TLC.

Adopted from a published method (12), the following procedure is used in our laboratory for separation of two to six aromatic ring adducts. In order for each sample to be chromatographed, attach by stapling a paper wick onto a 12.5 × 20-cm (laboratory-made) or 13.3 × 20-cm (commercial) PEI–cellulose plate as shown in Fig. 1B; use an 8-cm Whatman No. 3 wick if custom-made tall acrylic TLC tanks (18) are available for plate development and a 15-cm Whatman No. 1 wick if standard glass TLC tanks (12) are used. Using a No. 1 extra-soft pencil, mark a dot representing the origin where the sample is to be applied and two dashed lines, A and B (Fig. 1B), where the wick is to be cut off after D1 and D3 developments, respectively. Carefully spot 15 μl of the undiluted labeled solution onto the layer at the origin either manually or using a semiautomatic spotter (18). Develop the plate overnight (about 15 hr) in 1.7 *M* sodium phosphate (pH 6.0) in the D1 direction (Fig. 1B), with the wick staying within a tall acrylic tank (18) or protruding out of a standard glass TLC tank covered with protective plastic wrap (12). On the next day cut off the wick, while the sheet is still wet, at marked dashed line A with a pair of scissors and discard the wick in a radioactive waste container. Wash the sheets for 7 min in 500 ml of deionized water in stainless steel pans (500 ml), two plates per pan, with occasional stirring. Alternatively, washing of up to 28 sheets can be conveniently performed in a 10-gallon glass aquarium filled with deionized water, using a multiplate holder and a mechanical stirrer (18). Remove the sheets and air-dry under blowers with cool air (low setting) until dry, followed by warm air (medium setting) for 1–2 min. Alternatively, the sheets can be dried by placing them in a multiplate rack (18) in a mechanical convection oven (GCA, Precision Scientific Group, Chicago, IL) at 45°C for ~30 min.

Develop the sheets in the D3 direction (Fig. 1B) first in water to ~1 cm, then (without intermediate drying) in 85% of full-strength D3 solvent (diluted by mixing 85 ml of stock D3 and 15 ml of water) until the solvent reaches the top. The sheet may be cut along dashed line B (Fig. 1B) and the portion with the origin discarded, as adducts have now migrated out of the origin. Wash the sheets again in deionized water for 7 min, then dry as above.

Develop the sheets in the D4 direction (Fig. 1B) in water to ~1 cm, then in 80% of stock D4 solvent (phosphate–tris–urea or lithium chloride–tris–urea) until the solvent reaches the top. Wash the layers in deionized water for 7 min and air-dry as above.

The sheets may be given an additional development as follows to further remove unadducted material, although this step is not required for adducts present at levels of >1 in 10^8 N. Develop the sheets in the D5 direction (Fig. 1B) in 1.0 or 1.7 *M* sodium phosphate (pH 6.0) to 3–5 cm on a Whatman No. 1 wick attached at the top of the layer; the 1.0 *M* gives better purification, but some less aromatic adducts may be washed onto the wick. Remove the wick and discard it. Wash the layers in deionized water and dry as above before exposing to films (see "Autoradiography" below).

Mapping of Normal DNA Nucleotides

Spot 5 μl of the diluted samples onto a 12.5 × ~20-cm PEI-cellulose sheet (laboratory made) ~2 cm from the botttom 12.5-cm edge, leaving a 1-cm space between each sample. Develop the sheet in water to ~2 cm, then in 0.12 *M* sodium phosphate. (pH 6.0) to the top ~20 cm. Air-dry the sheet as above before autoradiography.

Mapping of dAp Samples

Equilibrate a 12.5 × ~20-cm PEI–cellulose layer (laboratory made) by soaking it in 200 ml of 0.1 *M* ammonium formate (pH 3.5) for 15–30 min. Dry the sheet in a current of cool air, followed by warm air for at least 2–3 min. Spot, in duplicate, 5-μl aliquots of the diluted postlabeled dAp samples onto this sheet at 2 cm from the bottom 12.5-cm edge and 1.5–2.0 cm apart. Develop the sheet in 1.1 *M* ammonium formate (pH 3.5) to 15–20 cm from the bottom edge. Dry the sheet before autoradiography.

Autoradiography

Normal Nucleotides and dAp Samples For subsequent alignment of the chromatograms with films, mark the bottom and top peripheries of the PEI–cellulose layers with two or three ^{99}Tc ink dots and the experiment number. In a darkroom with safety lamps, place the chromatograms in a film cassette and lay a Du Pont Cronex-4 X-ray film on top of the chromatogram. Place an intensifying screen over the film and close the cassette. Expose the film for 10–15 min at room temperature. Develop the film manually or in a standard X-ray film-processing machine (e.g., a countertop Kodak M35-A X-Omat Processor).

Adducted Nucleotides For subsequent alignment of the chromatograms with films, mark the left and top peripheries of the sheets with two or three dots of ^{14}C ink (for exposures >4 hr) or ^{99}Tc ink (for exposures <4 hr) and the experiment number. Assemble the chromatogram, Kodak XAR-5 X-ray film, and intensifying screen in a cassette as above. Develop the films after exposure at −80°C or 25°C for various lengths of time, depending on adduct levels (15): 1–2 min at 25°C for >100 adducts per 10^7 DNA nucleotides (N), 15 min to 2 hr at 25°C for one to 100 adducts in 10^7 N, and 15–40 hr at −80°C for fewer than one adduct in 10^7 N. Film sensitivity at −80°C is ~4-fold higher than at 25°C. Cronex-4 X-ray films are less expensive and three times less sensitive than Kodak XAR-5 films and may be used for higher adduct radioactivity.

Quantitation of Adducts

For measurement of radioactivity in ^{32}P-labeled nucleotide spots, circle the spots of interest on the film with a blue marking pen. Using a light box, place the chromatograms on the top of the films, matching the ink dots on the chromatograms with the complementary dots on the exposed film. Trace the location of the spots on the PEI–cellulose layer with a No. 1 extra-soft lead pencil. Cut out the spots with scissors and place each one into a Poly-Q vial with the layer side up. For background subtraction, cut out spots of equivalent area from blank sections adjacent to adduct spots and transfer them into vials. Also, cut out four ^{32}P-labeled dpAp spots (duplicate labeling and duplicate spotting) from the chromatograms. No background spot is taken for dpAp because of its high activity. Count the vials in a liquid scintillation counter without the addition of scintillator (Cerenkov counting). Two milliliters of ethanol may be added to each vial to prevent flipping of cutouts, which seems to influence the counting efficiency slightly (5–10%).

Alternatively, if large sections of the chromatograms must be counted (24), the layer is first wetted with absolute methanol or ethanol, then scraped with TLC scrapers (Alltech, Deerfield, IL) and transferred into a vial.

Data Analysis

Adduct levels are expressed as relative adduct labeling (RAL), which is calculated as follows. For calculations, the amount of DNA labeled is considered to be 10 μg, and 1 μg DNA = 3240 pmol of mononucleotides.

Determination of Specific Activity of [γ-^{32}P]ATP in cpm/pmol

A = pmol of dAp labeled = 10

B = volume of dAp labeling reaction = 10 μl

C = volume of diluted dAp solution applied to the TLC plate = 5 μl

$$D = \text{dilution factor} = \frac{\text{dilution volume}}{\text{volume used for dilution}} = \frac{375\ \mu\text{l}}{2\ \mu\text{l}}$$

$$= 1.875 \times 10^2$$

$$E = \text{pmol of } [5'\text{-}^{32}\text{P}]\text{dpAp applied to the TLC plate} = \frac{A \times C}{B \times D}$$

$$= \frac{10 \times 5}{10 \times 1.875 \times 10^2} = 2.667 \times 10^{-2}$$

$$F = \text{average cpm of } [5'\text{-}^{32}\text{P}]\text{dpAp spot}$$

$$G = \text{specific activity of } [\gamma\text{-}^{32}\text{P}]\text{ATP in cpm/pmol} = \frac{F}{2.667 \times 10^{-2}}$$

Determination of pmol of DNA Used for Adduct Analysis

$$H = \text{amount of DNA labeled} = 10\ \mu\text{g}$$

$$I = \text{volume of DNA labeling reaction (without apyrase)} = 20\ \mu\text{l}$$

$$J = \text{volume of labeled solution applied to the TLC plate} = 15\ \mu\text{l}$$

$$K = \text{pmol of dNp applied to the TLC plate}$$

$$= \frac{H \times J \times 3240}{I} = \frac{10 \times 15 \times 3240}{20} = 2.43 \times 10^4$$

Determination of RAL Values

$$\text{RAL} \times 10^7 = \frac{(\text{cpm in an adduct} - \text{cpm in background spot}) \times 10^7}{G \times K}$$

A value of n for (RAL $\times$ 10^7) corresponds to n adducts per 10^7 DNA nucleotides or $0.3 \times n$ fmol of adduct per μg of DNA, provided that the enzymatic and chromatographic recovery of adducts is quantitative.

COMMENTS

Interpretation of Results

Figure 2 A–C shows typical ^{32}P maps obtained when the described procedure is applied to the analysis of DNA adducts. DNA samples are from rat Zymbal glands exposed in culture to solvent control (Fig. 2A), benzo(*a*)pyrene (Fig. 2B), and dimethylbenz(*a*)anthracene (Fig. 2C). Extra spots present in treated samples but not in the control sample represent adducts. Spot patterns are carcinogen-specific. In Fig. 2D a typical ^{32}P map of normal nucleotides is shown. Normal nucleotide analysis is performed to ensure that there was an excess of ATP during labeling, as indicated by a strong ATP spot slightly above the origin, and that three enzymes (i.e., micrococcal nuclease, spleen phosphodiesterase, and nuclease P1) have effectively digested DNA and 3′-nucleotides, as shown by the absence of spots at the origin and at locations where normal nucleotides would migrate. These two conditions must be satisfied for quantitation of adducts. A typical map of ^{32}P-labeled dpAp is shown in Fig. 2E. Here, one expects to see two strong spots of dpAp and ATP, indicating the presence of excess ATP during labeling and efficient labeling of dAp, that is, conditions necessary for utilization of the [5′-^{32}P]dpAp spot for quantitative analysis.

Background Spots in Controls

Control DNA maps show weak or no background spots when analyzing adducts at levels >1 in 10^7 N. At lower adduct levels, however, significant amounts of background adduct spots are seen (25). These adducts, termed I compounds (25,26), are tissue, strain, and species specific and increase with aging of animals. These spots may comigrate with carcinogen-specific adducts and thus interfere in detection of the latter. Different TLC solvents (27; see below) or a monophosphate version of the nuclease P1 procedure (28,29) should be explored to resolve adducts of interest from I-compounds.

Application of Enzymatic Steps

In our experience micrococcal nuclease and spleen phosphodiesterase are found to be effective in digesting carcinogen-modified DNA to mononucleotide adducts (20,23), except for mycotoxin DNA, which seems to be incompletely digested, resulting in formation of adducted di- and trinucleotides (30). The use of nuclease P1 to enrich adducts and enhance sensitivity (Fig. 1A) depends on the resistance of adducted nucleotides to 3′-dephosphorylation by the enzyme. Adducts derived from structurally diverse chemical carcinogens, such as various polycyclic aromatic hydrocarbons (15), alkenylbenzene derivatives (15), benzene and its metabolites (31), and mitomycin C (15), as well as some small adducts such as thymine glycols (32) and ring-opened 7-methylguanine (33), are found to be resistant. Nuclease P1 enhancement has also been successfully applied for detection of aromatic adducts in humans exposed to complex mixtures (24,27,34,35). However, some adducts of aromatic amines (e.g., C-8 guanine derivatives of 4-aminobiphenyl and 2–acetylaminofluorene) are significantly dephosphorylated, resulting in low recovery (15,31,36). Nuclease S1 is as effective as nuclease P1 for adduct enrichment (37).

Application of the TLC Procedure

The PEI–cellulose TLC procedure described here is suitable for initial adduct purification derived from carcinogens containing two or more aromatic rings, since these adducts are retained on the PEI–cellulose layer during D1 chromatography in 1.7 *M* sodium phosphate (pH 6.0). Use of a higher concentration of sodium phosphate (e.g., 2.3 *M*) or development of D1 and D3 in the same direction allows the recovery of one aromatic ring adducts of safrole and benzene derivatives (29,31,38). However, reversed–phase TLC is more effective for purification of these adducts (23) or adducts from nonaromatic bulky carcinogens [e.g., mitomycin C (20)].

For resolution of adducts by two–dimensional PEI–cellulose TLC, the concentration of D3 and D4 solvents is adjusted, depending on the polarity or aromaticity of adducts; a range of 60% (i.e., prepared by mixing 60 ml of solvent with 40 ml of water) to 100% of full strength is appropriate for two or more aromatic ring adducts and 30–60% for one aromatic ring adducts.To prepare even stronger D3 and D4 solvents, as is required for some six aromatic ring adducts (e.g., those from dibenzoperylene) and for commercial plates because of their higher retention, the concentration of salts other than urea is increased. In addition to the change in ionic concentration, variation of pH and solvent compositions (24) improves resolution.

ACKNOWLEDGMENTS

Development of the ^{32}P-postlabeling assay for DNA adducts was supported by grants from the National Cancer Institute, Department of Health and Human Services (grants CA25590 and CA32157). The valuable contributions of Drs. R. C. Gupta and E. Randerath to the work described in this review are gratefully acknowledged, as is the support of Drs. C. A. Schreiner and C. R. Mackerer.

REFERENCES

1. E. C. Miller and J. A. Miller, *Cancer* **47,** 2327 (1981).
2. W. M. Baird, *in* "Chemical Carcinogens and DNA" (P. L. Grover, ed.), Vol. 1, p. 59. CRC Press, Boca Raton, Florida, 1979.
3. R. O. Rahn, S. S. Chang, J. M. Holland, and L. R. Shugart, *Biochem Biophys. Res. Commun.* **109,** 262 (1982).
4. K. Vahakangas, A. Haugen, and C. C. Harris, *Carcinogenesis* **6,** 1109 (1985).
5. M. C. Poirier, S. H. Yuspa, I. B. Weinstein, and S. Blobstein, *Nature (London)* **270,** 186 (1977).
6. R. Muller and M. F. Rajewsky, *Cancer Res.* **40,** 887 (1980).
7. R. M. Santella, L.-L. Hsieh, C.-D. Lin, and I. B. Weinstein, *Environ. Health Perspect.* **62,** 95 (1985).
8. D. E. G. Shuker, E. Bailey, S. M. Gorf, J. Lamb, and P. B. Farmer, *Anal. Biochem.* **140,** 270 (1984).
9. D. H. Fisher, J. Adams, and R. W. Giese, *Environ. Health Perspect.* **62,** 67 (1985).
10. M. V. Reddy, R. C. Gupta, and K. Randerath, *Anal. Biochem.* **117,** 271 (1981).
11. K. Randerath, M. V. Reddy, and R. C. Gupta, *Proc. Natl. Acad. Sci. U.S.A.* **78,** 6126 (1981).
12 R. C. Gupta, M. V. Reddy, and K. Randerath, *Carcinogenesis* **3,** 1081 (1982).
13. M. V. Reddy, R. C. Gupta, E. Randerath, and K. Randerath, *Carcinogenesis* **5,** 231 (1984).
14. R. C. Gupta, *Cancer Res.* **45,** 5656 (1985).

15. M. V. Reddy and K. Randerath, *Carcinogenesis* **7,** 1543 (1986).
16. R. A. Johnson and T. F. Walseth, *Cyclic Nucleotide Res.* **10,** 135 (1979).
17. K. Randerath and E. Randerath, *J. Chromatogr.* **22,** 110 (1966).
18. M. V. Reddy and G. R. Blackburn, *Carcinogenesis* **11,** 683 (1990).
19. R. K. Merrifield, *Anal. Biochem.* **167,** 400 (1987).
20. M. V. Reddy and K. Randerath, *Mutat. Res.* **179,** 75 (1987).
21. J. A. Marmur, *J. Mol. Biol.* **3,** 208 (1961).
22. R. C. Gupta, *Proc. Natl. Acad. Sci. U.S.A.* **81,** 6943 (1984).
23. K. Randerath, R. E. Haglund, D. H. Phillips, and M. V. Reddy, *Carcinogenesis* **5,** 1613 (1984).
24. E. Randerath, R. H. Miller, D. Mittal, T. A. Avitts, H. A. Dunsford, and K. Randerath, *JNCI, J. Natl. Cancer Inst.* **81,** 341 (1989).
25. K. Randerath, M. V. Reddy, and R. M. Disher, *Carcinogenesis* **7,** 1615 (1986).
26. K. Randerath, D. Li, and E. Randerath, *Mutat. Res.* **238,** 245 (1990).
27. E. Randerath, T. A. Avitts, M. V. Reddy, R. H. Miller, R. B. Everson, and K. Randerath, *Cancer Res.* **46,** 5869 (1986).
28. K. Randerath, E. Randerath, T. F. Danna, K. L. van Golen, and K. L. Putman, *Carcinogenesis* **7,** 1231 (1989).
29. M. V. Reddy, W. T. Bleicher, G. R. Blackburn, and C. R. Mackerer, *Carcinogenesis* **11,** 1349 (1990).
30. M. V. Reddy, R. T. Irvin, and K. Randerath, *Mutat. Res.* **152,** 85 (1985).
31. M. V. Reddy, G. R. Blackburn, C. A. Schreiner, M. A. Mehlman, and C. R. Mackerer, *Environ. Health Perspect.* **82,** 253 (1989).
32. M. V. Reddy, W. T. Bleicher, and G. R. Blackburn, *Cancer Commun.* **3,** 109 (1991).
33. K. Hemminki, *Carcinogenesis* **10,** 1761 (1989).
34. D. H. Phillips, K. Hemminki, A. Alhonen, A. Hewer, and P. L. Grover, *Mutat. Res.* **204,** 531 (1988).
35. M. V. Reddy, K. Hemminki, and K. Randerath, *J. Toxicol. Environ. Health* **34,** 177 (1991).
36. R. C. Gupta and K. Earley, *Carcinogenesis* **9,** 1687 (1988).
37. M. V. Reddy, *Carcinogenesis* **12,** 1745 (1991).
38. M. V. Reddy and K. Randerath, *Mutat. Res.* **241,** 37 (1990).

18 Genomic Hypomethylation

Vincent L. Wilson

INTRODUCTION

Whether the focus of the study is to determine the sensitivity of a selective human or other mammalian cell population to genotoxic damage, or to assess the toxic activities of various agents, DNA 5-methyldeoxycytidine (5mdC) levels are a useful indicator. Between 2 and 5% of deoxycytidine residues in mammalian DNA are methylated in the 5 position, forming 5mdC. This is an enzymatic process that takes place post-DNA synthesis, and is highly selective in regard to which deoxycytidine residues are methylated. Thus, the 5mdC patterns formed in DNA are species and cell type specific, and heritable. The progeny of cultured cells inherit these 5mdC patterns with high fidelity. Tumorigenic and immortal cells maintain a constant genomic 5mdC content through a large number of cellular generations, while normal mortal diploid cells lose 5mdC sites with each cell division (1). The rate of loss of DNA 5mdC sites is relatively constant in culture, is species dependent, and amounts to ~0.02% of the newborn genomic content per cell division in primary cultures of normal human cells (1,2). Primary cultured normal rodent cells, however, lose 5mdC sites at a much higher rate.

The genomic 5mdC content represents a genetic characteristic of a given cell population that is sensitive to perturbation by genotoxic agents. Previous studies have demonstrated the sensitivities of immortal mouse cells and primary cultures of normal human bronchial epithelial (NHBE) cells to carcinogen-induced decreases in genomic 5mdC content. These are short-term assays (24- to 72-hr exposures) and the decreases in 5mdC content were found to be dependent on both the dose and the exposure time. These genomic 5mdC decreases amounted to as much as 30% or as little as 4% (3,4). Although, these changes in 5mdC sites are small, they are significant. There are $\sim 2 \times 10^7$ 5mdC residues in the human genome, and the expression of a specific gene or the DNA binding of a transcription regulatory factor can be altered by the loss of a single 5mdC site.

Since 5mdC residues represent only ~1% or less of the total bases in DNA, and the observable changes in the genomic content of 5mdC may be as low as only 4%, the assay techniques must be exceedingly sensitive and precise. Numerous methods and techniques have been reported for the detection and

METHODS IN TOXICOLOGY, Volume 1B

quantitation of 5mdC. The most sensitive and most complex is the determination of specific 5mdC sites during sequencing analysis of DNA. However, high-performance liquid chromatography (HPLC) and ^{32}P-postlabeling techniques are more useful and more practical for short-term genotoxicity assays (4,5). The HPLC detection method reported by Kuo *et al.* (6) is a quicker assay than the postlabeling assay described here. However, the ^{32}P-postlabeling and nucleotide chromatographic assay is the most sensitive and precise technique available for 5mdC quantitation, requiring as little as 1 μg of DNA.

MATERIALS AND REAGENTS

Special Reagents and Supplies

Enzymes

Apyrase, potato, grade VI (Sigma, St. Louis, MO)
Micrococcal nuclease, staphylococcus aureus (Sigma)
Nuclease P1 (Sigma)
Phosphodiesterase II, calf spleen, 2 mg/ml, 2 U/mg (Boehringer Mannheim, Indianapolis, IN)
Proteinase K (Sigma)
T4 polynucleotide kinase, 5–15 U/μl (e.g., a 500 U vial, Amersham, Arlington Heights, IL) (Note: The T4 polynucleotide kinase is shipped in a 50% glycerol solution, and is very heat labile. T4 polynucleotide kinase is most stable when stored in 50% glycerol at -20°C or colder.)

Chemicals/Biochemicals

Adenosine-5′-triphosphate (ATP) (Sigma)
Adenosine-5′γ-[^{32}P]triphosphate ([γ-^{32}P]ATP), or [γ-^{32}P]GTP, >5000 Ci/mmol (Amersham)
Albumin, human serum (Irvine Scientific, Santa Ana, CA)
Aqueous scintillation fluid (e.g., Bio-Safe II, Research Products International, Mount Prospect, IL)
5-Azacytidine (Sigma)
Bicine (Sigma)
Deoxyadenosine-5′-monophosphate (dAMP) (Sigma)
Deoxycytidine-5′-monophosphate (dCMP) (Sigma)
Deoxyguanosine-5′-monophosphate (dGMP) (Sigma)
Deoxythymidine-5′-monophosphate (dTMP) (Sigma)
Dithiothreitol (Sigma)
Fibronectin (Collaborative Biomedical, Bedford, MA)

HEPES-buffered saline (HBS) (Biofluids, Rockville, MD)
Isobutyric acid (Sigma)
5-Methyldeoxycytidine-5′-monophosphate (5mdCMP) (Sigma)
Phenol, saturated and buffered solution, (Amresco, Solon, OH)
Spermidine (Sigma)
Vitrogen, human (Collaborative Biomedical)

Supplies and Equipment

Centrifuge (e.g., Model 12 Microfuge, Beckman, Fullerton, CA)
Cellulose thin-layer chromatography (TLC) plates, glass, 20 × 20 cm, 0.1-mm layer, without fluorescent indicator (Curtin Matheson, Denver, CO)
1.5-ml Eppendorf tubes, autoclaved (Brinkmann, Westbury, NY)
Heating block (e.g., Multi-Blok heater, Fisher Scientific, Pittsburgh, PA)
Liquid scintillation counter (e.g., Beckman)
Pipetteman, P20, P200, and P1000 (Rainin, Woburn, MA)
Pipette tips, autoclaved (Rainin) (Note: Wide-bore tips are necessary for viscous solutions of DNA and are prepared by cutting the end off of pipette tips prior to autoclaving.)
Plexiglas shielding (safety, β-blocking)
Speed Vac Concentrator (Savant I Farmingdale, NY)
TLC tanks, glass (Curtin Matheson)
Ultraviolet (UV) light source, 254 nm, hand held (for visualization of nucleotide spots) (e.g., Model UVG-11, UVP Inc., San Gabriel, CA)
X-Ray film (e.g., Kodak XAR-5, Eastman Kodak, Rochester, NY)

Solutions

DNA Isolation Solutions

Lysis buffer: 0.5% sodium dodecyl sulfate, 100 m*M* NaCl, and 10 m*M* EDTA (pH 8.0)
5 mg/ml proteinase K, dissolved in 10 m*M* Tris-HCl (pH 7.4), aliquoted in 0.5 ml in sterile Eppendorf tubes, and stored at −20°C
24 : 1 chloroform : isoamyl alcohol

DNA Digestion Solutions

Digestion buffer (10×): 12 m*M* $CaCl_2$ and 25 m*M* Tris-HCl (pH 8.8), sterile filtered, aliquoted in 0.5-ml volumes, and stored at 4°C
10 m*M* NaOH, sterile filtered and aliquoted in 0.5-ml volumes
0.1 *M* HCl, sterile filtered and aliquoted in 0.5-ml volumes
1 U/μl micrococcal nuclease, dissolved in sterile 1× digestion buffer, aliquoted in 0.5-ml volumes, and stored at −20°C

Postlabeling Solutions

Labeling buffer (10×): 100 m*M* $MgCl_2$, 100 m*M* dithiothreitol, 10 m*M* spermidine, and 100 m*M* bicine–NaOH (pH 9.5), sterile filtered, aliquoted in 0.5-ml volumes, and stored at 4°C

0.6 m*M* ATP (nonradioactive), dissolved in 10 m*M* Tris-HCl (pH 7.4), aliquoted in 0.5-ml volumes, and stored at −20°C

Neutral buffer (10×): 1 m*M* $ZnSO_4$ and 25 m*M* Tris-HCl (pH 7.4), sterile filtered, aliquoted in 0.5-ml volumes, and stored at 4°C

2 U/μl nuclease P1, dissolved in sterile 10× neutral buffer, aliquoted in 0.5-ml volumes, and stored at −20°C

1 U/μl apyrase, dissolved in sterile 1× neutral buffer, aliquoted in 0.5-ml volumes, and stored at −20°C

1 *M* sodium acetate (NaOAc), sterile filtered

3–6 U/μl T4 polynucleotide kinase; purchased enzyme solution is diluted by 50% with sterile water immediately before use

TLC Solvents

First dimension: isobutyric acid : H_2O : concentrated NH_4OH (66 : 20 : 1, v/v/v)

Second dimension: saturated $(NH_4)_2SO_4$: Isopropanol : 1 *M* NaOAc (80 : 2 : 18, v/v/v)

dNMP UV standard: 3–4 mg/ml each of dAMP, dCMP, dGMP, and dTMP, dissolved in sterile water and stored at −20°C in 0.5-ml aliquots

5mdCMP UV standard: 2.5 mg/ml of 5mdCMP, dissolved in sterile water and stored at −20°C in 0.5-ml aliquots

PROCEDURES

Tissue Culture, Treatment, Cell Harvest, and Micro-DNA Isolation

Cultures of mammalian cells of any type can be used in these assays with the appropriate media and culture conditions. Although immortal cell lines may be the easiest to work with, the use of primary cultures of NHBE cells is described here.

NHBE cell outgrowths (first passage) are obtained from freshly excised bronchial tissue from immediate autopsy donors and grown on surface-coated (10 μg/ml fibronectin, 10 μg/ml human serum albumin, and 30 μg/ml Vitrogen collagen) 100-mm plastic culture dishes with serum-free LHC-9 medium, as described (7). Second-passage cells are seeded at 2–5 × 10^5 cells per surface-coated T-75 flask. The use of screw-cap tissue culture flasks are especially recommended when the agent under study is volatile. Cell density is monitored by counting the cells in three randomly selected 1-mm^2 fields using a calibrated eyepiece grid and a light microscope. Logarithmic-phase cells at 0.8–1.2 × 10^4 cells/cm^2 of surface area are treated with the agent.

Only logarithmic-phase NHBE (or any other primary mammalian) cells at a set passage (e.g., second passage) should be used for these studies. The genomic 5mdC content of normal mammalian cells decreases with each population doubling (1). Thus, the age of the cells should be kept consistent during these analyses.

Many chemical compounds require solvents (e.g., dimethyl sulfoxide or ethanol) that may affect DNA 5mdC patterns or are otherwise toxic to mammalian cells. Thus, solutions of the test compounds of 100× or greater are prepared to minimize the effects of solvent exposure to the cells. Other agents are aqueous soluble and can be prepared in medium or buffered solutions. The positive standard control, 5-azacytidine solution, is made up as a 0.5 m*M* solution in HBS (pH 7.4) (7) or phosphate-buffered saline, immediately prior to treatment and filter sterilized. Treatment protocols should include an untreated control, a solvent control, and a 5 μ*M* 5-azacytidine positive control. A 24-hr exposure of NHBE cells to 5 μ*M* 5-azacytidine consistently induced a 30% decrease in genomic 5mdC content of these human cells.

The medium is aspirated and 5 ml of fresh medium is added to the T-75 flasks. The test chemical or control solution is added to the fresh medium just prior to feeding the cells. At preselected times later (e.g., 24 or, 48 hr) the cell density is again determined, the medium is drawn off, and the cells are gently washed twice with HBS. NHBE cells still attached are lysed directly on the flask by the addition of 1 ml of lysis buffer containing 0.1 mg/ml proteinase K (added to the lysis buffer just prior to use), and gently spreading the increasingly viscous solution over the growth surface of the flask. The flask is sealed and incubated at 45°C for 2–3 hr. The lysed solution is then gently transferred with a wide bore micropipette tip to two 1.5-ml Eppendorf tubes (0.5 ml into each) and extracted with an equal volume of phenol, followed by two chloroform : isoamyl alcohol extractions. Using a wide-bore pipette tip, carefully withdraw the aqueous phase (top phase) and place it in a fresh Eppendorf tube. Add 50 μl of 1 *M* NaOAc, followed by 2 vol (0.9–1.0 ml) of prechilled (−20°C) 95% ethanol, gently mix by manual inversion, and let stand for 10 min at 4°C. Pellet the DNA on the bottom of the tube by centrifugation at ≥12,000 rpm in a refrigerated microfuge (or a Beckman Model 12 Microfuge placed in a cold room (~4°C) or a refrigerated cabinet) for 10 min. If the DNA pellet is not visible, let the tubes stand at −20°C for 10 min and repeat the centrifugation. Gently remove all but the last 50 μl or so of supernatant, and add prechilled (−20°C) 70% ethanol, gently vortex, and let the tubes stand at −20°C for 10 min. Repeat the centrifugation procedure two or three times, letting the tubes stand at −20°C between spins. Gently remove all but the last 50 μl of supernatant and lyophilize the pellet in a Speed Vac Concentrator. With many cell lines, each tube will contain an adequate quantity of DNA. However, only between 1 and 5 μg of DNA is obtainable from each T-75 flask of NHBE cells by these procedures. Note also that it is not necessary to remove RNA for the subsequent analysis of 5mdC content.

DNA Digestion

To the dry DNA pellet add 9 μl of sterile water, 2 μl of digestion buffer, 2 μl of 10 m*M* NaOH, 2 μl of micrococcal nuclease solution, and 2 μl of phosphodiesterase II solution, vortex, and lightly centrifuge (2 sec at ~1000 rpm), and incubate in a heating block set at 37°C for 2 hr. Repeat the addition of micrococcal nuclease and phosphodiesterase II (at 2 μl each), vortex and lightly centrifuge, and incubate for an additional 2 hr at 37°C. The DNA digest is neutralized with the addition of 0.6 μl of 0.1 *M* HCl.

^{32}P Postlabeling

To 7 μl of the DNA digest add 1.2 μl of labeling buffer, 2 μl of T4 polynucleotide kinase (3–6 U/μl), 1 μl of 0.6 m*M* ATP to the top of the tube, and 3–4 μl (30–40 μCi) of [γ-^{32}P]ATP to the solution at the bottom of the tube, vortex and lightly centrifuge (2 sec at ~1000 rpm) to mix in the unlabeled ATP, and incubate in a heating block at 37°C for 1.5 hr. (Note that the T4 kinase stock solution is diluted to 25% glycerol before use, since glycerol will inhibit the labeling of the nucleotides. The concentration of glycerol should never be greater than ~7% in the final postlabeling reaction solution.) Add an additional 1 μl of T4 polynucleotide kinase (3–6 U/μl), vortex and lightly centrifuge, and incubate in at 37°C for an additional 1.5 hr. [Generally, labeling reactions with kinase are best performed with only [γ-^{32}P]ATP for an extended period, later followed by cold ATP to increase the concentration of ATP necessary to approach the K_m of the kinase reaction. However, the present method was found to provide a one-to-one labeling efficiency between methylated cytidine and unmodified cytidine residues (see Ref. 5).] Add 2 μl of 0.1 *M* HCl, 2 μl of nuclease P1, and 2 μl of apyrase, vortex and lightly centrifuge, and incubate at 37°C for 45–60 min. (Note that although apyrase type VII is more efficient in removing phosphates from ATP and ADP, it also has more dNMP activity than apyrase type VI.) Lightly centrifuge and spot directly onto prepared cellulose TLC plates, dividing the labeled sample between two plates (spotting ~11 μl of sample per plate).

TLC

TLC plates are prepared by spotting 3–4 μl of the UV standards (dNMP and 5mdCMP UV standards) at a location ~2 cm from each edge in the lower left-hand corner. The sample number is denoted by etching the cellulose in the upper left-hand corner of the plate. These standards not only provide for the UV

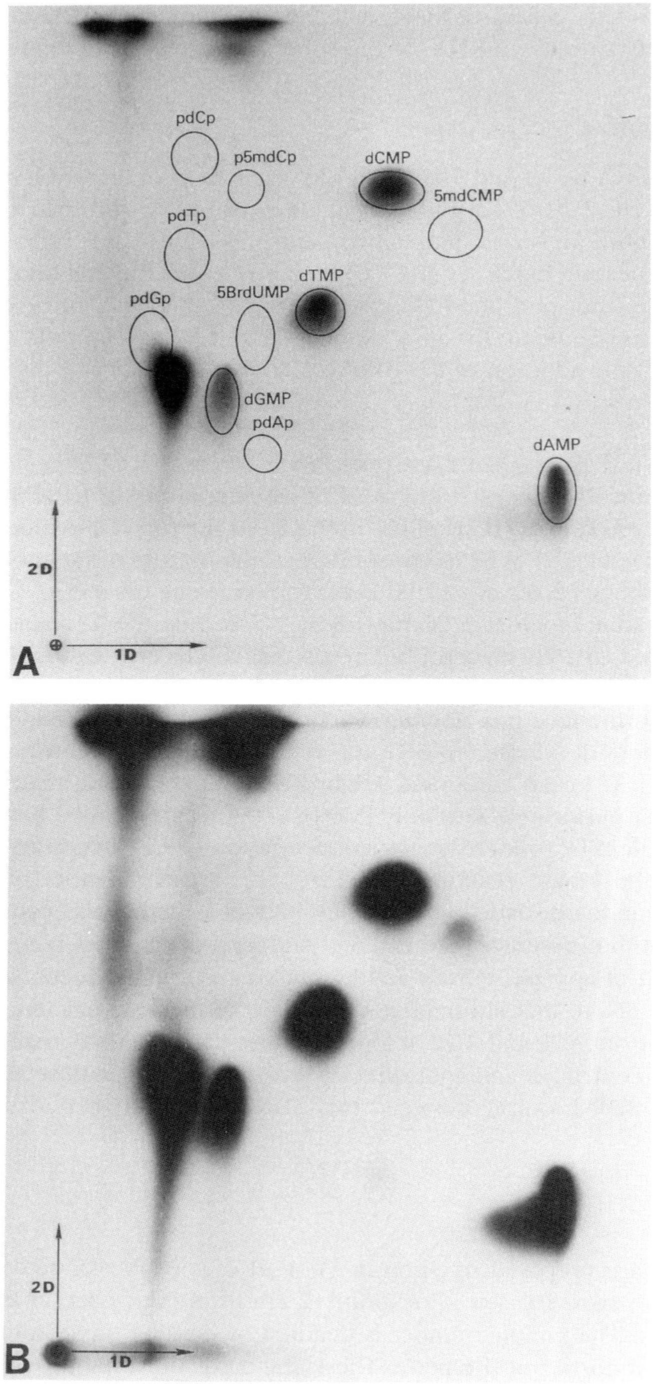
pdCp
p5mdCp
dCMP
5mdCMP
pdTp
dTMP
pdGp
5BrdUMP
dGMP
pdAp
dAMP
2D
1D
A
2D
1D
B

detection of the location of the labeled nucleotides, but also act as carriers for the exceedingly small amounts of labeled nucleotides. The spotting of standards and ^{32}P-labeled samples is facilitated by the use of a slide warmer heated to ~50°C, behind a β-shield (refer to "Safety," below). The plates are run in the first dimension twice before turning the plate 90° and running them in the second dimension (see Fig. 1). Each chromatographic run requires 5–8 hr for the solvent front to reach the top of the plate. All first-dimension chromatography must be carried out in an externally vented fume hood due to the strong odor of isobutyric acid. (Even then, fellow laboratory members may leave the area for a while!) Make sure that plates are dry between chromatographic runs. Upon completion of the second dimension, plates should be dried under a steady flow of air, such as that produced in the front portion of a fume hood, to avoid delicate $(NH_4)_2SO_4$ crystallization on the cellulose surface. Such crystallization is easily shaken off with radioactivity, causing the spread of contamination and the disruption of the subsequent quantitation of 5mdC levels.

With a No. 2 (or other soft-leaded) pencil gently circle the fluorescent spots detected under UV light (254 nm). These will be the dNMP and 5mdCMP standards as well as the ribonucleotides if RNA is present in the sample (Fig. 2). The relative chromatographic mobilities of many different nucleotides have been determined and are provided in Table I. Wrap the plates in plastic wrap and expose them to X-ray film for 1–4 hr (until the 5mdCMP spot can be detected). Use these autoradiograms to ensure that all of the radioactivity is encircled for the respective dCMP and 5mdCMP spots, and that adequate separation has been achieved. Using a sharp-edged spatula, carefully scrape each spot separately, as well as a blank region for background, and transfer powder to scintillation vials containing 2–4 ml of aqueous-based scintillation cocktail, cap, mix, and count each vial for 5 min in a liquid scintillation counter. The long counting time is important for the statistical accuracy of the percentage of 5mdC determinations. Some laboratories have used a computerized radioactive scanning instrument (such as a Beta Scanner Ambis, San Diego, CA) to quantitatively determine the radioactivity in each of the nucleotide spots on TLC plates. Scraping the nucleotide spots and counting is a less expensive alternative to the cost of this instrument.

Figure 1 Autoradiograms of the two-dimensional thin-layer chromatography analysis of ^{32}P-postlabeled DNA. The large oblong spot on the left side of dGMP is unreacted ATP. Apyrase was not used in the postlabeling of this sample. X-Ray film exposure times were (A) 10 min and (B) 4 hr. (Reprinted with permission from Ref. 5.)

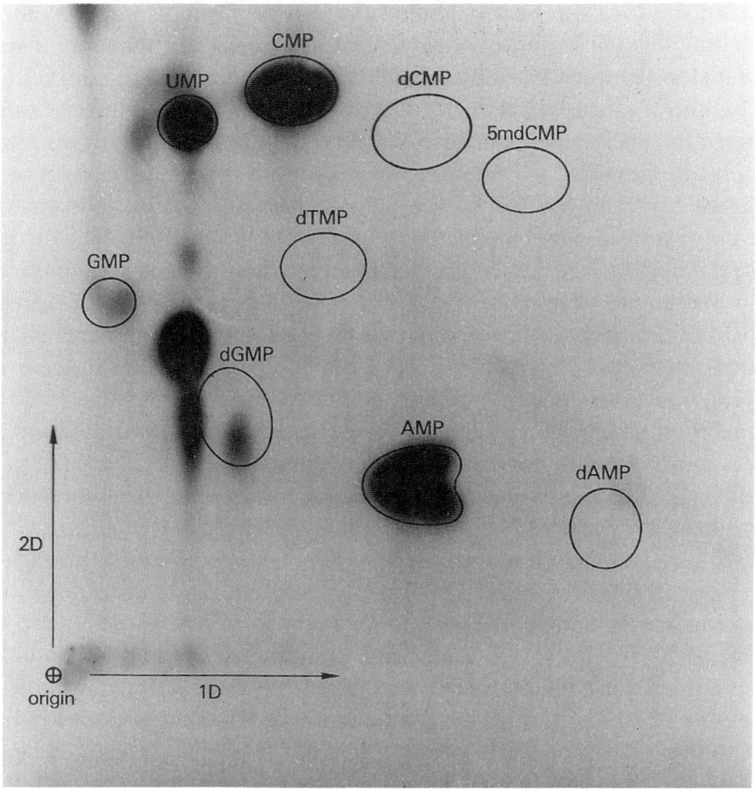

Figure 2 Autoradiogram of the two-dimensional thin-layer chromatography analysis of ^{32}P-postlabeled RNA. As in Fig. 1, apyrase was not used in the postlabeling of this sample. X-Ray film exposure time was 30 min.

Calculations

Subtract the background radioactivity from each of the counts of dCMP and 5mdCMP and calculate the percentage of total deoxycytidine residues methylated in the DNA, using the formula:

$$\%\ 5\text{mdC} = \frac{5\text{mdCMP}}{5\text{mdCMP} + \text{dCMP}} \times 100$$

Primary cultures of NHBE cells have been previously found to have a genomic 5mdC content of ~3.09% (4), although this level is also dependent on the age of the donor (2).

Table I Two-Dimensional TLC R_f Values for Standard Nucleotides[a]

Ribonucleotides										
5′-Monophosphate										
	CMP	UMP	GMP	AMP	N^7mGMP	N^6mAMP	5HUMP	1,N^6-Etheno-AMP	3,N^6-Etheno-CMP	
1D	0.34	0.20	0.10	0.54	0.43	0.68	0.10	0.34	0.57	
2D	0.83	0.80	0.48	0.33	0.74	0.35	0.85	0.37	0.51	
Deoxyribonucleotides										
5′-Monophosphate										
	5mdCMP	dCMP	dTMP	dGMP	dAMP	N^6 mdAMP	dUMP	5BrdUMP	5IodUMP	dIMP
1D	0.64	0.53	0.42	0.27	0.79	0.80	0.31	0.32	0.31	0.27
2D	0.65	0.72	0.53	0.40	0.24	0.23	0.73	0.51	0.40	0.52
3′,5′-Bisphosphate										
	p5mdCp	pdCp	pdTp	pdGp	pdAp					
1D	0.31	0.23	0.21	0.15	0.33					
2D	0.73	0.78	0.62	0.50	0.31					
3′-Monophosphate										
	p5mdC	pdC	pdT	pdG	pdA					
1D	0.62	0.51	0.40	0.26	0.70					
2D	0.66	0.73	0.54	0.43	0.34					

[a] The chromatographic location of each nucleotide was determined by applying UV-detectable levels of 5′ monophosphate nucleotides and/or by ^{32}P detection of the [5′-^{32}P]monophosphate nucleotide products of postlabeling analysis of polymers of oligonucleotides. (Reprinted with permission from Ref. 5.)

COMMENTS

General

The treatment time of 24, 48, or 72 hr has been chosen to ensure at least one cellular population doubling. The treatment of cells for a shorter period generally does not provide an observable effect on 5mdC levels. High doses of DNA-damaging agents will generally delay DNA synthesis and mitosis until sufficient repair has taken place. Although varying effects on 5mdC levels have been observed with doses of carcinogens that inhibit DNA synthesis, these doses are generally lethal to the cells. Thus, it is important to monitor population doublings of the cells during the treatment period. Decreases in population doublings greater than 50% should be suspect in the interpretation of genotoxic activity of the agent under study. Note, however, that the positive control, 5 μM 5-azacytidine, has multiple effects on NHBE cells and causes a greater than 50% decrease in NHBE cellular population doublings due to the induction of squamous differentiation (4,8).

A disadvantage in using primary cultures of epithelial cells, such as NHBE cells, is their sensitivity to the induction of terminal differentiation. Squamous differentiation of NHBE cells induced by serum, 12-*O*-tetradecanoylphorbol-13-acetate, transforming growth factor β, and weakly by 5-azacytidine, has also been associated with the loss of 5mdC sites (8). Thus, the morphology of these epithelial cells should be noted during these studies.

The damage produced by many agents that do not require metabolic activation will often be repaired during the time it takes for one cellular population doubling. However, the genomic 5mdC content of NHBE cells, but not murine BALB/3T3 cells, was found to be sensitive to the direct-acting carcinogen, *N*-nitroso-*N*-ethylurea, when incubated for a 24-hr treatment period (3,4). Thus, the cell type or cell line will impact on the usefulness of this assay to study their biological activity. Some carcinogens that require metabolic activation will not be picked up by this assay with cells that do not express activating enzymes, while other cells that are deficient in selective DNA repair capacities may be more efficient in detecting direct-acting carcinogens.

DNA damage produced by physical, alkylating, or arylating carcinogens is known to inhibit the complete digestion to individual nucleotides. The procedures used in the present protocol have been shown to be very effective, but may still be inhibited by some types of damage. A modification of these digestion procedures that may be useful in this work has been reported by Gorelick and Wogan (9).

Safety

Aside from the precautions that should be taken when using known or suspected carcinogens and other toxic agents (see *NIH Guidelines for the Labora-*

tory Use of Chemical Carcinogens, and the University of California, Berkeley, *Carcinogen Safety Directive*), extra care should also be used for the safe handling of the β-particle-emitting ^{32}P label. Plexiglas shielding ($\frac{3}{8}$-inch minimum thickness) should be used to protect individuals from direct exposure to this radioactivity. All postlabeling and TLC procedures should be performed behind Plexiglas shielding, and all TLC tanks should be behind shields. For further information regarding the safe handling of radioactivity, please refer to *The National Institutes of Health Radiation Safety Guide* [DHEW Publication No. (NIH) 79-18].

REFERENCES

1. V. L. Wilson and P. A. Jones, *Science* **220,** 1055 (1983).
2. V. L. Wilson, R. A. Smith, S. Ma, and R. G. Cutler, *J. Biol. Chem.* **262,** 9948 (1987).
3. V. L. Wilson and P. A. Jones, *Carcinogenesis* **5,** 1027 (1984).
4. V. L. Wilson, R. A. Smith, J. Longoria, M. A. Liotta, C. M. Harper, and C. C. Harris, *Proc. Natl. Acad. Sci. U.S.A.* **84,** 3298 (1987).
5. V. L. Wilson, R. A. Smith, H. Autrup, H. Krokan, D. E. Musci, N.-N.-T. Le, J. Longoria, D. Ziska, and C. C. Harris, *Anal. Biochem.* **152,** 275 (1986).
6. K. C. Kuo, R. A. McCune, C. W. Gehrke, R. Midgett, and M. Ehrlich, *Nucleic Acids Res.* **8,** 4763 (1980).
7. J. F. Lechner and M. A. LaVeck, *J. Tissue Cult. Methods* **9,** 43 (1986).
8. V. L. Wilson, T. Masui, R. A. Smith, and C. C. Harris, *Carcinogenesis* **9,** 2155 (1988).
9. N. J. Gorelick and G. N. Wogan, *Carcinogenesis* **10,** 1567 (1989).

19 DNA Degradation: Double-Strand Breaks

Andrew H. Wyllie, Mark J. Arends, Robert M. Hogg, and Alistair Nunn

INTRODUCTION

This chapter describes methods for studying the double-strand breaks that appear in genomic DNA during the process of apoptosis. In this mode of cell death, double-strand cleavage of DNA appears at internucleosomal sites throughout the genome, so that nuclear chromatin is reduced to fragments of various sizes (1). Although some of these are large, enough are of mono-, di-, and oligonucleosomal length to appear as a regular "ladder" in agarose gels. The presence of this ladder can therefore be used to confirm the presence of apoptotic cells within cell populations.

At the outset, however, it should be made clear that the appearance of such breaks is only one of the features of this process. Others include the morphological changes of chromatin condensation, compaction of cytoplasmic organelles, and explosive separation of the cell into membrane-bounded fragments (apoptotic bodies); the transient acquisition of high buoyant density; and expression of surface signals that permit phagocytosis by isogeneic macrophages (2). In some, but not all, circumstances apoptosis is inhibited by blockade of macromolecular synthesis. Thus, apoptosis may be recognized by a constellation of changes, of which DNA cleavage is only one. Moreover, although internucleosomal double-strand breaks are characteristic of apoptosis in many cell types, there appear to be some circumstances, albeit rare, in which they are absent. Such cells have been shown to have sustained double-strand DNA cleavage at more dispersed sites, detectable by electrophoresis of their DNA in pulsed-field gels (3). There are also specific situations in which such breaks occur physiologically in cells undergoing differentiation processes without death in the conventional sense, and without all of the other manifestations of apoptosis. The best example is erythrocyte maturation, in which a cytoplasmic remnant of the cell is retained in viable form for many months after loss and destruction of the nucleus. Terminal differentiation of lens cells shows similar features.

Apoptosis is a process whereby single cells are deleted from within living tissues. Because it is swiftly effected, and the apoptotic cells are subject to almost immediate phagocytosis by their neighbors, it is relatively inconspicuous in histological sections, even when it is responsible for a major reduction in tissue

METHODS IN TOXICOLOGY, Volume 1B

cell number. Apoptosis is the principal mode of involution of vertebrate embryonic cells because it is responsible for much of the extensive tissue remodeling that occurs throughout development. Endocrine-induced atrophy, cell death during selection of B and T cells in the development and maintenance of immunological competence, and the low-frequency cell death that balances cell proliferation in the homeostasis of renewing tissues are other circumstances in which apoptosis plays an important role. It is responsible for at least a proportion of immune cell killing, and for the cell death of vertebrate metamorphosis. Although similar strategies may be involved in invertebrate metamorphosis, there is good evidence that internucleosomal DNA cleavage is not involved here.

All of the above are essentially physiological processes, and there is a tendency to regard apoptosis as synonymous with physiological or even "programmed" cell death. Certainly, cells that die as a result of severe perturbation of their environment, for example, in severe hypoxia or exposure to respiratory poisons, tend to show an entirely different series of cellular changes (necrosis), in which discrete internucleosomal cleavage of DNA is not a feature. Apoptosis is also found, however, in the death induced in some cells by cytotoxic xenobiotics. In particular, many cancer chemotherapeutic agents can induce apoptosis when applied to appropriate target cells at suitable dosage (4). The capacity of these compounds to initiate apoptosis has little to do with their precise pharmacological mode of action, but appears critically dependent on the target cell. It is probable that the drugs are tapping into preexisting pathways in susceptible cells. There is good evidence that cellular susceptibility can be modulated by gene expression, leading to the concept that cells may switch from a state in which they are relatively resistant to apoptosis into one in which they are "primed" to enter the process on receipt of suitable stimuli. Several major cancer genes appear to be capable of effecting this switch in either direction, including c-*myc*, *bcl*-2, *p53*, *rb*, and the *ras* genes (4).

Study of double-strand cleavage of DNA can have three applications in the identification and analysis of apoptosis. First, it is often useful to extract the genomic DNA of dying cells to demonstrate that the characteristic internucleosomal cleavage has occurred, and so provide qualitative evidence for the initiation of apoptosis. Second, nuclei of viable cells can be incubated in suitable buffers to reveal whether they contain endogenous endonucleases capable of inducing internucleosomal cleavage. This type of analysis may have value in identifying cells that are primed for apoptosis, but as the effector proteins of apoptosis become defined, more specific means of identifying such cells will be available. Third, protein extracts of cells can be assayed against indicator DNA for the presence of double-strand endonucleases that might be responsible for apoptosis in their cells of origin. Methods of this type have been used to identify endonuclease activity during attempts to purify the endonucleases of apoptosis.

There are obvious constraints in the choice of this indicator DNA: If it is in the form of chromatin (and therefore competent to reveal the oligonucleosomal ladder), it must not be contaminated by endogenous endonucleases from its cell of origin. It is simpler to use a purified circular (plasmid) DNA. The protocols below give examples of these methods.

MATERIALS AND REAGENTS

Calcium Buffer A

150 m*M* NaCl
10 m*M* Tris (pH 7.4)
1.5 m*M* $CaCl_2$
3% Glycerol

Make up 100 ml, autoclave, and store at 4°C.

Calcium Buffer B

Buffer A plus 0.06% Nonidet P40

Make up 20 ml from buffer A stock and 10% autoclaved Nonidet stock; use immediately.

Calcium Buffer C

10 m*M* Tris (pH 7.4)
1.5 m*M* $CaCl_2$
25% Glycerol

Make up 100 ml, autoclave, and store at 4°C.

Tris–EDTA (TE) Buffer

10 m*M* Tris (pH 8.0)
0.5 m*M* EDTA

Store autoclaved 10-ml aliquots at 4°C.

Phosphate-Buffered Saline (PBS) Solutions

Dulbecco's PBS, without Mg or Ca, purchased from ICN–Flow Laboratories, High Wycombe, England)
PBS–EDTA is PBS supplemented with 0.02% EDTA

Autoclave and store PBS solutions at 4°C.

Tris–Borate Electrophoresis (TBE) Buffer

0.09 *M* Tris (pH 8.7)
0.08 *M* boric acid
0.1% EDTA

The buffer was purchased from Eastman-Kodak (Rochester, NY) as Buffereze Formula 3.

Hypotonic Lysis Buffer

10 m*M* Tris (pH 8.0)
20 m*M* EDTA
0.5% Triton X-100

Make up fresh from autoclaved stocks before use.

Triton X-100

10% Autoclaved stock in deionized distilled water

Bromphenol Blue Gel Loading Buffer

0.01% Bromphenol blue
2×TBE
20% Glycerol

RNase A

RNase A, 10 mg/ml stock (type 1-A, Sigma, St. Louis, MO)

Boil 1-ml aliquots in double-distilled water for 10 min to destroy DNase activity; store at −20°C.

EQUIPMENT

Vortex mixer (e.g., Stuart Scientific, Surrey, England)
Horizontal gel electrophoresis system (Northumbria Biologicals, Cramlington, England)
Microcentrifuge (e.g., Microcentaur, MSE Scientific Instruments, Crawley, England)
Ultraviolet (UV) gel transilluminator and recording system (e.g., UV Products, Cambridge, England)

UV fluorescence microscope (e.g., Ortholux2, Leica, England; a standard FITC filter, 450–490 nm, is acceptable for use with ethidium bromide)

PROCEDURES

Demonstration of Chromatin Cleavage in Apoptotic Cells

This method is suitable for demonstrating chromatin cleavage in apoptotic cells in suspensions, for example, cells harvested from culture vessels or thymocytes teased into isotonic buffered media.

1. Collect the cells by centrifugation (8 min at 800 rpm in a small bench centrifuge at room temperature; 120 *g*).
2. Discard the supernatant and resuspend the cells in 100 μl of PBS. Transfer to a 1.5-ml microfuge tube. To visualize a clear chromatin ladder, it is desirable to have $\sim 10^6$ cells in this volume.
3. Add 400 μl of hypotonic lysis buffer. Reflux gently through a 1-ml Eppendorf tip at room temperature.
4. Add 25 μl of 10% sodium dodecyl sulfate; reflux again.
5. Deproteinize by squential extraction in 1 ml of phenol, 1 ml of phenol : chloroform : isoamyl alcohol (25 : 25 : 1, v/v/v), 1 ml of chloroform: isoamyl alcohol (25 : 1, v/v). At each extraction, vortex mix the micofuge tube (for 10 sec), spin briefly (for 5 sec) at 9000 *g*, and collect the upper phase into a fresh tube.
6. Precipitate DNA from the last extract by addition of 50 μl of 4 *M* NaCl and 1 ml of absolute ethanol. Mix by inversion, place in a freezer at −20°C (for 30 min), and collect the pellet after centrifugation at 9000 *g* for 5 min. Decant ethanol and dry by standing at room temperatue for 30 min.
7. Resuspend in 50-μl TE buffer.
8. Take a 20-μl aliquot, add 5 ml of bromphenol blue gel loading buffer, and subject to electrophoresis in a 1.8% agarose gel (best if 18–20 cm long) made up in TBE buffer and including 1 μg/ml ethidium bromide, added just before pouring the gel.
9. Stop electrophoresis when the blue marker has migrated approximately two-thirds of the way down the gel (mono- and dinucleosomes run just ahead of the marker). Wash (for 20 min) in a large excess volume of distilled water. Photograph in UV light.

Comments

a. Depending on the cell preparation, it may be necessary to remove RNA prior to electrophoresis. This is most conveniently done by adding 5 μl of boiled RNase A and incubating at 37°C between steps 4 and 5.

b. In cell cultures apoptotic cells are most commonly found in the supernatant medium rather than within the monolayer. Even when not overlooked, they may fail to reveal convincing internucleosomal cleavage if allowed to accumulate over too long a period (e.g., overnight) because the chromatin fragments undergo progressive degradation. Under these circumstances, clear "ladders" can usually be obtained by harvesting the culture supernatant over consecutive 3-hr intervals, and pooling the recovered DNA at step 7 above.

c. This method seeks to display DNA from chromatin fragments of all sizes, including the very high-molecular-weight material from normal cells. The latter tends to be preferentially lost during the extraction steps, as it is viscous and clings to the insoluble material at the aqueous–organic phase interface. If there is so much high-molecular-weight DNA present in the sample that loading the gel is difficult, it is useful to insert an additional 9000 *g* (5-min at room temperature) centrifugation step between steps 3 and 4. The resulting supernatant contains only lower-order oligonucleosomes, whereas the high-molecular-weight chromatin is in the pellet and can be prepared for electrophoresis by mild shearing through a pipette tip and bringing into solution in 0.5% SDS in TE buffer.

Demonstration of Endogenous Endonuclease within Nuclei

This method is of value in distinguishing cells that are well endowed with endogenous endonuclease from those which are not. It can be made semiquantitative.

1. Ensure that the cells are in good condition prior to harvest. For cells cultured *in vitro*, select cells during log-phase growth, and refresh the medium overnight and again prior 3 hr to harvest.
2. Wash the cells gently twice in PBS–EDTA to remove any floating apoptotic cells and prepare a suspension from monolayer-cultured cells by exposure to 0.1% trypsin in PBS. Inactivate the trypsin by addition of an equal volume of growth medium (e.g., minimum essential medium) supplemented with 10% newborn calf serum, and prepare a cell pellet by centrifugation (150 *g* for 5 min at room temperature).
3. Resuspend the pellet in 3 ml of calcium buffer A and add an additional 3 ml of calcium buffer B to effect isotonic lysis . Reflux gently and let stand for 5–15 min at room temperature. Complete lysis can be confirmed by fluorescence microscopy of a single drop sample mixed with a drop of 2 μg/ml ethidium bromide in PBS. The dye will only enter the nuclei of cells whose membranes have been lysed.
4. Layer the lysed cells directly on top of 2 ml of calcium buffer C in a 12-ml centrifuge tube and centrifuge at 600 rpm (~100 *g*) for 20 min at 4°C. Decant

the supernatant and resuspend the nuclear pellet in 0.2 ml of calcium buffer A. Count a small sample and adjust the concentration to $\sim 10^7$/ml.

5. Set up pairs of microfuge tubes, each with 100 μl of nuclear suspension and 100μl calcium buffer A. To one member of each pair add 10 μl 40 mM $MgCl_2$. Incubate at 37°C for 1–16 hr (the time required for adequate digestion varies greatly among cell types).

6. Stop the reaction by addition of 100 μl of 1.5% Triton X-100, 60 mM EDTA, and 10 mM Tris (pH 8.0) followed by 15 μl of 10% SDS. Mix thoroughly.

7. Deproteinize, precipitate DNA, and subject to electrophoresis in 1.8% agarose as in steps 5–9 of the previous method.

Comments

a. The optimum concentration of Nonidet P40 in calcium buffer B varies among cell types.

b. Cation dependence can be demonstrated by using magnesium-based buffers in place of calcium buffers A and B, and adding $CaCl_2$ at step 5. The nuclei are unstable if no divalent cation is present during their isolation.

Demonstration of Double-Strand Cleavage Activity in Protein Extracts

This assay can be used to detect endonuclease activity in protein extracts from cells. The starting material can be crude eluates (e.g., in 0.3 M NaCl) from nuclei prepared as in steps 1–4 of the previous method, or from gradient fractions obtained from these. Nuclease activity in these samples is allowed to cleave a supercoiled covalently closed double-strand circular DNA substrate, which is then detected by electrophoresis in an agarose gel. This assay is extremely sensitive, as the migration of the uncleaved supercoiled circular substrate is much faster than that of the relaxed circular configuration that results from a just one single-strand cleavage event per molecule. Double-strand cleavage results in a linear configuration with a third, distinctly different, electrophoretic mobility, and if repeated at multiple sites, produces a smear. The assay can be made quantitative by densitometry of the gel, with calibration against micrococcal nuclease (Sigma), which must be used at very low concentrations ($\sim$100 ng/ml). Micrococcal nuclease and the apoptotic nucleases normally cut DNA to produce double-strand breaks, but at the low concentrations detected by this assay, may also show single-strand cleavage.

1. Purify any convenient plasmid DNA (we use SP64) by cesium gradient centrifugation and ethanol precipitation, by standard protocols. Suitable plasmids are also readily purchased from biotechnology firms. Freedom from protein contamination in this material is essential.

2. In a series of microfuge tubes, place 3 μl of test sample, 8 μl of assay buffer (20 mM Tris or acetate buffer, 0.1 mM $CaCl_2$, 0.1 mM $MgSO_4$, and 100 ng of plasmid DNA). The test sample can be prepared as a series of dilutions, and the pH and ionic concentrations can be varied, depending on the needs of the experiment. A matching tube containing 1 mM EDTA can be used to demonstrate dependence of cleavage on divalent cations.

3. Incubate at 37°C for 1hr, and stop the reaction by addition of 3 μl of gel loading buffer.

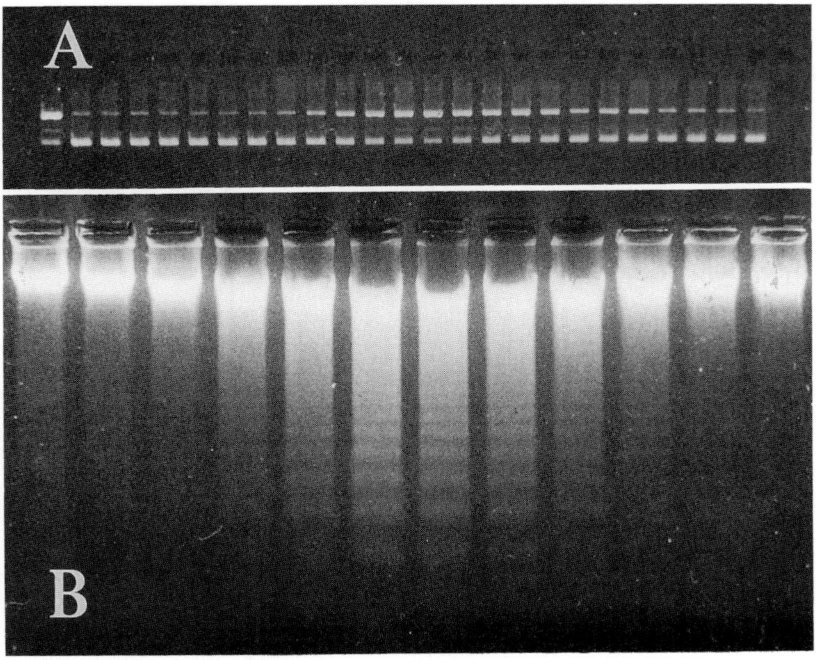

Figure 1 (A) Neutrophil endogenous endonuclease assayed for DNA cleavage activity *versus* plasmid SP64. The first track shows the effect of incubating the plasmid with unfractionated (active) nuclear eluate, as described in steps 1–5 of the method for demonstrating double-strand cleavage activity; all other tracks show the effect of serially collected column fractions prepared from this eluate. The lowest band in each track is supercoiled (uncut) DNA; the uppermost band is DNA, which has been subject to single-strand nicking and so adopts a relaxed circular configuration. The rare middle band, which appears only in the peak active fractions, is linear DNA which has sustained double-strand cleavage. (B) This agarose gel shows the effect of every second gradient fraction from (A) applied to neutrophil nuclei under conditions in which the nuclease normally associated with these nuclei has been quenched. Note the chromatin ladders in the active fractions.

4. Load directly and subject to electrophoresis on a 1% agarose gel in TBE buffer containing 1 μg/ml ethidium bromide.

5. View under UV light as in step 9 of the procedure for demonstrating chromatin cleavages.

Comments

a. Figure 1A shows an example of this assay applied to a series of gradient fractions of a human neutrophil extract. Note the change in relative intensity of the upper (nicked circle) and lower (supercoiled circle) plasmid bands in the fractions containing nuclease activity. Some of these fractions have also cleaved the plasmid to a just-visible full-length linear molecule. Figure 1B shows the effect of incubating every second fraction from Figure 1A with fresh neutrophil nuclei, prepared essentially as in steps 1–4 of the procedure for demonstrating endogenous endonuclease. A chromatin "ladder" is clearly visible in the active fractions.

b. The sensitivity of this assay is such that all tubes and reagents must be rendered nuclease free (by autoclaving) prior to use.

REFERENCES

1. M. J. Arends, R. G. Morris, and A. H. Wyllie, *Am. J. Pathol.* **136,** 593 (1990).
2. A. H. Wyllie, *Cancer Metastasis Rev.* **11,** 95 (1992).
3. P. R. Walker, C. Smith, T. Youdale, J. Leblanc, J. F. Whitfield, and M. Sikorska, *Cancer Res.* **51,** 1078 (1991).
4. C. Dive and A. H. Wyllie, *in* "Frontiers in Pharmacology—Cancer Chemotherapy" (J. A. Hickman and T. T. Tritton, eds.), pp. 21–56. Blackwell, Oxford, 1993.

20 Genotypic Mutation Analysis by RFLP/PCR

Fernando Aguilar and Peter Cerutti

INTRODUCTION

Somatic mutations have been detected in genes related to several forms of human disease, particularly in protooncogenes and tumor suppressor genes. In most cases somatic mutations in disease-related genes do not give rise to a functional change in the mutated cell which would allow its isolation or expansion *in vitro*. Therefore, selection of mutated cells on the basis of an altered phenotype must be replaced by biochemical separation and detection of the altered sequence of the gene of interest. Evidently, such "genotypic" mutation analysis requires large numbers of cells at the outset, since the expansion of mutated cells is avoided. Genotypic mutation systems are required because the actual mutability of a particular nucleotide sequence is expected to vary substantially for different genetic loci.

Genotypic mutation systems must possess analytical sensitivity which far exceeds the requirements for the detection of heterozygous or homozygous mutations in tissues from tumors or from patients with hereditary diseases (1). Average spontaneous mutation frequencies per base pair in human cells are estimated to be in the range of 10^{-8} to 10^{-10}, and these frequencies increase only 10- to 1000-fold upon exposure to a mutagen (2). Therefore, methods are required which allow the separation and/or distinction of a few altered DNA sequences from 10^5–10^{10} copies of the corresponding wild-type sequence in the presence of large quantities of cellular DNA. Ideally, genotypic mutation systems should allow the measurement of the type, frequency, and distribution of base pair changes, insertions, and deletions in any target gene. Genotypic mutation analysis has the advantage that there are no silent mutations which escape detection, in contrast to classical systems, which rely on the production of a selectable altered phenotype.

In this chapter we describe the restriction fragment-length polymorphism/polymerase chain reaction (RFLP/PCR) approach to genotypic mutation analysis, which measures mutations located in restriction enzyme recognition sites (3–7).

METHODS IN TOXICOLOGY, Volume 1B

PROCEDURES

Principal Steps of Genotypic Mutation Analysis by RFLP/PCR

The principal steps of the RFLP/PCR protocol are illustrated in Fig. 1 for the case of an arbitary *Msp*I endonuclease restriction site, CCGG. Base pair changes, and under certain conditions insertions and small delations, are measured which occur in restriction enzyme recognition sequences and render the mutated site resistant to cleavage by the corresponding endonuclease. The protocol includes the following steps. The cellular DNA from 10^7–10^9 cells is first enriched in the sequences of the gene of interest by nonspecific restriction and size fractionation. The DNA preparation is then exhaustively digested with the chosen restriction enzyme (i.e., *Msp*I in the present example), which cleaves the wild-type CCGG recognition sequences but leaves mutated *Msp*I sites intact. A known number of copies of "mutant standard" (MS) is added for later data calibration before or after digestion (see below). A second gel fractionation at this stage allows the purification of a short fragment population which is enriched in the mutated segment of the gene of interest. This DNA preparation then serves as the template for the amplification, under high-fidelity conditions, of the gene segment of interest. The resulting RFLP/PCR product is purified and directly sequenced by primer extension. Direct sequencing of the RFLP/PCR product allows the detection of predominant base pair changes. For more detailed analysis the amplified DNA is cloned into λ gt 10, and mutants are identified and quanti-

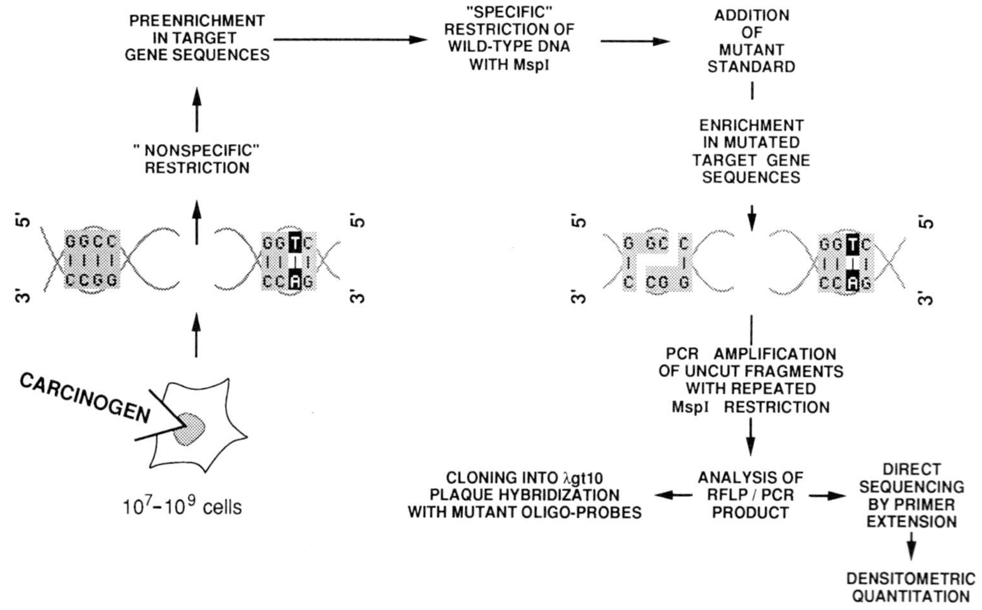

Figure 1 Genotypic mutation analysis by *Msp*I RFLP/PCR.

tated by oligonucleotide plaque hybridization. To facilitate cloning, primers are used which contain 5′tails with *Eco*RI recognition sequences in the final cycles of amplification. The mutant composition of the RFLP/PCR product is derived from quantitative sequence analysis together with λ-plaque hybridization.

While the initial number of cells and the quantity of DNA are known, the exact yields in the multiple steps of the RFLP/PCR protocol are subject to experimental variations. Therefore, direct sequencing or plaque hybridization of the RFLP/PCR product yields relative, rather than absolute, mutation frequencies. Absolute mutation frequencies are obtained by calibration with an internal MS, which is added at the outset of the experiment. The MS is homologous to the chosen gene fragment, but contains at least 1 bp change in the target restriction recognition sequence and one or more additional base pair changes outside of this sequence. The content of mutant standard in the final RFLP/PCR product allows data calibration and the estimation of absolute mutation frequencies (3,5–7).

*Msp*I RFLP/PCR Analysis of Hotspot Codon 248 of the Human *p53* Tumor Suppressor Gene

Experimental details of the RFLP/PCR protocol for genotypic mutation analysis are given using, as an example, *Msp*I/*Hpa*II site 14067–14070 of exon VII of the human *p53* gene. This restriction site covers hotspot codon 248 (CGG), which is preferentially mutated in several forms of cancer. Analogous experimental conditions can be applied to mutation analysis in any restriction recognition sequence of any gene of known sequence with only minor modifications.

Enrichment of Gene Fragments with Codon 248 Mutations

Because of the low frequencies of mutations in a specific base pair of the genome and because of the elimination of phenotypic selection and expansion of mutated cells in the RFLP/PCR protocol, DNA from a large number of cells must be analyzed for statistical reasons. Usually, DNA is extracted from 5–10 × 10^7 cells, and the DNA is first enriched in the gene of interest by size fraction on agarose gels. Typically, 400 μg of DNA was digested with *Bam*HI (3 U/μg of DNA) (Boehringer Mannheim, Rotkreuz, Switzerland) and seperated by electrophoresis on 1% agarose (run in 40 m*M* Tris base/20 m*M* sodium acetate/1 m*M* Na_2EDTA adjusted to pH 7.2). λ-DNA restricted with *Hin*dIII (Boehringer Mannheim) was used as the size marker. Gel slices containing DNA from ~6.5–9.4 kb which contain the *p53* gene were removed and the DNA was electroeluted in an Elutrap electroseparation system (according to the conditions outlined by the supplier, Schleicher & Schüell, Feldbach, Switzerland). The content of *p53* in enriched preparations was determined by Southern blotting using a nick-translated *Bam*HI 1.8-kb human *p53* probe extending from residues −130 to 1671 relative to the translation initiation site (8) (kindly provided by Dr. B. Vogelstein, Johns Hopkins Oncology Center, Baltimore, MD). Comparision of the intensities of the 7.8-kb bands on the blots for DNA before and after gel electrophoresis yielded the recovery of *p53* sequences. DNA samples containing 3–5 × 10^7 copies of the *p53* gene were then exhaustively digested with *Msp*I/*Hpa*II (12 U *Msp*I/μg of DNA and 5 U *Hpa*II/μg of DNA) as recommended by the supplier of the enzymes (Boehringer Mannheim). To these preparations a small number of copies of MS which possess a length of 462 bp (see below) were added for later data calibration. The ideal number of MS copies to be added depends on the expected mutation frequencies, but usually lies in the range of 10–50. The samples were then enriched in sequences with mutated *Msp*I/*Hpa*II site 14067–14070 by gel electrophoresis (Sub-cell DNA electrophoresis Cell, Bio-Rad Laboratories, Glattbrugg, Switzerland) on 2% agarose (Sigma, St. Louis, MO) in 40 m*M* Tris–borate (pH 8.2) and 1 m*M* Na_2EDTA, using *Hin*fI (Boehringer Mannheim) -digested pBR322 DNA as size markers. Wild-type *p53* sequences which were cleaved at this *Msp*I/*Hpa*II site gave rise to two short fragments and were eliminated. A gel slice containing a 380- to 500-bp fragment population was extracted with a Qiaex extraction kit (Qiagen, Studio City, CA) as specified by the supplier. The samples were again digested with *Msp*I/*Hpa*II and the DNA was precipitated with ethanol. These DNA preparations contained the predicted mutated 468-bp *p53* fragment which extends from the flanking 5′ *Msp*I site (13768) to the flanking 3′ *Msp*I site (14235) as well as the 462-bp MS fragments (unpublished observations, 1991).

High-Fidelity Amplification of a *p53* Exon VII Fragment Containing Codon 248

From the enriched DNA preparations described above, a 116-bp fragment spanning from residues 13999 to 14114 was amplified with *Pyrococcus furiousus* (*Pfu*) DNA polymerase (Stratagene, Zurich, Switzerland) for 35 cycles using sense primer 1 (5′ GTTGGCTCTGACTGTACCAC 3′, residues 13999–14018) and antisense primer 2 (5′ CCTGACCTGGAGTCTTCCAG 3′, residues 14114–14095). This type of oligonucleotide is available by custom synthesis from many companies worldwide. The amplification mixtures contained 20 pmol of each primer, 200 μ*M* dNTP's and 2.5 U of *Pfu* polymerase in 50 μl of amplification buffer consisting of 20 m*M* Tris-Cl (pH 8.2), 10 m*M* KCl, 6 m*M* $(NH_4)_2SO_4$, 2 m*M* $MgCl_2$, 0.1% Triton X-100, and 10 ng/μl nuclease free bovine serum albumin as recommended by the supplier of the polymerase (Stratagene). The amplification mixture was extracted with phenol–chloroform and the DNA was precipitated with ethanol. An aliquot of the resuspended DNA served as the template in an additional 15 cycles using primers 3 and 4 (5′ GTTGGCTCTGACTGTACCAC 3′, residues 13999–14018, and 5′ TCCAGTGTGATGATGGTGAG 3′, residues 14099–14080, respectively) (see Fig. 2) and *Taq*

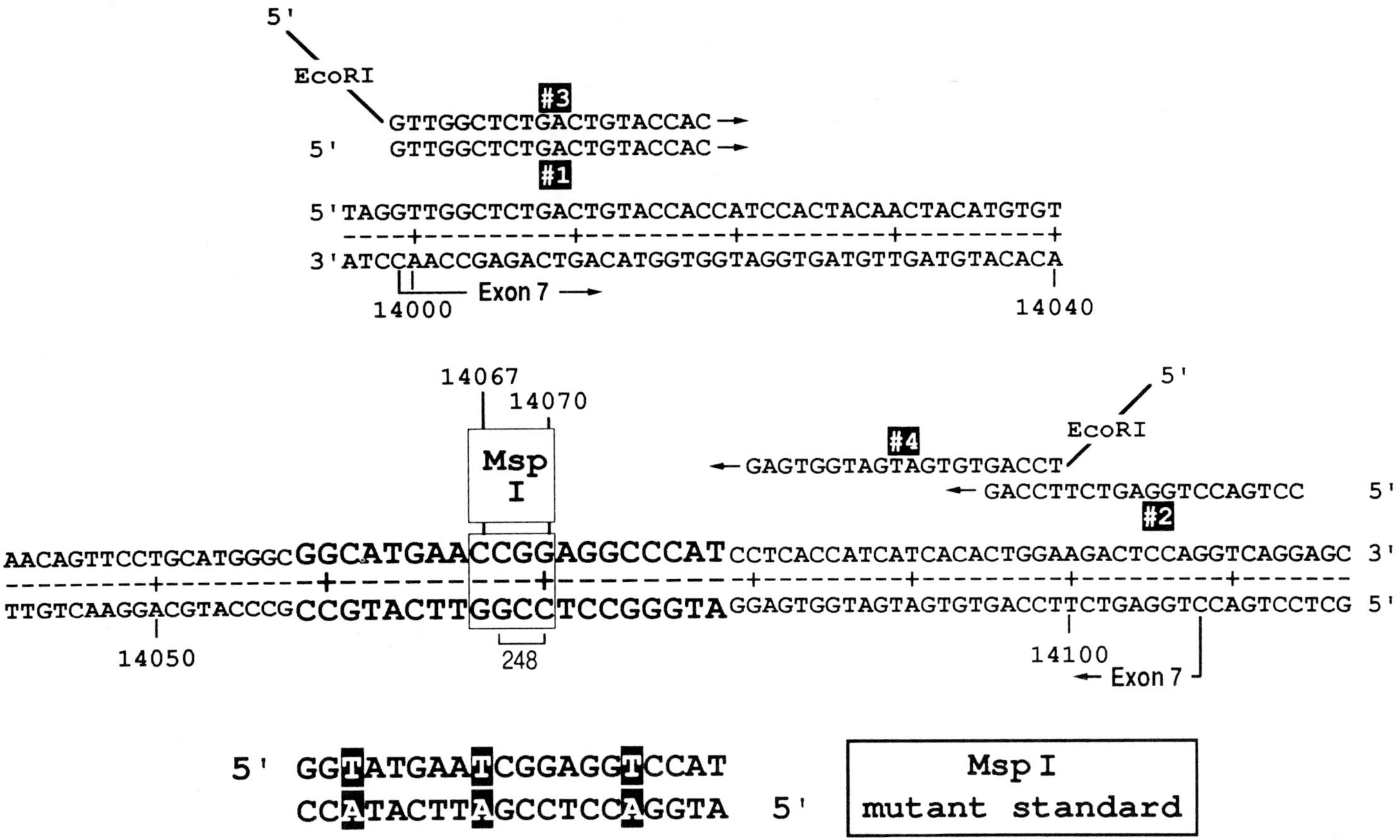

Figure 2 RFLP/PCR analysis of codon 248 of exon 7 of the human *p53* gene.

polymerase (Perkin-Elmer, Küsnacht, Switzerland) under the high-fidelity conditions defined by Eckert and Kunkel (9) [20 m*M* Tris-HCL (pH 7.3) at 70°C, 50 m*M* KCl, and 10 m*M* $MgCl_2$]. In addition to the sequences shown above, the second set of primers contained 5′ tails of 12 nucleotides with *Eco*RI recognition sequences in order to facilitate cloning (see Fig. 2). The temperature cycles consisted of 30 sec at 96°C and 1 min at 45°C for amplification with either polymerase. The amplifications were carried out in a Perkin-Elmer DNA Thermal Cycler 480. For basic information concerning PCR technologies, the reader is referred to recent monographs (10,11).

Preparation of Authentic Single Base Pair Mutants at *Msp*I Site 14067–14070 of Human *p53* and of Mutant Standard

All 12 possible single base pair mutations in the tetranucleotide CCGG of the *Msp*I recognition sequence (residues 14067–14070) of exon VII of the human *p53* gene were prepared using synthetic oligonucleotides and a PCR protocol (5,6) (see Fig. 2 for sequence information). Authentic constructs containing inserts with mutations in the restriction site of interest (here, *Msp*I site 14067–14070 of *p53*) are required for the determination of selective washing temperatures in the oligonucleotide filter hybridization procedure. Furthermore, they routinely serve as controls to ascertain the specificity of the hybridization conditions in each filter analysis of an RFLP/PCR product. Twelve different 19 mers corresponding to residues 14061–14079 of *p53* which contained single base changes in the CCGG sequence were used as antisense primers. These oligonucleotides were used with sense primer 3 (residues 13999–14018 plus a 12-nucleotide tail containing an *Eco*RI recognition sequence) in 35 PCR reactions with cloned wild-type *p53* DNA as template. The high-fidelity amplification conditions with *Taq* polymerase were as described above. The 12 resulting 92-bp fragments were purified on 2% agarose gels and then used as sense primers in a second round of amplifications with *Pfu* polymerase under the conditions described above, except that the amplification buffer contained 6% dimethyl sulfoxide. The common antisense primer 4 corresponded to residues 14099–14080 plus a 12-nucleotide tail containing an *Eco*RI recognition sequence. The resulting 125-bp fragments were precipitated with isopropanol, resuspended in 10 m*M* Tris-HCl (pH 7.4) and 1 m*M* Na_2 EDTA buffer, digested with *Eco*RI (Boehringer Mannheim), purified on 2% agarose gels (Sigma), and cloned into λgt 10 under standard conditions using commercially available λgt 10 arms and packaging mixture (Promega, Zurich, Switzerland).

All authentic mutant λgt 10 constructs were plaque purified on *Escherichia coli* C600 Hfl. For this purpose plaques were lifted onto Colony/Plaque Screen NEF-978 membranes (New England Nuclear–Dupont, Boston, MA) and probed with mutant-specific ^{32}P end-labeled oligonucleotides. Positive plaques were picked, and the phage was eluted from the agar and plated onto *E. coli* C600 Hfl. When confluent lysis had been achieved, the phage was collected in 5 ml of buffer [100 m*M* NaCl, 20 m*M* Tris-HCl (pH 7.4), and 10 m*M* $MgSO_4$], and after the addition of 100 μl of $CHCl_3$, the suspension was centrifuged at 10,000 rpm for 10 min 4°C. Mutant phage contained in the supernatant was titered and then stored at 4°C in the presence of 0.3% aqueous $CHCl_3$.

MS was prepared by an analogous PCR protocol, with the exception that the antisense primer corresponding to residues 14077–14058 in the first round of amplifications contained the 3 base changes indicated in Fig. 2 relative to wild-type *p53*. One of the changes is located at position 14067 (T replaces C) and renders the MS resistant to *Msp*I digestion. The two additional changes outside of *Msp*I site 14067–14070 were introduced in order to allow the distinction of MS from bona fide mutations in the RFLP/PCR products. MS was cloned into λgt 10 and the SP65 cloning vector as described above. It may be advantageous to construct an MS with a new restriction site which is not contained in the homologous wild-type sequence. This allows the removal of MS from the final RFLP/PCR product when it interferes with the quantitation of certain mutations.

We have taken the precaution to prepare the authentic mutant constructs and MS in a separate laboratory which is not being used for the preparation of cellular DNA or amplification. In view of the enormous sensitivity of RFLP/PCR analysis, even the smallest cross-contamination with these constructs must be painstakingly avoided.

Determination of Mutant Composition of RFLP/PCR Products by λ-Plaque Oligonucleotide Hybridization

The DNA of the amplification mixtures was precipitated with isopropanol and digested with *Msp*I (25 U) in order to digest *p53* fragments with wild-type restriction site 14067–14070. Following purification on Qiagen-tip 5 columns under the conditions outlined by the supplier (Qiagen), the samples were digested with *Eco*RI in order to produce staggered clonable ends with *Eco*RI recognition sequences. The DNA was further purified by electrophoresis on 2% agarose gels as described above. The DNA band corresponding to the expected amplified fragment of 117 bp was electroeluted onto a diethylaminoethyl–cellulose membrane NA 45 (Schleicher & Schuell) according to standard procedures (12), the eluate was extracted with phenol–chloroform, and the DNA was precipitated with ethanol. Aliquots of the purified DNA were ligated to λgt 10 arms, packaged under the conditions specified by the supplier (Promega), and used to infect *E. coli* C600 Hfl. Plaques were lifted onto Colony/Plaque Screen NEF-978 membranes. Oligonucleotide plaque hybridization was carried out with 12 end-labeled mutant-specific probes with single base pair changes in the *Msp*I site 14067–14070, a wild-type probe, and an MS probe according to standard conditions (12). Selective washing temperatures for each probe were determined in order to avoid nonspecific hybridization. For this purpose the λgt 10 constructs containing the *p53* inserts with authentic single base pair mutations in *Msp*I site 14067–14070 described in the preceding section were packaged and *E. coli* C600 Hfl was infected. The selective washing temperatures were then determined with the help of Colony/Plaque Screen NEF-978 membranes lifted from authentic mutant plaques and were found to lie in the range of 62–66°C.

In order to obtain statistically meaningful data, $1–3 \times 10^3$ plaques on 10–15 petri dishes (8.5 cm) were analyzed for each RFLP/PCR product with the 12 mutant-specific probes (for the 4 bp of the *Msp*I recognition sequence), the wild-type probe, and the MS probe. Care was taken that none of the plaques was counted more than once. The content in a particular mutation is expressed as a percentage of the total identified plaques. Usually, a small 10–30% of the plaques remained unidentified. Sequencing of the λ-inserts of unidentified plaques indicated the presence of small deletions and insertions which affect specific restriction as well as primer multimers.

Determination of Major Mutations by Quantitative Sequence Analysis

Major mutations in the RFLP/PCR product can be measured directly by quantitative sequence analysis. An aliquot of the RFLP/PCR product was used as the template for asymmetric amplification in order to produce preferentially noncoding strands using sense primer 3 and antisense primer 4 (see Fig. 2) at a ratio of 1 : 100 and *Taq* polymerase under the conditions described above. The amplification product was purified by precipitation with isopropanol and sequenced by extension of a 5′end-labeled primer corresponding to residues 14009–14028 with Sequenase version 2 T7 DNA polymerase (United States Biochemical/Lucerna Chemical, Lucerne, Switzerland) following the experimental conditions outlined by the supplier. The four lanes of the sequence autoradiograms were quantitatively evaluated by densitometry using a Zeiss (Oberkochen, Germany) MQ2 scanner connected to a Kontron (Zurich, Switzerland) Data System 450 multitasking version 2.

It is well known that band intensities in a particular lane depend on the position of the residues in the sequence, presumably because of conformational restraints of the DNA. However, these differences in band intensities are reproducible. Therefore, we normalized our data in each lane relative to reference residues located outside the selected restriction recognition sequence (6,7). For example, the bands of residues A14062 and A14077 were used for the normalization of mutant A bands in the *Msp*I site 14067–14070 of *p53*. Usually, two or three sequences derived from the same RFLP/PCR product are analyzed by densitometry and the data are statistically evaluated. Quantitative sequence analysis only yields reliable data for major mutations which represent at least 10% of the

RFLP/PCR product. When applicable, this method is rapid, economical, and amenable to automation (see Ref. 14).

Estimation of Absolute Mutation Frequencies by Data Calibration with MS

Plaque hybridization with mutant-specific oligonucleotide probes and quantitative sequence analysis determine the mutant composition of the RFLP/PCR products, rather than absolute mutation frequencies. Despite the fact that the amount of DNA and the number of gene copies at the outset of the experiment are known, absolute mutation frequencies can only be obtained by calibration with an internal MS, since the recoveries in the many experimental steps of the RFLP/PCR protocol are unknown. As already mentioned, MS consists of a fragment of the gene of interest which covers the restriction site chosen for mutation analysis. It contains a base pair change in the selected restriction site which renders it resistant to cleavage and two or more base pair changes outside of this site which allow its distinction in the RFLP/PCR product from bona fide mutations. The protocol for the construction of MS was described above. The sequence of the MS for *Msp*I site 14067–14070 of *p53* described here in detail is shown in Fig. 2. MS is added to the genomic DNA at the outset of the experiment before the enrichment of mutated sequences by agarose gel electrophoresis (see Fig. 1) and carried through the entire experiment. Although MS is identical to genomic DNA, with the exception of a few site-specific base pair changes, it should be ascertained that it is amplified with the same efficiency as the homologous wild-type sequence. Most reliable results are obtained when a constant number of initial gene copies and of MS copies is used in a series of related experiments.

The content of MS in the RFLP/PCR product is determined by quantitative sequence analysis or λ-plaque oligonucleotide hybridization, and a relationship can be established to the known number of MS copies which had been added to the cellular DNA at the outset of the experiment. This relationship allows the estimation of absolute mutation frequencies per base pair for single base pair changes from their content in the RFLP/PCR product (6,7). Since there is no guarantee that exact proportionality is maintained for the concentrations of *bona fide* mutations and MS in the final RFLP/PCR product, absolute frequencies obtained in this fashion have to be considered estimates rather than precise data.

COMMENTS: LIMITATIONS OF MUTATION ANALYSIS BY RFLP/PCR

The maximal sensitivity of the RFLP/PCR protocol is determined by the completeness of the removal of wild-type sequences and the inherent error rate at a particular base pair of the DNA polymerase used in the PCR. Repeated digestions with a large excess of restriction enzyme and gel fractionation are used to reduce uncut wild-type sequences to a minimum. However, even 0.1% intact sequences of the original 10^7–10^8 gene copies represents a large excess relative to mutant sequences. The application of the high-fidelity thermostable polymerase from *Pfu* (Stratagene) (13) has substantially increased the sensitivity of the assay (15). *Pfu* polymerase, unlike *Taq* polymerase, possesses a proofreading 3′–5′ exonuclease activity. The completeness of the initial restriction not only determines the level of polymerase-induced background mutations but also the content in wild-type sequences of the RFLP/PCR product. A large fraction of wild-type copies decreases the sensitivity of mutation analysis by quantitative sequencing as well as λ-plaque oligonucleotide hybridization. The content of wild-type sequences of the RFLP/PCR product varies for different restriction endonucleases and different restriction sites. For *Taq*I endonuclease site 2508–2511 of the human H-*ras 1* gene, it was below 0.1% (6,7); for *Pvu*II site 1727–1732, 14–23% (5); and for *Msp*I site 1695–1698, which covers hotspot codon 12, 35–40% (5). For *Msp* site 14067–14070 of exon VII of the human *p53* gene, which covers hotspot codon 248, the RFLP/PCR products contained 22–32% wild-type sequences (14, 15). The presence of residual wild-type sequences even after repeated digestions before and after amplification may be due to the formation of heteroduplexes between wild-type and mutant strands which are refractory to digestion. For *Taq*I RFLP/PCR products the wild-type content could be reduced to a minimum because *Taq*I endonuclease possesses high thermostability (the optimal activity of the enzyme lies at 65°C). Therefore, the enzyme was readded during PCR thermocycling, allowing the continuous removal of wild-type sequences from the amplification product (6,7).

RFLP/PCR can only be applied to sequences which harbor a restriction site. Therefore, the distribution of mutations in an entire gene cannot be determined even if many restriction sites are being analyzed. Because mutation frequencies per base pair are very low and the selectable target in the RFLP/PCR approach is limited to restriction recognition sequences of 4–6 bp, the DNA from large numbers of cells must be analyzed in order to rescue mutations at a reasonable rate. On the other hand, the RFLP/PCR protocol is highly sensitive and rapid when predominant mutations can be detected by direct sequencing of the amplified product.

ACKNOWLEDGMENTS

This work was supported by the Swiss National Science Foundation, the Swiss Association of Cigarette Manufacturers, and the Association for International Cancer Research.

REFERENCES

1. B. Rossiter and C. T. Caskey, *J. Biol. Chem.* **265,** 12753 (1990).
2. M. Mendelsohn and R. Albertini (eds.), "Mutation and the Environment. Part C: Somatic and Heritable Mutation, Adduction and Epidemiology." Wiley–Liss, New York, 1989.
3. J. Zijlstra, E. Felley-Bosco, P. Amstad, and P. Cerutti, *in* "Mutagens and Carcinogens in the Diet" (M. Pariza, ed.), p. 187 Wiley-Liss, New York, 1990.
4. J. Parry, M. Shamsher, and D. Skibinski, *Mutagenesis* **5,** 209 (1990).
5. E. Felley-Bosco, C. Pourzand, J. Zijlstra, P. Amstad, and P. Cerutti, *Nucleic Acids Res.* **19,** 2913 (1991).
6. M. Sandy, S. Chiocca, and P. Cerutti, *Proc. Natl. Acad. Sci. U.S.A.* **89,** 890 (1992).
7. S. Chiocca, M. Sandy, and P. Cerutti, *Proc. Natl. Acad. Sci. U.S.A.* **89,** 5331 (1991).
8. S. Baker, E. Fearon, J. Nigro, S. Hamilton, A. Presinger, J. Jessup, P. van Tuinen, D. Ledbetter, D. Barker, Y. Nakamura, R. White, and B. Vogelstein, *Science* **244,** 217 (1989).
9. K. Eckert and T. Kunkel, *Nucleic Acids Res.* **18,** 3739 (1990).
10. M. Innis, D. Gelfand, J. Sninsky, and T. White (eds.), "PCR protocols–A Guide to Methods and Applications." Academic Press, San Diego, 1990.
11. H. A. Erlich (ed.), "PCR Technology: Principles and Applications of DNA Amplification," p. 89. Stockton, New York, 1989.
12. J. Sambrook, E. Fritsch, and T. Maniatis (eds.), "Molecular Cloning: A Laboratory Manual." Cold Spring Harbor Laboratory, Cold Spring Harbor, New York, 1989.
13. K. Lundberg, D. Shoemaker, M. Adams, J. Short, J. Sorge, and E. Mathur, *Gene* **108,** 1 (1991).
14. S. P. Hussain, F. Aguilar, and P. Cerutti, *Oncogene*, in press (1994).
15. F. Aguilar, S. P. Hussain, and P. Cerutti, *Proc. Natl. Acad. Sci. U.S.A.* **90,** 8586 (1993).

21 Gluconeogenesis in Liver Cells

Richard G. Knowles and Chris I. Pogson

Inhibition of liver cell gluconeogenesis is an attractive paradigm for toxicological studies *in vitro*. This is because the optimal functioning of this pathway depends on relationships among cell membrane elements, mitochondria, and cytosol; any compromise of these components or of the cooperation among them is associated with loss of gluconeogenic capacity. This means, in addition, that gluconeogenesis will be affected not only by "specific" inhibitors and activators, but also by agents which have "non-specific" toxic effects on the cells. Further, because liver cells are responsible for much of the metabolism of xenobiotics, the potential exists for revealing the toxic effects not only of the parent compounds added, but also of their quantitatively important hepatic metabolites. Yet again, the quantity of liver cells obtained from one single preparation and the relative simplicity of the assay for glucose formation permit screening of large numbers of compounds for their toxic effects in a comparatively short time.

The sequence of reactions in gluconeogenesis is rather more complex than is shown in most textbooks. The liver cell plasma membrane is almost entirely impermeable to citric acid cycle intermediates (cf. kidney) so that the number of physiological substrates converted to glucose at an appreciable rate is limited to lactate, pyruvate, alanine, glutamine, proline, glycerol, and fructose. In herbivores (particularly ruminants) propionate is also an effective substrate.

There are considerable variations in the rates at which individual substrates are converted to glucose in different species. These variations are, in part, a consequence of differences in the paths of carbon flux caused by variation in the intracellular distribution of phospho*enol*pyruvate carboxykinase (EC 4.1.1.32) and the requirement for NADH and ATP (see Fig. 1). Thus, lactate (which is relatively reduced) generates cytosolic NADH directly and does not demand efflux of reducing equivalents from the mitochondria; pyruvate, on the other hand, requires mitochondrial output of malate, which can then give rise to NADH. Glucose synthesis from alanine differs again, in that urea synthesis is a parallel process.

The rate of gluconeogenesis in liver cells from any one species also depends on nutritional and hormonal status. In "fed" cells, the high rate of glycogenolysis makes it difficult to measure gluconeogenesis from other precursors; it is preferable, therefore, to use cells from livers depleted of glycogen by starvation. Expo-

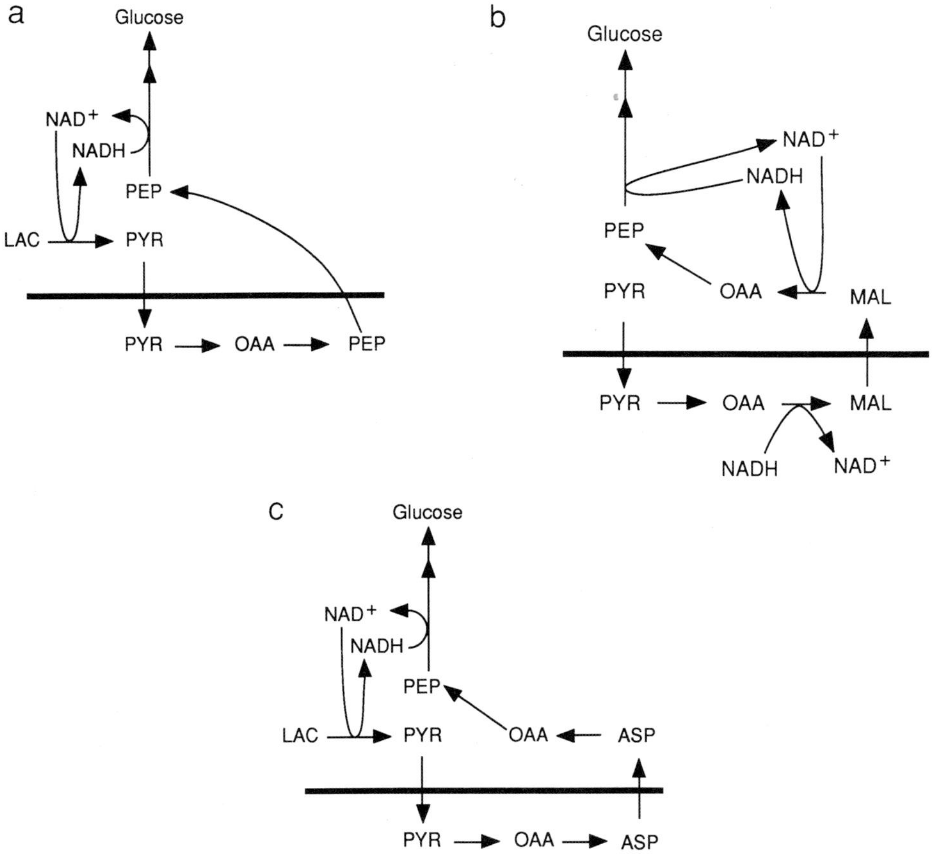

Figure 1 The pathways of gluconeogenesis from different substrates. (a) From lactate (LAC) as substrate with cytosolic phospho*enol*pyruvate carboxykinase (PEPCK). NADH derives from lactate through lactate dehydrogenase and carbon leaves the mitochondrion as aspartate (ASP). (b) From pyruvate (PYR) as substrate with cytosolic PEPCK. Both carbon skeleton and reducing equivalents come from the mitochondrion as malate (MAL). (c) From lactate as substrate with mitochondrial PEPCK. NADH derives, as in (a), from lactate, and the carbon leaves the mitochondrion as phospho*enol*pyruvate (PEP). (d) From pyruvate as substrate with mitochondrial PEPCK. The source of cytosolic NADH is not clear. Malate is possible, but this then leaves an "extra" carbon skeleton in the cytosol unless oxaloacetate (OAA) returns to pyruvate. Other nongluconeogenic pathways may generate NADH. (e) From alanine (ALA) as substrate with cytosolic PEPCK. One alanine goes to aspartate, which provides carbon for glucose synthesis and nitrogen for urea. A second alanine gives rise to oxaloacetate and ammonia; the "malate shuttle" then provides the cytosolic NADH required. FUM, fumarate; ARG, arginine; CIT, citrulline; ORN, ornithine; GLU, glutamate; OG, 2-oxoglutarate.

(*continued*)

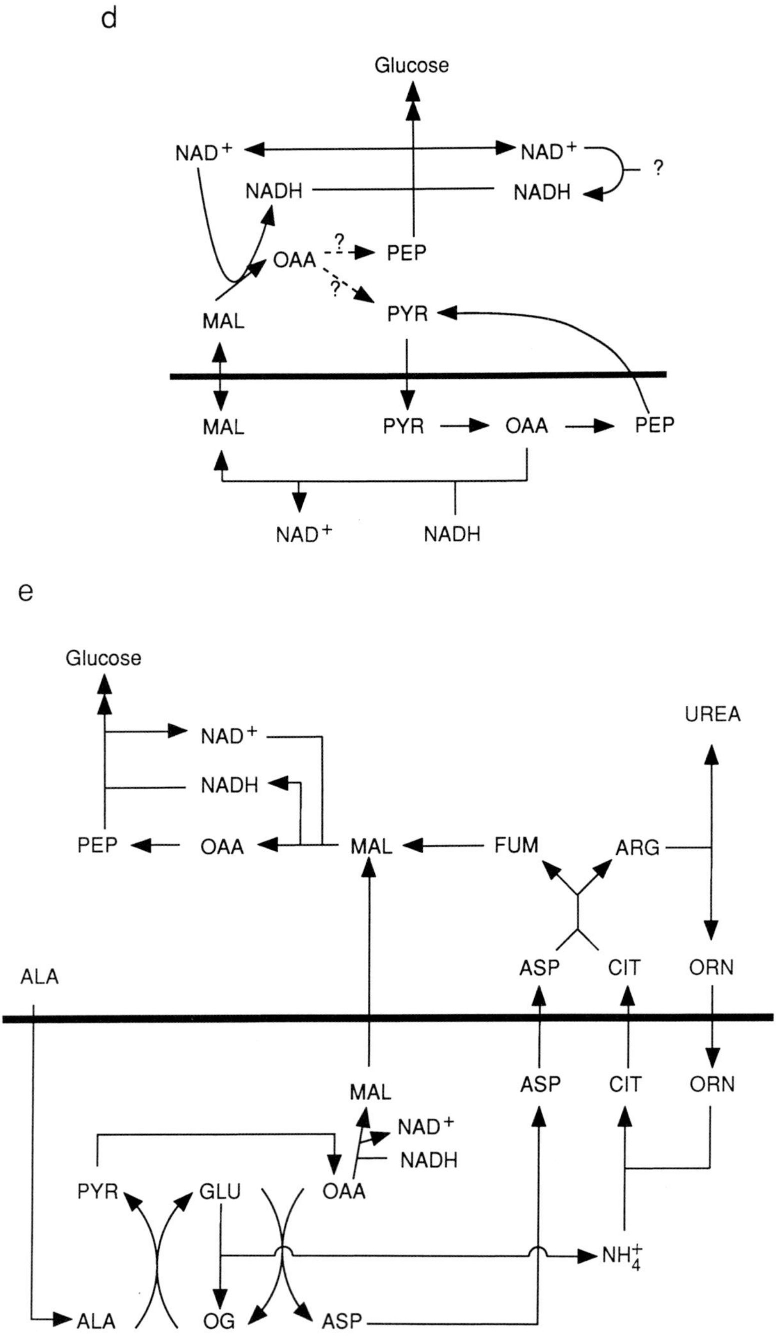

Figure 1 (*continued*)

sure of cells to hormones (e.g., glucagon) during incubation may affect the rate of gluconeogenesis. Equally, the availability of fatty acid in the medium may stimulate (as in the rat) or inhibit (as in the cat) glucose synthesis from lactate (1). It follows that care should be taken in defining the conditions for the assessment of gluconeogenesis in any species or conditions for incubation not previously well documented.

REGULATION OF GLUCONEOGENESIS

The control of gluconeogenesis is shared among several steps in the reaction sequence (2,3); the relative importance of each regulatory site varies as concentrations of hormones and effectors fluctuate. This means that the effects of inhibitors will also not be constant but change as the flux control coefficient for their target enzyme or transport protein changes.

CHOICE OF ASSAYS FOR GLUCONEOGENESIS IN LIVER CELLS

In principle, gluconeogenesis by liver cells from rats starved for 18–48 hr can be assayed either by determination of the amount of glucose formed from appropriate substrates (e.g., lactate) or by determination of the movement of a radioisotope from a labeled substrate to glucose. Studies of gluconeogenesis by liver cells from rats fed *ad libitum* can only be carried out using isotopic methods, because of the contribution of glycogenolysis to glucose formation. We would not recommend isotopic methods for toxicological studies, since the isotopic flux to glucose can be changed by agents affecting the specific activity of gluconeogenic intermediates, even in the absence of an effect on net glucose formation. We therefore describe here the methodology for measuring net production of glucose from gluconeogenic substrates such as lactate plus pyruvate by liver cells from fasted rats.

The most simple and convenient assays for the D-glucose formed by liver cells utilize glucose oxidase (GO, EC 1.1.3.4) to form D-gluconolactone and hydrogen peroxide. Peroxidase (PO, EC 1.11.1.7) is then used to react the hydrogen peroxide with a suitable reduced dye to form a colored product:

$$\text{D-glucose} + O_2 + H_2O \xrightarrow{\text{GO}} \text{gluconolactone} + H_2O_2$$
$$H_2O_2 + \text{reduced dye} \xrightarrow{\text{PO}} \text{dye} + H_2O$$

Although GO only oxidizes β-D-glucose, spontaneous mutarotation is sufficiently rapid for α-D-glucose to be converted during the assay. The most commonly used hydrogen donors are *o*-dianisidine [product absorbance measured at 437 nm (4)], 4-aminophenazone/phenol [product absorbance measured at 505 nm (5)], and aminobenzthiazoline sulfonate [ABTS, product absorbance measured at 405 nm (6)]. The protocol described below uses ABTS because of its relatively low toxicity and high stability in the assay reagent.

The assay is highly specific and relatively robust. High (millimolar) concentrations of some compounds, particularly reducing agents, can compete with the ABTS for hydrogen peroxide; for example, 5-hydroxytryptamine can substitute for the reduced dye and react without giving a colored product. These problems are apparent if appropriate controls are carried out with glucose standard plus the test compound. In such instances an alternative assay can be used which utilizes hexokinase (HK, EC 2.7.1.1) and glucose-6-phosphate dehydrogenase (G6PDH, EC 1.1.1.49) (7):

$$\text{glucose} + \text{ATP} \xrightarrow{\text{HK}} \text{glucose-6-phosphate} + \text{ADP}$$

$$\text{glucose 6-phosphate} + \text{NAD(P)}^{+} \xrightarrow{\text{G6PDH}} \text{gluconolactone 6-phosphate} + \text{NAD(P)H} + \text{H}^{+}$$

This assay is absolutely specific for glucose and is not as susceptible to inhibition as the GO assay, although it is less simple and convenient.

PROTOCOL FOR DETERMINATION OF LIVER CELL GLUCONEOGENESIS

Preparation and Incubation of Liver Cells

The methods for preparing liver cells by perfusion of the liver have been fully detailed elsewhere (8,9). Cell pellets (derived from perfusion of the livers of rats starved for 18–48 hr to deplete liver glycogen reserves) are weighed and the cells are resuspended in Krebs–Henseleit buffer/1.25 m*M* $CaCl_2$ at the required cell concentration (routinely 5 mg dry weight/ml), on the basis that 6 g of such a liver cell pellet contains ~1 g dry weight. This liver cell suspension is kept at room temperature under 95% O_2/5% CO_2 until the incubations are started (normally within 30 min).

For accurate determination of the liver cell concentration, 2-ml portions of the cell suspension are placed in preweighed tubes and centrifuged briefly, and the supernatants are removed. The cell pellets are then dried for determination of dry weight. One milligram dry weight is equivalent to 3.9 mg wet weight, or 0.39×10^6 cells (10).

For incubation, 2-ml portions of the cell suspension are placed in 25-ml polythene (or silicone-treated glass) scintillation vials containing substrates (routinely, lactate and pyruvate at final concentrations of 10 and 1 m*M*, respectively) and the compound(s) under study, dissolved in 20 μl of water or a solvent such as dimethyl sulfoxide or dimethyl formamide. The stock solution of lactate can be stored at −20°C at a concentration of 1 *M*; pyruvate solutions, however, are less stable and must be made up fresh, most conveniently by dissolution of solid to a final concentration of 0.1 *M* in the stock lactate. Rubber stoppers are placed loosely in the necks of the vials, and O_2/CO_2 is passed into the gas phase of each vial (through a syringe needle) for 2 min. The stoppers are then pushed home to effect a gastight seal. Vials are incubated at 37°C in a reciprocating water bath (100 cycles/min) for up to 90 min.

Incubations are terminated by addition of 0.2 ml of 20% (v/v) $HClO_4$, which precipitates all proteins. The resulting suspension is then transferred to microfuge tubes for storage at −20°C or for immediate centrifugation (5 min, 1000 *g*) and assay of glucose produced. Portions of some of these extracts may also be neutralized and stored at −20°C for subsequent assay of ATP content (11) as an index of the viability of the preparation (12). Metabolically viable liver cells from starved rats should contain ~9 nmol of ATP/mg dry weight; values below ~6 nmol/mg indicate a substantial proportion of damaged cells, and experimental results with such preparations should be treated with some reserve.

Glucose Assay

For the GO/PO assay the complete assay reagent is made by dissolving ABTS (final concentration, 0.5 m*M*), glucose oxidase (0.1 mg/ml of a suspension containing 100–150 U/mg from *Aspergillus niger;* e.g., type X-S from Sigma, St. Louis, MO), and peroxidase (0.1 mg/ml of a suspension containing 150–200 U/mg from horseradish; e.g., type II from Sigma) in 0.5 *M* phosphate (Na) buffer (pH 7.0). This reagent is stable for at least 3 weeks if kept in a foil-covered bottle at 4°C; 1 liter is sufficient for 1000 assays.

Suspensions in $HClO_4$ are thawed, mixed well, and then briefly centrifuged (e.g., 1 min, 10,000 *g*). Reagent (1 ml) is mixed with portions (25 μl) of the supernatant or 0–3.2 m*M* (0–80 nmol) glucose standard solutions, in 1-ml disposable plastic cuvettes. After incubation for 30 min at room temperature, the absorbance is determined within the next 60 min. The colored product can be measured spectrophotometrically at 405 nm (1 m*M* in the original sample gives a reading of ~1.0) or at a wavelength corresponding to the lower broad-absorbance peak at 650–750 nm (a glucose concentration of 2 m*M* in samples gives a reading of ~1.0). This assay can also be carried out in microtiter plates with 5 μl of sample plus 200 μl of reagent, with readings being taken of the differences in the absorbances at 405 and 450 nm. In either case the concentration of glucose in the samples is obtained by reference to the linear standard curve, which should be constructed from at least five glucose concentrations (25-μl volumes containing 0, 20, 40, 60, and 80 nmol of glucose) measured in duplicate.

For the HK/G6PDH glucose assay an assay buffer is prepared containing 150 mM triethanolamine (hydrochloride) and 10 m*M* magnesium acetate, adjusted to pH 7.0 with KOH. This is stable for several weeks at 4°C and for longer periods if frozen; 1 liter is enough for 1000 assays. On the day of the assay,

NAD^+ (final concentration, 0.5 mM), ATP (final concentration, 1.0 mM) and G6PDH [from *Leuconostoc mesenteroides;* suspension in $(NH_4)_2SO_4$, from Boehringer Mannheim; 1 μl/ml of buffer, giving a final concentration of 1 U/ml] are added to the assay buffer. Volumes (0.95 ml) of this reagent are mixed with 50-μl portions of supernatants derived from the suspensions in $HClO_4$ in 1-ml plastic disposable spectrophotometer cuvettes, and the initial absorbances at 340 nm are read. HK [from yeast; suspension in $(NH_4)_2SO_4$, from Boehringer Mannheim; 4 μl/ml of buffer, giving a final concentration of 5 U/ml] is then added, and the absorbances, when stable, are read again; this is typically 20–30 min after addition of HK. The concentrations of glucose in the samples are calculated from the changes in absorbance and the extinction coefficient of NADH (6220 M^{-1} cm^{-1}):

$$\text{concentration of glucose (m}M\text{)} = \frac{\text{absorbance change} \times \text{dilution } (1000/50)}{6220 \times 10^{-3}}$$

The rate of gluconeogenesis is expressed as nmol/hr mg dry weight of cells. With lactate plus pyruvate as substrates, the control rates of gluconeogenesis should be 200–300 nmol/hr mg dry weight (500–770 nmol/hr 10^6 cells).

COMMENTARY

Assay Methodology

The potential problem with inhibition of the GO/PO assay by extraneous compounds—added on purpose to incubations, or generated in them by phase I or other metabolism—dictates that studies of compounds that do appear to inhibit gluconeogenesis should be carefully controlled. For example, samples of the suspensions in $HClO_4$ can be reassayed after they have been "spiked" with a known amount of glucose. Alternatively, some glucose assays can be repeated with the HK/G6PDH assay as described above. If free of such problems, however, the GO/PO system is the easier (and cheaper) of the two for rapid screening exercises.

G6PDH from most sources is specific for $NADP^+$. Because NAD^+ is cheaper, we have used the enzyme from *Leuconostoc* which can use either nucleotide equally. Enzyme from other sources will work just as well, provided that $NADP^+$ is used.

It is possible to obtain both false-positives and false-negatives in screening numbers of compounds. First, serum albumin is often included in incubation media (although it is not necessary for the purpose described here); control rates may be higher than expected if the albumin has not been freed of bound fatty acids. More importantly, however, many nonphysiological compounds bind avidly to albumin, are thus effectively removed from contact with the cells, and hence appear inactive against gluconeogenesis. Second, many compounds are not readily soluble in water and require another solvent before addition to incubations. Ethanol is a common solvent, but should not be used in studies involving metabolic measurements. This is because it is a substrate for alcohol dehydrogenase and interferes by "pushing" all of the cytoplasmic NAD^+ to NADH. It is worth noting that a 1% (v/v) solution of ethanol is ~174 m*M*!

The timecourse of glucose synthesis from lactate and pyruvate is not entirely linear from zero time. There is a lag period of ~10 min, during which the cells reach "equilibrium." If truly linear rates are required, the measurements of glucose accumulation can be made for the 30- to 90-min period of incubation. Alternatively, the substrate can be omitted from the initial incubation and added after a preincubation period of 30 min. The deviation from linearity over the whole 90-min period, however, is not great, so that, conveniently for large numbers of incubations, reasonable estimates are obtained with measurements based from time zero.

We recommend that measurement of cellular ATP content is used to assess viability. This suffers from the drawback that such measurements cannot practically be done until after incubations are over. Assessment of fresh cells with trypan blue is of some use (see Ref. 8), but is not wholly reliable (13,14).

The rates of several metabolic processes in liver cell incubations vary with cell density (15). Gluconeogenesis is less sensitive to this parameter, but concentrations of cells below 2 mg dry weight/ml may give somewhat lower control rates, even with preparations with high ATP contents.

Inhibition of Gluconeogenesis

Gluconeogenic flux can be affected by either direct or indirect inhibition. Direct inhibitors include:

1. Quinolinate: An inhibitor of phospho*enol*pyruvate carboxykinase, this is a metabolite of tryptophan. It is a relatively weak inhibitor and is probably unimportant physiologically in most species other than rats, mice, and related species in which hepatic concentrations can be up to 5 m*M* (16).

2. 3-Mercaptopicolinate: This is related structurally to quinolinate, but is a much more potent inhibitor at the same site. It has been widely used experimentally (17). Care is needed to ensure that the compound has not undergone oxidation to the disulfide before use.

3. Aminooxyacetate (carboxymethoxylamine): This is an inhibitor of pyridoxal phosphate-dependent enzymes, although with varying affinity for each. It thus blocks aspartate aminotransferase (EC 2.6.1.1), hence the efflux of carbon skeletons from the mitochondrion when lactate or glutamine (for example) are substrates (see Fig. 1) (18).

4. Cyano-4-hydroxycinnamate: This compound is a very potent blocker of the transport of pyruvate across the inner mitochondrial membrane, hence its conversion to oxaloacetate and acetyl-CoA (19).

Indirect inhibitors are those which act on pathways and systems not usually thought of as part of the gluconeogenic sequence. As a first example, atractyloside and bongkrekic acid block the translocation of adenine nucleotide across the inner mitochondrial membrane and hence inhibit gluconeogenesis by decreasing cytosolic ATP concentrations. Second, it has been shown that gluconeogenesis is very sensitive to inhibitors of mitochondrial respiration (3). Third, 2-oxiranecarboxylates are converted to their CoA esters through the action of fatty acyl-CoA synthetase (EC 6.2.1.3); the acyl-CoAs so formed inhibit β-oxidation by direct interaction with carnitine palmitoyltransferase (EC 2.3.1.21). The decreased flux through β-oxidation leads to a decrease in the availability of acetyl-CoA, required as an activator of pyruvate carboxylase, important in the gluconeogenic pathway (20).

REFERENCES

1. H.-D. Söling and J. Kleineke, *in* "Gluconeogenesis: Its Regulation in Mammalian Species" (R. W. Hanson and M. A. Mehlman, eds.), p. 369. Wiley, New York, 1976.
2. A. K. Groen, C. W. T. Van Roermund, R. C. Vervoorn, and J. M. Tager, *Biochem. J.* **237,** 379 (1986).
3. H. J. Pryor, J. E. Smyth, P. T. Quinlan, and A. P. Halestrap, *Biochem. J.* **247,** 449 (1987).
4. H. A. Krebs, D. H. A. Bennet, P. De Gasquet, T. Gascoyne, and T. Yoshida, *Biochem. J.* **86,** 22 (1963).
5. P. Trinder, *Ann. Clin. Biochem.* **6,** 24 (1969).
6. W. Werner, H. G. Rey, and H. Wielinger, *Z. Anal. Chem.* **252,** 224 (1970).
7. H.-U. Bergmeyer, E. Bernt, F. Schmidt, and H. Stork, *in* "Methods in Enzymatic Analysis" (H.-U. Bergmeyer, ed.), p. 1196. Verlag Chemie, Weinheim, Germany, 1974.
8. P. O. Seglen, *Methods Cell Biol.* **13,** 29 (1976).
9. C. A. Tyson and J. M. Frazier (eds.), this series, Vol. 1, Part A.
10. E. A. Siess, D. G. Brocks, and O. H. Wieland, *in* "Metabolic Compartmentation" (H. Sies, ed.), p. 235. Academic Press, New York, 1982.
11. P. E. Stanley and S. G. Williams, *Anal. Biochem.* **29,** 381 (1969).
12. A. J. Dickson and C. I. Pogson, *FEBS Lett.* **83,** 27 (1977).
13. R. A. Page, K. M. Stowell, M. J. Hardman, and K. E. Kitson, Anal. Biochem. **200,** 171 (1992).
14. M. N. Berry, A. M. Edwards, and G. J. Barritt, *in* "Isolated Hepatocytes, Preparation, Properties and Applications: Laboratory Techniques in Biochemistry and Molecular Biology" (R. H. Burdon and P. H. van Knippenberg, eds.). Elsevier, Amsterdam, 1991.
15. R. R. Jurin and S. A. McCune, *J. Cell. Physiol.* **123,** 442 (1985).

16. C. I. Pogson, R. A. Muñoz-Clares, K. R. F. Elliott, E. A. Kean, P. Lloyd, and S. A. Smith, *in* "Short-Term Regulation of Liver Metabolism" (L. Hue and G. Van de Werve, eds.), p. 339. Elsevier/North-Holland, Amsterdam, 1981.
17. N. W. Di Tullio, C. E. Berkoff, B. Blank, V. Kostos, E. J. Stack, and H. L. Saunders, *Biochem. J.* **138,** 387 (1974).
18. R. Rognstad and J. Katz, *Biochem. J.* **116,** 483 (1970).
19. A. P. Halestrap and R. M. Denton, *Biochem. J.* **138,** 313 (1974).
20. L. Agius, D. Pillay, K. G. M. M. Alberti, and H. S. A. Sherratt, *Biochem. Pharmacol.* **34,** 2651 (1985).

22 Measurement of Protein Synthesis

Michael J. Meredith

Cellular response to toxic conditions produced by xenobiotic chemicals or alteration of nutritional status can be exhibited in a wide variety of forms. Outside of chemical overdose, rarely is acute toxicity induced by direct production of phenomena such as membrane damage (i.e., lipid peroxidation with lactate dehydrogenase leakage) or immediate cellular necrosis. Chronic effects are more often the result of some impaired biochemical function. Among these basic processes, protein synthesis is known to be altered by a number of agents. Moreover, the mechanisms by which protein synthesis is interrupted have been shown to be equally diverse. Heat shock (1) and glutathione oxidation (2) are known to block protein synthesis. As noted by Farber (3), such divergent chemicals as ethionine, carbon tetrachloride, galactosamine, and dimethylnitrosamine all produce the same measurable result, inhibition of amino acid incorporation into protein.

Measurement of protein synthesis *in vitro* has been used as a basic description of toxicity. As a methodological process protein synthesis can be assessed by techniques that fall into two major classes: quantitative determination and qualitative descriptions. Quantitative determination of protein synthesis is accomplished by measuring incorporation of labeled amino acids into protein, thus providing a measurable quantity differentiating newly synthesized and preexisting proteins. This is usually accomplished by measuring radioactive amino acid incorporation into precipitated proteins. Qualitative descriptions can be made by relying on imaging labeled proteins separated by some physical method. Autoradiography/fluorography of protein separated by polyacrylamide gel electrophoresis is the most common protocol for this method. This chapter presents methods for both procedures that have been useful in this laboratory and are representative of the methods used by others.

MEASUREMENT OF PROTEIN SYNTHESIS BY RADIOACTIVE AMINO ACID INCORPORATION

The procedure for measurement of protein synthesis by quantitation of incorporated amino acids can be broken down into three segments: (1) choice of a labeling compound, (2) sample precipitation, and (3) collection and counting of

METHODS IN TOXICOLOGY, Volume 1B

the sample. Since almost all radiolabeled amino acids are commercially available, the optimum labeling species can be used. The major concern in this choice is to select an amino acid that will represent newly synthesized protein. This means that the labeling amino acid should be uniformly represented in all proteins and should not be recycled extensively after proteolysis. The later point is more important for pulse–chase studies, but should be considered in all cases. The isotope for labeling must also be chosen with care. Tritium is the most commonly used isotope for this type of protein synthesis monitoring due to the high-specific-activity amino acids available and the lower cost of the compounds. Although ^{14}C and ^{35}S provide higher emission energies and counting efficiencies, when proteins are collected for counting this property is of less importance. Moreover, because methionine is not present in all proteins, some proteins may not be labeled (1). Culture medium for protein labeling should be prepared with the labeling amino acid omitted. This will provide a higher rate of incorporation, increasing the sensitivity of the method. For short-term labeling experiments (i.e., 1–3 hr) sufficient amino acid supplies are usually present as intracellular pools or from serum to support maximum rates of protein synthesis. Longer-term labeling experiments should be done only if it is certain that amino acid levels are sufficient to support protein synthesis. [^{3}H]Leucine (l-[4,5-^{3}H]leucine or l-[3,4,5-^{3}H]leucine), available from all major providers at specific activities ranging from 5 to 70 Ci/mmol, is the usual isotope of choice.

The following method has been applied successfully to several cell types, both substrate dependent and independent, including primary hepatocytes, epithelial cells, fibroblasts, and lymphoblasts.

Solutions and Materials

HEPES-buffered saline solution: 0.5 g/liter KCl, 8.3 g/liter NaCl, and 2.4 g/liter HEPES (pH 7.4)
100% Trichloroacetic acid (TCA) stock solution: 227 ml of water added to 500 g of TCA
15% and 5% (v/v) TCA
95% Ethanol
0.1 N NaOH

Equipment

Glass fiber filters (Reeve Angel 934AH, Whatman GF/B, or equivalent)
Vacuum filter manifold (Hoefer FH224V, FH125 filter holder, Hoefer, San Francisco, CA)
Scintillation fluid and counter (Beckman LS-500 scintillation counter with RPI BioSafe II fluid or equivalent equipment and material)

Cells can be maintained in either a T-flask or a culture dish, but for the most reproducible results cultures should be in log or early plateau growth phase. Culture medium is removed and the cells are washed twice with a buffered saline. This laboratory uses a HEPES-buffered saline instead of phosphate-buffered saline to prevent redistribution of mitochondrial glutathione (4,5).

Replace the growth medium with labeling medium containing the radioisotope. For general applications 2 μCi/ml [^{3}H]leucine will give a satisfactory amount of radiation incorporated to assess synthetic rate. Ideally, the volume of labeling medium should be the same as that of growth medium; however, to reduce cost and the volume of waste to be disposed of later, smaller volumes may be used. For 1- to 3-h labeling periods, up to a 50% reduction of volume may be used.

At the end point, labeling medium is removed and the cells are washed three times with ice-cold buffered saline. At this point two common methods are used to remove the protein from the plate and prepare the sample for counting.

Method A

Protein can be precipitated with TCA and counted directly after trapping on a glass fiber filter. The hygroscopic nature of TCA makes it impossible to keep TCA in a solid form for any length of time. To prepare solutions of TCA, make a 100% TCA stock by adding 227 ml of double-distilled (or better) water to 500 g from a freshly opened TCA. Dilute from this stock, which should be kept at 4°C (solutions referred to as "cold" should be at 4°C). For a 60-mm culture dish add 1.5 ml of cold 15% TCA and dislodge the cell material by a rubber policeman or a plastic scrapper. After soaking the glass fiber filter in cold 15% TCA, the filter is mounted in the vacuum manifold. Adjust the vacuum to move about 2 ml/min through the filter. Add the TCA extract to the filter reservoir and apply the vacuum. Rinse the plate and extract tube with an additional 1.5 ml of cold 15% TCA and apply to the filter. Wash the filter with 2 ml of cold 5% TCA and 2 ml of cold 95% ethanol to remove water and eliminate quenching. Allow air to be drawn through the filter to evaporate the ethanol. Transfer the dried filter to a scintillation vial (7 or 20 ml, glass or plastic) and add scintillation fluid. The opaque filter will become clear when the fluid is added, increasing the counting efficiency. Count the filters in a liquid scintillation counter, using manufacturer-suggested counting window settings for the isotope used. Counting time is dependent on the amount of radioactive material incorporated. A counting error of less than 10% is required. Increased counting time can decrease counting error. Although it is possible to construct a quench curve and obtain true disintegrations-per-minute information, for most purposes the uncorrected counts per minute (cpm) will prove sufficient. This procedure requires demonstration that counting efficiency is not altered among samples, either by sample channels ratio, external standard, or H-number for Beckman counters. Results obtained by this method are normalized to some previously selected standard, (i.e., cell number or cpm per dish). Method A has the advantage of supplying data rapidly. It suffers from the lack of an internal comparison standard and the possibility of incomplete removal of protein from the culture dish. For more precise determination of incorporated amino acids, method B provides better protein removal and a more accurate means of comparing samples.

Method B

Cultures labeled and washed as above are dissolved by adding 1 ml of 0.1 N NaOH to a 60-mm culture plate. The volume of NaOH can be varied proportionately with plate size. After 10 min at 37°C, the cells are removed by scraping and the NaOH is collected in centrifuge tubes. A small sample (10–50 μl) is taken for protein analysis[1] and the remaining sample is treated with 2 ml of cold 15% TCA. Precipitation is carried out for at least 45 min at 4°C. Proteins are then washed with 3 ml of cold 5% TCA with a 5-min centrifugation at 1500 *g* to pellet TCA insoluble material. Having been precipitated and washed to remove any residual labeling amino acid, protein pellets can be resuspended in cold 5% TCA, trapped and counted on glass fiber filters as described for method A, or redissolved in 1 ml of 0.1 N NaOH at 60°C for 30 min and counted directly (method B_1). Up to 1 ml of 0.1 N NaOH may be counted in 6 ml of fluid without significant chemiluminescence. If larger amounts are to be counted, samples can be stored at −20°C for 1 hr to reduce spurious counts. Results are then expressed as cpm/mg of protein. Of the two counting options, redissolving in NaOH produces more precise determinations of amino acid incorporation, as seen in Table I.

Table I Incorporation of [^{3}H]Leucine into ARL-15 Protein[a]

Time	Method A[b]	Method B[c]	Method B_1[c]
30	18,064 ± 3022	9275 ± 1052	109,843 ± 302
60	34,024 ± 7113	184,231 ± 1132	21,869 ± 498
120	60,329 ± 14,372	36,749 ± 1973	42,372 ± 835

[a] ARL-15 rat liver epithelial cells were labeled with 2 μCi/ml in Williams medium E [G. Williams and J. M. Gunn, *Exp. Cell Res.* **89**, 139 (1974)] prepared without leucine for the times shown. Results show the means ± SD of three 60-mm plates.
[b] Results are reported as cpm per 60-mm plate.
[c] Results are reported as cpm/mg of protein.

1 Analysis of protein in NaOH can be done by the BCA method (6). Preparation of protein standards in 0.1 N NaOH will correct for the modest inhibition of color formation by base.

Knowledge of acceptable data variability is helpful in selecting the appropriate method of protein synthesis evaluation. For example, heat shock is known to inhibit protein synthesis. In order to investigate the effect of glutathione depletion on protein synthesis after heat shock, the data in Table II were obtained by method A, the least refined of the precipitation methods (7). The precision is sufficient to show that glutathione depletion does not inhibit protein synthesis significantly, even after heat shock. As a general rule, if differences of more than 10% are expected between experimental samples, the precision allowed by method A is sufficient to discriminate between means, with a P value of greater than 0.05. Method B would be appropriate if small numbers of replicates are available or if a large standard deviation is anticipated.

EVALUATION OF PROTEIN SYNTHESIS BY ELECTROPHORESIS AND FLUOROGRAPHY

An alternative to determination of radioactive amino acid incorporation by scintillation counting is autoradiographically/fluorographically detected proteins. This protocol has the advantage of being able to assess synthesis of individual proteins as well as a general appraisal of protein synthesis due to the electrophoretic separation of labeled material. Several comprehensive collections of electrophoresis methods are available, but perhaps the most useful of these books are by Dunbar (8) and Walker (9). Both deal with the general aspects of electrophoresis and autoradiography as well as many advanced and specialized methodologies. In this chapter only the most elementary description of elec-

Table II Heat Shock Inhibition of Protein Synthesis

Temperature (°C)	Time (min)[a]	Protocol[b]	cpm[c]
37	15	DMSO	41,926 ± 5396
		DEM/BSO	51,240 ± 5100
43	15	DMSO	41,329 ± 950
		DEM/BSO	34,031 ± 1977
37	30	DMSO	167,742 ± 3950
		DEM/BSO	177,742 ± 18,198
43	30	DMSO	48,721 ± 4,561
		DEM/BSO	47,723 ± 5349
37	60	DMSO	415,233 ± 32,561
		DEM/BSO	411,107 ± 25,731
43	60	DMSO	109,594 ± 3764
		DEM/BSO	76,370 ± 5440

[a] Minutes of [^{35}S]methionine labeling (2 μCi/ml).
[b] Cells were treated for 1 hr with dimethyl sulfoxide (DMSO) or diethyl maleate/buthionine sulfoximine (DEM/BSO) to deplete glutathione prior to labeling.
[c] Means ± SD of four flasks.

trophoresis methods 15 made, but directions should be sufficient to allow the investigator to initiate this type of experimentation.

Proteins are labeled as described above. Tritium labeling is acceptable and produces high-quality images, but requires longer exposure times and enhancement by fluorographic techniques. ^{14}C and ^{35}S are both good choices, providing stronger β-emissions, but both are more expensive and, in the case of [^{35}S]methionine, could possibly produce incomplete labeling of all proteins. Consideration of the amount of label to be incorporated can determine the isotope used. If low levels of radiation are to be incorporated, the higher energies available from ^{14}C or ^{35}S could make these the materials best suited for the application.

Solution and Materials

30% Acrylamide and 2.7% bis-acrylamide (w/v): Dissolve acrylamide and bis-acrylamide in the best-quality water available, filter through Whatman No. 1 filter paper, and store at 4°C in the dark. Adding about 10 g of a mixed bed resin such as Amberlite MB per 100 ml of acrylamide solution is useful, preserving the quality of the acrylamide solution by remove acrylic acid formed over time. Acrylamide is know to be neurotoxic and readily absorbed through the skin. Gloves and eye protection are required, and weighing should be done in a fume hood. Polymerize any unused acrylamide solution and discard after 30 days

Separating gel buffer: 1.5 *M* Tris, pH 8.8 (20°C)—For 250 ml use 45 g of Tris base, adjusted to pH 8.8 with HCl

Stacking gel buffer: 0.5 *M* Tris, pH 6.8 (20°C)—For 250 ml use 15 g of Tris, adjusted to pH 6.8 with HCl

Running buffer: For 1 liter combine 14.4 g of glycine, 3 g of Tris, 1 g of sodium dodecyl sulfate (SDS); adjust to pH 8.3 if necessary. Running buffer can be prepared as a 5× stock for convenience

10% (w/v) SDS

10% (w/v) ammonium persulfate

Sample buffer (2×): For 10 ml combine 2 ml of glycerol, 1.5 g of Tris, 0.46 g of SDS, and 1 ml of 0.1% (w/v) bromphenyl blue solution. Titrate to pH 6.8 with HCl. Add 2–5% (v/v) β-mercaptoethanol immediately prior to use. Dithiothreitol (DTT) can also be used at concentrations of 200–500 m*M* in place of β-mercaptoethanol. DTT-containing sample buffer can be prepared and frozen in small aliquots prior to use. Unused sample buffer and be kept at 4°C for 24 hr. Do not refreeze DTT- or β-mercaptoethanol-containing sample buffer

N′,N′,N′,N′-Tetramethylethylenediamine (TEMED)

1 *M* sodium salicylate, pH 6.0

Slab Gel Electrophoresis Equipment

Glass plates
Spacers (0.75–1.0 mm)
Sample well formers ("combs" with eight to 12 wells per gel)
Casting stand
Buffer reservoir and gel holder
Power supply (output up to 500-mA constant current)

Gel equipment is available from a number of manufacturers. Bio-Rad (Richmond, CA) makes a very satisfactory minigel (7 × 8-cm gel format) apparatus. An additional advantage of the Bio-Rad equipment is the availability of an extensive line of equipment fitting the gel format, such as isoelectric focusing gels and electrophoretic transfer cassettes. Hoefer also produces good-quality equipment. Table III shows the reagents needed to prepare two minigels. The slab gel format is by far the most common, and the reagents listed above are for preparation of gels according to the method of Laemmli (10). Formulation of the gel (i.e., percentage of acrylamide) may vary from 7.5% to 15% or even a gradient of acrylamide. The best gel for the application should be determined based on separation needed and the size of the protein(s) of interest. The general references cited above (8,9) contain specific instructions for these variations.

To prepare the gel, assemble the gel form as per the manufacturer's instruction. Mark the height of the desired gel on the glass plate. In the minigel format a 5-cm separating gel height is sufficient and leaves enough room for the stacking gel. It is essential that the glass plates and spacers be clean and free of any material such as grease or residual acrylamide that might cause the plates to

Table III SDS–Polyacrylamide Gel Composition[a]

Stock	7.5%[b]	12%[c]	4% (Stacking gel)[d]
Water	4.85 ml	3.35 ml	6.10 ml
Separating gel buffer	2.50 ml	2.50 ml	
Stacking gel buffer	—	—	2.50 ml
10% SDS	100 μl	100 μl	100 μl
Acrylamide/bis-acrylamide	2.5 ml	4.0 ml	1.30 ml
10% Ammonium persulfate	50 μl	50 μl	50 μl
TEMED	5 μl	5 μl	5 μl

[a] SDS, Sodium dodecyl sulfate; TEMED, *N′*, *N′*, *N′*, *N′*-tetramethylethylenediamine.
[b] For proteins of 50–250 kDa.
[c] For proteins of 10–100 kDa.
[d] For use with all separating gels.

crack under the pressure of the plate holders. Combine the first five separating gel ingredients and degas under aspirator vacuum for about 10 min. Add TEMED and pipette the acrylamide mixture into the gel forms. Overlay with water-saturated *n*-butanol and allow the gel to polymerize for at least 45 min. When the gel is polymerized, *n*-butanol can be removed and the gel overlaid with 0.5× running buffer until needed. If the gel is not to be used for more than 12 hr, overlay, cover with Parafilm, and store at 4°C. Separating gels can be prepared in multigel casting apparatus. These gels can be stored for several days at 4°C in an air tight container. An overlayer of running buffer will prevent the gel from drying out. At the time of use, prepare the stacking gel as described in Table III, degas, and cast the stacking gel with sample well combs in place. Move the combs as necessary to remove bubbles. Since the stacking gel will shrink during polymerization, allow a larger sample well than needed for the volume of sample to be applied. After the stacking gel has been added, the completed gel should be used within a few hours to prevent diffusion of the pH discontinuity between stacking and separating gels.

Cells are labeled by the same procedures described above. Preparation of the protein sample for electrophoresis and autoradiography can be accomplished by several methods. It is essential that the sample be free of unincorporated radioactivity and that the protein content of the sample be known. This can be accomplished most expeditiously by a procedure similar to that previously described in method B. After washing, the cells are dissolved in a small volume of 0.1 N NaOH (0.1–1.0 ml) and a sample is then taken for protein determination. Addition of 3 vol of cold 15% TCA denatures proteins which are collected by centrifugation. The protein pellet is washed with cold ethanol and resuspended in a minimum volume of 1× sample buffer. Protein determination is done prior to precipitation, since it is assumed that TCA precipitation is quantitative. This allows resuspension to a known protein content for electrophoresis. Counting a small sample of the resuspended protein gives an exact figure for radiation content. Samples can now be run on the basis of constant protein or constant radiation content. Sample volume should be kept to a minimum for best protein separation results.

Samples are heated at 100°C for 4 min prior to electrophoresis to further denature and dissolve TCA precipitated proteins. Gels can then be run according to the manufacturer's recommendation. Prestained molecular weight standards should be run with each gel. For two 0.75-mm minigels standard electrophoresis conditions in this laboratory are 1 hr at 200 V constant voltage. Cooling is not usually required for small gels, but may be essential for larger gel formats. Cooling coils are usually built into the buffer reservoir. Cold water can be circulated through these cooling tubes. Buffer temperature should be kept under 20°C to prevent protein band distortion. However, buffer temperatures below 5°C can cause precipitation of SDS in the gels.

The terms "autoradiography" and "fluorography" are often, and incorrectly, used interchangeably. Detection of newly synthesized proteins by autoradiography is done without enhancers. Of the commonly used isotopes, only ^{35}S is sufficiently energetic to be effectively used without fluorography. Fluorography is necessary for ^{3}H- or ^{14}C-labeled proteins. By impregnating gels with fluor, a compound that converts radiochemical emission into light, it is possible to increase the sensitivity of the method by 5- to 10-fold, depending on the isotope. Earlier methods (11) relied on dimethyl sulfoxide to introduce the scintillant 2,5-diphenyloxazole (PPO) into gels. The method was technically demanding and somewhat unreliable. Commercially available enhancing fluors, such as EN^{3}HANCE (New England Nuclear—Dupont, Boston, MA), are available and are used successfully in many laboratories. Intensifying screens such as the Lightning Plus (Dupont Cronex) are very commonly used to increase the sensitivity of ^{32}P autoradiographs. Although these screens are not usually recommended for protein autoradiography, we have found that they do increase the sensitivity of ^{35}S detection slightly.

Sodium salicylate, a water-soluble compound (12), has largely replaced PPO. A brief water wash (30 sec) removes any surface radiation and excess detergent. The gel is then incubated for 30 min with mild agitation at room temperature in enough 1 *M* sodium salicylate, pH 6.0, to cover the gel. A final 30-sec water rinse eliminates excess salicylate and prevents surface crystallization that can distort the image of protein bands. The gel is then dried between sheets of cellulose or polystyrene before fluorography. Gel dryers are commercially available. Hoefer and Bio-Rad make dryers using heat and vacuum for drying gels as well as for drying membranes for autoradiography or fluorography.

The dried gel is placed directly on X-ray film, allowing the closest possible exposure. To transfer the position of the molecular weight standards to the X-ray film, place small pieces of phosphorescent tape over the prestained proteins. Cardboard and metal cassettes are commercially available in the most common sizes (8 × 10 and 5 × 7 inches) to hold the film and the gel during exposure. The only requirements for the cassette are that it must (1) be) lightproof and (2) hold the film and the dried gel motionless and flat at the −70°C temperature required for fluorographic exposure. Exposure time will vary from a few hours to several days, depending on the amount of radiation present in the gel. For ^{3}H-labeled proteins a good test exposure time is 12 hr at −70°C. Kodak (Rochester, NY) SB X-ray film is often recommended for fluorography, due to the sensitivity of the film at wavelengths produced by the fluor. However, Kodak X-Omat AR and RP have been used successfully in this laboratory. Both types of film are available from Sigma (St. Louis, MO) or other photographic suppliers.

Quantitative evaluation of protein synthesis by autoradiographic methods is possible if it is known that exposure of the film is in the linear range for all bands. The optical density of developed film is then proportional to the amino acids incorporated. Densitometry is possible with any of the currently available commercial units, such as the Hoefer GS300. These instruments provide a digital output that can be copied by a chart recorder, integrator, or computer. In addition, video densitometry, using a video camera to digitize and import the gel image into a computer and integration software to quantitate the bands, has become common. Image 1.44 (National Technical Service, Springfield, VA) is a public domain software package developed at the National Institutes of Health for this type of image manipulation.

All of these methods rely on conversion of film density into digitally comparable units. Total protein synthesis can be evaluated by summation of total film density. However, the most important property of the electrophoretic method is the ability to evaluate the synthesis of individual proteins.

Interpretation of results is dependent on how the samples were loaded onto the gels. If gels were loaded such that all lanes contained equal protein amounts, film density for individual bands, as well as for total protein, will be directly proportional to the rate of protein synthesis. If lanes were loaded with equal radioactivity, film density for individual bands is proportional to the synthesis of that specific protein. The later method of gel loading provides a means of examining translational effects on individual protein levels. Figure 1 shows the gels

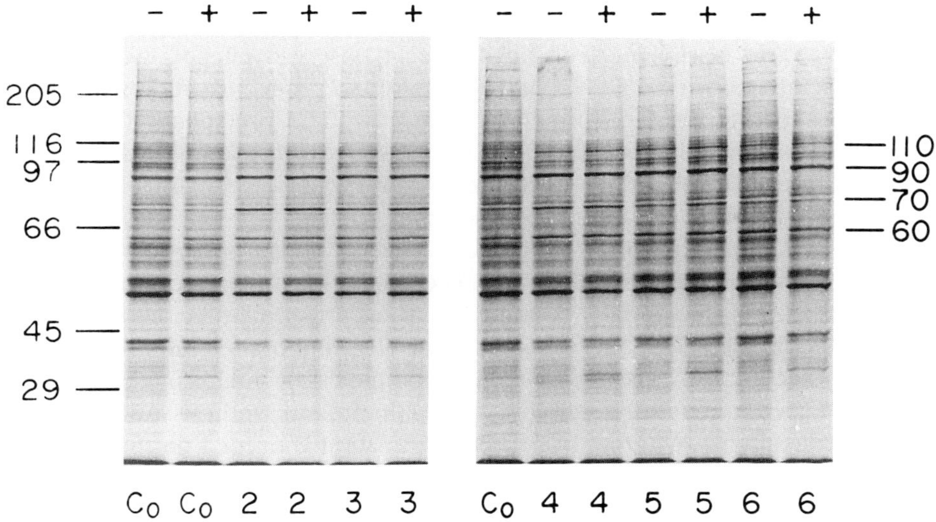

Figure 1 Fluorographic analysis of protein synthesis in Chinese hamster ovary cells after heat shock and glutathione depletion. After heating at 43°C, cells are incubated with or without buthionine sulfoximine to inhibit glutathione synthesis. [^{35}S]methionine (2 μCi/ml) was added with a medium change at the times shown (hr). Lanes labeled C_0 in the left panel are cells heated and immediately labeled with (+) or without (−) buthionine sulfoximine. The lane labeled C_0 in the right panel is an untreated control. [Reproduced from M. L. Freeman, M. J. Meredith, and A. Laszlo, *Cancer Res.* **48,** 7033–7037 (1988) by permission of the American Association of Cancer Research, Inc.]

from an experiment examining the effect of glutathione depletion on synthesis of heat shock proteins (7). Chinese hamster ovary cells were heated at 43°C for 15 min, then treated with the glutathione-depleting agent, diethyl maleate (DEM), for 1 hr, then, after washing out the DEM, cells were incubated with or without buthionine sulfoximine to block glutathione synthesis. After recovery times ranging from 2 to 6 hr, cells were labeled with 2 μCi/ml [^{35}S]methionine in methionine-free medium. Gels were loaded on an equal-protein basis. Beyond the synthesis of heat shock proteins at 70 and 90 kDa, these gels show that protein-synthetic capacity is reestablished by 4 hr after heat shock, independent of glutathione depletion. The information gained from this type of procedure both addresses total synthesis and allows detection of new proteins as well as shifts in translational specificity.

SUMMARY

The methods presented here to measure protein synthesis are those most commonly used. They have been compiled from many sources, and this chapter presents the modified protocols used in this laboratory. This is by no means an exhaustive list of methods, materials, or equipment. Examination of toxic effects expressed as altered protein synthesis can be done by *in vitro* translation experiments (13) to clarify mechanistic details of observed effects. Evaluation of protein synthesis *in vivo* is a far more complicated procedure. Although the ultimate procedures for measurement are the same, TCA precipitation or autoradiography/fluorography, *in vivo* analysis requires extensive knowledge of amino acid pool sizes, turnover rates, and amino acid-recycling mechanisms. Clearly, *in vitro* toxicity studies bypass these drawbacks.

Perhaps the most common error in experiments measuring protein synthesis is not experimental, but preparative. It is essential for the investigator to know what kind of information is to be gained from the experiment before choosing a method. Very often, the more complicated electrophoretic studies are done, when the technically easier TCA precipitation method would provide the information needed to monitor xenobiotic effects on protein synthesis. Autoradiography/fluorography is required only when information is needed on the synthesis of a specific protein. If the experimental goals are clearly understood, the appropriate methods can be chosen.

ACKNOWLEDGMENT

Research in this laboratory was supported by the National Institute of Environmental Health Sciences grant ES 03272.

REFERENCES

1. G. Borbely, G. Suranyi, A. Korcz, and Z. Palfi, *J. Bacteriol.* **161,** 1125 (1985).
2. N. S. Kosower and E. M. Kosower, *Lancet* **2,** 1343 (1970).
3. E. Faber, *Annu. Rev. Pharmacol.* **11,** 71 (1970).
4. M. J. Meredith, *Cell Biol. Toxicol.* **2,** 495 (1986).
5. M. J. Meredith and D. J. Reed, *J. Biol. Chem.* **257,** 3747 (1982).
6. P. K. Smith, R. I. Krohn, G. T. Hermanson, A. K. Mallia, F. H. Gartner, M. D. Provenzano, E. K. Fujimoto, N. M. Goeke, B. J. Olson, and D. C. Klenk, *Anal. Biochem* **150,** 76 (1985).
7. M. L. Freeman, M. J. Meredith, and A. Laszlo, *Cancer Res.* **48,** 7033 (1988).
8. B. S. Dunbar, "Two Dimensional Electrophoresis and Immunological Techniques." Plenum, New York, 1987.
9. J. M. Walker, "Methods in Molecular Biology," Vol. **1.** Humana, Clifton, New Jersey, 1984.
10. U. K. Laemmli, *Nature (London)* **227,** 680 (1970).
11. R. A. Laskey and A. D. Mills, *Eur. J. Biochem.* **56,** 335 (1975).
12. J. P. Chamberlain, *Anal. Biochem.* **98,** 132 (1979).
13. R. Reisbig, S. Olsnes, and K. Eiklid, *J. Biol. Chem.* **256,** 8739 (1981).

23 Measuring Collagen Synthesis

William J. Lindblad

INTRODUCTION

Extracellular matrix (ECM) deposition occurs in both normal and injured tissues. This deposition is a finely regulated balance between protein synthesis and degradation. Since a prominent phenotypic response of cells to injury is an enhanced deposition of ECM proteins, this response to injury may be considered a change in the homeostatic regulatory mechanisms of ECM production.

Whereas numerous proteins are present within the ECM, the protein composing the majority of its mass is collagen. Collagen is a triple-helical molecule containing extended arrays of repeating triplets of Gly–X–Y residues [where X = proline (Pro) and Y = hydroxy-L-proline (Hyp) generally] with over 13 types of collagen currently identified (1). Of these multiple collagen types, type I collagen is the predominant form of collagenous protein deposited following many forms of tissue injury, including hepatic injury. These various types of collagen are synthesized by a wide range of cell types, including those cells originating from all three embryonic germ layers (2).

Methods developed to quantitate collagen biosynthesis can be divided into biochemical and immunological methods. The latter approach requires the availability of type-specific collagen antibodies to recognize protein in radioimmunoassays, in enzyme-linked immunosorbent assays, or by immunoprecipitating radiolabeled collagenous proteins. These methods represent extremely powerful techniques to determine the synthesis of specific collagen types, particularly in cell cultures in which extracellular collagen cross-linking is minimal. However, if one is interested in the total amount of collagen produced by a system, the immunological approaches may be considered too specific, since it would be very difficult to specifically quantitate each of the numerous collagen types which may be synthesized by a given cell. Consequently, the biochemical measures are often used to obtain data on the total collagen biosynthetic rate.

Two methods dominate the biochemical techniques for collagen synthesis, namely, the bacterial collagenase digestion assay and the production of radiolabeled Hyp. The former method is based on the selective digestion of collagenous proteins by highly purified collagenase from *Clostridium histolyticum* (3). This enzyme, at 37°C, will specifically cleave the collagen-repeating triplet along

METHODS IN TOXICOLOGY, Volume 1B

the entire length of the molecule, producing soluble digestion fragments. The enzyme is insensitive to the length of the molecule or its triple helicity, thereby enabling one to determine all collagen produced in a cell culture, even if partially degraded.

The latter technique utilizes the unique production of Hyp by post-translational modification of Pro in the nascent collagen chain by the enzyme prolyl hydroxylase (4). Since this imino acid has such a restricted distribution among proteins, the quantitation of Hyp production is indicative of collagen synthesis. These two methods are described here in detail, using nonproliferating monolayers of adult rat hepatocytes as a representative culture system in which to measure collagen production.

MATERIALS AND METHODS

Collagenase Digestible Protein Assay

L-[5-^{3}H]Proline, 15–40 Ci/mmol (Amersham, Arlington Heights, IL)
Purified bacterial collagenase (Worthington, Freehold, NJ, code no. CLSPA)[1]: Highly purified collagenase free of nonspecific proteolytic activity, 0.7 μg/ml in enzyme buffer
Enzyme buffer, 50 m*M* Tris-HCl (pH 7.60) containing 5 m*M* $CaCl_2$
HEPES buffer, 1.0 *M*, (pH 7.20)
$CaCl_2$, 25 m*M*
N-Ethylmaleimide (NEM): Make up to 7.82 mg/ml in water
Trichloroacetic acid, crystalline (TCA): Make up to 5%, 10%, and 50% (w/v) in water
TCA/tannic acid: Freshly prepare a solution of 0.5% tannic acid in 10% TCA. Also prepare a 1 : 1 dilution using water

Equipment

Vortex mixer
Water bath capable of reaching 95°C
Refrigerated centrifuge capable of producing 10,000 *g*
Liquid scintillation counter

Protocol

1. Confluent hepatocyte cultures are labeled for 24 hr in serum-free medium containing 10 μCi of L-[^{3}H]proline per 60-mm dish in a temperature-controlled

[1] Since this reagent must be free of all contaminating neutral proteases, each lot of collagenase is further purified by chromatography over a gel filtration column (3).

incubator at 37°C under an air : CO_2 atmosphere.[2] When the culture dishes are removed from the incubator, they are immediately placed on ice to minimize proteolytic digestion of the newly synthesized collagen.

2. Cells are harvested by scraping the monolayer into the medium with a cell scraper, pipetting the suspension into a 50-ml round-bottomed centrifuge tube kept cold on ice, and washing the dishes two times with 1 ml of ice water. The washes are added to the cell suspension.

3. The tubes are placed into boiling water for 10 min to inactivate proteases present in the suspensions (5), then cooled on ice to 4°C.

4. Total proteins are precipitated by addition of one-fifth volume of ice-cold 50% TCA. The tubes are vortexed to ensure even mixing of the TCA and placed on ice for 30 min to allow the proteins to settle.

5. Centrifuge the tubes at 10,000 *g* for 10 min at 4°C, remove the supernatant, and resuspend the pellet in 5.0 ml of 5% TCA.

6. Repeat step 5 at least four times to eliminate free [^{3}H]Pro.[3]

7. Remove the final supernatant and let the tubes stand at room temperature for 10 min, then remove the TCA which is extruded from the pellet.

8. Dissolve the pellets in 0.5–1.0 ml of 0.2 N NaOH. This may require vigorous vortexing and heating at 37°C for 15–30 min.

9. From each sample remove the following aliquots and dispense into 3.0-ml conical tubes as indicated: 0.2-ml aliquot, tube marked "+"; 0.2-ml aliquot, tube marked "−". Save the residual sample for determination of DNA or protein.

10. To each tube add 0.3 ml of a solution prepared as follows: 100 μl of HEPES buffer, 10 μl $CaCl_2$, 20 μl of NEM, and 170 μl of water.

11. Adjust the pH of each tube to between 7.2 and 7.4, using no more than 20 μl of 1 N HCl or 1 N NaOH to achieve this pH.

12. Add 10 μl of neutral buffer to the "−" tubes and 10 μl of bacterial collagenase solution to each "+" tube, vortex to mix, and incubate at 37°C for 90 min.

13. Place the tubes on ice for 10 min and add 0.5 ml of TCA/tannic acid solution to each tube. Vortex and return to ice for 10 min to precipitate nondigested protein.

14. Centrifuge the tubes at 500 *g* for 10 min at 4°C. Remove the supernatant from each reaction tube and place it into liquid scintillation counting vials.

[2] The length of time required to label cells varies, depending on the total amount of collagen produced. Fibroblasts, which make over 2% of the total protein as collagen, may be effectively labeled after 4 hr.

[3] It is crucial that the cell pellets be washed sufficiently to remove all nonincorporated [^{3}H]Pro. Generally, this is accomplished with five TCA washes; however, some cells require as many as eight washes. The final TCA supernatant should contain $<$500 cpm.

15. Wash the pellet in each reaction tube by resuspending it in 0.5 ml of cold 5% TCA/0.25% tannic acid and centrifuging at 500 *g* for 10 min at 4°C. Add the supernatant to the respective liquid scintillation counting vials.

16. To each of the reaction tubes marked "+" add 0.5 ml of 5% TCA/0.25% tannic acid, vortex to resuspend, and transfer the contents to a separate liquid scintillation counting vial. Wash these reaction tubes with two 0.5-ml aliquots of 5% TCA/0.25% tannic acid and add to the respective liquid scintillation counting vials.

17. Prepare a "background" vial using 1.5 ml of 5% TCA/0.25% tannic acid. Add 10 ml of liquid scintillation fluid to each vial and count.[4]

Quantitation of 4-Hydroxy-L-proline

L-[U-^{14}C]Proline, >250 mCi/mmol[5]
TCA, 50%
HCl, 12 N and 1 N
7-Chloro-4-nitrobenz-2-oxa-1,3-diazole chloride (NBD-Cl) (Sigma, St. Louis, MO), 2.0 m*M* solution prepared in high-performance liquid chromatography (HPLC)-grade methanol
Potassium tetraborate buffer, 40 m*M*, (pH 9.5)
Dowex AG50W (Bio-Rad, Richmond, CA), 100–200 mesh, H^+ form

Equipment

HPLC system: Requirements are the ability to run a complex solvent gradient, a heated column compartment, and elution detection at 495 nm
Water bath capable of attaining 37°C
Refrigerated centrifuge capable of producing 10,000 *g*
Rotary concentrator/evaporator
Steam autoclave
Vortex mixer
Liquid scintillation counter

Protocol

1. Hepatocyte cultures are metabolically labeled for 24 hr in serum-free pro-free medium containing 3 μCi of L-[U-^{14}C]proline per 60 mm.

[4] Depending on the liquid scintillation fluid used, it may begin to turn yellow due to the tannic acid. This will significantly diminish the counting efficiency of the counter. Although other fluids may work, Ultima Gold (Packard Instrument Meriden, CT) works well for this application.

[5] Radiolabeled Pro often contains a significant amount of labeled Hyp. Prior to using a batch of labeled Pro, purify it by chromatographing on a small Dowex ion-exchange resin column (6).

2. Cells are harvested by scraping the monolayer into the medium using a cell scraper, pipetting the suspension into a 50-ml round-bottom centrifuge tube kept cold on ice, and washing the dishes two times with ice water. The washes are added to the cell suspension.

3. Total proteins are precipitated by addition of one-fifth volume of ice-cold 50% TCA. The tubes are vortexed and placed on ice for 30 min.

4. Centrifuge the tubes at 10,000 *g* for 10 min at 4°C, remove the supernatant, and resuspend the pellet in 5.0 ml of water. The supernatant will contain free [^{14}C]Pro as well as small fragments of collagen-containing [^{14}C]Pro which result from degradation of the newly synthesized collagen. Therefore, by quantitating the amount of isotope in this fraction, along with the precipitate, one can obtain a measure of both collagen synthesis and degradation. Add an equal volume of 12 N HCl to this supernatant and process as with the TCA-precipitated proteins, described as follows.

5. The suspension is transferred to a glass screw-top culture tube with the centrifuge tube rinsed twice with 1.0-ml aliquots of water and the rinses added to the suspension. An equal volume of 12 N HCl is slowly added to each tube to prevent excess heat production. The top of each tube is covered with a piece of Teflon tape, sealed with a screw cap containing a Teflon liner, and taped tightly around the outside of the cap.

6. The proteins are then hydrolyzed by autoclaving at 122°C for 16 hr.

7. Each hydrolysate is passed through a Pasteur pipette containing a plug of glass wool to remove particulate material and collected in a tube suitable for evaporation of the hydrolysates. The hydrolysates are then evaporated to dryness and reconstituted in 1.0 ml of 20 m*M* HCl.

8. Salts are removed from the samples by ion-exchange chromatography over minicolumns of Dowex AG50W. After application of the samples to the columns, salts are removed using a 10-ml water wash, with the amino acids released by addition of 5 ml of 1 N NH_4OH. The amino acids are then reconcentrated by evaporation, followed by reconstitution in 400 μl of water.

9. The samples are derivatized with NBD-Cl, which preferentially reacts with secondary amines, thus imparting the specificity of the reaction for Pro and Hyp (7). This involves reacting $\leq$100 μl of sample and 10 μl of *cis*-4-hydroxy-L-proline as internal standard (add water to make a final volume of 100 μl) with 100 μl of potassium tetraborate buffer and 100 μl of NBD-Cl for 20 min at 37°C in the dark.

10. The reaction is stopped by the addition of 50 μl of 1 N HCl and 150 μl of a 1 : 1 mixture of HPLC-grade methanol and water.

11. The sample is chromatographed by HPLC using two 4.6 mm × 25 cm columns in series, Zorbax-CN (MAC-MOD Analytical, Chadds Ford, PA) and Spherisorb 10 ODS (Spectra-Physics, Santa Clara, CA). The columns are maintained at 50°C with a flow rate of 1.0 ml/min. The imino acids are eluted with a

methanol gradient as follows: 0–5 min, 5% methanol; 5–30 min, 5–30% methanol; 30–40 min, 30–50% methanol; and 40–50 min, 50–5% methanol. The second solvent used to produce this methanol gradient is 1% acetic acid adjusted to pH 2.35. Eluting peaks are detected by absorbance at 495 nm.

12. Radiolabeled Hyp peaks are collected using a fraction collector connected with the HPLC. Aliquots of the collected fractions are counted by liquid scintillation spectrometry to determine the amount of radiolabeled Hyp that was synthesized (and degraded) by the cells in a 24-hr period.

COMMENTS

Collagenase Digestible Protein Assay

The procedure described here has been successfully applied to a wide variety of tissues and cell cultures, including hepatocytes, fibroblasts, smooth muscle cells, and leukocytes. For use in a unique tissue or cell culture, three parameters must be optimized for this assay to yield consistent results. These parameters are the length of metabolic labeling with L-[5-^{3}H]proline, the digestion time with bacterial collagenase, and the number of TCA washes to eliminate free isotope from the protein pellets. Generally, the length of time for protein labeling is directly related to the amount of collagen synthesized by the cells. Therefore, most mesenchymal cells can be readily labeled within 2–4 hr, whereas low collagen-producing parenchymal cells require overnight labeling times.

The rate of bacterial collagenase digestion will be influenced by several factors, most notably the accessibility of the collagen to the enzyme and the extent of collagen cross-linking (8). This is not generally a problem for cultured cells, since the collagen produced in culture is not extensively cross-linked.

The final parameter to be optimized for a particular cell culture is the washing of protein precipitates to remove free isotopes. This may be a problem for some cells which synthesize macromolecules that nonspecifically bind Pro, and therefore will slowly release the isotope. Multiple washes with TCA are essential, with the addition of a 20 m*M* Pro-containing TCA wash, if necessary, to competitively remove the isotope from the macromolecules.

Generally, the data are presented as relative collagen synthesis using the equation

$$\text{Relative collagen synthesis (\%)} = \frac{\Delta\text{cpm} \times 100}{\{[(\text{cpm P}) - \text{BK cpm}] \times 5.4\} + \Delta\text{cpm}}$$

where Δcpm = [(cpm +) − (cpm −)], cpm P = cpm in the pellet; and BK cpm = background cpm. By expressing the data in this manner, any treatment which may alter Pro transport, and thereby alter the labeling of the intracellular

Pro pools, will not influence this value, since both collagen and noncollagen protein-specific activity would be similarly affected. The factor 5.4 represents the relative enrichment of Pro in collagen compared to general proteins (9). However, expressing the data in this fashion may not accurately express the results if both the collagen synthetic rate and total protein synthesis are simultaneously affected by the culture treatment. Consequently, it is also important to calculate an absolute collagen synthetic rate, which is Δcpm per unit of protein or DNA. This point is exemplified in Table I, in which collagen synthesis in hepatocyte cultures was modulated by two experimental treatments.

Glucocorticoid steroids have been shown by numerous investigators to reduce relative collagen synthesis in hepatocytes (5) and fibroblasts (10). This is a dose-dependent effect. Additionally, hepatocytes are phenotypically very sensitive to the substratum used for coating the culture dishes (11). In hepatocytes plated onto native type I collagen, dexamethasone treatment decreased both absolute collagen synthesis and relative collagen synthesis (Table I). In this case the magnitudes of decrease in collagen synthesis expressed as relative (4.4-fold difference) or absolute (3.8-fold difference) are similar. However, when hepatocytes were cultured on denatured type I collagen, the relative collagen synthesis decreased by a factor of 5, but absolute collagen decreased by only 1.9. This difference results from a dramatic increase in noncollagen protein synthesis induced by dexamethasone in cells plated on denatured substratum. Therefore, to accurately represent the results, both calculations would be required to demon-

Table I Effect of Hepatocyte Substratum and Glucocorticoid Treatment on *in Vitro* Collagen Synthesis[a]

Treatment	cpm (collagen)	cpm Pellet (noncollagen)	Collagen synthesis: Relative (%)	Collagen synthesis: Absolute (dpm/mg of DNA)[b]
Denatured collagen substratum				
Vehicle control	ND	20,282	ND	ND
	223	13,651	0.30	498.5
Dexamethasone[c]	1288	308,991	0.08	338.9
	558	214,188	0.05	198.1
Native collagen substratum				
Vehicle control	1982	131,086	0.28	1016
	1956	86,821	0.42	1431
Dexamethasone	1679	400,912	0.08	338.6
	1206	290,565	0.08	309.9

[a] Primary cultures of adult rat hepatocytes were maintained on the indicated substratum for 8 days with or without dexamethasone. The cultures were then labeled for 24 hr with L-[5-^{3}H]proline prior to harvesting for analysis of collagen synthesis. DNA was determined by a fluorometric method (11). ND, Not detectable.

[b] From C. Labarca and K. Paigen, *Anal. Biochem.* **102,** 344 (1980).

[c] Dexamethasone was prepared as a 1×10^{-2} stock solution in dimethyl sulfoxide (DMSO), with 1 μl of stock added per milliliter of culture medium. Vehicle control cultures received 1 μl/ml of DMSO alone.

strate the responsiveness of the cells for increased noncollagen protein synthesis.

Quantitation of 4-Hydroxy-L-proline

The use of Hyp quantitation for routine collagen biosynthetic determinations is not as common due to the expense of the [^{14}C]Pro and the requirement for separating the radiolabeled Hyp and Pro by HPLC as described above, a technique which is not available in all laboratories. However, this method does enable one to independently confirm the bacterial collagenase method and also obtain a Pro-to-Hyp ratio for determination of the state of hydroxylation of the collagen produced. This method is also useful for quantitation of collagen degradation. In the experiment described in Table II, the ability of dexamethasone treatment on collagen degradation by hepatocytes was examined. For this application, the supernatant in step 4 was analyzed for free Hyp. Since the only mechanism for obtaining freely soluble Hyp is by the degradation of newly synthesized collagen, this value is a measure of overall collagen turnover in the culture. This analysis indicated that dexamethasone failed to significantly increase the amount of free Hyp in the media, which would be indicative of protein degradation.

Two procedures have been described to measure total collagen biosynthesis, since both methods have unique attributes. The bacterial collagenase method is a rapid procedure which readily accommodates multiple samples and does not require specialized chromatography instrumentation. The productivity of this method can be further enhanced by using a recently described application in which collagen synthesis was determined in 24-well cell culture plates (12). The measurement of radioactive Hyp also enables one to run multiple samples, although the isotope used is more expensive. It should be noted that ^{14}C is used for this method, due to the potential for tritium exchange from the Pro ring during acid hydrolysis. I have found a 2–5% exchange of tritium following a 16-hr

Table II Effect of 8 Days' Exposure to Dexamethasone on Formation of Soluble [^{14}C]Hydroxyproline by Hepatocyte Cultures[a]

Treatment	Soluble [^{14}C]hydroxyproline (dpm/μg of DNA)
Vehicle control	406.7 ± 104
Dexamethasone	
$1 \times 10^{-5}M$	238.0 ± 25
$1 \times 10^{-8}M$	239.6 ± 20

[a] Cultures, as described in the legend to Table I, were labeled with [^{14}C]proline using native collagen as a substratum. Values are the mean of duplicate determinations ± range. [Reprinted with permission from *Gastroenterology* **86,** 897 (1984).]

hydrolysis. Another consideration in selecting a specific radiolabeled Pro is the potential hydroxylation of the ring by prolyl hydroxylase which occurs on both the number 3 and 4 carbon atoms, albeit predominantly on the number 4 carbon. Therefore, it is advisable not to use a Pro precursor tritiated in the number 3 position. The strength of this second procedure is the ability to measure both synthesis and degradation.

REFERENCES

1. E. J. Miller and S. Gay, *in* "Wound Healing: Biochemical and Clinical Aspects" (I. K. Cohen, R. F. Diegelmann, and W. J. Lindblad, eds.), p. 130. Saunders, Philadelphia, 1992.
2. R. F. Diegelmann and W. J. Lindblad, *Fundam. Appl. Toxicol.* **5,** 219 (1985).
3. B. Peterkofsky and R. Diegelmann, *Biochemistry* **10,** 988 (1971).
4. S. Udenfriend, *Science* **152,** 1335 (1966).
5. P. S. Guzelian, W. J. Lindblad, and R. F. Diegelmann, *Gastroenterology* **86,** 897 (1984).
6. B. Peterkofsky and D. J. Prockop, *Anal. Biochem.* **4,** 400 (1962).
7. W. J. Lindblad and R. F. Diegelmann, *Anal. Biochem.* **138,** 390 (1984).
8. E. D. Harris, Jr., and M. E. Farrell, *Biochim. Biophys. Acta* **278,** 133 (1972).
9. R. F. Diegelmann and B. Peterkofsky, *Dev. Biol.* **28,** 443 (1972).
10. K. R. Cutroneo, R. Rokowski, and D. F. Counts, *Collagen Relat. Res.* **1,** 557, (1981).
11. W. J. Lindblad, E. G. Schuetz, K. S. Redford, and P. S. Guzelian, *Hepatology* **13,** 282 (1991).
12. R. F. Diegelmann, G. R. Bryson, L. C. Flood, and M. F. Graham, *Anal. Biochem.* **186,** 296 (1990).

24 Measurement of Macrophage Phagocytosis Using a Sheep Red Blood Cell Assay

Gregory L. Finch

INTRODUCTION

The importance of the ability of mononuclear cells to phagocytize foreign agents has been recognized for many years. Accordingly, investigators have developed a variety of *in vivo* and *in vitro* functional assays to measure this process and the way in which exposure to toxic materials may alter phagocytic ability. Generally, *in vitro* tests rely on the premise that measurements made on cells maintained in culture can be correlated with the *in vivo* performance of the cells. Therefore, toxicant-induced effects can be investigated by correlating the results of *in vitro* tests on cells obtained from unexposed animals (e.g., by bronchoalveolar lavage to obtain lung macrophages) with the results obtained on cells recovered from toxicant-exposed animals.

A variety of *in vitro* techniques can be used to quantitate phagocytosis. Direct techniques assess microscopically the ability of individual cultured cells to internalize test particles. Indirect techniques measure end points such as chemiluminescence, activity of phagocytized radiolabeled test particles (e.g., ^{51}Cr-labeled red blood cells), or a cellular physiological property (e.g., oxygen consumption) of the cell culture.

This chapter describes a direct *in vitro* phagocytosis assay that has been adapted from the work of Griffin *et al.* (1) and modified by other investigators (2–4). Phagocytic capacity is typically performed in parallel with other end points, such as cell killing and/or the release of intracellular enzymes or cytokines. The assay is performed under conditions that do not cause appreciable cell killing, so that effects on phagocytosis are a measure of cell function, rather than simply that of cell death. The investigator begins by obtaining pulmonary alveolar macrophages (PAMs) from unexposed experimental animals by bronchoalveolar lavage. The PAMs are placed into a monolayer culture and exposed to toxic agents or particles. After exposure, phagocytic capacity is measured by the light-microscopic determination of the extent of PAM internalization of sheep red blood cells (SRBCs). Here, as in the work cited above, the SRBCs are pretreated with a specific serum component (opsonin), such as complement proteins or immunoglobins, to enhance phagocytic uptake (5).

METHODS IN TOXICOLOGY, Volume 1B

Uptake of the SRBCs can then be quantified in terms of total phagocytic capacity, in which neither time nor the number of available test particles is limiting. Alternately, other parameters, such as phagocytic rate or the percentage of cells taking up test particles, can be measured (6). The uptake of SRBCs by toxicant-exposed PAMs is compared to that of control (unexposed) PAM cultures. Finally, statistical analyses are applied to estimate the influence of the agent on phagocytic capacity and to define dose–response relationships. Data from our previous work with beryllium metal-exposed PAM cultures (7) are used to illustrate the results obtained.

MATERIALS AND REAGENTS

- Cappel immunoglobulin G (IgG)-fraction rabbit anti-sheep red blood cell serum, (Cat. No. 0214-1322, Organon Teknika, West Chester, PA)
- RPMI 1640 medium (GIBCO, Grand Island, NY)
- Alsever's medium [20.5 g of dextrose, 4.2 g of NaCl, and 8.0 g of sodium citrate in 1000 ml of water; mix well and sterilize (8)]
- Dulbecco's phosphate-buffered saline (PBS), physiological concentration (e.g., ICN Biomedicals Cat. No. 18-600-54, Costa Mesa, CA)
- PBS, 2× physiological concentration
- Diff-Quik stain, (Fisher, Pittsburgh, PA)
- Distilled water
- Fresh sheep blood
- Refrigerated centrifuge
- Centrifuge tubes, polypropylene, 15- and 50-ml volume
- 96-Well round-bottomed microtiter plates
- Micropipette (Eppendorf or equivalent) and tips
- Humidified cell culture incubator with CO_2 gas inlet
- CO_2 tank
- Cytocentrifuge (e.g., Shandon Cytospin 2, Shandon, Astmore, Cheshire, England)
- Light microscope with lens immersion oil
- Microscope slides, coverslips, and Permount

PROCEDURES

Preparation of IgG-Opsonized SRBCs

The techniques for the preparation of the SRBC–IgG complex have been outlined by Griffin *et al.* (1) and by Harmsen and Jeska (2).

Preparation of SRBCs

Obtain fresh sheep blood from the jugular vein and place it into an equal volume of Alsever's medium. Separate SRBCs from the buffy coat (white blood cells) using standard blood separation techniques. Wash 10–20 ml of the pelleted SRBCs by diluting 1 : 1 with Alsever's medium, then centrifuge at 300 *g* for 10 at 4°C. Pour off the medium and plasma; wash three additional times in cold saline under the same centrifuge conditions. After the final wash, dilute the packed SRBCs to 1 : 100 and 1 : 10 (v/v) in cold RPMI 1640 medium. The 1 : 100, or 1%, solution will be used as described below; the 1 : 10 solution can be stored at 4°C for up to 1 month after preparation.

Determination of the Subagglutinating Titer

This procedure must be done only once upon first use of each batch of antiserum purchased. Begin by preparing a 1 : 16 dilution of antiserum in RPMI 1640 medium and placing 100 μl of this dilution in each of three wells in a 96-well round-bottomed microtiter plate. Continue by making serial 2-fold dilutions 11 times, ending with a 1 : 32,768 ($1:2^{15}$) dilution, each time placing triplicate 100-μl aliquots into the microtiter plate. To each well add 100 μl of the 1% solution of SRBCs in RPMI 1640 medium from above and mix well. Pipette tips should be changed when mixing samples of different dilutions to prevent cross-contamination. Incubate at room temperature (~20°C) for 30 min, then at 37°C for 30 min.

Following the incubation, examine each well for agglutination, which appears as a mat on the bottom of the well, as opposed to a small button of SRBC where no agglutination has occurred. The subagglutinating titer is defined as the highest dilution in which no agglutination occurs in any of the replicate wells, divided by 2. The antiserum can be refrozen or diluted with RPMI 1640 medium and refrozen for future use; we typically dilute the antiserum with RPMI 1640 medium to a volume of 20 ml, and freeze this in a 50-ml centrifuge tube for use in the next step.

Opsonization of the SRBCs

This step must be done each day the assay is performed. Thaw the antiserum/RPMI 1640 medium from above, add an equal volume of 1% SRBCs, and mix well by inverting the tube. Incubate for 30 min at room temperature and 30 min at 37°C. Centrifuge the suspension at 300 *g* for 10 min at room temperature, pour off the supernatant, and resuspend it with RPMI 1640 medium to a 1% concentration of SRBCs. Place the sensitized SRBC suspension on ice until it is used for that day's experiment.

Phagocytosis Assay

To examine variability within the assay, we recommend that all samples be run in triplicate. Following PAM culturing and *in vitro* toxicant exposure [typically, toxicant exposures are for 20 hr in our laboratory (see Ref. 7 for specific techniques)], begin the phagocytosis assay by removing the cells from the monolayer culture using trypsin or a rubber scraper. Cell recoveries are generally improved by trypsinization; one should be able to recover at least 75% of the cells if the exposure has not resulted in significant cell killing. Rinse the culture dish several times with RPMI 1640 medium to maximize cell recovery. Alternately, this assay can be used with cells exposed to toxicants in a suspension culture. Centrifuge the recovered PAMs (300 *g* for 10 min at 4°C), then resuspend the cell pellet in 1 ml of serum-free RPMI 1640 medium. Both total cell count and viability (using trypan blue dye exclusion) of the PAMs should be measured at this step. Our experience is that cell viability should be at least 50–60% to justify performing the phagocytosis assay. The cell suspension must be washed thoroughly two additional times with RPMI 1640 medium as above before proceeding. This ensures that the assay is run in serum-free conditions, so that phagocytosis is stimulated only through the IgG receptor sites. After removal of the medium from the last wash, add 1 ml of the SRBC preparation to each centrifuge tube for each 5×10^5 live PAMs, then incubate for 30 min at 37°C in a humidified atmosphere of 5% CO_2/95% air.

After incubation immediately place the tubes on crushed ice to stop phagocytosis. Centrifuge the cells as above, resuspend the pellet in 1 ml of distilled water for 20–30 sec, then immediately add an equal volume of the 2× normal concentration of PBS, and mix well to return the suspension to normal osmolarity. This hypotonic shock will lyse SRBCs external to the PAMs, but will not affect the PAMs and the phagocytized SRBCs, provided isotonicity is quickly restored. Prepare standard cytocentrifuge slides using 100- to 200-μl aliquots of the suspension, stain the slides in Diff-Quik, allow to air-dry, then affix glass coverslips to the top of the slides with Permount. The quality of staining is improved if cells are stained soon after the cytospin slides are prepared.

Analysis and Data Interpretation

Microscopic Evaluation

Count the number of SRBCs phagocytized by each of 100 PAMs under oil immersion light microscopy. The phagocytized SRBCs are easily recognized by their shape and a dark brown or rust color. It may be difficult to count the number of SRBCs in highly phagocytic cells; this problem may be somewhat alleviated by moving the microscope stage from slight underfocus to overfocus. A well-defined microscope stage movement strategy should be used to eliminate the possibility of recounting a particular field of cells.

Data Analysis

For a qualitative presentation one can simply present the percentage of phagocytic cells or the percentage phagocytizing certain numbers of SRBCs, (e.g., ≤ 1, 2–5, 6–9, and so on). Alternately, the investigator can report the percentage of cells phagocytizing at least 1 SRBC, although this could lead to an underestimation of effects of exposure if the number of particles per cell is reduced, but the number of cells having ≥ 1 SRBC is not.

For quantitative purposes the number of SRBCs per PAM should be determined on an individual cell basis, at least initially in a set of experiments, to examine potential alterations in the distribution of SRBCs per PAM. If the distribution is similar for control and experimental cultures, then one can more simply count the total number of SRBCs internalized by 100 PAMs and use the mean number of SRBCs per 100 PAMs to quantify phagocytosis. Alternately, if the distribution is changed by exposure (e.g., if a large fraction of cells phagocytize either zero or few SRBCs), then some parameter other than the mean should be used for quantitation. We have used the median number of SRBCs phagocytized to reduce the influence of differences in distribution observed in our studies of toxic beryllium particles (see Fig. 1, in which data are grouped for simplicity of presentation), because, as a measure of central tendency, the median is less sensitive to extreme values than is the mean (9). The distribution may be skewed because of decreased cell function or death, which underscores that this assay provides a more sensitive indicator of toxicity than cell viability assays, and is more useful when significant cell killing has not occurred.

Once calculated, the phagocytic ability of an exposed culture is expressed as a percentage of controls. This percentage is plotted on the y-axis against the logarithm of concentration of toxicant which is plotted on the x-axis. Various techniques exist to model the data; we have used both a probit procedure (SAS probit, SAS Institute, Cary, NC) and a simple linear fit (RSE software, BBN Corp., Cambridge, MA) to the portion of the curve where an effect on phagocytosis is expressed. The probit function is most useful when data at no-effect levels are included in the data set. If one selects a linear fit, it is common to perform a logarithmic transformation of the response variable to reduce the need to include weighting factors in the curve-fitting process; one then fits a function of the form:

$$y = \log (a + bx)$$

where x and y are the variables described above, a is the y-axis intercept, and b is the slope.

A value for EC_{50}, defined as the concentration that effectively decreases phagocytic capacity to 50% that of controls, can be calculated using either modeling method. During the fitting procedure it is important to include individual values from each replicate sample, rather than the mean value of all replicates,

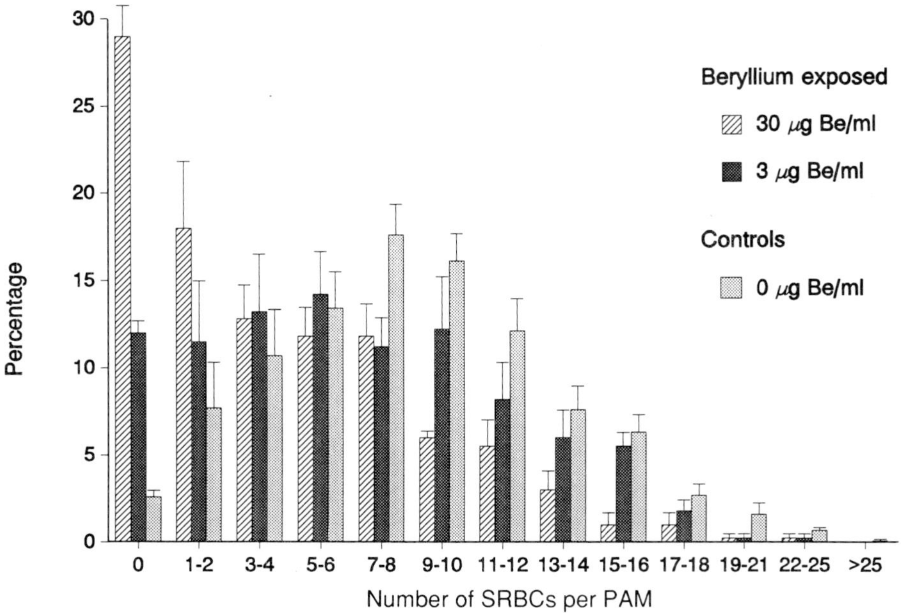

Figure 1 Percentage of pulmonary alveolar macrophages (PAMs) that phagocytized the indicated number of sheep red blood cells (SRBCs) in 1 hr. Data are taken from unexposed control cultures and cultures exposed to either 30 or 3 μg of beryllium (Be) metal particles per 1 ml of culture medium for 20 hr before the phagocytosis assay was performed. Error bars are +1 standard error (SE) for either seven (for control PAMs) or six (for Be-exposed PAMs) replicate cultures. Mean viabilities ± SE for the exposed cultures as a percentage of controls, were 90% ± 3% and 99% ± 2% for the 30- and 3-μg Be/ml exposures, respectively. A clear shift in distribution of the number of SRBCs phagocytized per PAMs resulted from Be exposure. [Data were adapted from (7).]

in order to estimate more realistically the error associated with the calculated parameter (in this case, the EC_{50}). Finally, the investigator should report the error, in terms of the upper and lower 95% confidence limits around the estimate of EC_{50}.

COMMENTS

We have found this assay to be a reproducible method that characterizes the *in vitro* effects of toxic materials on the function of cultured PAMs, at levels where no significant cell killing has occurred (7,10). The assay is relatively simple and can be mastered by individuals skilled in the basic techniques of cell culturing. It can also be used to assess the *in vivo* toxicity of inhaled particles to PAMs that are subsequently recovered by bronchoalveolar lavage (11). The utility of this assay is further exemplified by the fact that it provides a sensitive measurement of sublethal toxic effects regardless of whether it is used in conjunction with *in vivo* or *in vitro* exposures.

An important aspect of this assay is that only a fraction of the total cell population is needed, thus allowing other assays or end points to be examined in parallel. The use of hypotonic shock to lyse extracellular SRBCs has proved effective in our hands to ensure that only phagocytized SRBCs are counted. Finally, once quantified and expressed as a percentage of control cultures, rigorous statistical procedures can be used to describe the effects of toxic agents on the phagocytic capacity of PAMs.

One drawback, however, is the time-consuming nature of the microscopic analysis of the cell cultures. If possible, this assay should be used in experiments in which the toxicant is studied at sublethal concentrations, so that the assay is not used simply as a time-consuming indicator of cell death. Alternately, recent reports describe the measurement of the uptake of fluorescent particles using either computerized image analysis of culture cells (12) or flow cytometric analysis of cells in suspension (13), and represent means by which this assay might be streamlined.

An important precaution is understanding that decreased phagocytic capacity is not always a sign of toxicity. For example, in our *in vitro* exposure studies we routinely include negative control particles such as glass beads for comparison to the responses to toxic beryllium particles (7). Over the course of a 20-hr exposure to relatively high concentrations of glass beads, PAMs can become engorged with a large volume of the beads, thus decreasing their ability to internalize many SRBCs during the phagocytosis assay. Thus, the effect of previous phagocytosis of inert (or even relatively nontoxic) particles can result in an apparent decreased phagocytic capacity of PAMs because of volumetric, not toxic, considerations.

An investigator considering the use of this assay should realize that, as described, it provides a glimpse of total phagocytic capacity at only one point in time. If required for a specific application, the assay can be used at a variety of times after exposure to examine phagocytic rates. In this case it becomes more important to stop the phagocytic process at specific times, and the researcher should consider the use of chemical metabolic poisons (e.g., sodium azide) that would stop phagocytosis more quickly than would occur when cultures are simply chilled over crushed ice (4).

ACKNOWLEDGMENTS

This work was supported by the U.S. Department of Energy's Assistant Secretary for Defense Programs and the Office of Health and Environmental Research under Contract DE-AC04-76EV01013 in facilities fully accredited by the American Association for the Accreditation of Laboratory Animal Care. I thank members of the Inhalation Toxicology Research Institute's staff for their efforts in perfecting this assay and for their critical review of this chapter.

REFERENCES

1. F. M. Griffin, J. A. Griffin, J. E. Leider, and S. C. Silverstein, *J. Exp. Med.* **142,** 1263 (1975).
2. A. G. Harmsen and E. L. Jeska, *J. Reticuloendothel. Soc.* **27,** 631 (1980).
3. D. R. Shaw and F. M. Griffin, Jr., *in* "Methods for Studying Mononuclear Phagocytes" (D. O. Adams, P. J. Edelson, and H. Koren, eds.), p. 511. Academic Press, New York, 1981.
4. S. D. Wright, *in* "Methods in Enzymology" (G. Di Sabato and J. Everse, eds.), Vol. 132, p. 204. Academic Press, Orlando, Florida, 1986.
5. T. P. Stossel, *Semin. Hematol.* **12,** 83 (1975).
6. R. I. Kavet and J. D. Brain, *J. Reticuloendothel. Soc.* **27,** 201 (1980).
7. G. L. Finch, W. T. Lowther, M. D. Hoover, and A. L. Brooks, *J. Toxicol. Environ. Health* **34,** 103 (1991).
8. B. B. Mishell and S. M. Shiigi, "Selected Methods in Cellular Immunology," p. 453. Freeman, San Francisco, 1980.
9. R. D. Remington and M. A. Schork, "Statistics with Applications to the Biological and Health Sciences." Prentice Hall, Englewood Cliffs, New Jersey, 1970.
10. G. L. Fisher, K. L. McNeill, and C. J. Democko, *in* "Short-Term Bioassays in the Analysis of Complex Environmental Mixtures III" (M. D. Waters, S. S. Sandhu, J. Lewtas, L. Claxton, N. Chernoff, and S. Nesnow, eds.), p. 257. Plenum, New York, 1983.
11. P. J. Haley, G. M. Shopp, J. M. Benson, Y.-S. Cheng, D. E. Bice, M. I. Luster, J. K. Dunnick, and C. H. Hobbs, *Fundam. Appl. Toxicol.* **15,** 476 (1990).
12. C. O. Odeyale and G. R. Hook, *J. Leukocyte Biol.* **48,** 403 (1990).
13. J. A. Steinkamp, J. S. Wilson, G. C. Saunders, and C. C. Stewart, *Science* **215,** 64 (1982).

25 Cell Function Studies Using Fluorescent Ca^{2+} Indicators

Andrew P. Thomas

INTRODUCTION

Normal cells maintain cytosolic free Ca^{2+} concentrations ($[Ca^{2+}]_i$) on the order of 100 n*M*, despite the presence of millimolar levels of Ca^{2+} in the extracellular fluid. This low level of $[Ca^{2+}]_i$ and the large concentration gradient across the plasma membrane allows $[Ca^{2+}]_i$ to function as a rapidly changing intracellular messenger. In one form or another, $[Ca^{2+}]_i$ probably plays a messenger role in almost all types of mammalian cells. Among the important processes regulated by $[Ca^{2+}]_i$ are muscle contraction, neurotransmitter release, both endocrine and exocrine secretion, metabolism, and cellular locomotion. Investigation of $[Ca^{2+}]_i$ changes in studies of toxicology can be important in a number of ways. Cellular damage may result in elevation of $[Ca^{2+}]_i$ due to nonspecific increases in leakage at the level of cellular membranes, or to more direct effects on specific components involved in maintaining cellular Ca^{2+} homeostasis. Since high levels of $[Ca^{2+}]_i$ can activate a range of degradative pathways and induce damage to organelles, Ca^{2+} has the potential to play a role in cell killing and the induction of cellular abnormalities. In addition, toxic agents may act by perturbing normal $[Ca^{2+}]_i$ signaling mechanisms, leading to a variety of consequences from modifications of normal function to cell death. A number of methods are available for measuring $[Ca^{2+}]_i$, but at present the use of Ca^{2+}-selective fluorescent indicators is by far the most prevalent. This reflects the versatility of the approach and ease which the technique can be applied using standard equipment. Fluorescent Ca^{2+} indicator techniques allow temporal and spatial information to be obtained from living cells, with a minimum of perturbation of cell function. This chapter discusses theoretical and methodolical aspects of the application of these techniques.

PRINCIPLES OF FLUORESCENT Ca^{2+} INDICATOR USE

The fluorescent Ca^{2+} indicators were first developed by Tsien (1), who designed a series of molecules based around the highly selective binding site of EGTA for Ca^{2+}. EGTA has a Ca^{2+} affinity that is more than 10^5 higher than for

METHODS IN TOXICOLOGY, Volume 1B

Mg^{2+}, and a dissociation constant (K_D) for Ca^{2+} close to the physiological $[Ca^{2+}]_i$. The first group of compounds synthesized by Tsien and co-workers utilized the basic Ca^{2+} binding site structure of EGTA, but incorporated additional groups that resulted in changes in spectral properties when Ca^{2+} was bound. These new Ca^{2+} chelators also had a reduced pH sensitivity relative to EGTA, the Ca^{2+} affinity of which changes very markedly over the physiological pH range. The most successful of the initial group of Ca^{2+} chelators was quin2, which incorporated a fluorescent group that gave a substantial enhancement in fluorescence yield on binding Ca^{2+}. Since Ca^{2+} binds to quin2 in a simple one-to-one manner, the concentration of quin2–Ca complex at equilibrium is determined by the free $[Ca^{2+}]$, the total amount of dye, and the K_D under apporpriate conditions of pH and ionic composition of the medium. This relationship may be described by the mass action equation

$$K_D = \frac{[\text{quin2}] * [Ca^{2+}]}{[\text{quin2–Ca}]} \tag{1}$$

This can be rearranged to give $[Ca^{2+}]$ in terms of the relative amounts of Ca^{2+}-bound and Ca^{2+}-free quin2:

$$[Ca^{2+}] = K_D * \frac{[\text{quin2–Ca}]}{[\text{quin2}]} \tag{2}$$

The Ca^{2+}-free form of quin2 gives a certain fluorescence yield, while an equivalent concentration of the Ca^{2+}-bound form yields a larger fluorescence signal. Therefore, the difference between the signal when all of the dye is unbound (F_{min}) and the measured fluorescence intensity at any given $[Ca^{2+}]$ (F) is proportional to the concentration of quin2–Ca. The concentration of unbound quin2 may be obtained by subtraction of the calculated [quin2–Ca] from the total dye concentration. Total dye is determined from the fluorescence signal at saturating $[Ca^{2+}]$ (F_{max}). Thus, Eq. (2) can be expressed in terms of the fluorescence intensity of quin2, yielding the following relationship, as first described by Tsien *et al.* (2):

$$[Ca^{2+}] = K_D * \frac{(F - F_{min})}{(F_{max} - F)} \tag{3}$$

Although the units of dye concentration cancel out in this expression, it is important to realize that the values of F_{min} and F_{max} are specific for a particular dye concentration. Therefore, these values must be determined for the actual concentration of dye being used. Furthermore, in spatially resolved measurements, any heterogeneity in dye distribution or sample thickness would require that the values of F_{min} and F_{max} be determined on a point-by-point basis. This is inherently difficult and can easily be invalidated if the dye redistributes, leaks from the cell, or bleaches during the course of an experiment.

To overcome this problem, Tsien's group developed a series of fluorescent $[Ca^{2+}]_i$ indicator dyes that respond to Ca^{2+} binding with shifts in their fluorescence spectra, rather than just altering fluorescence intensity (3). Spectral shifts with Ca^{2+} can take the form of Ca^{2+}-induced changes in either the excitation (e.g., fura 2) or emission spectra (e.g., indo 1). The net result is that measurements can be made at two separate wavelengths where the effects of Ca^{2+} binding on fluorescence intensity occur in opposite directions (or remain static at one wavelength). This permits $[Ca^{2+}]_i$ to be calculated from the ratio of fluorescence intensities at the two wavelengths in a manner that is essentially independent of the intracellular concentration of the dye. In essence, the ratio of fluorescence intensities at the two wavelengths is proportional to the ratio of the two forms of the indicator (Ca^{2+} bound/Ca^{2+} free). With appropriate correction parameters to account for the relative fluorescence yields of the bound and free forms of the dye at each wavelength, together with measurements of the limiting fluorescence ratio values, an equation can be derived which has a similar form to Eq. (3):

$$[Ca^{2+}] = K_D * \frac{(R - R_{min})}{(R_{max} - R)} * \frac{S_{f2}}{S_{b2}} \qquad (4)$$

where R is the ratio of the fluorescence signal obtained at the wavelength where the Ca^{2+}-bound dye predominates, divided by the fluorescence signal at the wavelength where the Ca^{2+}-free form predominates. R_{max} and R_{min} are the fluorescence ratio values under saturating and Ca^{2+}-free conditions, respectively. The ratio S_{f2}/S_{b2} is the ratio of fluorescence values for Ca^{2+}-bound/Ca^{2+}-free indicator measured at the wavelength used to monitor the Ca^{2+}-free indicator (the denominator wavelength of R). These are all unitless values, which depend only on the chemical properties of the indicator and the relative sensitivity of the instrument at the two wavelengths being measured. Because the parameters are measured as ratios, their absolute values are independent of dye concentration. As a result, the ratio approach to obtaining $[Ca^{2+}]$ information is amenable to measurements in which the dye is heterogeneously distributed or in which its effective concentration changes with time. As with the single-wavelength method, calibration measurements at zero and saturating levels of Ca^{2+} must still be carried out to determine the constants R_{max}, R_{min}, and S_{f2}/S_{b2} for the particular experimental conditions.

Apart from the introduction of fluorescent Ca^{2+} indicator dyes that offer the possibility for carrying out ratio measurements of $[Ca^{2+}]$, there have been a number of other improvements in the properties of available indicators compared to quin2. Almost all of the Ca^{2+} indicator dyes developed recently have much higher fluorescence yields than quin2, allowing lower intracellular concentrations to be used. Many also have moderately lower Ca^{2+} affinities, which increases the $[Ca^{2+}]$ range over which the dyes can give useful information. In addition, while the earlier dyes required excitation with ultraviolet (UV) light, there is now a broad range of Ca^{2+} indicator choices which vary in optimal excitation wavelength from UV almost to the red part of the visible light spectrum. This has increased the potential for using these indicators in a wide variety of instrument types.

The contribution of Tsien and co-workers (2,4) in designing new molecules suitable for Ca^{2+} measurement was complemented by their development of a method for loading these dyes into living cells. This was achieved by esterifying the carboxylic acid groups of the Ca^{2+} chelators with acetoxymethyl groups, so that these highly charged molecules became sufficiently lipophilic to easily penetrate biological membranes. Once inside a cell, these acetoxymethyl groups are cleaved by endogenous esterase activities. Thus, the esterified dye can be loaded into cells without disruption of the cell membrane. The intracellular formation of nonpermeant dye results in accumulation of dye within the cells, even when relatively low concentrations of the ester form are added to the bathing medium. The fact that this dye-loading strategy could be applied to whole populations of cells in a relatively straightforward manner made the measurement of $[Ca^{2+}]_i$ in living cells a widely available technique for the first time. However, as discussed below, in many cases there are significant advantages in introducing the free acid forms of the dyes directly by microinjection or related techniques.

RELATIVE ADVANTAGES OF FLUORESCENT Ca^{2+} INDICATORS COMPARED TO OTHER TECHNIQUES

There are a variety of other potential methods for measuring $[Ca^{2+}]_i$ in living cells, and it is worth briefly comparing the relative merits of these with the fluorescent Ca^{2+} indicator technique. Other methods that have been used to obtain information about $[Ca^{2+}]_i$ in living cells include (a) nuclear magnetic resonance (NMR) measurements of fluorine-containing Ca^{2+} chelators, (b) Ca^{2+}-sensitive dyes that change absorbance on Ca^{2+} binding, (c) Ca^{2+}-sensitive photoproteins, (d) Ca^{2+}-selective microelectrodes, and (e) indirect assessment of $[Ca^{2+}]_i$ changes by measurement of other Ca^{2+}-sensitive processes (e.g., Ca^{2+}-activated Cl^- channels). Apart from the fluorinated Ca^{2+} indicators for use in NMR, only the fluorescent Ca^{2+} indicators are available in an esterified form that can be loaded noninvasively. Some indicators can be scrape-loaded into cells, but this is not always successful and may result in significant damage to cell function. Thus, the ability to load the fluroscent Ca^{2+} indicators as the acetoxymethyl ester makes them most appropriate for cell population measurements. An additional advantage of the ester-loading technique is that it is amenable to very small cells (e.g., platelets) or organelles (e.g., mitochondria), which are difficult to access directly with injection pipettes or microelectrodes. In terms of signal response, fluorescent Ca^{2+} indicators have better signal to noise than photoproteins and substantially higher temporal resolution than ion-selective microelectrodes or NMR. Of particular significance for toxicology measurements, Ca^{2+} indicators offer the most sensitive and accurate approach to measuring resting levels of $[Ca^{2+}]_i$. Furthermore, no other technique can compare with these indicators for spatially resolved measurements of $[Ca^{2+}]_i$.

There are some potential disadvantages associated with using the fluorescent Ca^{2+} indicators. As with any reporter agent, these dyes must bind Ca^{2+} in order to give a signal related to its concentration. The presence of excess Ca^{2+} binding sites can result in buffering of $[Ca^{2+}]_i$ changes that alter both the kinetics and the absolute amplitude of the changes. In the case of the fluorescent dyes, buffering of $[Ca^{2+}]_i$ can be quite, significant, especially if high loading levels are used. In this respect Ca^{2+}-sensitive photoproteins appear to be less perturbing because they have lower Ca^{2+} affinity and are generally used at relatively low intracellular loads. Least perturbing to $[Ca^{2+}]_i$ are approaches that utilize an endogenous reporter, such as Ca^{2+}-activated Cl^- or K^+ channels. However, these only give information about $[Ca^{2+}]_i$ in their local environment, close to the plasma membrane. It should also be noted that the fluorescent Ca^{2+} indicators are limited in temporal resolution to about 5 msec, and so may not respond sufficiently rapidly to follow the fastest cellular $[Ca^{2+}]_i$ changes, such as those occuring in contracting skeletal muscle. Most of the other disadvantages of using fluorescent Ca^{2+} indicators are associated with the problems of ensuring that the signal is derived exclusively from the cytosolic compartment, that the dye does not leak from the cells, and that the excitation light does not damage the cells. These problems are addressed in depth later in this chapter.

PROPERTIES OF AVAILABLE Ca^{2+} INDICATORS

Over the last few years a substantial number of fluorescent Ca^{2+} indicators have become available commercially. Unfortunately, most of these are restricted to the single-wavelength variety. However, the newly developed dyes offer the benefits of a broader range of usable wavelengths, substantial variations in Ca^{2+} K_D, and a variety of chemical properties that allow them to interact in somewhat differing ways with cells. Table I lists some of the key spectral data on several of these dyes, together with their reported K_Ds for Ca^{2+}. It should be noted, however, that the Ca^{2+} affinity of these dyes is sensitive to the ionic composition of the medium and may also be affected by viscosity (higher in the cytosol than physiological buffers) or by binding to proteins. All of the dyes listed in Table I

Table I Properties of Fluorescent Ca^{2+} Indicators[a]

	Optimal wavelengths for measurement (nm)		K_D for Ca^{2+} (μM)	Extinction coefficient[b]
	Excitation	Emission		
Single wavelength				
Quin2 · Ca	340	495	0.12	5 (332)
Quin2/AM	340	430		5 (339)
Fluo3 · Ca	505[c]	525	0.40	83 (506)
Fluo3/AM	NF			23 (464)
Rhod2 · Ca	550	575	1.00	80 (553)
Rhod2/AM	550	575		80 (550)
Calcium green-1 · Ca	505[c]	535	0.19	74 (506)
Calcium green-1/AM	NF			28 (302)
Calcium green-2 · Ca	505[c]	530	0.57	93 (506)
Calcium green-2/AM	NF			28 (302)
Calcium green-5N · Ca	505[c]	530	3.30	79 (506)
Calcium green-5N/AM	NF			46 (302)
Calcium orange · Ca	550	575	0.33	80 (555)
Calcium orange/AM	540	570		80 (540)
Calcium crimson · Ca	590	610	0.21	108 (588)
Calcium crimson/AM	583	610		100 (583)
Dual wavelength				
Fura2	380	510		30 (362)
Fura2 · Ca	340	510	0.22	35 (335)
Fura2/AM	370	480		30 (369)
Indo1	340	485		34 (349)
Indo1 · Ca	340	405	0.25	34 (331)
Indo1/AM	360	480		34 (361)
Fura red (Ca^{2+} free)	490[c]	650		29 (472)
Fura red (Ca^{2+} insensitive)	435	650	0.13	41 (436)
Fura red/AM	460	600		35 (458)

[a] Data are from: G. Grynkiewicz, M. Poenie, and R. W. Tsien, *J. Biol. Chem.* **260,** 3440 (1985); R. P. Haugland, "Handbook of Fluorescent Probes and Research Chemicals." Molecular Probes, Eugene, Oregon, 1992; and A. Minta, J. P. Y. Kao, and R. Y. Tsien, *J. Biol. Chem.* **264,** 8171 (1989). NF, Not fluorescent.

[b] Extinction coefficients ($cm^{-1} mM^{-1}$) were determined at the wavelength shown in parentheses.

[c] These dyes can also be excited with an argon ion laser 488-nm line.

Figure 1 Excitation and emission spectra of fluorescent Ca^{2+} indicators. Spectra of commercial preparations of free acid forms of the Ca^{2+} indicators were obtained in a buffer composed of 120 mM KCl, 20 mM HEPES, 10 mM NaCl, and 0.5 mM $MgCl_2$, with Ca^{2+} buffered to the indicated concentrations with 1 mM EGTA at pH 7.2. For spectra at which [Ca^{2+}] was not varied, the concentration was set to 400 nM. Conditions with saturating Ca^{2+} (Sat) were obtained with 1 mM excess $CaCl_2$. [Reproduced from A. P. Thomas and F. Delaville, *in* "Cellular Calcium—A Practical Approach" (J. G. McCormack and P. H. Cobbold, eds.), p. 1. Oxford University Press, Oxford, 1991.]

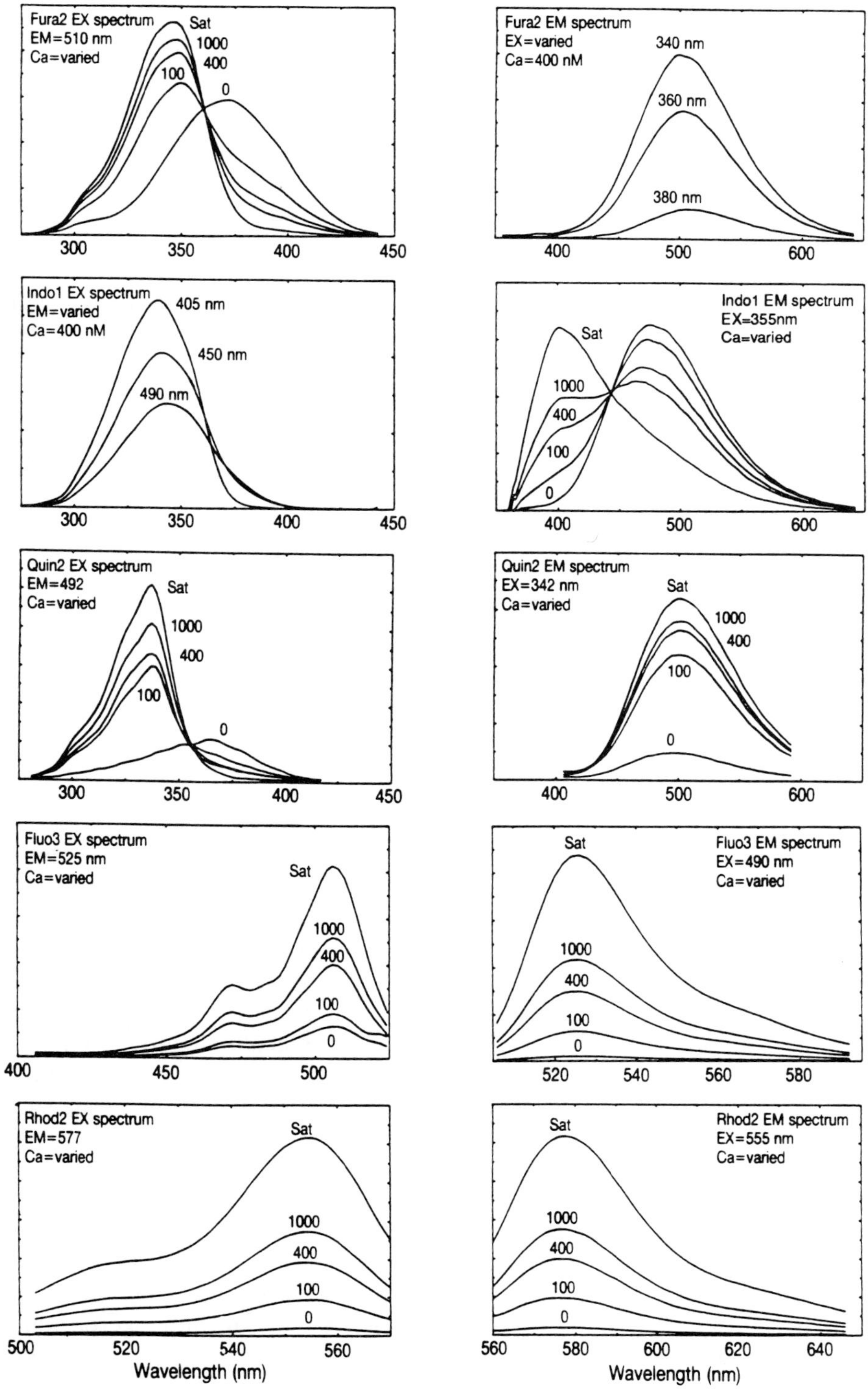

Fura2 EX spectrum
EM=510 nm
Ca=varied
Sat
1000
400
100
0
300
350
400
450
Fura2 EM spectrum
EX=varied
Ca=400 nM
340 nm
360 nm
380 nm
400
500
600
Indo1 EX spectrum
EM=varied
Ca=400 nM
405 nm
450 nm
490 nm
300
350
400
450
Indo1 EM spectrum
EX=355nm
Ca=varied
Sat
1000
400
100
0
400
500
600
Quin2 EX spectrum
EM=492
Ca=varied
Sat
1000
400
100
0
300
350
400
450
Quin2 EM spectrum
EX=342 nm
Ca=varied
Sat
1000
400
100
0
400
500
600
Fluo3 EX spectrum
EM=525 nm
Ca=varied
Sat
1000
400
100
0
400
450
500
Fluo3 EM spectrum
EX=490 nm
Ca=varied
Sat
1000
400
100
0
520
540
560
580
Rhod2 EX spectrum
EM=577
Ca=varied
Sat
1000
400
100
0
500
520
540
560
Wavelength (nm)
Rhod2 EM spectrum
EX=555 nm
Ca=varied
Sat
1000
400
100
0
560
580
600
620
640
Wavelength (nm)

can currently be purchased as acetoxymethyl esters, so that they can readily be introduced into cells. They are also all available in the free acid form necessary for microinjection and for *in virto* calibration. Excitation and emission spectra of dyes used to date in this laboratory are shown in Fig. 1. These spectra were obtained in a KCl-based buffer to mimic cytosolic composition (120 m*M* KCl, 10 m*M* NaCl, and 0.5 m*M* $MgCl_2$, buffered to pH 7.2 with 20 m*M* HEPES). Ca^{2+} concentrations were set with Ca^{2+}–EGTA buffers. Together with the data in Table I, the spectra in Fig. 1 can be utilized to assess the useful wavelength ranges for fluorescence measurements. The dyes developed to date have in common the property that they bind many divalent heavy metal ions (e.g., Mn^{2+}, Zn^{2+}, and Fe^{2+}), which generally quench dye fluorescence. However, all of the dyes have good selectivity for Ca^{2+} over Mg^{2+} at physiologically relevant concentrations of the two ions. This section briefly describes some of the distinct properties of the dyes.

Single-Wavelength Indicators

For most purposes quin2 has now been superseded by newer dyes with greater fluorescence yield, better selectivity for Ca^{2+}, and higher Ca^{2+} K_Ds. However, for some purposes quin2 may still have advantages. It can be loaded into cells at very high levels (several millimolar) as the acetoxymethyl ester, which makes it ideal for buffering $[Ca^{2+}]_i$ and at the same time giving some measure of the extent of $[Ca^{2+}]_i$ change in the buffered cells (i.e., it can act as both Ca^{2+} buffer and reporter). Of the higher wavelength dyes, fluo3 has been the most widely used. It is readily excited using standard fluorescein filter sets and can be used with the 488-nm line of an argon ion laser (e.g., in confocal microscopy). Fluo3 gives a very large fluorescence enhancement on Ca^{2+} binding (starting from almost zero fluorescence in the absence of Ca^{2+}). This property allows even small $[Ca^{2+}]_i$ changes at the low end of the sensitivity range to give a significant magnitude of change in the fluorescence signal. Another useful property of fluo3 is that the acetoxymethyl ester form is essentially nonfluorescent, eliminating some of the problems that can arise from compartments of unhydrolyzed dye in some cells. An atypical property of fluo3 is that Mn^{2+} binding does not quench its fluorescence; instead, the Mn^{2+}-saturated dye has an intermediate fluorescence between the Ca^{2+}-free and -bound forms. Rhod2 was introduced at the same time as fluo3, but has been used much less because it has a lower fluorescence yield and a smaller Ca^{2+}-dependent change in fluorescence. It does have the advantage of having a lower Ca^{2+} affinity than most other dyes (K_D = 1 μM), which can be advantageous for measuring relatively high $[Ca^{2+}]_i$ levels.

A new group of fluorescent Ca^{2+} indicators was recently introduced by Molecular Probes (Eugene, OR), with excitation optima in the range of 500–600 nm (5). These dyes, calcium greens (-1, -2, and -5N), calcium orange, and calcium crimson, all have properties similar to those of fluo3, although only the calcium green dyes show the property of having near-zero fluorescence in the Ca^{2+}-free state and no fluorescence when esterified with acetoxymethyl groups. The calcium green dyes are more fluorescent than fluo3 (as much as 5-fold higher under Ca^{2+} saturating conditions) and these dyes are said to be less sensitive to photobleaching. Calcium green-5N has the highest K_D for Ca^{2+} of any of the available dyes (3.3 μM). Calcium orange and calcium crimson can be used when multiple fluorescent dye signals are to be monitored and these dyes are also useful for certain laser-based instruments. In addition, the higher-excitation wavelengths used for these dyes are likely to be less harmful to the cells and limit the amount of cellular autofluorescence that contributes to the measured signal. One major use of the high-wavelength dyes has been for $[Ca^{2+}]_i$ measurements in cells during photoactivation of caged compounds [e.g., caged Ca^{2+}, caged Ins(1,4,5)P_3]. The available caged compounds must be activated with near-UV light, which makes it impractical to monitor $[Ca^{2+}]_i$ using dyes that require UV excitation.

Ratio Indicators

Fura2 has been used most widely for ratiometric $[Ca^{2+}]_i$ measurements. This dye undergoes a significant shift in its excitation spectrum on Ca^{2+} binding, from a maximum at ~370 nm to 335 nm. The two wavelengths most often used for fura2 measurements are 340 nm, at which Ca^{2+} increases the fluorescence about 3-fold, and 380 nm, at which there is an ~15-fold decrease in fluorescence on Ca^{2+} binding. When these data are expressed in terms of the ratio of 340 nm/380 nm, this gives a dynamic range of 40- to 50-fold change in the measured ratio. Fura2 has an isoflorescence point at ~360 nm, which is useful for monitoring Ca^{2+}-independent fluorescence changes, such as quenching by heavy metal ions, loss of dye through bleaching or leakage, and changes in autofluorescence. Since $[Ca^{2+}]_i$ studies with fura2 involve fluorescence measurements with two seperate excitation wavelengths, it is necessary to provide a light source with alternating wavelengths. Simultaneous accumulation of the two signals can only be approximated by rapid wavelength changes. This is not a problem with indo1, which can be excited at a single wavelength because its emission, rather than excitation, spectrum is shifted by Ca^{2+} binding. The Ca^{2+}-bound and -free species of indo1 are generally monitored at 405 and 485 nm, respectively. Indo1 is excellent for following rapid $[Ca^{2+}]_i$ changes with some form of dual-detector system (T-format fluorometer or microscope photometer), because it can monitor both signals simultaneously. However, indo1 is somewhat more difficult to use in imaging studies as compared to dual-excitation dyes such as fura2. This is because the calculation of $[Ca^{2+}]_i$ images depends on accurate coregistration of the pairs of images prior to calculation of the ratio. If seperate detectors are used to acquire the pair of images, any inhomogeneity in terms of spatial distortion or light sensitivity will give rise to artifacts in the calculated $[Ca^{2+}]_i$ image. By contrast, with dual-excitation dyes, the same detector is used for both wavelengths, eliminating this problem. One other available ratio dye is fura red, which can be excited with visible light. When excited at 490 nm and monitored at 650 nm, the fluorescence of fura red *decreases* on Ca^{2+} binding. While there is no suitable wavelength at which Ca^{2+} binding causes an opposing signal change, it is possible to obtain a second set of measurements using 435 nm excitation, at which the fluorescence is insensitive to Ca^{2+} changes. This can be used to calculate a ratio as a means to determine $[Ca^{2+}]_i$ independent of dye distribution. One problem with using fura red is that it is much lower in fluorescence than the other dyes currently in general use.

FLUORESCENCE MEASUREMENT SYSTEMS

It is possible to obtain some information about how $[Ca^{2+}]_i$ changes in response to a stimulus using almost any research-level fluorometer for cell populations. However, to obtain a more accurate assessment of absolute $[Ca^{2+}]_i$, a fluorometer system with some option to collect dual-wavelength information is required. A serious drawback with fluorometer measurements of cell populations is that the population may not behave homogeneously either in its basal state or in response to treatment. This may be particularly problematic in toxicology studies, in which cells may respond to test agents with different time courses and to varying extents. In addition, when dye leaks from cells in a closed cuvette system, the fluorometer signal does not distinguish dye leakage from slow changes in $[Ca^{2+}]_i$, nor can it differentiate between a slow leak from all cells and spontaneous rapid dye loss occurring as individual cells in the population breakdown. To overcome these problems, a system that provides cell-by-cell information is preferable.

Fluorometer Systems

The fluorescence intensity obtained with most cell populations loaded with Ca^{2+} fluorescent indicators is more than adequate to give sufficient signal for measurement with a standard research fluorometer. Much of the noise in these signals is likely to come from light scattering by the cells themselves, so it is often preferable to limit the cell density. For most work a stirring device will be required to maintain the cells in suspension and ensure rapid mixing of added agents. It may also be necessary to thermostat and gas the cuvette chamber appropriately. In some cases, adherent cells can be monitored by fixing a coverslip or slide in the cuvette at a 45° angle to the excitation light path. While single-wavelength fluorometers can give a useful signal, some form of dual-wavelength capability is preferable for calculation of $[Ca^{2+}]_i$ changes. Many modern fluorometers offer the option to slew monochromators between to wavelengths. This is relatively slow and may cause premature wearing of the monochromator drives. For dual-emission measurements (e.g., with indo1) an excellent solution is a T-format fluorometer, in which two photomultipliers detect fluorescence at separate wavelengths resulting from a common excitation wavelength. These have the fastest response and are relatively simple in design. A number of commercial dual-excitation systems are also available. These rely on some form of rapid optical switching between two excitation light sources (most often a single light source split between two monochromators). Dual-excitation systems have relatively complex light paths that may somewhat attenuate light throughput. However, the most sophisticated instruments can provide temporal resolution on the order of a few milliseconds, more than adequate for most requirements. A dual-excitation instrument trends to be more flexible than a dual-emission fluorometer, since multiple excitation also lends itself to measurements with multiple dyes.

Microscope Imaging and Photometer Systems

Imaging and photometer systems differ in that the latter only gives fluorescence data from a single location at each time point. This can be an individual cell, a region within a cell, or a group of cells. By contrast, imaging measurements are spatially resolved (usually two-dimensional) data sets, which are generally collected at sufficiently frequent intervals to yield time course information. Imaging measurements can provide $[Ca^{2+}]_i$ time courses from multiple individual cells in the same microscope field, and/or provide information about the subcellular localization of $[Ca^{2+}]_i$ changes within a single cell. In addition, by collecting the raw fluorescence information, imaging allows a separate determination of the rate at which fluorescent dye signal is lost from individual cells and allows cell viability to be monitored simultaneously.

For both microphotometry and single-cell fluorescence imaging, an appropriate microscope equipped for epifluorescence is required. Inverted microscopes are most suited for living specimens; the high numerical aperture objectives required to obtain adequate fluorescence signal are not available with sufficient working distance to allow use with an upright microscope while maintaining the cells in physiological medium. In fact, the objective is probably the most important element in the microscope for imaging fluorescent Ca^{2+} indicators. A high numerical aperture is essential, since this will determine the relationship between illumination intensity and fluorescence signal. Light transmission through an objective is proportional to the square of the numerical aperture. In epifluorescence both the excitation light and the emission light pass through the objective, so for a given illumination strength, the fluorescence signal increases with the fourth power of the numerical aperture. It should also be noted that special glasses or quartz are required to transmit sufficient light in the near-UV region where fura2 and indo1 are excited. The microscope should also include suitable optics for locating and viewing cells under study. This is often a compromise with the efficiency of the epifluorescence system. Phase-contrast objectives cause a modest loss of light due to the phase rings, while polarizers, etc., in differential interference-contrast optics are generally incompatible with direct fluorescence measurements. However, these may be removable for fluorescence measurement, or in some configurations can be located outside of the fluorescence path. Other important microscope elements include a stable stage and vibration-free table, a long working distance condenser to allow manipulation of cells on inverted microscopes, and an appropriate cell incubation chamber. In general, cells are grown on coverslips that can be fitted into some form of thermostatically regulated chamber on the microscope stage. It may also be preferable to provide a laminar flow gassing manifold to maintain physiological conditions. In systems with immersion objectives, the objective itself can provide a substantial heat sink. This problem can be minimized by warning the objective with a coiled tube containing appropriately warmed circulating water (excessive heating may damage the objective).

Most epifluorescence microscopes are available with either mercury or xenon arc lamps for excitation. The xenon lamp is preferable because it offers a smoother spectrum, especially in the UV region where fura2 is excited. However, for a system to be used only with indo1, a mercury lamp may be suitable, since it has two major lines in the 335- to 365-nm range. For dual-emission systems the standard excitation lamp with an appropriate filter may be all that is required. However, in dual-excitation systems a synchronized (generally computer-controlled) wavelength changer is required. This may take the form of a complex chopper system with monochromators similar to that discussed above for fluorometer measurements, or can be a simpler mechanical device to exchange between two or more optical filters. It is generally a good idea to include a shutter at the level of the excitation light controller, since this can be used to limit the exposure of the cells to the period when data are being collected. A shutter can also be used to eliminate stray light or other artifacts during the exchange of filters. The speed of operation of the filter changer or other wavelength-switching device is likely to be one of the limiting factors in setting the maximum data acquisition rate of the system. A rate of one pair per second or better would be good. The other optical components of the epifluorescence system are a dichroic reflector, which will separate the excitation light from the returning fluorescent light by reflecting one (usually excitation) and passing the other, together with an appropriate emission filter. The emission filter will often be selected with a relatively broad band width to ensure maximum throughput of emission light, although it is necessary that it completely excludes any stray light at the excitation wavelength.

A wide array of integrated imaging systems are now available commercially. It is beyond the scope of this chapter to survey all of the potential options. The most important component in an imaging system is likely to be the detector. At present there are three basic types of camera available: (a) a silicone-intensified target camera, (b) an intensified charge-coupled device (CCD) camera, and (c) a cooled CCD camera with digital readout. The former two generate a standard video signal which can be digitized by a wide variety of computer boards, while the latter signal is digitized at the level of the detector electronics and is read into the computer directly. At present the video-based systems are faster and in some ways more versatile, while the cooled CCD systems have a substantial advantage in signal to noise. For a more detailed discussion of imaging hardware, see the work of Thomas and Delaville (6). In addition to camera-based imaging devices, a number of laser scanning fluorescence confocal microscopes are currently available. In these instruments the excitation light is provided by a laser that is scanned through the objective over the sample in two dimensions, while the fluorescence is recorded with a photomultiplier (in most cases two emission channels can be provided). With a confocal microscope the range of fluorescent Ca^{2+} dyes that can be used is likely to be limited by the available laser. Most systems come standard with only a visible light laser (e.g., argon ion with blue and green lines). As a result most confocal microscopy studies of $[Ca^{2+}]_i$ are uncalibrated in absolute concentration terms, although the ability to obtain an optical slice with the confocal microscope can reduce problems associated with variations in cell thickness. See the work of Lemasters *et al.* (7) for further discussion of the use of the confocal microscope in this way.

Once image data have been digitized by any of the fluorescence imaging detectors mentioned above, it is necessary to process the data and extract relevant information using some form of image analysis software. This should include facilities to subtract appropriate background signals and carry out corrections for inhomogeneity in the detector. It should also provide standard image-processing functions to smooth noise and extract features. An important feature of the imaging system is the ability to construct images of $[Ca^{2+}]_i$ using the ratio method described above on a pixel-by-pixel basis (a pixel is a picture element equal to one digitized point in the image). The software should also provide a simple facility to extract $[Ca^{2+}]_i$ time courses from user-selected regions (e.g., individual cells or subcellular regions) of the image and plot these for analysis. In cases in which motile cells are to be studied, some form of cell tracking may be required. Ideally, the computer running the image-processing software should have sufficient memory to retain an entire data set in RAM, since this will speed the processing operations.

METHODS FOR LOADING DYES INTO CELLS

The most common method for loading fluorescent Ca^{2+} indicators into cells is in the form of the acetoxymethyl ester. Intracellular hydrolysis of the ester groups causes accumulation of the active dye beyond the level in the extracellular medium, so it is not necessary to use very large quantities. For most of the dyes, a concentration of 1–10 μM is sufficient, although more will be required for quin2 or fura red. The density of cells also affects the loading level; with higher densities more dye is required. With cells in monolayer culture, in which cell density can be very low, a higher proportion of dye to cells may be required to achieve the same level of intracellular loading. In cell suspensions the loading efficiency tends to be on the order of 10–40%, and a final load of about 0.1–0.4 nmol of dye per 1 mg of cell protein is appropriate. Loading is generally carried out in a standard physiological buffer. Incubation at 37°C gives the most rapid loading, but the extent of compartmentalization of the dye is often less at 25–30°C. Inclusion of serum albumin can aid in the dispersion of the hydrophobic dye, and it is also useful to mix or agitate the cells during loading. Once the cells are loaded (15–60 min), the excess dye is washed off and the cells are immediately ready for study. Most of the dyes tend to leak slowly from cells over a period of a few hours (faster in some cases). Therefore, cells should either be loaded with indicator as required, or with some preparations they may be stored on ice once loaded and warmed for a few minutes prior to carrying out the measurements. In some cases in which dye loss from the cells is a significant problem, it can be reduced by including the anion transport inhibitor sulfinpyrazone (8).

The other major methods for loading cells with fluorescent Ca^{2+} indicators are microinjection and intracellular perfusion from a patch-clamp pipette in the whole-cell configuration. The advantage of these methods is that the free acid form of the dye is used, so that compartmentation due to penetration and cleavage of the ester form in noncytosolic compartments is avoided. However, these approaches are limited to single-cell measurements. Usually, an intracellular dye concentration of 30–100 μM is optimal. This may be achieved by microinjection of ~ 1% cell volume with 3–10 mM indicator dye. A further advantage of microinjection is that other agents can also be introduced together with the dye.

CALIBRATION OF Ca^{2+} SIGNALS

Calibration of the signals derived from fluorescent Ca^{2+} indicators involves determination of the parameters required by Eq. (3) or (4) under appropriate conditions and measurement of fluorescence signals not derived from cytosolic dye (e.g., compartmentalized dye, autofluorescence, and detector dark currents). If the fluorescence data are stored digitally in a computer, it is possible to transform the raw fluorescence data directly to plots of $[Ca^{2+}]_i$ through time, or images of the spatial distribution of $[Ca^{2+}]_i$ by direct application of the calibration equations. There are two ways in which the calibration parameters for a particular experiment configuration can be obtained. They may be measured *in situ* using the cytosolic dye within intact cells, or they may be measured in free solution under the same instrument configuration used to acquire cell fluorescence data. The former approach is preferable, since it preserves most of the interactions of the dye with endogenous constituents and retains a physiological ionic milieu. However, it is often difficult to achieve the conditions necessary to fully interconvert intracellular dye between Ca^{2+}-bound and -free forms without damaging the cells. As a result it is common to determine fluorescent parameters after lysing the cells or in the complete absence of cells. For a similar reason most investigators use Ca^{2+} K_Ds for the fluorescent Ca^{2+} indicators derived from measurements carried out in free solution. In some cases the K_D values have been calculated for a specific cell by Ca^{2+} titration in the presence of ionophore in an intact cell (9). These measurements can yield significantly different K_D values, although the measured K_D could be distorted if Ca^{2+} equilibration across the cell membrane is incomplete. The following sections describe the major steps involved in calibration both single- and dual-wavelength Ca^{2+} indicators. Examples of all of the calibration procedures described can be found elsewhere (6).

Determination of Fluorescence Contributions from Extracellular Dye

In most cell population measurements there is some contribution from extracellular dye. This contributes to the total measured signal and may change if extracellular Ca^{2+} is modified in the submicromolar range. This contribution can be determined for most dyes by adding a small amount (100 μM) of $MnCl_2$ to quench the extracellular dye. The Mn^{2+} can be chelated by adding the heavy metal chelator diethylenetriaminepentaacetic acid (DTPA; see Ref. 10) immediately after the rapid signal change due to extracellular dye quench. A 3-fold molar excess of DTPA is sufficient to completely reverse the initial dye quench. The rapid decrement in fluorescence following Mn^{2+} addition can be subtracted from the fluorescence data prior to calculating $[Ca^{2+}]_i$. However, the Mn^{2+} quench in fluorescence is not appropriate to subtract from fluorescence values obtained under conditions in which extracellular Ca^{2+} changes occur in the range where the dye is sensitive to Ca^{2+} (e.g., when high EGTA levels are used to determine F_{min} or R_{min}). Under these conditions only the fraction of extracellular dye fluorescence resulting from the relevant dye form should be subtracted. For example, a single-wavelength Ca^{2+} indicator may give 20% of the Ca^{2+}-bound fluorescence signal when Ca^{2+} is removed. Thus, if extracellular dye contributions are measured by Mn^{2+} quench in the presence of normal (millimolar) Ca^{2+}, fluorescence values measured in the presence of excess EGTA would only need to be corrected by subtracting 20% of the Mn^{2+}-induced fluorescence decrement. The relative magnitudes of correction for Ca^{2+}-bound and -free extracellular dye can be determined using solutions of the indicator. Similar correction factors are needed for each wavelength when using dual-wavelength indicators. In this case, the two Mn^{2+}-induced decrements of fluorescence measured under saturating Ca^{2+} conditions will be corrected in opposite directions under Ca^{2+}-free conditions (e.g., the signal at the wavelength at which fluorescence is highest under Ca^{2+}-free conditions will be corrected by a factor greater than 100% of the Mn^{2+} quench at the wavelength).

An alternative approach to account for extracellular dye signal is to add excess EGTA to cells in medium containing physiological Ca^{2+}. The amplitude of fluorescence changes due to the interconversation of the extracellular dye between Ca^{2+}-bound and -free forms can be used to calculate the total fluorescence signal contributed by this dye using correction factors obtained in free solution experiments, as described above for Mn^{2+} quenching. However, when single-wavelength dyes are used, it is sufficient to determine only the Ca^{2+}-sensitive component of extracellular dye fluorescence. This can then be subtracted from all fluorescence values obtained in the presence of extracellular Ca^{2+}, while values measured with zero extracellular Ca^{2+} are not corrected. In this approach the Ca^{2+}-insensitive fluorescence of extracellular dye is simply included as part of the measured value of F_{min}. A similar approach is not appropriate for dual-wavelength indicators. In this case the entire fluorescence signal due to extracellular dye at each wavelength must be subtracted before the ratio can be calculated.

Corrections for Cellular Autofluorescence

Autofluorescence of cells varies considerably. In some cases it is sufficiently small that its contribution to the total measured fluorescence signal is negligible, although in other cells it can represent as much as 50% of the total fluorescence. Autofluorescence can be estimated easily using a preparation of cells not loaded with the dye. If autofluorescence contributes significantly, it is most readily measured by quenching all ion-sensitive dye fluorescence with Mn^{2+} in the presence of ionomycin (a nonfluorescence divalent cation ionophore). Residual fluorescence under these conditions is composed of autofluorescence and any signal due to Ca^{2+}-insensitive forms of the dye (e.g., unhydrolyzed ester). Clearly, this correction can be obtained in concert with the measurement of extracellular dye, by adding Mn^{2+} followed by ionomycin. Even if autofluorescence is minimal, it is important to check for Ca^{2+}-insensitive dye with Mn^{2+} plus ionophore. However, it should be noted that some dyes may bind Mn^{2+} and Ca^{2+} with lower affinity when the acetoxymethyl ester groups are only partially removed.

Corrections for Compartmentalized Dye

The most difficult correction to make in a satisfactory manner is the correction for compartmentalized dye. Depending on cell type, indicator species, and loading protocol, this can vary from a negligible contribution to greater than 50% of total cellular dye. Most protocols that correct for compartmentalized fluorescent Ca^{2+} indicators do so by accessing the cytosolic compartment specifically. This can be achieved using digitonin to make the plasma membrane permeable. When digitonin is used at limiting concentrations, most intracellular organelles remain intact (11). Therefore, the residual fluorescence when cells are treated briefly with Mn^{2+} after digitonin permeabilization can be subtracted as compartmentalized dye (this signal also contains much of the cellular autofluorescence and unhydrolyzed dye signal). In single-cell measurements it is not necessary to use Mn^{2+} to quench the cytosolic fluorescent indicator released by digitonin, since this can be washed out rapidly.

Calibration of Single-Wavelength Data

Calibration of single-wavelength data requires determination of the values of F_{min} and F_{max} [Eq. (3)]. Since these terms are directly dependent on the actual dye concentration, they must be measured with the endogenous dye load in each cell preparation. This can be achieved either by manipulating $[Ca^{2+}]_i$ in intact cells or by releasing the dye from the cells into the extracellular medium, where it is easily manipulated between Ca^{2+}-saturated and unbound forms. The cell lysis calibration is not valid for configurations in which the release dye may redistribute out of the light path (e.g., single-cell or monolayer studies), but can work effectively in fluorometer studies with cells in suspension in a well-mixed cuvette. For both methods it is essential to eliminate contributions of fluorescence signals due to extracellular dye, as described above. However, provided that autofluorescence does not change during the experimental or calibration period, this fluorescence component need not be subtracted separately from all values, since it cancels out in both the numerator ($F - F_{min}$) and the denominator ($F_{max} - F$) of Eq. (3).

For the cell lysis approach a plasma membrane-specific detergent such as digitonin or saponin is best, since these can be used in such a way as to leave compartmentalized dye relatively undisturbed (11). After completion of cell lysis (check for 100% trypan blue-positive cells), F_{min} and F_{max} are determined by addition of excess EGTA and excess Ca^{2+}, respectively. When EGTA is added in the presence of physiological Ca^{2+} (1–2 mM), it is necessary to alkalinize the medium to ensure that the EGTA completes effectively for Ca^{2+} with the fluorescent Ca^{2+} indicator. This is achieved by adding sufficient Tris base to give a final pH of >8.0. For physiological buffers containing 1 mM $CaCl_2$, addition of 10 μl/ml of a stock solution containing 400 mM EGTA and 3 M Tris base at pH 8.7 is sufficient to chelate Ca^{2+} to a point close to F_{min}. An example of a single-wavelength calibration by cell lysis is shown in Fig. 2, where $MnCl_2$ has also been used to estimate the contribution of extracellular indicator. In some preparations cell lysis can result in marked changes in autofluorescence or light scattering, which may yield erroneous values for F_{min} and F_{max}. This problem should be assessed by carrying out the calibration procedure using cells not loaded with the fluorescence Ca^{2+} indicator.

Calibration of single-wavelength measurements *in situ* uses essentially the same steps described above, except that the cell membrane is made specifically permeable to Ca^{2+} using an ionophore. In this way the dye remains in its cellular environment. Ionomycin is used most commonly, with concentrations in the range of 1–20 μM being appropriate for most cell preparations. A23187 is fluorescent with excitation in the 200- to 430-nm range (12), but Br-A23187 is nonfluorescent and can be used with UV dyes. The value of F_{max} can be obtained simply by adding ionomycin in physiological Ca^{2+} medium, while F_{min} is obtained in the presence of excess EGTA at alkaline pH, as described above. In some cases the ionophore-mediated equilibration of $[Ca^{2+}]_i$ with medium Ca^{2+} occurs so slowly at the extremes of saturating and zero Ca^{2+} that it limits the usefulness of the *in situ* calibration approach. F_{min} is best determined before F_{max}, to minimize the amount of Ca^{2+} that must be removed from the cell. Attainment of F_{max} can be accelerated by adding supraphysiological Ca^{2+} levels (10–20 mM) if necessary. An alternative approach to obtain the value of F_{min} is

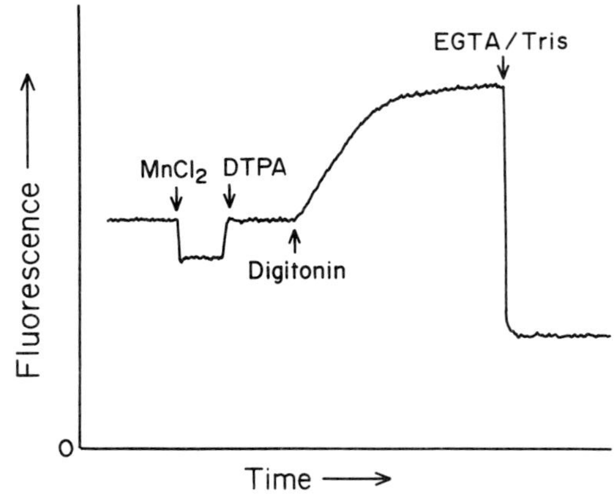

Figure 2 Single-wavelength calibration by cell lysis in a cell suspension $[Ca^{2+}]_i$ measurement. An initial addition of $MnCl_2$ (50 μM) followed by its chelation with diethylenetriaminepentaacetic acid (DTPA) (200 μM) is used to measure the fluorescence contribution from extracellular indicator. Subsequent addition of digitonin causes a time-dependent permeabilization of cell plasma membranes, allowing saturation of the dye by high Ca^{2+} in the medium. This gives F_{max} after subtraction of signal due to extracellular dye. Finally, excess EGTA is added to chelate all medium Ca^{2+}, giving F_{min}.

to use excess Mn^{2+} to quench intracellular dye. Since the fluorescence due to Ca^{2+}-free dye is a fixed proportion of that due to Ca^{2+}-saturated dye, F_{min} can be calculated from the Ca^{2+}-sensitive component of F_{max} (6). When $[Ca^{2+}]_i$ values are calibrated *in situ*, it is difficult to correct for signals derived from compartmentalized dye.

Calibration of Dual-Wavelength Data

Dual-wavelength $[Ca^{2+}]_i$ data can be calibrated using either the cell lysis or *in situ* methods described above to obtain values for R_{min} and R_{max}. However, autofluorescence does not cancel out in Eq. (4) (assuming that it is different at each wavelength). Therefore, autofluorescence must be measured separately at each wavelength and subtracted from all of the data and calibration values before calculating the ratios. It is also necessary to subtract signals due to extracellular dye if this contributes significantly, using one of the protocols described above. R_{min} is determined from the ratio of fluorescence at the two wavelengths in the presence of excess EGTA, and R_{max} is calculated from the fluorescence ratio at saturating Ca^{2+}. The additional constant S_{f2}/S_{b2} represents the relative fluorescence yields of the Ca^{2+}-free and -bound dyes at the wavelength used to monitor the Ca^{2+}-free form. Since S_{f2} and S_{b2} are directly proportional to the dye-dependent fluorescence signals of Ca^{2+}-free and -bound dyes, respectively, the ratio of these measurements (the denominators of R_{min} and R_{max}) is equal to the constant S_{f2}/S_{b2}. Figure 3 shows an example of a calibration of dual-wavelength data carried out using an ionophore to manipulate $[Ca^{2+}]_i$ and obtain values for R_{min}, R_{max}, and S_{f2}/S_{b2} *in situ.*

Unlike single-wavelength calibrations, dual-wavelength data calibrated using the ratio approach are independent of the absolute dye concentration. As a result these data can be calibrated directly from ratios obtained in free solution in the absence of cells (with the caveat that the properties of the dye may not be identical in the intact cell). The calculated values of R, R_{min}, R_{max}, and S_{f2}/S_{b2} are dependent on the exact wavelengths used and the efficiency of the instrument at each wavelength. Therefore, these parameters must be determined under conditions that are as identical as possible to the experimental measurements under which $[Ca^{2+}]_i$ is measured with intracellular dye. The values measured *in vitro* should not, of course, be corrected for autofluorescence or other cell-dependent fluorescence signals, but should be corrected in the same way as the cell data for any instrument-specific background signals (e.g.,dark current of detector). While it is not possible to mimic the intracellular milieu in all aspects, the *in vitro* determination of R_{min} and R_{max} should be carried out in a buffer with similar ion composition to the cytosol (e.g., high K^+, low Na^+, and 0.5 m*M* Mg^{2+} at pH 7.2). It has also been suggested that increasing the viscosity of the medium may yield calibration parameters that relate more closely to those in the cytosol of intact cells (13).

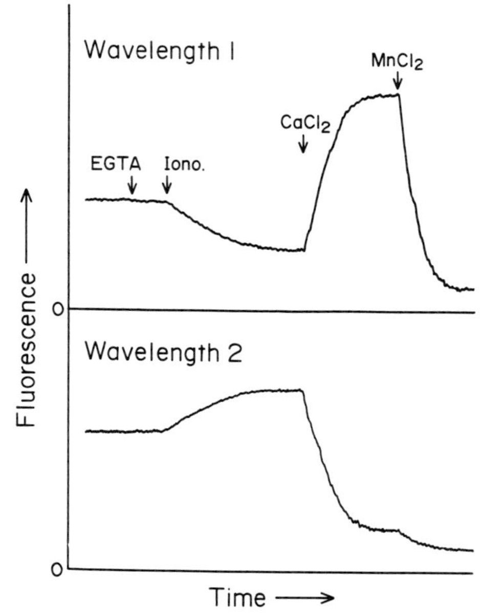

Figure 3 Dual-wavelength calibration using an ionophore (Iono.) to manipulate [Ca^{2+}] within the intact cell. EGTA is added, either with Tris base or in medium containing low Ca^{2+}, to clamp extracellular Ca^{2+} close to zero. Subsequent addition of ionophore causes depletion of intracellular Ca^{2+} and conversion of the cytosolic fluorescent Ca^{2+} indicator entirely to the Ca^{2+}-free form. As a consequence of the decrease in $[Ca^{2+}]_i$, fluorescence at wavelength 1 (derived primarily from the Ca^{2+}-bound dye form) decreases, while fluorescence at wavelength 2 (predominantly resulting from the Ca^{2+}-free dye form) increases. The point where the two signals stabilize as $[Ca^{2+}]_i$ reaches its minimum is used to calculate R_{min} (after subtraction of autofluorescence, etc.). Addition of $CaCl_2$ in excess of the initial EGTA addition causes Ca^{2+}-saturation of the intracellular dye (fluorescence increases at wavelength 1 and decreases at wavelength 2). The steady-state fluorescence values under this condition are used to calculate R_{max}. The constant S_{f2}/S_{b2} is the ratio of background-subtracted fluorescence signals at wavelength 2 (zero Ca^{2+}/high Ca^{2+}). Finally, in this calibration, an excess of $MnCl_2$ is added to quench the Ca^{2+}-sensitive dye, allowing an estimation of the other contributions to the fluorescence signal at each wavelength.

POTENTIAL DIFFICULTIES IN THE USE AND INTERPRETATION OF Ca^{2+} INDICATOR DATA

Fluorescence Signals Not Derived from Cytosolic Indicator

In addition to cytosolic Ca^{2+} indicator, contributions to the fluorescence signals can also include (a) extracellular dye, (b) compartmentalized dye, (c) incompletely hydrolyzed dye, and (d) autofluorescence. Suitable corrections for these fluorescence contributions were discussed in the section on calibration. Some of these problems can be minimized by modifying the conditions used to load the cells with Ca^{2+} indicator. Extracellular dye, Ca^{2+}-insensitive dye forms, and to a large extent compartmentalized dye are eliminated when cells are loaded by injection of the free acid form of the fluorescent Ca^{2+} indicator. When acetoxymethyl ester loading is used, the proportion of dye that ends up in the correct chemical form and cytosolic location can often be increased by reducing the incubation temperature. Incubation at 25–30°C is usually sufficient for cytosolic esterase activity to fully activate the dye. It may also be helpful to use longer loading periods with lower esterified dye concentrations, at which the cytosolic esterases have a greater opportunity to activate the dye before it penetrates other organelles.

As noted above, loss of dye from the cells can be a significant problem in calibration. If substantial dye loss occurs during an experiment, it is very difficult to determine the appropriate correction of the data. In many cells the major pathway of dye loss is through a nonselective anion transporter that can be blocked with sulfinpyrazone (8). A concentration of 200 μM can be used for this (stock solutions must be dissolved at alkaline pH). Where dye loss cannot be blocked, it may be possible to correct time course data if the indicator is released to the medium at an essentially constant rate. Once the rate of dye release to the medium has been determined, the contribution at any given time point can be back-calculated based on a direct determination of extracellular dye at the end of each experiment. When measurements of $[Ca^{2+}]_i$ are obtained from dual-wavelength ratio calibrations, dye loss from the cells is relatively unimportant if the dye redistributes in such a way that it no longer contributes significantly to the measured fluorescence signal (e.g., in cell perfusion or single-cell measurements by fluorescence microscopy). However, if dye released into the medium remains in the light path and continues to contribute a similar magnitude of fluorescence signal, it must be subtracted. Otherwise, there will be an apparent time-dependent $[Ca^{2+}]_i$ change (a drift upward in $[Ca^{2+}]_i$ if the extracellular medium contains physiological Ca^{2+}).

Data obtained using fluorescent Ca^{2+} indicators can be corrected for autofluorescence in a relatively straightforward manner under most conditions, as described above. However, if the autofluorescence changes during an experiment, and this represents a significant component of the total fluorescence signal, it may present problems in calibrating the data in terms of $[Ca^{2+}]_i$. One way to get a round this problem is to carry out parallel measurements in the presence and absence of the Ca^{2+} indicator dye. This may not be appropriate for single-cell $[Ca^{2+}]_i$ measurements, however, since $[Ca^{2+}]_i$ responses are often quite heterogeneous from cell to cell. An alternative approach is to monitor fluorescence at a wavelength at which the dye fluorescence does not change with Ca^{2+} binding (isofluorescence wavelength). An excitation wavelength of

~360 nm is suitable for both fura2 and quin2, and appropriate Ca^{2+}-insensitive wavelength also exist for indo1 and fura red. Depending on the source of the autofluorescence, it may also be possible to minimize this contribution by judicious selection of Ca^{2+} indicator dye. For example, in many cells the major autofluorescence component is derived from reduced pyridine nucleotides, which are excited in the near-UV range where quin2, fura2 and indo1 are excited. These compounds do not contribute to fluorescence signals obtained with the higher-excitation wavelengths used for the visible light Ca^{2+} indicators.

Photobleaching

The use of high illumination intensities can result in photobleaching of the fluorescent Ca^{2+} indicators. In general this does not occur in population measurements with cell suspensions in a fluorometer, in which the excitation light is relatively diffuse and cells are well mixed within the beam. However, in single-cell microscope photometer or imaging studies, in which signal strength is often a limiting factor, the use of high levels of excitation light can result in significant rates of photobleaching. Photobleaching is difficult to distinguish from leakage of dye from the cells, unless the appearance of the dye in the medium is measured. In single-wavelength studies photobleaching of most dyes will result in an apparent time-dependent decline in $[Ca^{2+}]_i$. When dual-wavelength indicators are used to calculate $[Ca^{2+}]_i$ by the ratio method, the effect of photobleaching cancels out of the $[Ca^{2+}]_i$ calculation. In these measurements photobleaching is not a major problem, provided that the total intracellular dye concentration does not decline to a level at which accurate $[Ca^{2+}]_i$ measurements cannot be made. It should be noted, however, that photobleaching may result in the formation of toxic chemical components. The best way to deal with photobleaching is to reduce the illumination intensity as far as possible. In single-cell measurements carried out at relatively low data acquisition rates, it is helpful to limit the exposure of the cells to excitation light to just those periods when fluorescence data are being acquired. This can be achieved using a computer-controlled shutter on the excitation lamp.

In single-wavelength $[Ca^{2+}]_i$ measurements in which it is not possible to eliminate photobleaching, it may be possible to correct the data. Photobleaching of $[Ca^{2+}]_i$ indicator dyes generally follows a simple exponential decay. Thus, if the photobleach rate is estimated using a separate cell preparation not treated with any test agents, fluorescence data can be back-corrected before calculating $[Ca^{2+}]_i$, essentially as described above for correction of dye leakage. An alternative approach to discriminate photobleaching from true $[Ca^{2+}]_i$ changes is to measure the fluorescence at a Ca^{2+}-insensitive wavelength.

Cell-Motility and Shape Change

For the most part changes in cell shape do not affect the total flourescence signal derived from a cell. However, in spatially resolved $[Ca^{2+}]_i$ measurements carried out by digital imaging flourescence microscopy, any shift in cell shape, thickness, or position can lead to artifacts in the calculated image of $[Ca^{2+}]_i$ distribution. Provided that the morphological changes are slow relative to the data acquisition rate, they are unlikely to distort $[Ca^{2+}]_i$ images calculated by the ratio method. However, any static measurements such as autofluorescence or compartmentalized dye cannot be subtracted on an image-by-image basis if the cell does not remain in the same spatial configuration throughout the experiment.

Interactions of Fluorescent Ca^{2+} Indicators with Other Ions

The fluorescent Ca^{2+} indicators are relatively insensitive to monovalent cations or pH in the physiological range and have a high selectivity for Ca^{2+} over Mg^{2+}. However, as with EGTA, all of the indicator dyes have high affinities for binding certain divalent metal ions. These include Ba^{2+}, Sr^{2+}, Mn^{2+}, Ni^{2+}, Zn^{2+}, Co^{2+}, Cd^{2+}, Fe^{2+}, Pb^{2+}, and La^{3+}. The relative affinities of these ions compared to Ca^{2+} varies considerably among different Ca^{2+} indicator dyes. In general, Ba^{2+} and Sr^{2+} have slightly higher K_Ds compared to Ca^{2+}, while many of the transition metal ions bind with higher affinity than Ca^{2+}. There is also considerable variation among dyes in the effects of these ions of flourescence, which varies from complete quenching, to some cases in which the metal-dye complex has a higher fluorescence yield than the Ca^{2+}-dye complex. Thus, it is necessary to determine the potential interference of any divalent cation of interest independently for each dye. This will be most important when the toxic effects of metal ions are to be investigated, or when these ions are used to block physiological processes (e.g., to block Ca^{2+} channels). In the case of Mn^{2+}, its high-affinity quenching of flourescent Ca^{2+} indicators has been used to monitor plasma membrane Ca^{2+} influx pathways, by using the ion as a Ca^{2+} surrogate and measuring the quench of intracellular dye (see, e.g., Refs. 14 and 15). One caution with this approach, however, is that it has been found that Mn^{2+} can further penetrate some intracellular membranes on Ca^{2+} channels such as the Ins(1,4,5)P_3-activated receptor channel in the endoplasmic reticulum (15,16). As a result any indicator compartmentalized within these organelles can be quenched when the relevant Ca^{2+} channel is activated.

Many of the metal ions that bind with high affinity to the Ca^{2+} indicator dyes are also normal constituents of healthy cells (e.g., Mn^{2+}, Zn^{2+}, and Fe^{2+}). These ions are tightly associated with proteins and are present only at low concentration within cells. However, in some cases a significant fraction of intracellular flourescent Ca^{2+} indicator can become associated with these ions. In this case the calibration parameters obtained using EGTA (which also binds these ions) may be distorted. In addition, the flourescence signal may be severely limited as a result of the Ca^{2+} indicator dye binding significant concentrations of other ions. The extent of endogenous metal ion interference can be assessed using the cell-permeant heavy metal ion chelator *N, N, N′, N′*-tetrakis (2-pyridylmethyl)-ethylenediamine (TPEN) (10,17). Any flourescence signal change when TPEN (10–50 μM) is added would suggest interference from other ions. Since TPEN does not appear to affect most cell functions or interfere with normal $[Ca^{2+}]_i$ homeostasis, it is possible to include this chelator throughout an experiment. However, since the endogenous metal ions bound by TPEN (or the flourescent Ca^{2+} indicators) may play implortant roles in normal cell function, it is important to determine whether the cell physiology and biochemistry under investigation is perturbed by the chelators introduced into the cells.

Effect of Flourescent Ca^{2+} Indicators on Normal Cell Function

In order to report $[Ca^{2+}]_i$, the flourescent Ca^{2+} indicators must bind Ca^{2+} in the cytosol of cells. Since intracellular indicator concentrations on the order of 30–300 μM are commonly used, while $[Ca^{2+}]_i$ is on the order of 0.1–1 μM, it might be thought that the indicators would greatly distort the $[Ca^{2+}]_i$. However, almost all cells have relatively large amounts of cytoplasmic fixed Ca^{2+} binding sites that are in dynamic equilibrium with $[Ca^{2+}]_i$. These include specific Ca^{2+}-binding proteins such as calmodulin, and nonspecific sites such as anionic phospholipids, metabolites, and nucleic acids. At physiological levels of $[Ca^{2+}]_i$, the ratio of $[Ca^{2+}]_i$ to bound Ca^{2+} in the cytoplasm is in the range of 10^{-2} to 10^{-3} (18). Thus, the contribution of the flourescent Ca^{2+} indicators to total cytosolic Ca^{2+} buffering is significant, but not overwhelming. The cell membrane pumps and channels that are responsible for setting the level of $[Ca^{2+}]_i$ are all regulated primarily by the *free* cytoplasmic Ca^{2+} concentration. Therefore, under steady-state conditions, even quite high cytosolic loads of the flourescent Ca^{2+} indicator dyes are unlikely to perturb $[Ca^{2+}]_i$. However, during transient changes in $[Ca^{2+}]_i$, the additional Ca^{2+} buffering may modify the normal response. This can be manifest as a slower rate of $[Ca^{2+}]_i$ change, a reduced peak amplitude, or inhibition of normal Ca^{2+} feedback effects. For example, in electrically stimulated cardiac myocytes, increasing the load of Ca^{2+} indicator dye first reduces the rate at which Ca^{2+} transients decay, and at very high loads interferes with the process of Ca^{2+}-induced Ca^{2+} release that links sarcolemmal depolarization with Ca^{2+} release from the sarcoplasmic reticulum (19,20).

MEASUREMENTS OF Ca^{2+} CHANGES DURING CELL INJURY

In this section one example of the use of flourescent Ca^{2+} indicators for toxicology studies is described. In a recent study (21) we investigated the role of $[Ca^{2+}]_i$ in the cytotoxic effects of an oxidative stress imposed on hepatocytes by incubation with *tert*-butyl hydroperoxide (TBHP). Treatment of hepatocytes in primary culture with 0.5 m*M* TBHP results in loss of cell viability markers, with a half-time of about 45 min. The loss of viability is associated with an increase in $[Ca^{2+}]_i$, which has been suggested to play a causal role in cell killing. The loss of cell viability is a rapid event at the level of individual cells, but is spread out over a relatively prolonged period for the cell population as a whole. Therefore, the relationship between cell killing and $[Ca^{2+}]_i$ was examined at the single-cell level in fura2-loaded hepatocytes, using a digital imaging flourescence microscopy system based on a cooled CCD camera (22,23). A time series of image pairs (340 and 380 nm excitation, 460- to 580-nm emission) was accumulated, starting shortly before TBHP addition and continuing for ~60 min. A low magnification was used to obtain measurements over a microscope field containing a large number of cells (typically 25–100 cells). The time courses of flourescence change at each wavelength for individual cells were extracted by an image-processing program and used to calculate the cell-by-cell changes in $[Ca^{2+}]_i$ over time.

Figure 4A shows representative data from a single cell. There was an initial $[Ca^{2+}]_i$ spike within 1–3 min of adding TBHP (in some cells as many as five $[Ca^{2+}]_i$ spikes were observed). The upper panels of Fig. 4A show the reciprocal flourescence changes at 340 and 380 nm, while the bottom panel depicts the $[Ca^{2+}]_i$ signal calculated from these. We have recently determined that the initial $[Ca^{2+}]_i$ spikes induced by TBHP are secondary to the oxidation of cellular glutathione, and represent a specific modification of the Ins(1,4,5)P_3 receptor that causes Ca^{2+} release from intracellular hormone-sensitive Ca^{2+} stores (23,24). Following the initial $[Ca^{2+}]_i$ spikes $[Ca^{2+}]_i$ returned to basal levels for 10–20 min, before beginning to rise slowly to a new plateau, close to the maximum observed during the $[Ca^{2+}]_i$ spiking phase. Finally, there was a further rapid $[Ca^{2+}]_i$ rise to a point where the dye became Ca^{2+} saturated, presumably as cellular Ca^{2+} permeability barriers were broken down. However, complete loss of cell viability did not occur until 10–15 min after this drastic $[Ca^{2+}]_i$ rise. The loss of cell viability was manifest as a sudden precipitous disappearance of flourescence from the cells. This occurred ~50 min in the example of Fig. 4A. Calculation of $[Ca^{2+}]_i$ from the ratio of flourescence intensities has no meaning after the total loss of dye from the cell. The residual flourescence signal was largely due to cellular autoflourescence and compartmentalized fura2, which was subtracted prior to calculation of $[Ca^{2+}]_i$ at earlier time points. Thus, exper-

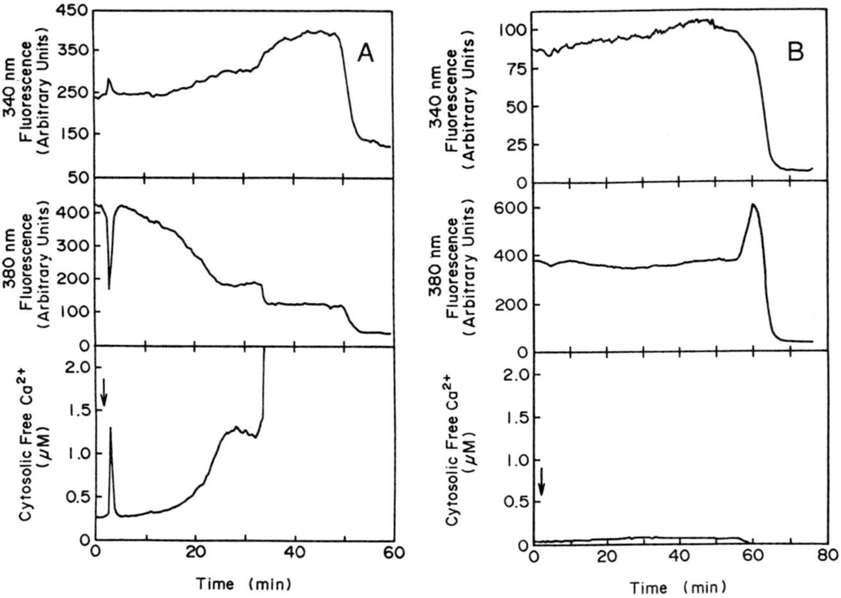

Figure 4 Effects of *tert*-butyl hydroperoxide (TBHP) on fura2 fluorescence and calculated $[Ca^{2+}]_i$ in single hepatocytes. Fura2 loaded hepatocytes in primary culture were treated with 0.5 m*M* TBHP at the arrows. Fluorescence was monitored using excitation at 340 nm (top panels) and 380 nm (middle panels). The ratio of the signals at these two wavelengths was used to calculate $[Ca^{2+}]_i$ (bottom panels). Left panels (A) demonstrate the response of a typical cell incubated in physiological medium containing 2 m*M* $CaCl_2$. Right panels (B) show a typical response for a cell incubated under similar conditions, but with 3.5 m*M* EGTA present throughout. In both cases a precipitous loss of dye after 50–60 min represents the point at which cells finally lose viability, as judged by the ability to retain the fura2 in the cytosol. [Reproduced from I. Sakaida, A. P. Thomas, and J. L. Farber, *J. Biol. Chem.* **266,** 717 (1991) by permission of the American Society for Biochemistry & Molecular Biology.]

iments of this type give information on the relative time courses of $[Ca^{2+}]_i$ change and loss of cell integrity, and also reveal unexpected complexities in the pattern of $[Ca^{2+}]_i$ change following treatment with toxic agents such as TBHP.

The data in Fig. 4A are consistent with a model in which early $[Ca^{2+}]_i$ increases are responsible for the subsequent cell killing by TBHP. However, in the same study we showed that incubation of cells with TBHP in the absence of Ca^{2+} completely eliminated all of the phases of $[Ca^{2+}]_i$ increase, but did not prevent TBHP-induced cell killing. Ca^{2+} depletion was achieved by prolonged incubation of the cells with excess EGTA in the extracellular medium. The response of a typical single cell to TBHP under these Ca^{2+}-depleted conditions is shown in Fig. 4B. TBHP (added at the arrow and present throughout) did not cause any changes in $[Ca^{2+}]_i$, but still led to a loss of cell viability manifest as the sudden decrease in dye flourescence at both wavelengths. Interestingly, there was a large *decrease* in $[Ca^{2+}]_i$ shortly before the final loss of cell viability. This presumably reflects the same loss of the plasmalemmal Ca^{2+} permeability barrier that underlies the large $[Ca^{2+}]_i$ increase observed in cells incubated with TBHP in medium containing physiological Ca^{2+} (Fig. 4A). Thus, experiments of the type shown in Fig. 4 allowed us to characterize the temporal relationship between $[Ca^{2+}]_i$ and cell damage, and to carry out experiments that dissociated the los of cell viability from the elevation of $[Ca^{2+}]_i$ induced by TBHP (for more details see Ref. 21).

ACKNOWLEDGEMENT

This work was supported by U.S. Public Health Service Grants DK-38422, AA-07186, and DA-06290.

REFERENCES

1. R. Y. Tsien, *Biochemistry* **19,** 2396 (1980).
2. R. Y. Tsien, T. Pozzan, and T. J. Rink, *J. Cell Biol.* **94,** 325 (1982).
3. G. Grynkiewicz, M. Poenie, and R. W. Tsien, *J. Biol. Chem.* **260,** 3440 (1985).
4. R. Y. Tsien, *Nature (London)* **290,** 527 (1981).
5. R. P. Haugland, "Handbook of Fluorescent Probes and Research Chemicals." Molecular Probes, Eugene, Oregon, 1992.
6. A. P. Thomas and F. Delaville, *in* "Cellular Calcium—A Practical Approach." (J. G. McCormack and P. H. Cobbold, eds), p. 1. Oxford University Press, Oxford, 1991.
7. J. J. Lemasters, E. Chacon, G. Zahreblski, J. M. Reece, and A-L. Nieminen, *in* "Optical Microsocopy: Emerging Methods and Applications" (B. Herman and J. J. Lemasters, eds.), p. 339. Academic Press., San Diego, 1993.
8. F. DiVirgilio, C. Fasolato, and T. H. Steinberg, *Biochem. J.* **256,** 959 (1988).
9. D. A. Williams, K. E. Fogarty, R. Y. Tsien, and F. S. Fay, *Nature (London)* **318,** 558 (1985).
10. R. Y. Tsien and T. Pozzan, *in "Methods in Enzymology"* (S. Fleischer and B. Fleischer, eds.), Vol. 172, p. 230. Academic Press, San Diego, 1989.
11. A. L. Nieminen, G. J. Gores, T. L. Dawson, B. Herman, and J. J. Lemasters, *J. Biol. Chem.* **265,** 2399 (1990).
12. D. R. Pfeiffer, P. W. Reed, and H. A. Lardy, *Biochemistry* **13,** 4007 (1974).
13. M. Poenie, *Cell Calcium* **11,** 85 (1990).
14. J. E. Merritt and T. J. Hallam, *J. Biol. Chem.* **263,** 6161 (1988).
15. M. C. Glennon, G. S. J. Bird, C.-Y. Kwan, and J. W. Putney, Jr., *J. Biol. Chem.* **267,** 8230 (1992).
16. G. Hajnoczky, E. Gao, T. Nomura, J. B. Hoek, and A. P. Thomas, *Biochem. J.* **293,** 413 (1993).
17. P. Arslan, F. DiVirgilio, M. Beltrame, R. Y. Tsien, and T. Pozzan, *J. Biol. Chem.* **260,** 2719 (1985).

18. S. K. Joseph, K. E. Coll, R. H. Cooper, J. S. Marks, and J. R. Williamson, *J. Biol. Chem.* **258,** 731 (1983).
19. A. P. Thomas, M. Selak, and J. R. Williamson, *J. Mol. Cell Cardiol.* **18,** 541 (1986).
20. B. O'Rourke, D. K. Reibel, and A. P. Thomas, *Am. J. Physiol.* **259,** H230 (1990).
21. I. Sakaida, A. P. Thomas, and J. L. Farber, *J. Biol. Chem.* **266,** 717 (1991).
22. T. A. Rooney, E. J. Sass, and A. P. Thomas, *J. Biol. Chem.* **264,** 17131 (1989).
23. T. A. Rooney, D. C. Renard, E. Sass, and A. P. Thomas, *J. Biol. Chem.* **266,** 12272 (1991).
24. D. C. Renard, M. B. Seitz, and A. P. Thomas, *Biochem. J.* **284,** 507 (1992).

26 Ca^{2+}-Bioluminescent Indicators

André B. Borle

INTRODUCTION

Oxidative stress and toxic agents are known to disrupt intracellular Ca^{2+} homeostasis and to cause cell injury and cell death. There is a vast literature showing that toxic chemicals, CCl_4, $HgCl_2$, menadione, cystamine, as well as chemical anoxia induced by cyanide and iodoacetate, hypoxia, and simple anoxia under nitrogen trigger an increase in cytosolic free Ca^{2+} (Ca_i^{2+}) in heart, liver, kidney, brain, and other tissues. The link between the increase in Ca_i^{2+} and cell injury is still debated. Although Ca^{2+} activates hydrolytic enzymes such as phospholipase A_2, proteases, and endonucleases and promotes free radical formation by converting xanthine dehydrogenase to xanthine oxidase, an elevation in Ca_i^{2+} may or may not be directly involved in the sequence of events leading to toxic injury. Indeed, despite the large number of articles reporting an increase in Ca_i^{2+} caused by toxic agents or oxidative stress, a few investigators have observed an elevation in Ca_i^{2+} without cell injury, membrane damage preceding the rise in Ca_i^{2+}, or cell death without an increase in Ca_i^{2+}. Nevertheless, the elevation in Ca_i^{2+} has been measured by a wide variety of direct or indirect methods: with Ca^{2+}-sensitive fluorescent indicators, bioluminescent probes, Ca^{2+}-sensitive microelectrodes, nuclear magnetic resonance (NMR), and by measurements of phosphorylase *a* activity.

The measurement of Ca_i^{2+} is an important part of any study related to the development of cell injury. This chapter describes the method developed to measure Ca_i^{2+} in mammalian cells with bioluminescent Ca_i^{2+} indicators. Of the two most widely used Ca^{2+}-sensitive photoproteins, aequorin and obelin, the former is the more commonly used. Several articles dealing with the technical aspects of intracellular Ca^{2+} measurements with aequorin have already been published (1–5). They describe in great details the photoprotein source, properties, preparation, assay,incorporation into cells, instrumentation, advantages and disadvantages, and comparison with other Ca^{2+} indicators. Aequorin is a photoprotein isolated from the marginal photocytes of the jellyfish *Aequorea forskalea*. When it binds Ca^{2+}, it emits photons in proportion to the concentration of ionized Ca^{2+}, and the light intensity can be detected by a suitable photomultiplier tube.

METHODS IN TOXICOLOGY, Volume 1B

METHOD

Materials

Aequorin is available from J. R. Blinks, Friday Harbor Photoprotein, (Friday Harbor, WA). It is supplied as 1 mg of photoprotein lyophilized in 150 m*M* KCl and 5 m*M* HEPES buffer (pH 7.6). Chelex-100 used in the columns to decontaminate all solutions that will contain aequorin is purchased from Bio-Rad (Richmond, CA). EDTA, HEPES, and Triton X-100 can be purchased from Sigma (St. Louis, MO). Ultrapure solutions of $CaCl_2$ are obtained from BDH Ltd., (Pool, England) and of $MgCl_2$ are obtained from Johnson Matthey (England). EGTA is obtained from Fluka (Buchs, Switzerland).

Ca^{2+} Decontamination

The luminescent reaction of photoproteins with Ca^{2+} is irreversible so that aequorin can be rapidly inactivated by small amounts of calcium contamination. The success of the method rests largely on the care used in avoiding Ca^{2+} contamination. It is crucial that the Ca^{2+} concentration of every solution that comes in contact with aequorin be less than 10^{-8} *M*. Consequently, they must be thoroughly decontaminated of all traces of Ca^{2+} by passage through Chelex columns (4). Moreover, laboratoryware that is to be in contact with aequorin must be made of plastic and also must be decontaminated. This is achieved by several washes with 10 m*M* EDTA followed by six to ten rinses with distilled water decontaminated through Chelex columns.

Aequorin Stock Solution

The aequorin lyophilized powder is stored at $-50°C$ until needed. It is reconstituted by adding 1 ml of deionized Chelexed water, and 0.1-ml aliquots are placed in to 10 separate plastic 1.5-ml microcentrifuge tubes and frozen at $-50°C$. One 0.1-ml aliquot contains enough aequorin for five to 10 experiments and the tube can be stored at normal freezer temperature ($-20°C$) between experiments.

INTRACELLULAR INCORPORATION OF AEQUORIN

Many techniques can be used to introduce photoproteins into cells: microinjections (6,7), cell hybridization (8), membrane permeabilization to aequorin by incubation of cells or tissue in EGTA (9), brief incubations in a hypoosmotic medium (10,11), scrape loading (12), and gravity loading (13).

Aequorin Incorporation by Gravity Loading

Gravity loading is the fastest and easiest method for aequorin incorporation. It has been successfully used in a large number of cell types: cultured monkey kidney (LLC-MK_2), cells, Madin–Darby canine kidney cells, rabbit renal tubules, rat and human hepatocytes, Kupffer cells, rat myocytes, aortic smooth muscle cells, human fibroblasts, rat Sertoli cells, RAW-264 macrophages, neutrophils, and BALB/c 3T3 cells. Cultured cells or cells freshly isolated from various tissues are kept in suspension. They are washed twice in GKN (a Na^+, K^+ saline solution containing glucose and buffered with phosphate: 137 m*M* Na^+, 4 m*M* K^+, 0.51 m*M* Na_2HPO_4, 0.15 m*M* NaH_2PO_4, and 11 m*M* glucose, and once briefly in GKN containing 1 m*M* EGTA to remove all traces of Ca^{2+} bound to the cells' glycocalyx. Centrifuge the cells at 200 *g* for 2 min at 25°C, decant the GKN and EGTA, and resuspend the cells in 0.5 ml of a buffered saline containing 140 m*M* NaCl, 3 m*M* HEPES, and 10–20 μg/ml of aequorin. Incubate them on ice for 10 min and then centrifuge at 200 *g* for 30 sec at 25°C. Discard the supernatant and resuspend the cells in Krebs–Henseleit bicarbonate buffer (KHB) at 37°C, equilibrated with 95% O_2, 5% CO_2, as previously defined (11).

Aequorin Incorporation by Scrape Loading (Cell Cultures)

Scrape loading has been used to incorporate aequorin into cultured cells (12). When the cells have established a confluent monolayer, decant the growth medium and wash the monolayer three times with cold (4°C) GKN. Dissolve aequorin (10–20 μg) in 4 ml of a buffered solution at 4°C [140 m*M* K^+, 3 m*M* K_2H_2ATP, and 3 m*M* HEPES (pH 7.0)] then pipette this solution on the monolayer and briefly swirl to cover all of the cells. Then scrape the cells off the plastic surface with a soft rubber policeman. Transfer the cell suspension to a plastic centrifuge tube and rinse the culture flasks several times with small amounts of GKN that are added to the cell suspension. Centrifuge the cells at 200 *g* for 1 min at 25°C, wash the pellet several times with cold KHB, and finally resuspend the cells in 0.5 ml of KHB and incubate at 37°C for 1 hr with a gas phase of 90% O_2/5% CO_2.

Aequorin Incorporation by the HOST Method

The HOST method (for hypoosmotic shock treatment) was initially used to load the photoprotein obelin in red blood cells (14) and was later modified to incorporate aequorin in small mammalian cells. (10,11). In this laboratory the method has been abandoned in favor of gravity loading. Wash isolated cells (cultured cells or cells isolated with collagenase from fresh tissues) two or three times with cold (4°C) GKN. Separate the cells from their suspending medium by centrifugation at 200 *g* at 25°C. After the last centrifugation, resuspend ~0.3 ml of packed cells in 2 ml of HOST medium at 4°C. The HOST medium (osmolarity, 20 mOsm) contains 3 m*M* MgATP, 3 m*M* HEPES (pH 7.4), and 10–15 μg/2.3 ml of aequorin. The cells suspended in the hypotonic HOST medium are gently stirred for exactly 2 min at 4°C. After 2 min restore normal osmolarity by adding to the 2.3 ml of cell suspension 0.175 ml of a 2*M* KCL solution containing 3 m*M* HEPES (pH 7.4). Incubate the cells in this isotonic medium for 15 min at 4°C. Then wash the cells with 3 ml of KHB and incubate at 37°C for at least 1 hr to allow the cells to resume a normal steady state. The washing of the cells and their subsequent incubation in a medium containing 1.3 m*M* calcium remove or consume all of the aequorin which is not sequestered inside the cells. The viability of some types of cells, (e.g., cardiomyocytes) is improved by raising the calcium concentration of the incubating medium stepwise, every 10–15 min from 0 to 0.1, 0.5, and finally 1.3 m*M*.

Aequorin Incorporation by Microinjection

This technique is the most demanding and requires special skills and equipment, which are described in detail elsewhere (1,6). It has been used successfully to measure Ca_i^{2+} in single cells: salivary glands, oocytes, fibroblasts and hepatocytes (7,15,16).

Distribution of Aequorin within the Cells

There has been no systematic study on the distribution of the photoprotein within the cell. However, from single-cell experiments, aequorin appears to spread in an apparently uniform fashion throughout the cytoplasm of cells into which aequorin is injected (2). Moreover, the photoprotein is excluded from the sarcoplasmic reticulum and from mitochondria (17,18).

MEASUREMENT AEQUORIN LUMINESCENCE

Instrumentation

There is no commercially available very sensitive photometer dedicated to the measurement of aequorin luminescence. Different light-detecting systems can be custom built depending on the type of cells, the size of the tissue strip, whether the cells are attached or free, or whether one studies a single cell or a large population of cells. For single cells image intensifiers or photomultiplier tubes attached to a photon counting system have been used successfully (6,17). An apparatus capable of measuring both tension and very low light intensity from muscle strips injected with aequorin has been described by Blinks (19).

An aequorin luminescence photometer modified from Blinks' apparatus was built by this laboratory to measure light signals from perfused cells embedded in agarose gel threads (4). Both utilize a low-noise photomultiplier tube with a high quantum efficiency close to the aequorin λ_{max} of 469 nm, attached to a light-gathering system consisting of two hemiellipsoidal mirrors (4,19).

Cell Attachment for Continuous Perfusion of Aequorin-Loaded Cells

Cultured cells attached to a coverslip are placed into a cuvette and continuously perfused. Alternatively, attachment to a fiberglass matrix is also suitable for cells that readily attach to glass substrates. However, the best method is to cast the cells in agarose gel threads (20). Suspend the aequorin-loaded cells, equivalent to 0.5 ml of packed cells, in 0.5 ml of KHB at 37°C containing 1.2% agarose (type VII, low gelling temperature, from Sigma). The liquid cell suspension is gently forced with a 1-ml tuberculin syringe through a 0.5-mm inner diameter plastic catheter which is coiled in an ice bath, and the extruded gel threads are collected in 2 ml of KHB in the cuvette to be perfused at 37°C.

Conversion of the Measured Aequorin Light Signal to Ca_i^{2+}

The conversion of the light signal L recorded as current to intracellular free Ca^{2+} concentration is done by interpolating the experimental values on a calibration curve according to the method of Allen and Blinks (21). The Ca^{2+}-dependent luminescence recorded from aequorin-loaded cells depends not only on Ca_i^{2+} but also on the amount of photoprotein incorporated in the cells. Aequorin incorporation must be determined for each experiment, since it may vary from experiment to experiment. The amount of aequorin incorporated is measured at the end of each experiment to give the value L_{max}. To do so, lyse the cells *in situ* in the cuvette by perfusing a solution containing the membrane detergent Triton X-100 [2% (w/v)], 10 m*M* $CaCl_2$, 120 m*M* KCl, and 3 m*M* HEPES (pH 7.4). The resulting flash of light, L_{max} is carefully integrated by an amplifier-integrator. It is usually five to six orders of magnitude larger than L (milliamperes versus nanoamperes). To convert the original data recorded as current (in nanoamperes) to intracellular Ca^{2+} concentration, each experiment data point L is normalized with L_{max} as fractional luminescence and its negative logarithm ($-\log L/L_{max}$) is interpolated on the appropriate calibration curve.

Calibration Curve

The method of calibration relies on a few assumptions about the intracellular concentrations of Mg^{2+}, K^+, and pH, since the composition of the assay solutions must mimic the intracellular milieu. The curve is generated by the rapid mixing of known concentrations of Ca^{2+} with fixed amounts of aequorin in an assay photometer. Below 10^{-5} *M*, Ca^{2+} can be set by a Ca–EGTA buffer system. Since the aequorin light signal or luminescence (L) depends not only on the Ca^{2+} concentration but also on the total amount of aequorin present in the cuvette, this total amount of aequorin must be determined by letting the photoprotein react with supramaximal concentrations of Ca^{2+} which give the maximal luminescence (L_{max}). The signal L is then normalized as the fractional luminescence L/L_{max}. L_{max} is obtained by injecting 10 μl of the same solution of aequorin into a cuvette containing 10 m*M* Ca^{2+}. To draw the calibration curve, the negative logarithm of the fractional luminescence is plotted against the negative logarithm of the Ca^{2+} concentration pCa (Fig. 1). The log versus log plot and the sigmoid shape of the curve mask the sensitivity of the method at physiological intracellular Ca^{2+} concentrations ranging between 50 and 600 nM. Figure 2 shows the relationship between the net signal current and Ca^{2+} in a linear plot at a constant L_{max}. This shows that the signal intensity is fairly linear with respect to Ca^{2+} throughout this range. Several standard curves should be made at different Mg^{2+} concentrations (0, 0.5, 1.0, or 2 m*M*) unless the precise concentration of cytosolic Mg^{2+} (Mg_i) of the particular cell population under study is known with certainty. Finally, the aequorin–Ca^{2+} reaction is temperature sensitive, so that the calibration curve and the experimental data must be obtained at the same temperature.

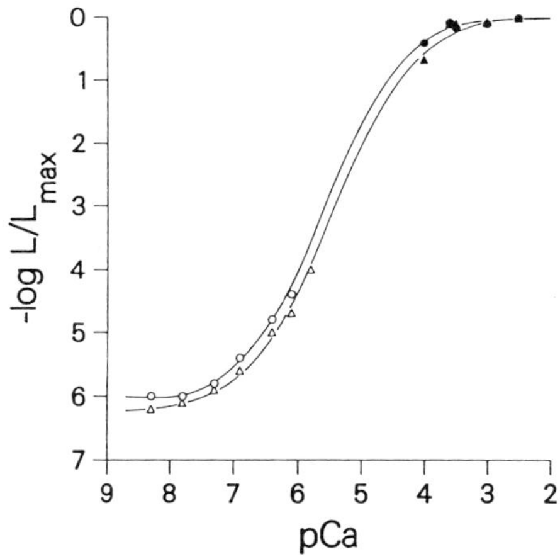

Figure 1 Aequorin calibration curve obtained in 140 m*M* KCl and 20 m*M* HEPES (pH 7.4) and 0.5 or 1.0 m*M* $MgCl_2$. The data points expressed by closed symbols were obtained by simple dilution of solutions containing ultrapure $CaCl_2$. The data points represented by open symbols were obtained with Ca–EGTA buffer solutions. Circles show a curve obtained with 0.5 m*M* Mg^{2+}; triangles show a curve obtained in the presence of 1 m*M* Mg^{2+}. pCa, negative logarithm of the ionized Ca^{2+} concentration. (Reproduced from Snowdowne and Borle with permission from *American Journal of Physiology* **247**, C396–C408, 1984. Copyright © 1984 by the American Physiological Society.)

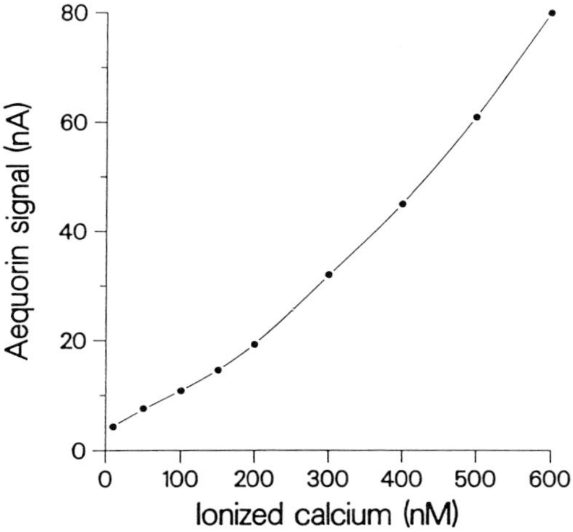

Figure 2 Relationship between the aequorin light signal and the concentration of ionized Ca^{2+}, assuming an intracellular free Mg^{2+} of 1 m*M* and a constant L_{max}. (Reproduced from Snowdowne and Borle with permission from *American Journal of Physiology* **247**, C396–C408, 1984. Copyright © 1984 by the American Physiological Society.)

Conversion of the Aequorin Light Signal

The conversion of the aequorin current signal to absolute values of Ca^{2+} concentration rests on several assumptions regarding Mg_i^{2+}, the intracellular pH (pH_i), the homogeneity of the cell population, and the uniform distribution of both cytosolic Ca^{2+} and aequorin, assumptions that can rarely be documented.

Like most Ca^{2+} indicators, aequorin is Mg^{2+} sensitive. Mg^{2+} reduces the rate of spontaneous photon emission by aequorin and decreases the photoprotein affinity for calcium, which results in a lower light emission. Thus, for a given free calcium concentration, Mg^{2+} will reduce the aequorin signal, and the higher the Mg^{2+}, the lower the signal. Unless Mg_i^{2+} is measured with a reliable method in the particular cell population under study and under the same experimental conditions, the conversion of current to Ca^{2+} must rely on the best educated guess. Since Ca^{2+} and Mg^{2+} have reciprocal effects on the aequorin luminescence, changes in Mg_i^{2+} may themselves influence the aequorin signal. However, only very large decreases in Mg_i^{2+} could be wrongly interpreted as an increase in Ca_i. If Mg_i^{2+} is unknown, one must assume a reasonable value to interpolate the experimental data on the appropriate calibration curve. Figure 1 shows that Mg^{2+} produces a shift of the calibration curve to the right. Even when Ca^{2+} is too low to be detected, Mg^{2+} will lower the level of Ca^{2+}-independent fractional luminescence ($Ca^{2+} < 10^{-8}$ *M*).

The Ca_i^{2+} values should also be corrected for large changes in pH_i which may occur for instance during anoxia (22). Although the aequorin signal is relatively insensitive to changes in pH within the physiological range, a large decrease in pH_i may cause a reduction in the light emission from aequorin (23): in heart cells, for instance, a ΔpH of 0.8 units causes a ΔpCa of 0.2 units (24).

Finally, under some experimental conditions, Ca_i^{2+} may be elevated to very high levels for prolonged periods. As a result significant amounts of aequorin are consumed, since the reaction of Ca^{2+} with aequorin is irreversible. In such cases the aequorin luminescence signal should be integrated throughout the experiment, and the calculation of Ca_i^{2+} at each time point must be referred to the final maximal luminescence (L_{max}) plus the integrated amount of photoprotein consumed after that time.

Because Mg^{2+} and pH influence aequorin luminescence, and because the current is not linearly related to the Ca^{2+} concentration, the relative changes in current from the aequorin light signal cannot be interpreted as a direct reflection of Ca^{2+}. The nonlinearity precludes a direct quantitative interpretation of the aequorin light signal and its fluctuations without interpolation on a calibration curve. Furthermore, if the intracellular Ca^{2+} concentration is not homogenous throughout the cell population under study, the light signal emanating from cells with high Ca_i^{2+} will predominate and small Ca^{2+} changes in that population will be exaggerated because the relationship between Ca^{2+} and the current signal has a steeper slope at higher Ca^{2+} concentrations. Within physiological limits, however (i.e., between 50 and 600 n*M* Ca_i^{2+}), this relationship is almost linear, as shown in Fig. 2, and the problem is relatively minor, but at higher Ca^{2+} concentrations ($>10^{-6}$) the slope becomes significantly steeper. High Ca^{2+} concentrations also consume and inactivate significant amounts of aequorin. Ca_i^{2+} concentrations between 10^{-5} and 10^{-4} M would consume all of the aequorin present in the cell between 4 and 10 sec, depending on the Mg_i^{2+} concentration. Below Ca_i^{2+} of 10^{-6} *M*, however, the current signal *L* is only an insignificant fraction of the total signal L_{max} measured at the end of each experiment, even when the aequorin signal *L* is integrated for several hours. The five to six orders of magnitude difference between *L* and L_{max} indicates that less than 1% of the aequorin incorporated is consumed during a 2- to 3-hr experiment.

APPLICATIONS

Cytosolic Free Ca^{2+} in Anoxic or Toxic Cell Injury

The increase in Ca_i^{2+} and its importance in anoxic or toxic cell injury are still controversial. Orrenius and collaborators, as well as our group, believe that a sustained increase in cytosolic Ca^{2+} is linked to the onset of cytotoxicity (25–27). Lemasters' and Farber's groups, on the other hand, challenge both the existence and the importance of a rise in Ca^{2+} as factors in cell damage (28–

30). The evidence that Ca_i^{2+} increases in toxic or anoxic cell injury is overwhelming. A rise in Ca_i^{2+} evoked by anoxia has been documented in heart (30–34), liver (22,26,35–39), kidney (10,13,40–42), and brain (43–48) with completely different techniques: Ca^{2+}-sensitive microelectrodes, NMR, aequorin, quin2, fura2, indo1, and phosphorylase *a* activity. For example, Fig. 3 shows an aequorin luminescence tracing documenting the biphasic increase in Ca_i^{2+} obtained during 2-hr of anoxia in perfused rat hepatocytes. The first Ca_i^{2+} peak is caused by a release of Ca^{2+} from mitochondria, while the second arises from an influx of Ca^{2+} from the extracellular fluids, presumably on the Na^+–Ca^{2+} antiporter operating in the reverse mode (22,26). In contrast, a few investigators failed to see any increase in Ca_i^{2-} during anoxia in both liver and kidney cells when fura2 was used as a Ca^{2+} indicator (27,28,49).

The reason for the discrepancy is still obscure. One can only speculate why fura2 would sometimes fail to document an increase in Ca_i^{2+} during simple or chemical anoxia. First, it has been shown by many investigators that fura2 is not restricted to the cytosol: It enters mitochondria (50–55) and other subcellular organelles (28,56), it accumulates in the nucleus (57), and possibly as much as 85% of the dye may be in the protein-bound form (58,59). Consequently, the mixed signals from a rising Ca^{2+} activity in the cytosol and from a falling Ca^{2+} concentration in the organelles may blur or completely mask an increase in the

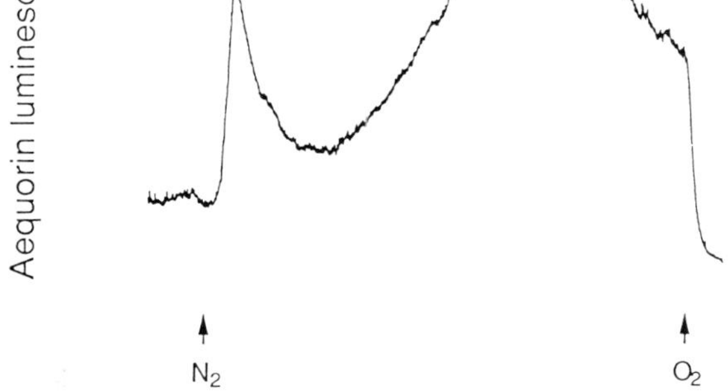

Figure 3 Effect of 2 hr of anoxia on the aequorin luminescence of hepatocytes isolated from fed rats, loaded with aequorin incorporated by gravity, cast in agarose gel threads, and perfused with a Krebs-Henseleit bicarbonate buffer containing 1.3 m*M* Ca^{2+} and 5 m*M* glucose. Anoxia was produced by shifting the gas phase of the perfusate from 95% O_2/5% CO_2 to 95% N_2/5% CO_2, as indicated by the arrows.

cytosolic free Ca^{2+} concentration (56). Second, EGTA and its derivatives, quin2 and fura2, have been shown to inhibit the Na^{+}–Ca^{2+} antiporter operating in the reverse mode (60–64), which may inhibit the influx of Ca^{2+} responsible for the major increase in Ca_i^{2+}. Third, Ca^{2+}–EGTA, Ca^{2+}–quin2, and Ca^{2+}–fura2 complexes act as a substrate for the Ca^{2+} ATPase-dependent Ca^{2+} pump and have been shown to activate the Ca^{2+} pump (65). Fourth, when aequorin is incorporated together with quin2 in a cell population, or with fura2 in a single cell, the peak Ca_i^{2+} measured with the fluorescent dyes is, respectively, 10 and 100 times smaller than that measured with aequorin (66,67). Several investigators have warned that these various aspects of the fluorescent Ca^{2+} indicators may compromise their function as a general cytosolic Ca^{2+} probe (50,63).

COMPARISON OF TWO CLASSES OF Ca^{2+} INDICATORS

Several reviews have been published comparing the properties and the relative advantages and defects of various Ca^{2+} probes tetracarboxylate fluorescent indicators, biazometallochromic indicators, bioluminescent protein indicators, and the various ligands used in Ca^{2+}-sensitive microelectrodes (2,5,68). In this short review only the two types of Ca^{2+} indicators most commonly used are compared: the bioluminescent photoproteins and the fluorescent dyes.

Bioluminescent Ca^{2+} Indicators

The photoproteins aequorin and obelin have many assets. Aequorin is a 20-kDa apoprotein which is a natural intracellular component of the hydromedusan *Aequorea* and, as such, is not toxic to the cell. It appears to spread uniformly throughout the cytosol (2) and to be excluded from both mitochondria and sarcoplasmic reticulum (17,18). It is the most sensitive of all Ca^{2+} indicators: 10^{-14} *M* aequorin is enough to detect Ca^{2+} luminescence down to 10^{-8} *M*. Besides its great sensitivity, aequorin has practically no Ca^{2+} buffering action: With a dissociation constant K_{Ca} of 10^{-5} *M* (1), a cytosolic free Ca^{2+} of 10^{-7} *M*, and an intracellular concentration of aequorin estimated at less than 10^{-8} *M*, the binding of Ca^{2+} to the photoprotein is less than 10^{-10} *M*. Within physiological limits aequorin is insensitive to changes in Na^{+}, K^{+}, and osmolarity and relatively insensitive to changes in pH. It is not sensitive to volume or viscosity changes, and its response time is relatively fast (τ = 5 msec). On the negative side, as noted above, aequorin is sensitive to changes in Mg^{2+}, the relationship between light emission and Ca^{2+} is not linear, and the reaction between the photoprotein and Ca^{2+} is irreversible. Finally, there is no commercially available highly sensitive photometer dedicated to the aequorin method, and each investigator usually builds his own instrument according to his specific cell model and his special needs.

Tetracarboxylate Fluorescent Ca^{2+} Indicators

Quin2, fura2, indo1, and fluo3 are all derived from the Ca^{2+} chelator EGTA and have a K_d ranging from 125 to 450 n*M*. They have an excellent selectivity against H^+, Na^+, and K^+ and are easy to use. Their incorporation as membrane-permeable acetoxymethyl esters is efficient and well recognized. Their calibration and the calculation of Ca_i^{2+} are relatively simple with dual-excitation/dual-emission spectrofluorometers. However, there are also many problems associated with these fluorescent probes. Because of their high affinity for Ca^{2+} (on the same order of magnitude as EGTA), they have a significant Ca^{2+}-buffering action. They are also sensitive to changes in Mg^{2+}. The selectivity of fura2 for Ca^{2+} over Mg^{2+} is slightly inferior to that of aequorin: Its discrimination ratio K_dCa^{2+}/K_dMg^{2+} is ~25,000, compared to 10^5 for aequorin (5). As with aequorin, the relationship between fluorescence and Ca^{2+} is not linear; but although aequorin measurements are biased toward high Ca_i^{2+} values, the fluorescent dyes are biased toward low Ca_i^{2+} values. Tetracarboxylate Ca^{2+} indicators are not inert. The by-products of the deesterification of the acetoxymethyl esters groups are toxic to the cells, and the dyes affect a wide variety of cellular functions (5; see above). They are not restricted to the cytosol and are taken up by subcellular organelles. Finally, there are spectral shifts and changes in K_d as a function of viscosity, pH and polarity, dye leakage from the cells, photobleaching, photochemical alterations, and phototoxicity (28).

Each Ca^{2+} probe has its share of technical pitfalls and every method has its great assets and its limitations. The selection of an appropriate Ca^{2+} indicator does not depend on its characteristics alone but, more importantly, on a good match between its properties and the type of cell or the toxicological problem under study.

REFERENCES

1. J. R. Blinks, P. H. Mattingly, B. R. Jewell, M. Van Leeuwen, G. C. Harrer, and D. G. Allen, *in* "Methods in Enzymology" (M. A. DeLuca, ed.), Vol. 57, p. 292. Academic Press, New York, 1978.
2. J. R. Blinks, W. G. Wier, P. Hess, and F. G. Prendergast, *Prog. Biophys. Mol. Biol.* **40**, 1 (1982).
3. J. R. Blinks, *in* "Bioluminescence and Chemiluminescence: Instrument and Applications" (K. Van Dyke, ed.), Vol. II, p. 185. CRC Press, Boca Raton, Florida, 1985.
4. A. B. Borle and K. W. Snowdowne, *in* "Methods in Enzymology" (P. M. Conn, ed.), Vol. 124, p. 90. Academic Press, Orlando, Florida, 1986.
5. A. B. Borle, *in* "Calcium and Cell Function," (W. Y. Cheung, ed.), Vol. 7, p. 160. Academic Press, Orlando, Florida, 1987.
6. P. H. Cobbold, K. S. Cuthbertson, M. H. Goyns, and V. Rice, *J. Cell Sci.* **61**, 123, (1983).

7. N. H. Woods, K. S. Cuthbertson, and P. H. Cobbold, *Nature (London)* **319**, 600, (1986).
8. A. K. Campbell and K. G. Hallet, *J. Physiol. (London)* **338**, 537 (1983).
9. J. P. Morgan and K. G. Morgan, *Pfluegers Arch.* **395**, 75 (1982).
10. A. B. Borle and K. W. Snowdowne, *Science* **217**, 252 (1982).
11. K. W. Snowdowne and A. B. Borle, *Am. J. Physiol.* **247**, C396 (1984).
12. P. L. McNeil and D. L. Taylor, *Cell Calcium* **6**, 83 (1985).
13. A. B. Borle, C. C. Freudenrich, and K. W. Snowdowne, *Am J. Physiol,* **251**, C323 (1986).
14. A. K. Campbell and R. L. Dormer, *Biochem. J.* **152**, 255 (1975).
15. B. Rose and W. R. Loewenstein, *Science 190*, 1204 (1975).
16. N. M. Woods, K. S. R. Cuthbertson, and P. H. Cobbold, *Biochem. J.* **246**, 619 (1987).
17. B. Rose and W. R. Loewenstein, *J. Membr. Biol. 28*, 87 (1976).
18. J. R. Blinks, R. Rüdel, and S. R. Taylor, *J. Physiol. (London)* **277**, 291 (1978).
19. J. R. Blinks, *in* "Techniques in the Life Sciences, Physiology Section" (P. F. Baker, ed.), Vol. P1, Part II, p. 126, Elsevier, Amsterdam, 1982.
20. D. L. Fox, J. S. Cohen, and J. B. Mitchell, *Exp. Cell Res.* **154**, 521 (1984).
21. D. G. Allen and J. R. Blinks, *in* "Detection and Measurement of Free Ca^{2+} in Cells" (C. C. Ashley and A. K. Campbell, eds.), p. 159, Elsevier, Amsterdam, 1979.
22. A. Gasbarrini, A. B. Borle, H. Farghali, C. Bender, A. Francavilla, and D. Van Thiel, *J. Biol. Chem.* **267**, 6654 (1992).
23. D. G. Moisescu and C. C. Ashley, *Biochim. Biophys. Acta* **460**, 189 (1977).
24. D. G. Allen and C. H. Orchard, *J. Physiol. (London) 335*, 555 (1983).
25. S. Orrenius, D. J. McConkey, G. Bellomo, and P. Nicotera, *Trends Pharmacol. Sci.* **10**, 281 (1989).
26. A. Gasbarrini, A. B. Borle, H. Farghali, A. Francavilla, and D. Van Thiel, *J. Biol. Chem.* **267**, 7545 (1992).
27. J. J. Lemasters, J. DiGiuseppi, A. L. Nieminen, and B. Herman, *Nature (London)* **325**, 78 (1987).
28. J. J. Lemasters, G. J. Gores, A. L. Nieminen, T. L. Dawson, B. E. Wray, and B. Herman, *Environ. Health Perspect* 84, 83 (1990).
29. J. L. Farber, *Environ. Health Perspect* **84**, 107 (1990).
30. P. H. Cobbold and P. K. Bourne, *Nature (London)* **312**, 444 (1984).
31. K. W. Snowdowne, R. J. Ertel, and A. B. Borle, *J. Mol. Cell. Cardiol.* **17**, 233 (1985).
32. C. Steenbergen, E. Murphy, L. Levy, and R. E. London, *Circ. Res.* **60**, 700 (1987).
33. H. C. Lee, R. Mohabir, N. Smith, M. R. Franz, and W. T. Clusin, *Circulation* **78**, 1047 (1988).
34. Y. Koretsune and E. Marban, *Am. J. Physiol.* **258**, H9 (1990).
35. R. J. Sharma, L. M. Rodrigues, P. D. Whitton, and D. A. Hems, *Biochim. Biophys. Acta* **630**, 414 (1980).
36. P. Nicotera, P. Hartzell, C. Baldi, S. A. Svensson, G. Bellomo, and S. J. Orrenius, *J. Biol. Chem.* **261**, 14628 (1986).
37. A. L. Nieminen, G. J. Gores, B. E. Wray, Y. Tanaka, B. Herman, and J. J. Lemasters, *Cell Calcium* **9**, 237 (1988).
38. P. Nicotera, H. Thor, and S. Orrenius, *FASEB J.* **3**, 59 (1989).
39. I. Sakaida, A. P. Thomas, and J. L. Farber, *J. Biol. Chem.* **266**, 717 (1991).

40. K. W. Snowdowne, C. C. Freudenrich, and A. B. Borle, *J. Biol. Chem.* **260,** 11619 (1985).
41. M. S. Goligorsky and K. A. Hruska, *Miner. Electrolyte Metab.* **14,** 58 (1988).
42. C. E. McCoy, A. M. Selvaggio, E. A. Alexander, and J. H. Schwartz, *J. Clin. Invest.* **82,** 1326 (1988).
43. J. D. Johnson, W. G. Conroy, and G. E. Isom, *Toxicol. Appl. Pharmacol.* **88,** 217 (1987).
44. D. Uematsu, J. H. Greenberg, M. Reivich, and A. Karp, *Ann. Neurol.* **24,** 420 (1988).
45. R. A. Kaupinen, H. McMahon, and D. G. Nicholls, *Neuroscience* **27,** 175 (1988).
46. D. Uematsu, J. H. Greenberg, W. F. Hickey, and M. Reivich, *Stroke* **20,** 1531 (1989).
47. J. H. Greenberg, D. Uematsu, N. A. Araki, W. F. Hickey, and M. Reivich, *Stroke* **21,** (Suppl. 4), 72 (1990).
48. I. A. Silver and M. Erecinska, *J. Gen. Physiol.* **95,** 837 (1990).
49. W. R. Jacobs, M. Sgambati, G. Gomez, P. Vilaro, M. Higdon, P. D. Bell, and L.J. Mandel, *Am. J. Physiol.* **260,** C545 (1991).
50. S. F. Steinberg, J. P. Bilezikian, and Q. Al-Awqati, *Am. J. Physiol.* **253,** C744 (1987).
51. M. H. Davis, R. A. Altschuld, D. W. Jung, and G. P. Brierly, *Biochem. Biophys. Res. Commun.* **149,** 40 (1987).
52. G. L. Lukacs and A. Kapus, *Biochem. J.* **248,** 609 (1987).
53. M. Reers, R. A. Kelly, and T. W. Smith, *Biochem. J.* **257,** 131 (1989)
54. J. G. McCormack, H. M. Browne, and N. J. Dawes, *Biochim. Biophys. Acta* **973,** 420 (1989).
55. T. E. Gunter, D. Restrepo, and K. K. Gunter, *Am. J. Physiol.* **255,** C304 (1988).
56. T. T. DeFeo, G. M. Briggs, and K. G. Morgan, *Am. J. Physiol.* **253,** H1456 (1987).
57. D. A. Williams, K. E. Fogarty, R. Y. Tsien, and F. S. Fay, *Nature (London)* **318,** 558 (1985).
58. M. Konishi, A. Olson, S. Hollingworth, and S. M. Baylor, *Biophys. J.* **54,** 1089 (1988).
59. H. Karaki, *Trends Pharmacol. Sci.* **10,** 320 (1989).
60. P. F. Baker, *in* "Calcium and Cellular Function" (A.W. Cuthbert, ed.,) p. 96. St. Martin's, New York, 1970.
61. P. F. Baker and P. A. McNaughton, *J. Physiol. (London)* **259,** 103 (1976).
62. T. J. A. Allen and P. F. Baker, *Nature (London)* **315,** 755 (1985).
63. G. J. Kaczorowski, M. L. Garcia, V. F. King, and R. S. Slaughter, *Handb. Exp. Pharmacol.* **83,** 163 (1988).
64. P. Blanco, A. Martinez-Serrano, E. Bogònez, and J. Satrùstegui, *Cell Calcium* **11,** 25 (1990).
65. M. R. James-Kracke, *J. Gen. Physiol.* **99,** 41 (1992).
66. P. C. Johnson, J. A. Ware, P. B. Cliveden, M. Smith, A. M. Dvorak, and E. W. Salzman, *J. Biol. Chem.* **260,** 2069 (1985).
67. N. Suda and S. Kurihara, *Jpn. J. Physiol.* **41,** 277 (1991).
68. R. Y. Tsien, *Annu. Rev. Biophys. Bioeng.* **12,** 91 (1983).

27 Measurement of Receptor-Activated Accumulation of Inositol Phosphates as an Index of Phospholipase C Activity

Stephen B. Shears

INTRODUCTION

In intact cells receptor-activated PtdIns(4,5)P_2[1] hydrolysis by phospholipase C is not usually measured by directly assaying changes in the levels of the lipid itself. This approach is of limited value because one of the consequences of receptor occupation is a stimulation of PtdIns(4,5)P_2 resynthesis to ensure a continuing supply of substrate for phospholipase C. Thus, during the course of the cell activation, levels of PtdIns(4,5)P_2 tend to decrease only transiently, returning to or even exceeding basal levels within seconds (see, e.g., Ref. 1).

Changes in the mass levels of the two products that are formed from PtdIns(4,5)P_2—Ins(1,4,5)P_3 (2) and 1,2-diacylglycerol (3)—can be measured with commercially available kits. However, both of these approaches will greatly underestimate phospholipase C activity, since each product is rapidly metabolized; it is therefore necessary to also record the accumulation of downstream metabolites. This is an onerous goal as far as diacylglycerol is concerned, because of the difficulties involved in accurately accounting for its rapid deacylation and its phosphorylation and reincorporation back into inositol lipids (4). Receptor-dependent diacylglycerol turnover is also difficult to measure against its high background involvement in intermediary metabolism. Furthermore, diacylglycerol release by the action of phospholipase C is supplemented by hydrolysis of phosphatidylcholine, particularly during prolonged cell activation (4). It is difficult to distinguish between the two lipid sources of diacylglycerol. This leaves measurements of changes in inositol phosphate levels as the preferred means of studying receptor-coupled phospholipase C activity.

[1] Inositol lipids and inositol phosphates are abbreviated according to International Union of Pure and Applied Chemistry nomenclature; for example, Ins(1,4,5)P_3 = D-inositol-1,4,5-trisphosphate and PtdIns(4,5)P_2 = Phosphatidylinositol-4,5-bisphosphate.

METHODS IN TOXICOLOGY, Volume 1B

MATERIALS

High-performance liquid chromatography (HPLC) system (e.g., Waters–Millipore, Milford, MA; Beckman, Columbia, MD; or Gilson, Middleton, WI), including an on-line radioactivity detector (e.g., Beckman or Packard, Downers Grove, IL) or a fraction collector

Adsorbosphere SAX 5-μm HPLC column (the replaceable cartridge setup is cheaper than the columns), plus guard column and Pre-Sat silica precolumn (Alltech, Deerfield, IL)

Microcentrifuge for small multiple samples with the capacity to spin at $\sim$10,000 *g*.

1 kg of ion-exchange resin, AG 1-X8 200–400 mesh, formate form, plus 500 Poly-Prep columns (Bio-Rad, Melville, NY). Bio-Rad also supplies small racks for holding multiple samples, but most research departments should have the facilities to construct Plexiglas racks.

[2-^{3}H]Inositol [New England Nuclear (NEN)–Dupont, Boston, MA; Amersham, Arlington Heights, IL; or American Radiolabeled Chemicals, St. Louis, MO]. NEN and Amersham sell the widest range of [^{3}H]-labeled inositol phosphates, which can be used as standards to calibrate ion-exchange columns: Ins1P, Ins4P, Ins(1,4)P_2, Ins(1,4,5)P_3, Ins(1,3,4)P_3, Ins(1,3,4,5)P_4, and InsP_6

The remaining reagents can be made up from chemicals which are widely available from, for example, Sigma (St. Louis, MO), Fluka (Ronkonkoma, NY), and Aldrich (Milwaukee, WI):

Lithium chloride (100 ml, 2–5 *M*)

100 ml of 100 m*M* NaOH plus 0.1% (v/v) Triton X-100

100 ml of either (a) 2 *M* perchloric acid containing 1 mg/ml InsP_6, or (b) 0.6 *M* perchloric acid containing 0.2 mg/ml InsP_6 (dissolve the InsP_6 in water before adding the acid)

100 ml of 1.2 *M* KOH, 75 m*M* HEPES, and 20 m*M* EDTA (do not adjust the pH)

1000 ml of 0.06 *M* ammonium formate

1000 ml of 0.18 *M* ammonium formate

1000 ml of 0.4 *M* ammonium formate/0.1 *M* formic acid

1000 ml of 0.8 *M* ammonium formate/0.1 *M* formic acid

1000 ml of 1.05 *M* ammonium formate/0.1 *M* formic acid

1000 ml of 1.2 *M* ammonium formate/0.1 *M* formic acid

1000 ml of 2 *M* ammonium formate/0.1 *M* formic acid

1000 ml of 0.85 *M* ammonium dihydrogen phosphate, pH 3.35 with phosphoric acid

USE OF [^{3}H]INOSITOL TO MEASURE LEVELS OF [^{3}H]INOSITOL PHOSPHATES IN ISOLATED CELLS AND TISSUE SLICES

It is possible to directly assay the mass levels of a number of inositol phosphates in extracts of isolated cells and tissue preparations (5), although the complexity of both the method and the equipment required, and the associated expense, have not led to its widespread use. Thus, levels of inositol phosphates in cells are most usually studied after first labeling them with radioactive inositol. In discussing the details of this goal, it is assumed that the experimenter has already developed appropriate conditions for preparing and maintaining viable preparations of cells or tissue slices.

Either [2-^{3}H]- or [U-^{14}C] inositol can be used, since in either case there does not seem to be significant exchange of label out of the inositol moiety. While [^{3}H]inositol is by far the cheaper alternative, the quantities that must be used in an experiment still necessitate substantial expenditure; negotiations with competing suppliers may prove to be rewarding. In general, the higher the specific activity of the radiolabeled inositol added to the incubations, the greater the proportion of label that can be incorporated into the inositol lipids (6)—and hence also into Ins(1,4,5)P_3 and its closely related metabolites. Thus, it is the usual practice to keep the *mass* of inositol to the absolute minimum that the cells can accommodate. The precise amount of radioactivity added is ultimately constrained by one's budget, but it is not unusual to use ~10–20 μCi/ml. Even higher amounts (100 μCi/ml or more) are sometimes used, usually when data are to be analyzed by HPLC, and particularly when there is a need to resolve some of the smaller peaks. Higher levels of radioactivity are also sometimes needed to compensate for the relatively low counting efficiency that results in mixtures of scintillant and high-salt HPLC eluates.

Unfortunately, some mammalian cells incorporate exogenous inositol only poorly (platelets, for example), thereby obliging some experiments to rely on labeling with [^{32}P]P_i. Of course, ^{32}P will not be specifically incorporated into inositol phosphates, so techniques must be used that preferentially extract the ^{32}P-labeled inositol phosphates; these are described elsewhere (7).

In tissue slices, or in preparations of either isolated cells or cells in culture, the inositol lipids, Ins(1,4,5)P_3, and its closely related metabolites en route to free inositol, can all be labeled within 24 hr to a steady state. While isotopic equilibrium will not always have been achieved, it is still reasonable to believe that changes in levels of radioactivity associated with a particular metabolite reflect changes in actual total cellular concentration. Most workers restrict their analysis to *relative* rather than *absolute* levels of inositol phosphates. Some will extrapolate further, using the specific activity of exogenous inositol to calculate intracellular amounts of the various inositol phosphates. This procedure sometimes yields values for Ins(1,4,5)P_3 in resting cells that greatly exceed that required to fully mobilize cellular Ca^{2+} stores (8). In general, the apparent high levels of Ins(1,4,5)P_3 have been confirmed with mass assays; why then do such cells have a normal low basal [Ca^{2+}]? It appears that some cells can accumulate a portion of total cellular Ins(1,4,5)P_3 into an as yet undefined subcellular compartment (8). Nevertheless, the moral here is that the possibility of cellular compartmentalization of inositol phosphate pools, and maybe the differential labeling of such pools, should always be considered to be potentially compromising indirect estimates of inositol phosphate mass. There may also be intracellular concentration gradients of inositol phosphates (8).

While a labeling peroid of at least 24 hr is often used to ensure incorporation of [^{3}H]inositol to a steady state, this can exceed the time during which one can maintain the viability of both tissue slices and freshly isolated cell preparations. In such cases an alternative procedure is to prelabel to a pseudo steady state, such that within the time frame of the experimental manipulations, the specific activity of the radiolabeled inositol phosphates remains relatively constant. The usual procedure is to label cells with [^{3}H]inositol for the maximum amount of time that retention of cell viability will permit. Then the suspension medium is changed and replaced with medium containing non radioactive inositol. Usually, there will then be a subsequent period of 30 min or so during which there will not be a substantial change in the specific activity of the inositol phosphates.

Once released into the cell, Ins(1,4,5)P_3 is rapidly metabolized, both by a 5-phosphatase to Ins(1,4)P_2 and by a 3-kinase to Ins(1,3,4,5)P_4 (Fig. 1). Once these metabolites are themselves completely dephosphorylated to free inositol—and this occurs very quickly—they are "lost" from the assay. It is therefore a common practice to inhibit the metabolic flux to inositol by using lithium as a metabolic trap. This cation achieves this effect by inhibiting Ins(1,4)P_2/Ins(1,3,4)P_3 1-phosphatase and inositol monophosphatase (8).

A small volume of a concentrated stock lithium solution is usually added to incubations some time before the agonist; a widespread procedure is to add a final concentration of 10 m*M* lithium (as LiCl), some 10–20 min before the experimental protocol begins. It is wise to be aware of some complications that can arise from the use of lithium. For example, different cells accumulate lithium at different rates and to different extents, both of which can impact the efficiency of lithium as an inhibitor. It is a good idea to empirically determine the lithium treatment that leads to the maximum accumulation of inositol phosphates. It is also often forgotten that only rarely will lithium *near-totally* prevent the recycling of inositol phosphates to inositol; indeed, the extent of the usually unknown "leak" past the lithium block can be significant. A control experiment that can be indicative of the extent of this leakage is to reverse the action of the agonist with an antagonist and monitor the time course of the decay in inositol phosphate levels. However, this is not always a practical approach.

Lithium is also an unusual inhibitor in that it acts noncompetitively (8). This means that its efficacy increases with substrate concentration. In other words,

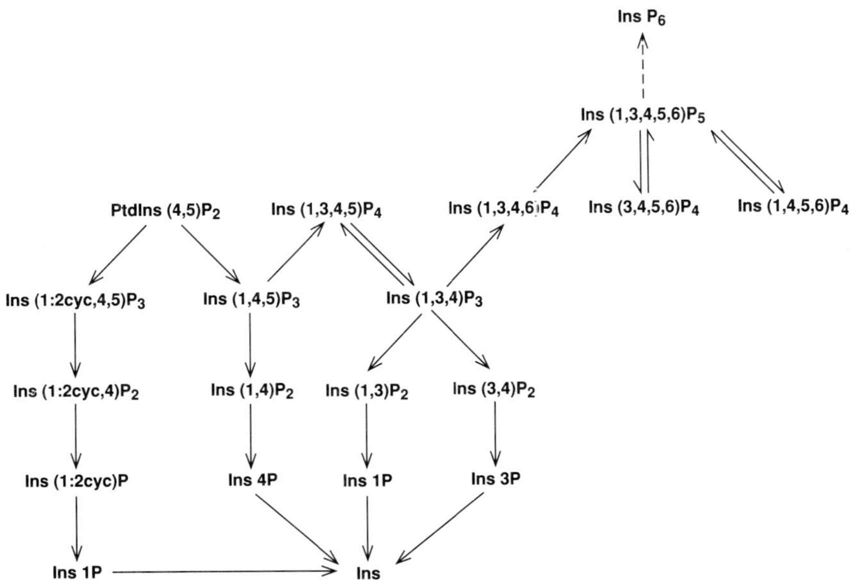

Figure 1 Inositol phosphate metabolism. Occupation of cell surface receptors activates the release of Ins(1,4,5)P_3 from PtdIns(4,5)P_2, usually accompanied by the release of very small amounts of Ins(1 : 2cyc,4,5)P_3. The further metabolism of these inositol phosphates is shown. For access to the enormous literature on this topic, see Refs. 8 and 15. The broken arrow that links Ins(1,3,4,5,6)P_5 to InsP_6 is meant to convey not only the rather slow kinetics with which this reaction proceeds, but also the possibility that Ins(1,3,4,5,6)P_5 may be distributed between more than one cellular pool, with differential ability to act as a precursor for InsP_6. While the direct hydrolysis of PtdIns4P and PtdIns is not shown here, these reactions should be considered potential contributors to receptor-dependent inositol phosphate turnover, at least in some circumstances.

lithium can have a graded effect, being most effective in stimulated cells and less so under basal conditions. Nevertheless, some degree of inhibition is usually still seen in the basal condition; lithium will slowly increase levels of inositol phosphates even in the absence of agonist. In other words, the experiment's baseline will shift during the course of an experiment. Thus, it is important to compare the *time course* for changes to inositol phosphate levels in *both* resting and stimulated cells. Yet another problem with lithium is that its actions on cells may not be specifically directed at inhibition of inositol phosphate phosphatases. For example, in some cells lithium can perturb receptor-dependent increases in levels of Ins(1,4,5)P_3 and Ins(1,3,4,5)P_4 (9) (the mechanism of this nonspecific effect is not yet clear). Lithium may also perturb the action of some GTP-binding proteins, which of course can also impact on signal transduction (10).

Despite all of the difficulties that may be encountered in the use of lithium, phospholipase C activity cannot be assayed with any degree of accuracy unless the cation is present to limit the dephosphorylation of inositol phosphates to free inositol. If the appropriate precautions described above are taken, then, in general terms, useful data will be obtained. On the other hand, if it is necessary to measure any real, physiologically relevant, levels of individual inositol phosphates, lithium cannot be used.

METHODOLOGY FOR QUENCHING INCUBATIONS AND EXTRACTING THE SOLUBLE INOSITOL PHOSPHATES

Having decided on a satisfactory radiolabeling protocol and planned a series of experimental manipulations, the investigator must now choose a method to rapidly quench the incubations. A number of quench media have been used, but some have potential pitfalls. Media based on a mixture of chloroform and methanol should be avoided since there can sometimes be problems with recovery of inositol polyphosphates (11), and it can also lead to the nonphysiological production of methyl-Ins(1,4,5)P_3 (12). Therefore, incubations are most frequently quenched with either trichloroacetic acid or perchloric acid. Whichever of these two acids is used, the extracts must subsequently be neutralized; otherwise, the acid will react with the chromatographic resins that are used to separate individual inositol phosphates. Trichloroacetic acid-quenched samples are frequently neutralized by repeated washes with diethyl ether (in which the acid is soluble). Despite the widespread use of this method, it is, in my opinion, a laborious procedure, and in any case the use of diethyl ether is a safety hazard.

My recommendation is to quench incubations with perchloric acid: 0.4 vol of 2 *M* acid plus 1 mg/ml $InsP_6$—the latter aids recovery of inositol phosphates through the extraction and neutralization procedures. In those cases in which cells are not in suspension, but instead are attached to culture cell plates, the incubation medium can be aspirated and then quickly replaced with a minimum volume of 0.6 *M* perchloric acid plus 0.2 mg/ml $InsP_6$ (the precise volume will depend on the diameter of the tissue culture well). Quenched samples are then placed on ice for 20–30 min to aid precipitation of protein, which is then subsequently removed by centrifugation at 0–4°C (10,000 *g*, 5 min). The supernatant is then saved and neutralized. The perchlorate-precipitated pellet should also be saved, for analysis of levels of [^{3}H]inositol lipids (see below).

There is a choice of procedures for neutralizing the perchlorate. This can be achieved using a mixture of freon and octylamine (13). However, the well-known environmental implications arising from the use of fluorocarbons impose a responsibility on us to seek alternatives. Thus, it is preferable to neutralize (i.e., to an approximate pH of 6.5–7.5) with an appropriate volume of medium containing 1.2 *M* KOH, 75 m*M* HEPES, and 20 m*M* EDTA. The precise volume can be predetermined by processing "blank" assays. In samples to be chromatographed on small gravity-fed columns, the efficiency of neutralization can be checked with the addition of 5 μl of universal indicator. However, if the samples are to be analyzed by HPLC, the indicator should be avoided since, after multiple runs, it will saturate the HPLC column. In any case careful pipetting will obviate the necessity to check that every sample is appropriately neutralized. After neutralization the extracts should be placed on ice for at least 1 hr to maximize the precipitation of the potassium perchlorate, and then centrifuged (10,000 *g*, 5 min, 0–4°C). Samples are then stored at 0–4°C and are stable for at least 2–3 weeks; they should not be lyophilized, since this can sometimes artificially generate diphosphoinositol polyphosphates ("inositol pyrophosphates") (14) (this artifact should not be confused with the physiologically relevant accumulation of genuine diphosphoinositol derivatives of $InsP_5$ and $InsP_6$ (14,15).

It should be noted that a very small proportion of the inositol lipids that are hydrolyzed by phospholipase C yield inositol phosphates containing a 1,2-cyclic diester. The cyclic bond is unstable in acid conditions; an acid-quenched sample that originally contained Ins(1 : 2cyc,4,5)P_3 will have this compound converted to Ins(2,4,5)P_3 plus Ins(1,4,5)P_3. Workers who are interested in quantifying cyclic inositol phosphates should use a neutral phenol/chloroform quench medium and dedicated HPLC separation procedures (16).

BATCH ELUTION OF INOSITOL PHOSPHATES FROM GRAVITY-FED ION-EXCHANGE COLUMNS

If the degree of phospholipase C activity is the main parameter under investigation, and assays of individual inositol phosphates are not important, cell extracts can be analyzed by gravity-fed anion-exchange chromatography. The resin of choice is made by Bio-Rad: the AG 1-X8 200–400 mesh (formate) form is particularly suitable. It is supplied in a dry form, and the only preparation needed is to wash it twice with distilled water, while also removing any "fines" that float to the surface. The resin is stored as a slurry in a refrigerator in a dark bottle. Some batches of resin are particularly prone to turning green when exposed to sunlight (!). At least in our laboratory there has not been an investigation as to whether greened resin has altered elution properties; we do, however, avoid it by covering the beaker with foil when washing the resin.

The optimal column size and the best elution conditions should both be established for every batch of resin. Usually, a resin bed volume of 0.6–0.8 ml is used. Bio-Rad supplies custom-made polypropylene column supports which can hold not only the resin but also a reservoir of ~10 ml. These columns may appear to be surprisingly expensive, and in this laboratory the problem with reusing them is that the frit at the base of the column gets irreversibly blocked with repeated use. A much cheaper alternative that some workers still use is to make homemade supports by packing a bolus of glass wool into the constriction of a Pasteur pipette, adding the resin, and then constructing a reservoir by fixing the end of the glass pipette to a plastic syringe barrel via a piece of silicone tubing. From personal experience this can be said to be an unsafe procedure; the Pasteur pipettes can break as the tubing is attached and the resultant jagged end can impale one's hand. It is best to bear the cost of the Bio-Rad supports.

Care should be taken to prepare a series of identically sized columns to enhance the reproducibility of the chromatographic procedures. To this end, a slurry of resin in water is prepared that is ~25% greater than the final wet packed volume of the column. When pipetting aliquots from the stock slurry, it should be continuously stirred, and it is advisable to cut the last few millimeters from the end of the pipette tip to avoid a biockage from forming. However, none of these precautions can substitute for taking the time to check that all bed volumes are actually the same.

Newly made columns should be washed with 10 ml of water and not allowed to dry out until the analysis is completed. Neutralized cell extracts are added to the column diluted ~10-fold with water. In practice this is achieved by first adding 9–10 ml of water to the column, immediately followed by the neutralized extract. The [^{3}H]inositol, being uncharged, is not bound by the column. However, the radioactivity in [^{3}H]inositol will greatly exceed the radioactivity in the ^{3}H-labeled inositol phosphates. Therefore, it is advisable to next wash the column with sufficient additional water to remove residual [^{3}H]inositol. Then [^{3}H]glycerophosphoinositol must be eluted from the column, typically with 10–15 ml of 0.06 *M* ammonium formate. Again, it is important to check each batch of resin, using appropriate standards.

To analyze an experiment in which cells were labeled for 2–4 hr, the small amount of label incorporated into $InsP_5$ and $InsP_6$ can be ignored. [The rate of phosphorylation of Ins(1,4,5)P_3 through Ins(1,3,4,6)P_4 to $InsP_5$ (see Fig. 1) is relatively slow, while the accumulation of [^{3}H]$InsP_6$ is even slower.] To separately assay InsP, $InsP_2$, $InsP_3$, and $InsP_4$, the following elution protocol would be a good starting point when setting out to characterize a new batch of resin: 10–15 ml of 0.18 *M* ammonium formate for InsP, followed by 10–15 ml of 0.4 *M* ammonium formate/0.1 *M* formic acid to remove $InsP_2$, then 10–15 ml of 0.8 *M* ammonium formate/0.1 *M* formic acid for $InsP_3$, and finally 10–15 ml of 1.2 *M* ammonium formate/0.1 *M* formic acid for $InsP_4$. Fine adjustments to optimize resolution can take the form of altering either the volume of the eluant or the concentration of the ammonium formate; the elution characteristics should be checked with appropriate standards. Resolution is optimized if each individual eluant is added as three equal aliquots. In other words, three 4-ml aliquots would work better than simply using a single dose of 12 ml. It is also best to apply each addition down the inside wall of each column, thus minimizing disturbance to the resin bed. If it is only necessary to measure levels of total inositol phosphates, then this could be achieved in a single step with 10 ml of 1.2 *M* ammonium formate/0.1 *M* formic acid (after first eluting both inositol and glycerophosphoinositol; see above).

Longer-term labeling experiments (and certainly those continued for 12 hr or more) must account for ^{3}H incorporation into $InsP_5$/$InsP_6$. In the elution procedure described above, [^{3}H]$InsP_5$ and [^{3}H]$InsP_6$ will elute with [^{3}H]$InsP_4$ in the 1.2 *M* ammonium formate eluate. Reducing the concentration of ammonium formate in the "$InsP_4$" eluate to 1.05 *M* will usually eliminate contamination from $InsP_5$/$InsP_6$ (e.g., $InsP_4$ may be eluted from a 0.8-ml column with ~15 ml of 1.05 *M* ammonium formate/0.1 *M* formic acid, and then $InsP_5$ can be eluted with 3 ml of 2 *M* ammonium formate/0.1 *M* formic acid). However, an additional problem accompanies the incorporation of radiolabel into $InsP_5$, since levels of its own metabolites—Ins(3,4,5,6)P_4 and Ins(1,4,5,6)P_4 (15)—will also naturally increase. Furthermore, receptor-activated dephosphorylation of [^{3}H]$InsP_5$ to [^{3}H]Ins(3,4,5,6)P_4 inevitably accompanies activation of phospholipase C, independently of [^{3}H]Ins(1,4,5)P_3 metabolism (15). The batch elution procedures described above will not resolve $InsP_4$ isomers. Thus, Ins(1,4,5,6)P_4 and [^{3}H]Ins(3,4,5,6)P_4 which are not markers for phospholipase C activity will contaminate [^{3}H]Ins(1,3,4,5)P_4 and [^{3}H]Ins(1,3,4,6)P_4, the levels of which (see Fig. 1) are required for the assay of phospholipase C. The only way to avoid interference from [^{3}H]Ins(3,4,5,6)P_4 and/or [^{3}H]Ins(1,4,5,6)P_4 is by HPLC analysis, which in any case is also essential if individual isomers of any other inositol phosphates are to be resolved.

HPLC ANALYSIS OF INOSITOL PHOSPHATES

The minimum hardware requirements for an HPLC system are an injector, two pumps, a gradient controller, and either a fraction collector or an on-line radioactivity detector. Usually, the setup is computer controlled. Titanium pumps have superior solvent resistance compared to those using stainless steel. Pump seals should be changed at adequate intervals to maintain accurate flow rates.

The most commonly used HPLC columns are silica based, and the silica will dissolve in water and certain buffers, causing loss of retention and increasing back-pressure, and eventually a void or channel will form in the column. These difficulties can be prevented by saturating the mobile phase with silica, by placing a silica saturation column (e.g., Alltech) between the pumps and the injector.

No ion-exchange chromatographic system will reliably resolve all of the inositol phosphates. One reason for this is that naturally occurring enantiomeric pairs [e.g., Ins3P and Ins1P, or Ins(3,4,5,6)P_4 and Ins(1,4,5,6)P_4; see Fig. 1] can only be separated by chiral methodology. A more empirical difficulty is that HPLC columns that provide good resolution of lower phosphates are less successful with the higher phosphates and vice versa. The maximum amount of information will be obtained from a sample that has been split between two alternative but complementary HPLC systems.

A method that preferentially resolves lower phosphates has been described elsewhere (17). The HPLC system most often used in this laboratory is the 5-μm Adsorbosphere SAX column supplied by Alltech. This has been reported to resolve the following isomers: Ins4P, Ins1P/Ins3P, Ins(1,4)P_2, Ins(3,4)P_2, Ins(1,3)P_2, Ins(1,4,5)P_3, Ins(1,3,4)P_3, Ins(1,3,4,6)P_4, Ins(1,3,4,5)P_4, Ins(3,4,5,6)P_4/Ins(1,4,5,6)P_4, $InsP_5$, and $InsP_6$ (see Ref. 18). The usual target in this laboratory is to forgo the resolution of individual isomers of InsP and $InsP_2$ and concentrate on separating naturally occurring inositol phosphate isomers with three or more phosphates (except, of course, for enantiomeric pairs). The motive behind setting this limited goal arises from a number of factors, some unavoidable, which conspire to prevent an ideal resolution, particularly with regard to the lower phosphates; some of these difficulties are not restricted to the Adsorbosphere column.

One problem, despite there being little evidence that ^3H in [2-^3H]inositol can exchange into other compounds, is that cells labeled for 24 hr or more do sometimes accumulate a number of soluble ^3H-labeled compounds, some of which are not inositol phosphates, and which impair the resolution of genuine ^3H-labeled inositol phosphates. For example, substantial amounts of [^3H]glycerophosphoinositol are usually present, and this compound elutes very close to the inositol monophosphates, making it difficult to quantify Ins4P and Ins1P individually.

It is always a worrying possibility that there may be unexpected contaminants in some preparations of [^3H]inositol. While these may be present as a very small proportion, it is conceivable that they could be preferentially incorporated into cellular molecules. To further investigate this possibility, I have occasionally chromatographed commercial [^3H]inositol with an internal standard of [^{14}C]inositol on a carbohydrate separation column (18): A surprising amount of ^3H sometimes failed to coelute with [^{14}C]inositol (nearly 50% in the worst case, albeit with a batch of [^3H]inositol which had been sitting in the refrigerator for some time—which is itself a further warning that [^3H]inositol does not have the properties of Methuselah). A further potential problem is that some of the additional unidentified ^3H-labeled compounds may, depending on the cell type, represent unexpected inositol phosphate isomers not depicted in Fig. 1.

The HPLC column resolution will also suffer from some batch-to-batch variation, and will also tend to decrease as the column ages. One way to compensate for this is to make the salt gradient more shallow by extending its length. Another useful manipulation that helps to retain column resolution is to progressively decrease the maximum concentration of buffer that the column sees at the end of each gradient, in 3–5% stages every 10–15 runs or so. In general terms, the less salt the column experiences, the longer it can successfully be used. Nevertheless, the column does have a limited useful life.

The Adsorbosphere columns are supplied in methanol, which must first be washed out with ~60 ml of water, applied at a flow rate of 1 ml/min. A typical gradient has a flow rate of 1 ml/min and is constructed from a mixture of water (buffer A) and 0.85 *M* ammonium dihydrogen phosphate, pH 3.35 with phosphoric acid (buffer B): For a new column, 0–5 min, B = 0%; 5–110 min, B increases linearly to 100%; 110–115 min, B = 100%; 116 min, B returns to 0%. There should then be a 15-min wash with water before the next run begins. Both buffers A and B should utilize HPLC grade water and should be filtered. Degassing of solutions can be achieved by vacuum filtration and can be maintained by sparging them with either helium or argon. If the latter is not practicable, the HPLC pumps will need priming every 12–24 hr to eliminate air locks.

It is best to preequilibrate the HPLC column with a "blank" run before checking elution properties with standards. With careful use it can cope adequately with more than 50 runs; between analyses the column can be stored in methanol (60 ml is applied to the column after first washing with 60 ml of water). If the column is only to be "stored" overnight, it may save time in the long run to apply blank runs.

The [^{3}H]inositol phosphate profiles that are obtained for each sample are frequently calibrated so as to compensate for the inevitable variation that results both within and between samples. The best common denominator as far as assays of phospholipase C is concerned is the level of ^{3}H incorporated into total inositol lipids. In other words, the levels of each ^{3}H-labeled inositol phosphate in a particular sample are expressed as a percentage with reference to radioactivity in the lipids. [^{3}H]Lipid levels can be obtained from the perchlorate-precipitated pellet which was produced when cell incubations were quenched (see above). The pellets are washed twice with an appropriate volume of ice-cold 0.6 *M* solution of perchloric acid and recentrifuged, and after removal of the supernatant the pellet can be dissolved in 100 m*M* NaOH plus 0.1% (v/v) Triton X-100. Samples are stored overnight at 0–4°C to ensure complete digestion, and aliquots are then counted for radioactivity the next day.

REFERENCES

1. B. P. Perret, M. Plantavid, H. Chap, and L. Douste-Blazy, *Biochem. Biophys. Res. Commun.* **110,** 660 (1983).
2. S. Palmer, K. T. Hughes, D. Y. Lee, and M. J. O. Wakelam, *Cell. Signalling* **1,** 147 (1989).
3. J. Preiss, C. R. Loomis, W. R. Bishop, R. Stein, J. E. Niedel, and R. M. Bell, *J. Biol. Chem.* **261,** 8597 (1986).
4. S. B. Shears, *Pharmacol. Ther.* **49,** 79 (1991).
5. G. W. Mayr, *Biochem. J.* **254,** 585 (1988).

6. V. Prpic, P. F. Blackmore, and J. H. Exton, *J. Biol. Chem.* **257,** 11315 (1982).
7. L. R. Stephens and C. P. Downes, *Biochem. J.* **265,** 435 (1990).
8. S. B. Shears, *Adv. Second Messenger Phosphoprotein Res.* **26,** 63 (1992).
9. E. D. Kennedy, R. A. J. Challis, and S. R. Nahorski, *J. Neurochem.* **53,** 1652 (1989).
10. S. Avissar, G. Schreiber, A. Danon, and R. H. Belmaker, *Nature (London)* **331,** 440 (1988).
11. K. A. Wreggett, L. R. Howe, J. P. Moore, and R. F. Irvine, *Biochem. J.* **245,** 933 (1987).
12. J. E. Brown, M. Rudnick, A. J. Letcher, and R. F. Irvine, *Biochem. J.* **253,** 703 (1988).
13. E. D. Sharpes and R. L. McCarl, *Anal. Biochem.* **124,** 421 (1982).
14. G. W. Mayr, T. Radenberg, U. Thiel, G. Vogel, and L. R. Stephens, *Carbohydr. Res.* **234,** 247 (1992).
15. F. S. Menniti, K. G. Oliver, J. W. Putney, and S. B. Shears, *Trends Biochem. Sci.* **18,** 53 (1993).
16. N. S. Wong, C. J. Barker, S. B. Shears, C. J. Kirk, and R. H. Michell, *Biochem. J.* **252,** 1 (1988).
17. N. M. Dean and M. A. Beaven, *Anal. Biochem.* **183,** 199 (1989).
18. T. Balla, A. J. Baukal, G. Guillemette, and K. J. Catt, *J. Bio. Chem.* **263,** 4083 (1988).
19. L. R. Stephens, P. T. Hawkins, and C. P. Downes, *Biochem. J.* **262,** 727 (1989).

28 Covalent Binding to Proteins

Sidney D. Nelson

INTRODUCTION

In the late 1940s the Millers (1,2) reported that the administration of *N,N*-dimethyl-4-aminoazobenzene (butter yellow) to rats resulted in the covalent binding of metabolites of this carcinogen to hepatic proteins. Results of subsequent studies led to the hypothesis that the covalent binding of reactive metabolites of many chemicals to DNA served to initiate processes that lead to carcinogenesis (3–6). This hypothesis was soon extended to suggest that covalent binding of reactive metabolites to other tissue macromolecules may initiate processes such as cellular necrosis, blood dyscrasias, teratogenesis, and hypersensitivity reactions (7–10).

Widespread use of methods to assay the covalent binding of chemicals and their metabolites to proteins commenced after the appearance in the literature of a series of papers in 1973 on acetaminophen-induced hepatic necrosis (11–14). The method was clearly described for studies both *in vivo* (12) and *in vitro* (13), and excellent correlations were obtained between covalent binding of reactive metabolites of radiolabeled acetaminophen to target tissue hepatocytes and necrosis in these hepatocytes under a variety of conditions that modulated these two parameters as well as concentrations of hepatic glutathione (15–17). These results, coupled with results of metabolism studies, provided enough information about the nature of the reactive metabolite of acetaminophen, and its role in the pathogenesis of toxicity, that treatment intervention in clinical cases of acetaminophen overdose were immediately begun that has saved many lives annually (18–20).

This chapter focuses on the use of radiodetection methods to determine the extent of covalent binding of chemicals and/or their metabolites to proteins, and does not cover less widely applied but extremely useful methods based on immunodetection. Three different procedures that we have used for measurements of covalent binding by radiodetection are described. The final section of this chapter compares these methods and discusses the overall merits and limitations of the methodology in general.

METHODS IN TOXICOLOGY, Volume 1B

MATERIALS

Radiolabeled Compounds

All methods described here use radiolabeled drugs or other chemicals that are either administered to animals or used as a substrate in incubations of tissues, cells, subcellular fractions, or proteins. Both the chemical and radiochemical purities of the compound should be as high as possible, because even a minor impurity can skew the results if only a small fraction of the dose covalently binds to macromolecules. In most cases high-performance liquid chromatography (HPLC) purification of a radiolabeled compound shortly before use will suffice to obtain chemical and radiochemical purities of >98%. (Note: This level of purity may not be sufficient for some studies.) If a reversed-phase system is used for the purification, a normal phase system should be used to verify the purity. If this is not possible, a different reversed-phase system should be used for the purity check.

All of the radiolabels (^{14}C, ^{3}H, and ^{35}S) that are normally used in covalent binding assays can become incorporated into amino acids if they end up in 1-carbon pools (^{14}C and ^{3}H), water (^{3}H), or sulfate (^{35}S). Most investigations use ^{14}C as the tracer, because it often can be incorporated into the chemical of interest in relatively high specific activity in a nonlabile position. Although ^{3}H can provide much higher specific activities, it often must be incorporated into positions in which a fraction of it is lost and becomes incorporated into water or nucleotide pools. This is not to say that ^{3}H should not be used, but rather that sites of incorporation should be judiciously chosen. How to differentiate covalent binding of radiolabel to proteins from incorporation into amino acids of proteins is discussed under "Comments." The specific activity to be used depends on the level of binding of the compound and the amount of tissue to be sampled. As a starting point we have used ~250 dpm/nmol for experiments *in vivo* and 500 dpm/nmol for experiments *in vitro.*

Solvent Extraction Method

This method uses plain glass conical centrifuge tubes, heavy duty, 10–15-ml capacity. One tube is required for each sample to be assayed; that is, if proteins from three tissues are to be assayed in quadruplicate, 12 tubes are needed. Centrifugation can be carried out in any tabletop or other centrifuge that has a holder or rotor that will accept the tubes used and develops forces of ~1000–2000 *g*. Use of a refrigerated centrifuge leads to more complete protein precipitation after solvent washes, but is not mandatory.

A small narrow stainless steel spatula is used to break up compacted protein and a vortexer is used to mix the protein with the solvent. Tubes may be capped with any material that is not affected by acids, bases, and the solvents used. Parafilm is appropriate in most instances.

Typical precipitants are 70% (w/v) perchloric acid, 0.5–3.0 *M* trichloroacetic acid, 100% ice-cold methanol, and 100% ice-cold acetone. Typical washing solvents are 80–90% (w/v) methanol, 3 : 1 (v/v) ethanol/diethyl ether, 4 : 1 (v/v) acetone/chloroform, and 3 : 1 (v/v) acetonitrile/ethyl acetate. Washed proteins are commonly dissolved in 1 N NaOH which is then neutralized with 1 N HCl or 1 N acetic acid (HOAc) prior to counting in a scintillation cocktail such as Aquasol-2 (New England Nuclear, Boston, MA). All of the above solutions can be made up in relatively large volumes and stored in glass jars with adjustable dispensers for adding solutions to the test tubes containing protein.

Solvent Filtration Method

A modification to the solvent extraction method is to apply the initially precipitated protein to 0.45-μm high-vacuum hydrophobic filters loaded on a Millipore sampling manifold. Both the filters and the manifold are available from Millipore, Bedford, MA. The protein on the filters is then washed with solvents used in the solvent extraction method.

Equilibrium Dialysis Method

This method uses sodium dodecyl sulfate (SDS) (final concentration 2%) to denature proteins, followed by equilibrium dialysis of the denatured protein solution in dialysis tubing with a molecular weight cutoff of ~3–4 kDa (e.g., Spectra/Por 3 from Spectrum, Los Angeles, CA). The dialysis buffer used is 0.01 *M* sodium phosphate (pH 7.0) containing 0.1% (w/v) SDS.

PROCEDURES

The procedures described have been applied to tissues excised from laboratory animals at various times after treatment with radiolabeled drugs or other chemicals, and to incubations of these radiolabeled compounds with tissue slices, isolated suspensions of cells, microsomes or other subcellular fractions, and individual proteins obtained from various sources. Animals are often treated with other agents that modulate concentrations, total amounts, and/or activities of various enzymes. Cofactors, cosubstrates, inhibitors, trapping agents, and many other substances are often added to incubation media. It is not the purpose of this chapter to describe all of these permutations. The following descriptions relate to the procedures used to assess covalent binding of radiolabel from the radiochemical that has been either administered to animals or used as a substrate *in vitro.*

Solvent Extraction Method

The procedure may be somewhat different with different compounds and is dependent on the solubility characteristics of the compound and its metabolites. A common procedure that covers most organic substrates is to homogenize tissues in 3 vol of ice-cold water (or appropriate buffer if other analyses are to be carried out that require a special buffer). For tissue samples taken from animals dosed with compound, proteins are precipitated by the addition of 2 ml of 10% trichloroacetic acid (~0.9 *M*) to 1 ml of homogenate (equivalent to ~0.5 g of protein). The precipitate is centrifuged at ~1000 *g* for 10 min and the supernatant is removed by aspiration into a flask. The various supernatants may be either discarded according to radiation safety guidelines or saved for other analyses. The precipitate is then successively washed with one 3-ml portion of 10% trichloroacetic acid, two 3-ml portions of 90% methanol, two 3-ml portions of ethanol/diethyl ether [3 : 1 (v/v)], and two 3-ml portions of 90% methanol. Alternative precipitants and solvent mixtures were described under "Materials."

A modification to this procedure, for samples taken from incubations that normally contain smaller amounts of protein (1–10 mg per incubation sample), is to initially precipitate the protein with 3 *M* trichloroacetic acid. For example, it is common to add 0.8 ml of 3 *M* trichloroacetic acid to 3 ml of incubate that contains 6 mg of protein. The remaining washing procedures are the same as those listed above.

Some additional suggestions and precautions for the precipitation and washing procedures are the following: (a) The samples should not be stored in the precipitated form or in suspensions other than 80–90% methanol at 4–15°C. Otherwise, they may form hard pellets that are difficult to suspend. (b) Sometimes trichloroacetic acid forms rubbery precipitates. In these cases 70% perchloric acid (0.5 ml/3 ml of protein suspension) may yield a finer more granular precipitate that is easier to wash. (c) Centrifugation times, in order to precipitate as much of the protein as possible, may vary with the solvents and centrifugal force used. (d) When vortexing the samples, the spatula may be left in the tube to aid in breaking up the protein. This requires a little practice so that the sample is not splashed out or the tubes are not broken. (e) If diethyl ether is used in the washing procedure, care must be taken to avoid sparks or flames as they occur in some centrifuges. (f) The use of latex gloves, goggles, and all other safetywear and bench-covering materials is required for working with radiolabeled substances to avoid contamination.

When the last wash has been completed, and the protein has been compacted by centrifugation, an aliquot (0.5–1.0 ml) of the supernatant is removed and the residual radioactivity is determined by scintillation counting. Additional washes are usually carried out if this sample contains counts above background (30–50 dpm under most circumstances). It should be noted that fewer washes than those noted above may be sufficient to give the desired background. In some cases the addition of relatively high concentrations of unlabeled drug and/or metabolites may decrease the number of washes needed to achieve background.

Finally, the extracted protein is solubilized in 0.5–1.0 ml of 1 N NaOH by heating the tubes containing protein and NaOH solution at ~60°C for 5–60 min, depending on the amount and source of the protein. An aliquot (50–90% of the sample) is added to an equal amount of 1 N HCl or 1 N HOAc in a scintillation vial, and scintillant is added for counting. In some cases samples require cooling at 4–15°C in a refrigerator to decrease chemiluminescence. Duplicate aliquots of the sample (10–100 μl) are removed for determination of protein concentration by any of the methods routinely available.

Solvent Filtration Method

This method works best when ~2 mg of protein is suspended in 8 ml of 90% hot methanol and allowed to slowly precipitate over a 45-min period. The suspension then is applied to an high-vacuum hydrophobic filter (0.45 μm) in a Millipore sampling manifold that is under vacuum (~15–30 mm Hg house vac line or aspirator vacuum). Samples are then sequentially washed with 5-ml aliquots of various solvents and solvent mixtures as described previously, and the washings are collected in test tubes which are sampled as described above to determine when background levels of radioactivity are achieved. The filter membranes are then transferred to scintillation vials that contain 1 ml of 1 N NaOH. Note that the filter membranes should be wet before the transfer process in order to avoid loss of dry protein caused by static. These samples are analyzed for protein concentration and radioactivity as previously described.

Equilibrium Dialysis Method

Protein samples are boiled for 10 min in a solution of SDS (final concentration 2%). Aliquots of the protein solution (1–2 ml) are transferred to Spectra/Por 3 dialysis bags dialyzed against 1 liter of 0.01 *M* sodium phosphate buffer (pH 7.0) containing 0.1% (w/v) SDS. Dialysis can be achieved in sealed flasks by attaching the bag via nylon string to a magnetic stir bar so that the bag is at least 2 inches below the surface of the buffer, or by using a multidialysis chamber (e.g., CMA Microdialysis Chambers, Bioanalytical Systems, West Lafayette, IN). Time to reach equilibrium is determined by removal of aliquots from the dialysis bag and dialysis buffer for calculations of total radioactivity. When these do not change, covalent binding is calculated as the total amount of radioactivity that remains in the dialysis bag minus the amount in an equal volume of dialysis buffer. The time to reach equilibrium varies with the compound used and the nature of the sample, although it is usually less than 8 hr.

COMMENTS

The measurement of covalently bound chemicals to macromolecules is not inherently difficult, and relies on the use of either radiochemical or immunochemical techniques to detect and quantitate bound adducts. Each method has advantages and disadvantages. The major advantages and disadvantages of the radiochemical techniques are described below. The major advantages of immunochemical methods are that radiolabeled chemicals do not need to be used, which provides not only a possible safety factor but also allows for studies on tissues from humans undergoing normal drug treatment or who have been exposed to some chemical. The major disadvantage of immunoassay techniques is that they usually do not detect all adducts formed because of epitope selectivity or inaccessibility of some adducts to the antibodies used. The immunoassay techniques also require time for the production and characterization of antibodies.

Comparison of the Different Radiochemical Techniques

Of the three techniques described, the solvent extraction method has been the most widely applied. This method requires the least elaborate and expensive equipment, and is readily adaptable in most laboratory settings. The solvent filtration method is a semiautomated modification of the sample extraction method which takes less time ($\sim$4 hr compared to 6 hr) than the solvent extraction method, but requires costlier equipment and supplies.

The major disadvantage of both methods is the loss of some lower-M_r($<$20-kDa) proteins during the washing procedures which may skew results if a particular reactive metabolite selectively reacts with these proteins to cause toxicity. In this case the equilibrium dialysis method would provide covalent binding levels that would correlate better with indicators of toxicity. This method has the disadvantages that it requires two to five times more radiolabeled sample (because of sample dilution), and rather detailed time course studies on the approach to dialysis equilibrium must be carried out for each compound. An advantage of the method is that after dialysis, the proteins can be analyzed by additional techniques, such as SDS–polyacrylamide gel electrophoresis.

Merits and Limitations of Covalent Protein Binding Assays

In general, covalent protein binding is an easily obtainable experimental parameter that serves as a quantitative index of the exposure of tissue proteins to reactive metabolites formed from drugs and other chemicals. With some limiting assumptions, covalent binding is a measure of the area under the curve of reactive metabolites in a tissue and is dependent on (a) the proportion of the dose of a chemical that is converted to reactive metabolites, (b) the proportion of reactive metabolites that become covalently bound, and (c) the proportion of the bound metabolites that are not lost from the tissue by secretion and/or repair (21,22).

The major utility of covalent binding measurements is assessment of the role that reactive metabolites may have in the pathogenesis of acute lethal cell injury. Thus, changes in the covalent binding of reactive metabolites that parallel changes in the incidence or severity of toxicity provide evidence that the reactive metabolites initiate events that lead to the observed toxic insult. Experimentally, various inducers, inhibitors, activators, repressors, etc., of enzymes that metabolize chemicals are either administered *in vivo* or added *in vitro* to modulate rates of enzymatic reactions, and the effects on covalent binding of radiolabel to tissue proteins are measured in parallel with measurements of toxicity. These studies are most useful when the time courses of both covalent binding and parameters of cellular or tissue injury are determined.

Two major criticisms/limitations of the methods' usefulness are that the role of covalent binding in tissue injury is not clear and that the method does not prove that a covalent adduct of protein and reactive metabolite has formed. The first of these issues has yet to be answered for any chemical that forms reactive metabolites that covalently bind to cellular proteins and causes toxicity. The strongest case at present for a relationship between covalent binding and toxicity is that of the metabolism of hexane to a γ-diketone that binds to neurofilaments and causes a peripheral neuropathy (23,24).

It is clear that the relationship of covalent binding to total tissue protein and tissue damage is not simple. At the organ level, one area or cell type may be damaged and/or sustain adduct formation, while others may not. At the cellular level some subcellular fractions may be damaged and/or sustain adduct formation, while others may not. At the macromolecular level one protein may be more critical to cell viability than another, even though both may form adducts with the reactive metabolite. Moreover, different reactive metabolites may interact in different ways with a single protein that may lead to completely different effects on the function of that protein. These issues have been discussed at length elsewhere (25,26).

The second major question that is not answered by the methods described is whether or not the binding measured represents a covalent adduct between proteins and reactive metabolites of the chemical. In only a few cases have the structures been determined of reactive metabolite adducts to amino acid residues in proteins from target tissues for toxicity (27–32). In addition, antibodies directed against only a few protein-bound drug metabolites have been used to detect reactive metabolite protein adducts in cells of target tissues for toxicities caused by the drug (32–37).

Although an important goal is to characterize proteins that form adducts with reactive metabolites and determine the effects of adduct formation on protein function, such a goal often is not achievable within the time and budgetary constraints of most studies. In order to more rigorously ensure that the binding observed is due to a covalent adduct to protein and not to high-affinity reversible binding, two procedures can be used. The first is to use high concentrations of the parent drug (and metabolites if available) in washing or dialysis procedures to compete off any reversibly bound radiolabeled material. The second is to dissolve the protein in base, followed by reprecipitation with acid and additional washes of the reprecipitated protein with solvents. In our experience we have not found that these procedures significantly change the covalent binding "concentration," but do decrease overall protein yields. However, when studies are carried out with a new compound, these additional steps provide added confidence that the binding measured is not high-affinity reversible binding. It should be noted that some covalently bound adducts may be hydrolyzed under the conditions of dissolution in base and acid reprecipitation.

The most problematic issue that should be addressed in covalent binding studies is that of possible incorporation of radiolabel from the chemical under investigation into the amino acid pool. This issue has been discussed at length by others (38,39) and in the case of proteins is addressed experimentally (a) by incorporation of the radiolabel into nonlabile positions (chemically and metabolically) on the molecule under study and (b) by complete hydrolysis of the protein fraction into its constituent amino acids, and radiometric analysis of the amino acids obtained after their chromatographic separation (e.g., two-dimensional thin-layer chromatography with autoradiography).

In spite of the rather crude nature of the covalent binding assay and its inherent limitations, the method is easily set up in any laboratory approved to handle small quantities of radiolabeled compounds. As long as the limitations of the method are understood and some possible pitfalls are addressed, covalent binding assays can provide, in a timely fashion, very useful dispositional and mechanistic information about reactive potentially toxic metabolites.

REFERENCES

1. E. C. Miller and J. A. Miller, *Cancer Res.* **7,** 468 (1947).
2. E. C. Miller, J. A. Miller, R. W. Sapp, and G. M. Weber, *Cancer Res.* **9,** 336 (1949).
3. E. C. Miller and J. A. Miller, *Pharmacol, Rev.* **18,** 805 (1966).
4. P. N. Magee and J. M. Barnes, *Adv. Cancer Res.* **10,** 163 (1967).
5. J. A. Miller, *Cancer Res.* **30,** 559 (1970).
6. J. H. Weisburger and E. K. Weisburger, *Pharmacol. Rev.* **25,** 1 (1973).
7. R. O. Recknagel, *Pharmacol. Rev.* **19,** 145 (1967).
8. B. B. Brodie, W. D. Reid, A. K. Cho, I. G. Sipes, G. Krishna, and J. R. Gillette, *Proc. Natl. Acad. Sci. U.S.A.* **68,** 160 (1971).
9. J. R. Mitchell, W. Z. Potter, J. A. Hinson, W. R, Sondgrass, J. A. Timbrell, and J. R. Gillette, *Handb. Exp. Pharmacol.* **27,** 383 (1975).

10. S. D. Nelson, M. R. Boyd, and J. R. Mitchell, *ACS Symp. Ser.* **44,** (1977).
11. J. R. Mitchell, D. J. Jollow, W. Z. Potter, D. C. Davis, J. R. Gillette, and B. B. Brodie, *J. Pharmacol. Exp. Ther.* **187,** 185 (1973).
12. D. J. Jollow, J. R. Mitchell, W. Z. Potter, D. C. Davis, J. R. Gillette, and B. B. Brodie, *J. Pharmacol. Exp. Ther.* **187,** 195 (1973).
13. W. Z. Potter, D. C. Davis, J. R. Mitchell, D. J. Jollow, J. R. Gillette, and B. B. Brodie, *J. Pharmacol. Exp. Ther.* **187,** 203 (1973).
14. J. R. Mitchell, D. J. Jollow, W. Z. Potter, J. R. Gillette, and B. B. Brodie, *J. Pharmacol. Exp. Ther.* **187,** 211 (1973).
15. W. Z. Potter, S. S. Thorgeirsson, D. J. Jollow and J. R. Mitchell, *Pharmacology* **12,** 129 (1974).
16. D. J. Jollow, S. S. Thorgeirsson, W. Z. Potter, M. Hashimoto, and J. R. Mitchell, *Pharmacology* **12,** 251 (1974).
17. D. C. Davis, W. Z. Potter, D. J. Jollow, J. R. Mitchell, *Life Sci.* **14,** 2099 (1974).
18. J. R. Mitchell, S. S. Thorgeirsson, W. Z. Potter, D. J. Jollow, and H. Keiser, *Clin. Pharmacol. Ther.* **16,** 676 (1974).
19. L. F. Prescott, R. W. Newton, C. P. Swainson, N. Wright, A. R. W. Forrest, and H. Matthew, *Lancet* **1,** 588 (1974).
20. M. J. Smilkstein, G. L. Knapp, K. W. Kulig, and B. H. Rumack, *N. Engl. J. Med.* **319,** 1557 (1988).
21. J. R. Gillette, *Biochem. Pharmacol.* **23,** 2927 (1974).
22. J. R. Gillete, *in* "Biological Reactive Intermediate III" (J. J. Kocsis, D. J. Follow, C. M. Witmer, J. O. Nelson, and R.. Synder, eds.), p. 63. Plenum, New York, 1986.
23. L. M. Sayre, L. Autilo-Gambetti, and P. Gambetti, *Brain Res. Rev.* **10,** 69 (1985).
24. M. B. Genter, G. Szakal-Quin, C. W. Anderson, D. C. Anthony, and D. G. Graham, *Toxicol. Appl. Pharmacol.* **87,** 351 (1987).
25. C. V. Smith, B. H. Lauterburg, and J. R. Mitchell, *in* "Drug Metabolism and Disposition: Considerations in Clinical Pharmacology" (G. R. Wilkinson and M. D. Rawlins, eds.), p. 161. MTP Press, Lancaster, England, 1985.
26. S. D. Nelson and P. G. Pearson, *Annu. Rev. Pharmacol. Toxicol.* **30,** 169 (1990).
27. M. C. Dyroff and R. A. Neal, *Cancer Res.* **41,** 3430 (1981).
28. A. P. DeCaprio, E. J. Olajos, and P. Weber, *Toxicol. Appl. Pharmacol.* **65,** 440 (1982).
29. K.-J. Hoffmann, A. J. Streeter, D. B. Axworthy, and T. A. Baillie, *Mol. Pharmacol.* **27,** 566 (1985).
30. P. E. Weller and R. P. Hanzlik, *Chem. Res. Toxicol.* **4,** 17 (1991).
31. D. E. Slaughter and R. P. Hanzlik, *Chem. Res. Toxicol.* **4,** 319 (1991).
32. J. A. Hinson and D. W. Roberts, *Anu. Rev. Pharmacol. Toxicol.* **32,** 471 (1992).
33. H. Satoh. Y. Fukuda, D. K. Anderson, V. J. Ferrans, J. R. Gillette, and L. R. Pohl, *J. Pharmacol. Exp. Ther.* **233,** 857 (1985).
34. J. B. Bartalone, K. Sparks, S. D. Cohen, and E. A. Khairallah, *Biochem. Pharmacol.* **36,** 1193 (1987).
35. D. W. Roberts, N. R. Pumford, D. W. Potter, R. W. Benson, and J. A. Hinson, *J. Pharmacol. Exp. Ther.* **241,** 527 (1987).
36. J. Neuberger and R. Williams, *Gut* **30,** 315 (1989).
37. N. R. Pumford, J. C. Davila, T. G. Myers, and L. R. Pohl, *Toxicologist* **12,** 253 (1992).
38. J. R. Gillette and L. R. Pohl, *J. Toxicol. Environ. Health* **2,** 849 (1977).
39. P. N. Magee, *J. Toxicol. Environ. Health* 883 (1977).

29

Glutathione, Oxidized Glutathione, and Mixed Disulfides in Biological Samples

Evan P. Gallagher, Terrance J. Kavanagh, and David L. Eaton

INTRODUCTION

The critical role played by intracellular glutathione (γ-glutamylcysteinylglycine, or GSH) in a variety of cellular regulatory functions has been well documented (1–4). Of interest in toxicological studies is the participation of GSH in the detoxification and modification of a wide variety of drugs and chemicals. In this regard GSH may serve either as a cofactor for glutathione *S*-transferases (GSTs) during the conjugation of electrophilic agents or as a reductant for GSH peroxidase-mediated hydroperoxide removal (2). In cells the oxidation of GSH as a result of oxidative stress or exposure to chemicals may lead to the formation of glutathione disulfide (GSSG) and mixed disulfides (GSSR), which may be freely soluble (e.g., GSS–CoA) or bound to proteins (e.g., GSS–albumin) (1,2,4). Because changes in GSH status may ultimately reflect the mechanism of toxicity of a compound and, to some degree, the health status of the biological component of study (e.g., cell, blood, and tissue), quantitation of GSH status is of interest.

Numerous methods, including enzymatic, chromatographic, and flow-cytometric approaches, have been developed to determine the GSH and GSSG content of biological samples. While all analytical methods share advantages and disadvantages, the existence of such a plethora of methods reflects the interest in the topic as well as the sample types for which GSH quantitation is important. Many of the methods are extremely sensitive but necessitate the use of expensive specialized equipment. Others suffer from complicated sample preparation procedures which affect sample processing time. Detailed in this chapter are four methods for determination of GSH and, in certain cases, related thiols and/or GSSG. When viewed collectively, these methods cover a wide range of experimental applications. Ultimately, the assay of choice will be dependent on the needs of the researcher (e.g., assay sensitivity and specificity, biological matrix, cost, and sample processing time) as well as the availability of specialized laboratory equipment.

While somewhat outside the scope of this chapter, it should be mentioned that a thorough understanding of the effects of a chemical on redox status of a biological system necessitates assessment of thiols in addition to GSH. In this re-

METHODS IN TOXICOLOGY, Volume 1B

gard most procedures do not have the flexibility to simultaneously evaluate all oxidized and reduced nonprotein thiol components of biological samples [with the possible exception of ion pair high-performance liquid chromatography coupled with electrochemical detection (HPLC–ECD); see method III, below].

SAMPLE PREPARATION

Samples must be processed rapidly to minimize metabolic reactions occurring in tissues which may result in artifactual GSH and GSSG values (5,6). This is a particular problem in blood, in which significant amounts of GSH may oxidize to form GSSG and GSSR after 3–4 min of collection (5). Because GSH oxidizes rapidly at pH values above 7.0 (7) , it is necessary to acid-precipitate the samples to maintain proper thiol : disulfide redox status. Despite such precautions, however, some disulfide exchange may still occur after acid homogenization (5). In addition to maintaining GSH : GSSG redox status, sample acidification allows for the precipitation of proteins and ensures cell lysis and the subsequent release of free thiols and disulfides. Tissues with high γ-glutamyl transpeptidase (GGT) activity (kidney, epithelium of the small intestine, pancreas, and biliary ductules) must be homogenized rapidly and acid-precipitated to avoid GGT-catalyzed degradation of GSH (6). GSH degradation is a particularly severe problem in the kidney, which contains high GGT and dipeptidase activities.

While various acids have been used for deproteinization, 5-sulfosalicylic acid [5-SSA; 5% (w/v)] and picric acid [1% (w/v)] are of choice for protein precipitation. Perchloric, metaphosphoric, and trichloroacetic (TCA) acids may not maintain true GSH : GSSG ratios (4). However, because certain acids interfere with subsequent enzymatic reactions or chromatographic procedures, selection of acid precipitate is also dependent on the experimental system. For example, 5-SSA and TCA may cause chromatographic interference of low-molecular weight-thiols and disulfides using electrochemical detection (7). Furthermore, both picric and perchloric acids present a serious explosive hazard if not stored and used properly. The autoxidation of GSH in neutralized samples can also be prevented by the derivatization of GSH with either *N*-ethylmaleimide (NEM) (5,8) or 2-vinylpyridine (9). However, excess NEM must be removed from reaction mixtures due its interference with some assay procedures (9).

As more than 95% of total glutathione (reduced plus oxidized) content in healthy cells is present in the reduced form (GSH), most investigators elect to simply measure either GSH or total glutathione without analyzing the contribution of GSSG. To determine total glutathione content of a tissue, glutathione present in GSSR must first be released by the reduction of disulfide bonds prior to measurement. This may be accomplished by reduction with 2% sodium borohydride (incubated at 40°C for 30 min in Tris-HCl, pH 7.4) or dithiothreitol (DTT; 100 m*M* containing 10% Triton X-100) incubated for 30 min at room temperature (10). However, DTT and sodium borohydride will cleave thioesters as well as disulfides (11). Specific cleavage of disulfides can be achieved using hydroxylamine in the presence of NEM to block released thiols (11). GSS-protein-bound mixed disulfides may also be cleaved with performic acid (12). In addition, some GSSR can be analyzed directly by HPLC–ECD (method III) without prior reduction by DTT or sodium borohydride.

The optimal procedure for preparation of cell extract varies with cell type. Thiol oxidation is a particular problem when preparing cell extracts for GSH analysis. High-purity buffers such as Tris and HEPES are generally preferred, and the use of chelating agents such as EDTA can prevent iron-mediated formation of peroxides in the presence of oxygen.

METHOD I: DETERMINATION OF GSH AND GSSG BY ENZYMATIC RECYCLING

GSH and GSSG are readily measured with a kinetic assay which utilizes the continuous glutathione reductase-catalyzed reduction of the sulfhydryl reagent 5,5′-dithiobis-2-nitrobenzoic acid (DTNB; Ellman's reagent) to the chromophoric product 2-nitro-5-thiobenzoic acid [reactions (1) and (2)] (8,9).

$$2\ \mathrm{GSH} + \mathrm{DTNB} \longrightarrow \mathrm{GSSG} + \mathrm{TNB} \qquad (1)$$

$$\mathrm{GSSG} + \mathrm{NADPH} + \mathrm{H}^{+} \xrightarrow{\text{GSSG reductase}} 2\ \mathrm{GSH} + \mathrm{NADP}^{+} \qquad (2)$$

Detection of the chromophore is monitored spectrophotometrically at 412 nm. Quantitation is achieved by comparison with a standard curve of known GSH concentrations carried out in parallel. Because this assay responds to both GSH and GSSG, selective quantitation of reduced and oxidized forms of glutathione requires derivatization of GSH by 2-vinylpyridine. The procedure detailed below is that of Griffith (9), which is a modification of the original procedure by Tietze (8).

Materials and Reagents

Stock buffer and solutions

125 m*M* sodium phosphate containing 6.3 m*M* EDTA (pH 7.5)
- Solution A: 1.70 g of KH_2PO_4 (monobasic) plus 0.234 g of disodium EDTA per 100 ml of deionized water; store at 0–4°C for <2 weeks
- Solution B: 2.175 g of K_2HPO_4 (dibasic) plus 0.234 g of disodium EDTA per 100 ml of deionized water; store at 0–4°C for <2 weeks
- For assay buffer add solution A to solution B in the presence of a pH meter until pH 7.5 is attained; make up assay buffer fresh daily

20 m*M* NADPH in 0.5% $NaHCO_3$: NADPH 18 mg/ml; prepare fresh daily and store on ice
6 m*M* DTNB (Sigma Cat. No. D-8130, St. Louis, MO): 119 mg of DTNB per 50 ml of deionized water; prepare fresh daily in stock buffer and store in a lightproof container or wrap with foil
GSSG reductase 50 U/ml (type IV, Sigma Cat. No. G-4759): Dilute in stock buffer daily and store in ice; vortex 3–5 sec prior to addition to the reaction mixture
5% (w/v) 5-SSA: 5 g of 5-SSA (American Chemical Society reagent grade, Sigma Cat. No. S-0640) per 100 ml of deionized water
GSH standard: Dilute daily from frozen stock solution of 10 m*M* GSH (free acid, Sigma Cat. No. G-4251) in 5% 5-SSA (30.7 mg GSH/10 ml), typically diluted to 1–10 nmol GSH/ml

Additional reagents, if determining GSSG

2-Vinylpyridine (Aldrich Cat. No. 13,229-2, Milwaukee, WI): Use undiluted and store at −20°C
GSSG standards (Sigma Cat. No. G-9027): 5 m*M* stock in 5% 5-SSA (GSSG 30.6 mg/10 ml) typically diluted to 50–500 pmol GSSG/ml
Triethanolamine (free base, Sigma Cat. No. T-1377), undiluted liquid
pH test strips

Additional reagents, if determining GSH concentrations in blood

500 m*M* Na_4EDTA: 19.01 g of Na_4EDTA per 100 ml of deionized water
10% (w/v) 5-SSA: 10 g of 5-SSA per 80 ml of deionized water; bring up to 100-ml final volume

Equipment

Tissue homogenizer
UV/visible spectrophotometer
pH meter
Low-speed centrifuge (10,000-*g* capacity)

Sample Preparation

Plasma

One to five milliliters of blood is collected into a glass beaker containing 25 μl of 500 m*M* Na_4EDTA (pH 7.0) and gently swirled. Two 700 μl aliquots of the EDTA-treated blood are transferred to microtubes and centrifuged at 10,000 *g* for 1.5 min. A 100-μl aliquot of the plasma is then quickly mixed with 50 μl of cold 5-SSA [5% (w/v)] and vortexed. It is important that the preceding steps are carried out through the addition of acid in less than 4 min from the time that the blood is withdrawn. The sample is centrifuged for 5 min at 5000 *g* at 4°C, and the supernatant is retained and either assayed directly for total glutathione or derivatized with 2-vinylpyridine (see below) for selective analysis of GSSG.

Tissues

Tissues (~100 mg) are rapidly removed, rinsed in saline, blotted dry, and homogenized in 9 vol of cold 5% 5-SSA. The acidified homogenates are then centrifuged in a microfuge (10,000 *g*) for 5 min, and stored at 4° C until assayed. As with other samples, selective determination of GSSG requires derivatization of GSH by 2-vinylpyridine.

Procedures

Determination of Total (Reduced and Oxidized) Glutathione

Phosphate buffer (700 μl), DTNB solution (100 μl), water (150 μl), NADPH (20 μl), and sample or GSH standard (20 μl) are added to the cuvette (1-cm light path) and mixed. After equilibration of cuvettes to 25°C, 10 μl of GSSG reductase is added (10 μl of buffer added to reference) with mixing, and the formation of 2-nitro-5-thiobenzoic acid is monitored spectrophotometrically at 412 nm. A sample blank lacking GSH is run separately and the resulting background rate of product formation is subtracted from the sample values prior to GSH quantification. Alternatively, if a dual-beam instrument is used, background formation of the product is automatically subtracted from the sample. The total GSH content of the sample ("total glutathione" is used here to indicate the sum total of freely soluble GSH and GSSG, and does not reflect glutathione present as mixed disulfides) is determined by comparison of the rate observed from a standard curve generated with known amounts of GSSG prepared in buffer. Values are reported in GSH equivalents as micromoles per gram for tissues, micromolar for plasma, or micromoles μl per 10^6 cells.

Comments

For samples containing more than 0.5 nmol GSH, the rate of DTNB production is linear throughout the absorbance range. However, the most linear portion of the curve is generally between absorbance values of 1.0 and 2.0.

Advantages

The GSSG reductase recycling asssay is highly specific due to the substrate preference of GSSG reductase for GSH. In addition, the assay is highly sensitive (detection limit of ~32 pmol of GSH equivalent to the GSH in ~5 μg of normal liver tissue) and applicable to tissues, blood, and cells grown in culture. If discrimination of GSH and GSSG is not required, sample processing time is fairly rapid. In addition, the only specialized equipment needed for this procedure is a visible spectrophotometer.

Disadvantages

The selective determination of GSSG requires derivatizing GSH with 2-vinylpyridine (see below), which markedly increases sample processing time. Also, since quantitation is dependent on comparison of sample values with an accurate standard curve, standards must be prepared under identical conditions as the sample. In addition to GSH and GSSG content, the reaction rate is also dependent on the GSSG reductase activity in the sample cuvette. Therefore, to avoid underestimation of GSH content, care must be taken to use freshly prepared enzyme concentrations and to be certain that the reaction mixtures are free of enzyme inhibitors such as phenylmethylsulfonyl fluoride.

GSSG Determination

To selectively measure GSSG, the GSH present in the sample must be derivatized as follows: 500 μl of acidified sample or standard is mixed with 10 μl of 2-vinylpyridine in a 1.5-ml microtube. Triethanolamine (30 μl) is added to the inside of each microtube above the level of the liquid and vortexed vigorously for 5 sec (final pH 7.0–7.5). Check the sample pH with a pH test strip; if the final pH exceeds 7.5, rederivatize using less triethanolamine. Let samples stand at 25 °C for 60 min. The amount of GSSG is assayed as described above with the exception that 100 μl of the derivatized sample is added to the reaction cuvette, and the amount of water added is reduced to 70 μl (final reaction volume of 1.0 ml).

Comments

2-Vinylpyridine is sparingly soluble in aqueous solutions and will remain as small globules on the inside of the microtubes. However, these residues will not interfere with the recycling assay and they ensure saturation of the solution with the reagent.

Advantages

In contrast to other derivatizing agents such as NEM, 2-vinylpyridine does not cause significant inhibition of GSSG reductase. Therefore, lengthy cleanup steps for its removal are not necessary. When used in conjunction with the above procedure for total glutathione, the GSSG concentration of a sample can be subtracted from total glutathione content to give the amount of GSH present.

Disadvantages

Complete derivatization of GSH by 2-vinylpyridine takes 20–60 min, thus allowing for some artifactual production of GSSG from the oxidation of GSH. Also, since GSSG standards and samples must be simultaneously carried through the derivatization and neutralization process, sample throughput time is fairly slow. Alternatively, tissues or blood may be homogenized directly in 10 m*M* NEM, centrifuged, and passed through a C_{18} Sep-Pak (Waters Associates, Framingham, MA) cartridge according to the method of Adams *et al.* (13). The eluates can then be assayed using the above DTNB enzyme-recycling assay. The limitations of low sample throughput can be overcome by using modifications of the recycling assay to accommodate flow injection analysis (14) or a microplate reader with compatible software (15). The use of flow injection analysis increases the sensitivity of the assay (14).

METHOD II: MONOBROMOBIMANE LABELING OF GSH FOLLOWED BY HPLC/FLUORESCENCE DETECTION

The halogenated bimanes constitute a family of a reagents which have been utilized for the characterization of low-molecular-weight thiols (16). These compounds exhibit high reactivity and specificity toward sulfhydryls, forming stable and fluorescent thioethers (16). Monobromobimane (3,7-dimethyl-4-bromomethyl-6-methyl-1,5-diazobicyclo-octa-3,6-diene-2,8-dione) (mBBr) is particularly useful for the analysis of a variety of low-molecular-weight thiols, primarily because it is itself weakly fluorescent but forms stable thioethers which are highly fluorescent and amenable to a variety of chromatographic separations. In addition, mBBr passes easily through biological membranes (17), allowing for derivatization of intracellular thiols without membrane disruption.

There are a variety of methods using mBBr–thiol derivatization followed by HPLC/fluorescence analysis (10,16,18–20). Detailed below is the method of Hamel *et al.* (20) which describes an *in situ* thiol derivatization procedure coupled with HPLC separation and fluorescence detection of GSH and cysteine bimane adducts. While the basis for derivatization of thiols was developed by Fahey *et al.* (18), the method presented here offers the added flexibility of quantifying γ-glutamylcysteine synthetase (GCS) and glutathione synthetase (GS) activities, the two principal enzymes of GSH biosynthesis (21), by simply varying assay incubation conditions. The simultaneous quantitation of GCS and GS activities with GSH content requires somewhat different sample preparation than determination of GSH alone, but only the procedure for GSH is detailed here. The experimentor should consult the original reference if quantification of GSH biosynthetic enzymes is desired.

Materials and Reagents

0.9% Saline: 900 mg of NaCl per 100 ml of deionized water
200 m*M* 5 SSA: 10.9 g per 250 ml of deionized water
25 m*M* mBBr (thiolyte, Calbiochem Cat. No. 596105, San Diego, CA) in acetonitrile: 100 mg of mBBr per 14.75 ml of acetonitrile; store in a lightproof bottle at 4°C
200 m*M* potassium hydroxide (KOH): 1.12 g of KOH per 100 ml of deionized water; dilute 1:10 for 20 m*M* KOH
0.2 *M* *N*-ethylmorpholine (NEMP; Sigma Cat. No. E-0252) in 20 m*M* KOH (2.3 ml of NEMP per 100 ml of 20 m*M* KOH)
10 m*M* stock GSH standard: 30.7 mg/10 ml 5-SSA; dilute for linear range of sample (typically 50–1000 μM GSH for tissues, 10–750 μM GSH for cells)

HPLC solvents

Solvent A:1 m*M* tetrabutylammonium phosphate adjusted to pH 3.0 with 10% phosphoric acid
Solvent B: 100% methanol (HPLC grade)

Additional reagents, if analyzing for GSH in cell preparations

2 m*M* KOH: 1:100 dilution of 200 m*M* KOH (see above)
20 m*M* *N*-ethylmorpholine in 2 m*M* KOH: 0.23 ml of NEMP per 100 ml of 2 m*M* KOH)
1 m*M* mBBr in acetonitrile (8 mg of mBBr per 7.38 ml of acetonitrile): Store in a lightproof bottle at 4°C
Phosphate-buffered saline (PBS): 800 mg of NaCl, 20 mg of KCl, 144 mg of Na_2HPO_4, and 24 mg of KH_2PO_4 in 80 ml of deionized water; adjust the pH to 7.4 with HCl and add water to bring the volume to 100 ml
20 m*M* 5 SSA (1.09 g/250 ml of deionized water)

Equipment

pH test strips
Tissue homogenizer
Microcentrifuge or low-speed centrifuge (10,000-*g* capacity)
Ternary gradient HPLC
15 × 0.5-cm C_{18} reversed-phase column
Fluorescence detector
Computing integrator or digital data collection hardware and software

Additional equipment, if analyzing for GSH in cell preparations

Ultrasonicator
Low-speed centrifuge

Sample Preparation

Tissues

Tissues are removed, rinsed in cold 0.9% saline, and homogenized in 4 vol of cold 200 m*M* 5-SSA. The homogenate is centrifuged at 10,000 *g* for 5 min at 4°C to remove precipitated proteins.

Isolated Cells

Cell suspensions (25,000–800,000 cells) are transferred to a 15-ml polypropylene tube and centrifuged at 200 *g* for 5 min at room temperature to separate the cells from the medium. The medium (supernatant) is removed and the pellet is washed once in PBS buffer, transferred to a 1.5-ml microtube, and recentrifuged. The PBS wash (supernatant) is removed and the cellular pellet is resuspended in 125 μl of 20 m*M* 5-SSA. Cellular GSH is released by sonication, using two successive 10-sec blasts. The sonicated samples are centrifuged for 2 min at room temperature at 10,000 *g* and the supernatatants (containing free GSH) are placed on ice for derivatization and analysis (see below).

Procedure for Free GSH and Other Low-Molecular-Weight Thiols

Tissues

The pH of a 100-μl sample (or standard) aliquot is brought to 7.0–8.0 by the addition of 100 μl 0.2 *M* NEMP/20 mM KOH. Check the sample pH with a pH test strip and adjust the volume of NEMP solution if the pH is not above 8.5. GSH is then derivatized by the addition of 20 μl of mBBr in acetonitrile and incubation at room temperature for 20 min, shielded from light. The reaction is terminated by the addition of 180 μl of 200 m*M* 5-SSA. The samples are then vortexed for 5 sec and centrifuged at 10,000 *g* at room temperature for 2 min prior to HPLC analysis. The acidified thiol–bimane conjugates are stable for 24–48 hr when protected from light, and for at least 2 weeks if stored at −20°C.

Cells

Add 50 μl of acidified cellular supernatant to 100 μl of 20 m*M* NEMP/2 m*M* KOH in a 500-μl microtube. Free cellular GSH is then derivatized by the addition of 10 μl of 1 m*M* mBBr and incubation at room temperature for 20 min.

The reaction is terminated by the addition of 100 μl 20 mM 5-SSA. The samples are then vortexed for 5 sec and centrifuged at 10,000 *g* at room temperature for 2 min prior to HPLC analysis.

HPLC Analysis

Aliquots of the supernatant (20–50 μl for tissues, 100–150 μl for cells, depending on GSH content) are analyzed using HPLC and a C_{18} reversed-phased column maintained at ambient temperature. HPLC separation of glutathione–mBBr (GS–mBBr) adducts is carried out at a flow rate of 1.5 ml/min. The solvent profile is as follows: 95% A/5% B maintained for 0.5 min, followed by a linear gradient of 80% A/20% B at 1 min, 70% A/30% B at 10 min, and 40% A/60% B at 12 min. The solvent mixture is maintained at 40% A/60% B from 12 to 14 min. The column is re-equilibrated to starting conditions (95% A/5% B) using a gradient program between 15 and 20 min. In small tissue samples or in samples with low GSH content (including cells), fluorescence detection should be used, with excitation at 375 nm and emission at 475 nm. Alternatively, UV detection at 375 nm works well for tissue samples with GSH concentrations greater than ~1 m*M*. Quantitation is achieved by integration of peak areas and conversion to GSH equivalents, using a standard curve of GSH standards carried through the identical procedure.

Comments

To measure GSSG and other low-molecular-weight disulfides, tissues are extracted in the presence of thiol-blocking agents such as NEM, and the disulfide or thioester is converted to its corresponding thiol by incubating the sample (100 μl) with 100 m*M* DTT and 10% (v/v) Triton X-100 (5 μl) for 30 min (10). Once reduced, the thiol is labeled with mBBr as described above.

Advantages

The assay is highly sensitive (5 pmol of GSH by fluorescence detection) and yields excellent chromatographic separation of GS–mBBr adducts (retention time, ~11.4 min) from breakdown products of mBBr (retention time, ~8.8–9.0 min), as well as bimane adducts of cysteine (~7 min) and γ-glutamylcysteine (12.4 min). As previously mentioned, a modification of the procedure can be used to allow for simultaneous quantitation of GCS and GS activities of biological samples (20).

Disadvantages

A principal disadvantage of this assay is the relatively slow processing rate for individual samples, as each analysis requires ~20 min of HPLC time. However, since GSH–mBBr adducts are stable for 24–48 hr at room temperature, a sample autoinjector will easily overcome this deficit. Also, as mBBr does not react with disulfides and other oxidized forms of sulfur, this method cannot be used to directly determine free GSSG. However, this limitation may also be overcome using variations in sample preparation (see comments below). Although mBBr preferentially reacts with thiols, it also reacts slowly with amines and other nucleophiles to form fluorescent products. Thus, there is the possibility of some chromatographic interference in samples containing high concentrations of these compounds. Interferences can be minimized by using high-purity buffer components of low nucleophilicity to minimize the formation of fluorescent impurities. Finally, erroneous thiol values may occur if the photosensitive bimane derivitives are not shielded from light (18,20).

METHOD III: HIGH-PERFORMANCE LIQUID CHROMATOGRAPHY WITH DUAL ELECTROCHEMICAL DETECTION

(HPLC–ECD) is an extremely sensitive and specific method for the analysis of a number of biologically important thiols and disulfides (7,22–24). HPLC–ECD methods typically utilize isocratic separation of thiols and disulfides by reversed phase ion pair HPLC, followed by dual electrochemical detection using two Au/Hg thin-layer electrodes in series. The disulfides are reductively cleaved to thiols at the upstream electrode, and subsequent detection of all thiols is carried out by electrochemical oxidation at the downstream electrode, which is set at a thiol–specific potential. Detailed here is a slight modification of the HPLC–ECD method reported by Stein *et al.* (7), which has been validated for a number of thiols and disulfides in various biological matrices. The original method reported the use of alternative equipment for performing reductions at the upstream electrode, thus eliminating some of the expense involved for HPLC–ECD analysis. However, the use of a commercially available dual electrochemical detector will also provide satisfactory results.

Materials and Reagents

HPLC solvent

Mobile phase

96.5% Monochloroacetic acid (MCA) buffer (0.1 *M* MCA containing 3.3 m*M* 1-heptanesulfonic acid (HSA) adjusted to pH 2.6 using freshly made sodium hydroxide solution (MCA and HSA are available from Kodak, Rochester, NY). Prepare MCA buffer using deionized water and purify through a 0.45-μm filter prior to use)

3% (v/v) methanol (HPLC grade, Fisher, Fair Lawn, NJ)

0.5% Ultrapure *N,N*-dimethylformadine (Alvers, Danvers, MA) (note: the mobile phase should be refluxed at 50–55°C and continuously sparged with helium to remove oxygen)

Stock standards

0.25 *M* ultrapure perchloric acid (Alvers, Danvers, MA)

10 m*M* GSH (30.7 mg/10 ml) and 10 m*M* GSSG (61.2 mg/10 ml) in 0.25 *M* ultrapure perchloric acid stored at −80°C. Working standards of 200 μ*M* GSH and 25 μ*M* GSSG are prepared daily from the stock standard solution and are further diluted in HPLC solvent to give final GSH concentrations similar to those of the samples

Equipment

HPLC apparatus

pump
5-μm C_{18}, stainless steel column
50 × 4.6-mm C_{18} guard column
Thermoregulated water jacket
Computing integrator
Electrochemical detector

Sample Preparation

Tissues

After excision, tissues (~100 mg) are rinsed in ice–cold 0.85% (w/v) NaCl. Liver and kidney samples are homogenized in 9 vol of 0.25 *M* ice-cold perchloric acid. Samples are centrifuged at 10,000 *g* for 10 min at 4°C and analyzed directly or stored at −80°C. If necessary, the supernatants can be diluted (1:50 for rat liver) with HPLC solvent immediately prior to analysis.

Plasma

Fresh heparinized whole blood (200 μl) is centrifuged at 2000 *g* for 10 min at 4°C. The plasma is removed and diluted (1 : 1) with 0.25 *M* perchloric acid prior to analysis.

HPLC–ECD

The amalgram is prepared by placing triple–distilled mercury onto the highly polished gold surface and after 2–3 min removing the excess mercury with the edge of a card. The surface should be wiped clean with a laboratory tissue and all air must be removed from the detector cell prior to use. Separations are carried out using a 5-μm, C_{18} column (250 mm × 3.9 mm) with a thermoregulated water jacket maintained at 35°C. The analytical column is protected by a guard column (50 × 4.6 mm). Compounds are eluted with a flow rate of 1.0 ml/min and detected using a dual electrochemical detector consisting of two thin circular gold electrodes positioned in series. The reference electrode is positioned directly opposite the downstream electrode. The upstream Au/Hg electrode is set at a potential of −1.0 V versus Ag/AgCl to reductively cleave disulfides to the corresponding thiols. All thiols are detected by monitoring the current (nA) at the downstream electrode, which is set at a thiol-specific potential of +0.15 V versus Ag/AgCl. The resultant profiles are quantitated on the basis of peak areas computed daily from external standards.

Comments

The detector response for a variety of thiols and disulfides is linear from 7.8 to 1000 pmol, the coefficients of correlation being >0.996 (7). The reported limits of detection for thiols and disulfides are ~3.5 and 6.0 pmol per 10-μl injection. Because the retention times of thiols are affected by temperature changes, a thermoregulated water jacket must be applied to the column to maintain optimum temperature in a laboratory prone to temperature fluctuations. Baseline noise can be reduced by surrounding the detector cell and reference electrode with a well–grounded copper Faraday cage. All lines passing through the cage should be electrically insulated. Stainless steel tubing should be used between the mobile-phase reservoir and pump to prevent oxygen from entering the mobile phase.

Advantages

The HPLC–ECD assay is highly sensitive and thiol specific, and is applicable to measuring a variety of low-molecular-weight thiols and disulfides (all eluting within 20 min) from different biological matrices. Therefore, this method is particularly useful when quantification of SH/SS groups other than GSH is of interest. The chromatographic conditions described above allow for simultaneous quantification of GSH and its degradation products without interference from coeluting compounds, which was a recurrent problem with earlier HPLC–ECD methods. Because disulfides are determined directly, the autooxidation of thiols as a result of sample processing and storage is avoided. Also, because sample derivitization is not necessary, processing is straightforward and rapid (20 min per HPLC run). The use of an automated sample injector greatly increases the number of samples that can be analyzed using the above procedure.

Disadvantages

Electrochemical detectors are highly sensitive to interference from pulses generated by HPLC pumps, to oxidation of solvents and lines, and to temperature fluctuations at the electrodes. Therefore, adequate shielding is necessary to minimize interferences generated when working at high sensitivities. Also, the cost of a dual electrochemical detector may be prohibitive to some laboratories. Since the usable life span of an electrode is ~200–400 injections, periodic repolishing and resurfacing of the electrode are necessary to avoid loss of linearity and detector response.

METHOD IV: FLOW-CYTOMETRIC EVALUATION OF GLUTATHIONE

In recent years there has been increasing use of flow cytometry to acquire information on heterogeneity of various physiological and pathophysiological parameters within and among cell populations. Several fluorescent indicators to measure GSH content on an individual cell basis using flow cytometry have been developed (25–28). Most of these thiol stains react with thiols in general, and thus are not specific for GSH. However, because most of the nonprotein sulfhydryl pool consists of GSH under normal physiological conditions, results from such measurements are generally indicative of GSH content.

In contrast, monochlorobimane (MCB) can be used to selectively measure changes in GSH status in viable individual normal and tumor cells (29). The specificity of MCB for GSH is based on its role as a substrate for GSTs (see below) and its relatively low nonenzymatic reactivity toward GSH and other thiols (30). MCB has very low fluorescence, but when conjugated to GSH it is converted to the fluorescent GSH–bimane product (29). More recently, Poot *et al.* (26) used 5–chloromethylfluorescein diacetate (CMFDA) as an intracellular GSH stain. This dye, once deesterified and conjugated to GSH, has excitation and emission characteristics similar to those of fluorescein, so that simultaneous GSH and DNA content (using Hoechst 33342) can be determined for individual viable cells. Since both MCB and CMFDA will generally give satisfactory results, dye selection can reflect the selective needs of the experimentor.

Materials and Reagents

MCB or CMFDA stock (Molecular Probes, Eugene, OR): 5 m*M* in dimethyl sulfoxide. Final concentrations should not exceed 1% of the cell suspension. MCB and CMFDA stock solutions can be stored at 4°C in the dark for up to 1 month

Equipment

Flow cytometer equipped with a UV light source (typically a mercury arc lamp or 5-W argon-ion laser) for MCB analysis. CMFDA analysis is performed with a flow cytometer equipped with an argon-ion laser tuned to 488 nm

Procedure

Cell Staining

MCB

Cell suspensions (typically 1×10^6 cells/ml) are thoroughly mixed with MCB stock solution (50 μM MCB for rodent cells, 1 mM for human cells) and the tubes are placed in a 37°C water bath for 10–15 min protected from light. Stained suspensions are then placed on ice and protected from light until analysis (usually within 1 hr of staining).

CMFDA

As with MCB, the appropriate CMFDA concentrations, times, and temperatures required to achieve faithful representation of the GSH content of cells are expected to be specific to cell type. In general, cells are stained with a 50 μM CMFDA solution (final concentration) for 10 min (or longer, if nonspecific esterase activity is low) at 37°C. If the cells are to be stained in culture medium, care should be taken to minimize or exclude serum in the medium, because serum contains variable esterase activity that will convert the reagent extracellularly to a cell-impermeant form.

Analytical

Cells are gated from debris based on electronic volume, forward-angle light scatter, or right-angle light scattering characteristics. GSH analyses on instruments utilizing forward-angle light scatter can be corrected either by gating on a specific cell size or by subtracting log forward scatter from log fluorescence for each cell. Excitation of the glutathione–bimane conjugate is carried out at 351–362 or 375 nm and emission is detected at 475 nm. Excitation of the glutathione–methylfluorescein conjugate is at 488 nm and emission is detected at 530 nm. Simultaneous acquisition of GSH-dependent fluorescence and electronic cell volume yields data which can easily be adjusted for cell volume bias in GSH content (31). Most commercial flow cytometry software packages provide for some form of volume/size discrimination.

Comments

Because cells regulate their GSH *concentration* (as opposed to absolute *content*), it is important to account for cell volume effects on the MCB signal. GST isozyme expression is heterogeneous among cells, and GST isozyme classes show different reactivity toward MCB (32,33). In addition, specificity of CMFDA can also vary with cell type. Therefore, calibration of flow-cytometric data using biochemically based assays of GSH (preferably on split samples) is an essential part of MCB/flow-cytometric analyses.

Advantages

The use of flow cytometry allows for elucidation of cellular or tissue heterogeneity in GSH content. In addition, simultaneous use of specific cell surface markers allows for the quantitation of GSH in low cell numbers (<1000 cells). Since the reaction of MCB with GSH is dependent on glutathione *S*-transferase-mediated catalysis, MCB is highly specific for GSH. As previously mentioned, staining cells with CMFDA has the advantage of allowing for simultaneous quantitation of DNA and GSH content.

Disadvantages

The use of flow cytometry has only recently been exploited by toxicologists, primarily due to the high cost of initial setup and to technical difficulties that can be encountered during analyses. Therefore, many institutions utilizing flow cytometry have found it advantageous to dedicate full-time operators to assist in analyses, further increasing analytical cost. Regarding cell staining, CMFDA has been reported to be less specific for GSH than MCB (26). In addition, conditions required to adequately stain cells for GSH content with MCB depend on several factors, including dye concentration, staining time/temperature, and the constitutive presence of sufficient GST activity to ensure that the fluorescence signal is proportional to GSH content, not GST activity. Excessive concentrations of MCB may also result in nonspecific staining of protein thiols.

OTHER METHODS

In earlier studies nonprotein thiols were typically determined by stoichiometric reaction with DTNB (Ellman's reagent) (34). Although the aforementioned procedure is both straightforward and rapid, it does not allow the experimentor to discriminate GSH from other low-molecular-weight thiols (e.g., cysteine, cysteinylglycine, and ergothioneine) which can substantially contribute to the total nonprotein thiol content of many biological samples. Another chromophore, *o*-phthaldehyde (OPT), has also been used to derivatize thiols (35). However, OPT undergoes a pH-dependent reaction with primary amines (36). As a result, GSSG assays involving the reaction of OPT with GSSG at high pH may produce artifactually high GSSG values (36). Keller and Menzel (37) described a modified OPT procedure for simultaneous assay of oxidized and reduced forms of glutathione and cysteine using ion–exchange chromatography and post-column derivatization with OPT and 2-mercaptoethanol. HPLC analysis also can be used to separate a variety of oxidized and reduced sulfur-containing amino acids or their derivatives after initial formation of *S*-carboxymethyl derivatives of free thiols followed by conversion of free amino groups to 2,4-dinitrophenol derivatives (38). Enzymatic determinations of GSH have also been accomplished using glyoxylase (5) and GSTs (39).

REFERENCES

1. D. J Reed and P. W. Beatty, *in* "Biochemical Toxicology" (E. Hodgson, J. Bend, and R. Philpott, eds.), Vol. 2, p. 213. Elsevier, Amsterdam, 1980.
2. N. S. Kosower and E. M. Kosower, *Int. Rev. Cytol.* **54,** 109 (1978).
3. N. S. Kosower and E. M. Kosower, *in* "Functions of Glutathione: Biochemical, Physiological, Toxicological, and Clinical Aspects" (A. Larsson, ed.), p.307. Raven New York, 1983.
4. A. Meister and M. Anderson, *Annu. Rev. Biochem.* **52,** 711 1983.
5. P. M. Akerboom and H. Sies, *in* "Methods in Enzymology" (W. B. Jakoby, ed.), Vol. 77, p. 373. Academic Press, New York, 1981.
6. M. E Anderson, *in* "Methods in Enzymology" (A. Meister, ed.), Vol. 113, p. 548. Academic Press, Orlando, Florida, 1985.
7. A. F. Stein, R. L. Dills, and C. D. Klaasen, *J. Chromatogr.* **381,** 259 (1986).
8. F. Tietze, *Anal. Biochem.* **27,** 502 (1969).
9. O. W Griffith, *Anal. Biochem.* **106,** 207 (1980).
10. I. A. Cotgreave and P. Moldeus, *J. Biochem. Biophys. Methods* **13,** 231 (1986).
11. S. S. Fenton and R. C. Fahey, *Anal. Biochem.* **154,** 34 (1986).
12. A. Spector, G. M. Wang, and R. R. C. Huang, *Curr. Eye Res.* **5,** 47 (1986).
13. J. D. Adams, B.H. Lauterburg, and J. R. Mitchell, *J. Pharmacol. Exp. Ther.* **227,** 749 (1983).
14. F. A. M. Redgegeld, M. A. J. van Opstal, E. Houdcamp, and W.P. van Bennekom, *Anal. Biochem.* **174,** 489 (1988).
15. M. A. Baker, G. J. Cerniglia, and A. Zaman, *Anal. Biochem.* **190,** 360 (1990).
16. R. C Fahey, and G. L. Newton, *in* "Methods in Enzymology" (W. B. Jakoby and O. Griffith, eds.), Vol. 143, p. 85. Academic Press, Orlando, Florida, 1987.
17. N. S. Kosower, E. M. Kosower, G. L. Newton, and H. M. Ranney, *Proc. Natl. Acad. Sci. U.S.A.* **76,** 3382 (1979).
18. R. C. Fahey, G. L. Newton, R. Dorian, and E. Kosower, *Anal. Biochem.* **111,** 357 (1981).
19. G. L. Newton, R. Dorian, and R.C. Fahey, *Anal. Biochem.* **114,** 383 (1981).
20. D. M. Hamel, C. White, and D. L. Eaton, *Toxicol. Methods.* **1,** 273 (1992).
21. E. D. Mooze and A. Meister, *in* "Methods in Enzymology" (H. Tabor and C. W. Tabor, eds.), Vol. 17, p. 483. Academic Press, New York, 1971.
22. E. G. DeMaster and B. Redfern, in "Methods in Enzymology" (W. B. Jakoby and O. Griffith, eds.), Vol. 143, p. 110. Academic Press, Orlando, Florida, 1987.
23. J. P. Richie, Jr., and C. A. Lang, *Anal. Biochem.* **163,** 9 (1987).
24. L. A. Allison, and R.E. Shoup, *Anal. Chem.* **55,** 8 (1983).
25. R. E. Durand and P. E. Olive, *Radiat. Res.* **95,** 456 (1983).
26. M. Poot, A. Verkerk, J. F. Koster, and J. F. Jongkind, *Biochim. Biophys. Acta.* **883,** 580 (1986).
27. J. Treumer and G. Valet, *Exp. Cell Res.* **163,** 518 (1986).
28. M. Poot, T. J. Kavanagh, H. C. Kang, R. P. Haugland, and P. S. Rabinovitch, *Cytometry* **12,** 184 (1991).
29. G. C. Rice, E. A. Bump, D. C. Shrieve, W. Lee, and M. Kovacs, *Cancer Res.* **46,** 1 (1986).
30. A. E. Radkowsky and E. M. Kosower, *J. Am. Chem. Soc.* **108,** 4257 (1986).

31. T. J. Kavanagh, G. M. Martin, M. H. El-Fouly, J. E. Trosko, C. Chang, and P. E. Rabinovitch, *Cancer Res.* **47,** 6046 (1987).
32. J. A. Cook, S. N. Iype, and J. B. Mitchell, *Cancer Res.* **51,** 1606 (1991).
33. G. A. Ublacker, J. A. Johnson, F.L. Siegel, and R. T. Mulcahey, *Cancer Res.* **51,** 1783 (1991).
34. G. L Ellman, *Arch. Biochem. Biophys.* **82,** 70 (1959).
35. V. H. Cohn and J. Lyle, *Anal. Biochem.* **14,** 434 (1966).
36. E. Beutler and C. West, *Anal. Biochem.* **81,** 458 (1977).
37. D. A Keller and D. B. Menzel, *Anal. Biochem.* **151,** 418 (1985).
38. D. J. Reed, J. R. Babson, P.W. Beatty, A. E. Brodie, W. W. Ellis, and D. W. Potter, *Anal. Biochem.* **106,** 55 (1980).
39. K. Asaoka and K. Takahashi, *J. Biochem. (Tokyo)* **90,** 1237 (1981).

30 Thiobarbituric Acid Assay Reactants

Steven D. Aust

INTRODUCTION

Numerous toxins are thought to be toxic through their ability to cause lipid peroxidation. Chemicals such as paraquat, Adriamycin (Adria, Chicago, IL), and carbon tetrachloride can cause lipid peroxidation, and as such lipid peroxidation is often referred to as the "mechanism of toxicity." Lipid peroxidation is also thought to occur, and perhaps cause, cell death by toxins that indirectly affect some biochemical function or activity that in turn affects lipid peroxidation. An example of a more indirect mechanism would be by toxins that affect glutathione (GSH) metabolism, as GSH is required for the metabolism of hydrogen peroxide and lipid hydroperoxides by glutathione peroxidase and for the maintenance of protein thiols (1). Upon depletion of GSH, protection from lipid peroxidation is lost (2). Bromobenzene (3) and paracetamol (4) are toxins that can cause liver necrosis by depleting tissue GSH levels, and their toxicity can be decreased by *N*-acetylcysteine, a precursor to cysteine which is required for the synthesis of GSH (5–7). Lipid peroxidation can also occur as a consequence of tissue damage, perhaps contributing to cell death.

There is considerable interest lately in the role of iron in lipid peroxidation (8). Therefore, chemicals that may affect the chemistry or biochemistry of cellular iron may in turn cause lipid peroxidation. Iron metabolism might be affected either directly or indirectly. For example, chemicals that enter redox reactions to generate superoxide and their respective organic radicals, both of which will release iron from ferritin, although the organic radicals are much more efficient than superoxide, can cause lipid peroxidation (9,10). Secondly, upon tissue damage iron may become uncontrolled; for example, hemorrhage and red blood cell hemolysis releases hemoglobin which can catalyze lipid peroxidation (11,12). A number of biological chemicals are good reductants of iron and can therefore catalyze lipid peroxidation given a source of iron. The classic example is ascorbic acid. Ascorbic acid and iron are frequently used in model lipid peroxidation studies (13,14). Many other reductants of cellular origin can be used, including biogenic amines (15). Normally, these reactions would be controlled by efficient compartmentalization of at least one of the reactants (i.e., iron is stored in ferritin). The possibility therefore exists for the loss of this control by compartmentalization upon tissue damage, resulting in lipid peroxidation.

METHODS IN TOXICOLOGY, Volume 1B

The interesting observation is that iron itself is toxic (16,17). The toxicity of iron is difficult to study because it does not exist alone in solution as the free ion but is complexed with various chelating agents and in different oxidation states. However, the toxicity and even carcinogenicity of iron (18) are hard to deny. And there are extremely good correlations between iron status and other health problems, such as arteriosclerosis, thought to be related to the oxidation of low density lipoproteins (19).

ASSAYS FOR LIPID PEROXIDATION

Many methods can be used to detect or measure lipid peroxidation, especially *in vitro* (20–22). The measurement of lipid peroxidation *in vivo* is a totally different subject. Some of the methods can be used to get an indication of the occurrence of *in vivo* lipid peroxidation but very few can be used to quantitate *in vivo* lipid peroxidation. And the absence of positive results cannot be used as evidence against the involvement or occurrence of lipid peroxidation.

Of the many assays that might be used *in vitro* the thiobarbituric acid (TBA) assay for determination of malondialdehyde (MDA) formation (or levels), is probably most popular, perhaps because of the ease and sensitivity of the methods. MDA results from the decomposition of lipid endoperoxides, during lipid peroxidation and/or during the TBA assay, as follows (23) (where *x* and *y* are the carboxyl and aliphatic ends of fatty acids):

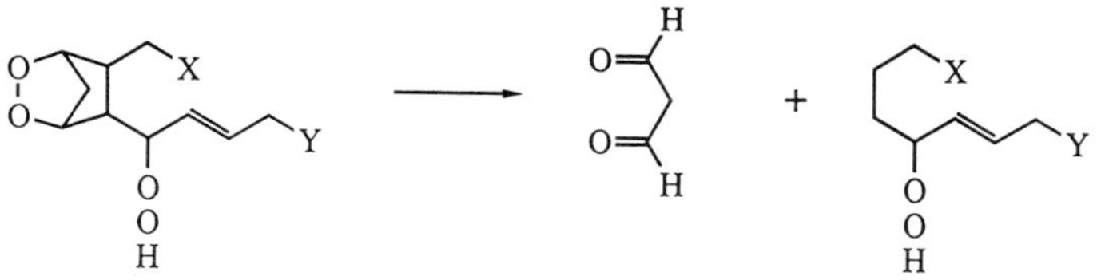

The formation of MDA can occur both during lipid peroxidation (probably catalyzed by transition metals such as iron) and during the quantitation of MDA by TBA. The assay involves heat and acid and there would always be transition metals available during heating biological samples in acid. However, if desired, the formation of MDA during the assay can be prevented by the inclusion of an antioxidant. The usual way this is done is to include butylated hydroxytoluene (BHT) in the TBA assay (24,25). If no antioxidants are included, the assay is more sensitive, as both preformed MDA and substances that can give rise to MDA (e.g., lipid hydroperoxides) are quantitated. Also, the difference between the data obtained with and without BHT would be an estimate of the amount of lipid hydroperoxides present in the sample.

The lack of specificity of the TBA assay for MDA is a potential problem (26) and a basis for frequent criticism of it. However, most of the other substances that react with the TBA reagent still arise from lipid peroxidation. Fortunately, the MDA adduct (shown below) has a rather unique absorption maximum at 535 nm (27). If specificity is of concern, it is best to determine the absorption spectrum of the reaction product. Methods have also been developed to extract the adduct and to analyze for the MDA adduct by high-performance liquid chromatography (HPLC) (28). However, since most of the non-MDA- but TBA-reactive products usually are derived from lipid peroxidation, it is frequently unnecessary to be overly concerned about the nature of the product, especially for *in vitro* lipid peroxidation assays, and the product is simply referred to as TBA-positive or -reactive material (20). Otherwise, it is important to determine whether there are other substances besides lipid in the samples of interest that might also give rise to MDA (e.g., deoxyribose) (29).

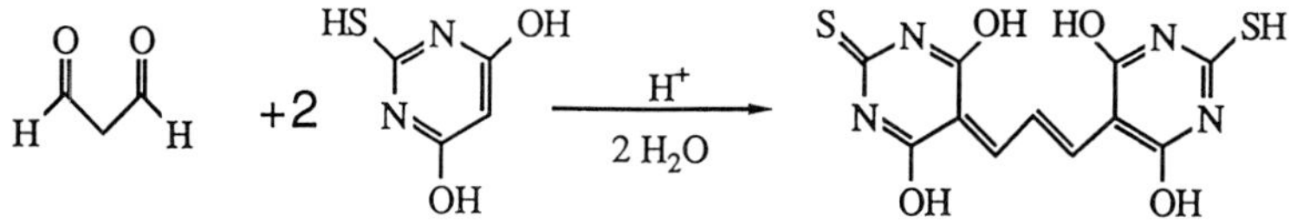

MECHANISM OF LIPID PEROXIDATION

Lipid peroxidation had long been recognized and studied in the food industry. Many analytical methods were developed to study the rancidity of foods. The occurrence of lipid peroxidation in biological systems came much later. The exact mechanism by which lipid peroxidation occurs in biological systems has been argued almost since the day it was originally observed. It was discovered almost simultaneously by Paul Hochstein (30,31), working in the laboratory of Professor Lars Ernster, and by Beloff-Chain et al. (32). They had observed NADPH- and ADP-dependent oxygen uptake with the microsomal fraction of liver. Since they had just read all of the new and exciting developments in the field of oxidative phosphorylation, in which NADH was used as the electron donor, they naturally thought that they had discovered an NADPH-dependent oxidative phosphorylation in the endoplasmic reticulum. Both groups found, upon further investigation, no phosphorylation of ADP; moreover, they discovered that the requirement for ADP was really a requirement for iron, which was a contaminant in the ADP (31). But more importantly, Hochstein et al. (31) proposed that the mechanism of lipid peroxidation directly involved this iron. We (24) and others (33) have confirmed that iron is indeed required for lipid peroxidation. Many investigators have proposed that the iron is involved in generation of the hydroxyl radical, which is the actual initiator of lipid peroxidation (34). The controversy surfaced again when we (35) and others (36) proposed that both ferrous and ferric iron were required for lipid peroxidation in many systems, including one dependent on hydrogen peroxide (37) and one occurring in peribacteroid membranes from French bean nodules (38).

The bottom line is that a transition metal, most frequently iron, is required for most *in vitro* lipid peroxidation systems. And therein lies a potential problem. Frequently, *in vitro* lipid peroxidation studies are conducted with little or no regard for iron, although sometimes there are very complete investigations of the role of iron in lipid peroxidation (39,40). The other side of the coin is that lipid peroxidation occurs in some *in vitro* systems because iron is a contaminant in buffers, water, and many reagents, and biochemical iron reductants exist in most *in vitro* systems.

Related to this subject is the general misconception that polyunsaturated fatty acids and other biomolecules autoxidize. There have been frequent proposals that the autoxidation of various biochemicals results in the production of superoxide and hydrogen peroxide. The classic example is probably with ascorbate (41,42). However, the direct reaction of molecular oxygen with organic molecules, true autoxidation, is spin forbidden (43). Frequently, when "autoxidation" is observed, metals are involved. Ascorbic acid is a good chelator of iron as well as a good reductant of iron. The iron is reduced and autoxidizes to set up a redox cycle in which ascorbic acid is oxidized and oxygen is reduced, giving the appearance of ascorbic acid autoxidation (42). However, the true autoxidation in this situation is that of ferrous iron. Therefore, ascorbic acid will catalyze lipid peroxidation in which the reduced iron is involved in the lipid peroxidation, not oxygen radicals produced by ascorbic acid "autoxidation." This can be demonstrated by showing that lipid peroxidation does not occur when there is excess ascorbic acid, even though it is undergoing rapid oxidation and reduced species of oxygen are being produced (44). The same general phenomenon is observed with numerous biochemicals, such as the biogenic amines (15).

It is therefore important to be cognizant of the probable presence of iron and the reactions that it can cause and enter in all *in vitro* toxicity systems in which lipid peroxidation is a possible mechanism of toxicity. In general, iron metabolism is tightly controlled *in vivo*. The question arises, however, as to whether it is always tightly controlled in *in vitro* studies. A good test for the presence of iron in buffers and reagents was devised by Garry Buettner, who reasoned that adventitious iron probably is not a problem when ascorbic acid does not oxidize (42). This is an excellent simple test that can be done in the laboratory in several ways, including measuring oxygen consumption, the formation of reduced iron species, and electron paramagnetic resonance spectroscopy. Another excellent way directly related to *in vitro* lipid peroxidation studies is to show either that iron is absolutely required for lipid peroxidation or that iron somehow becomes available for lipid peroxidation. This can be done by addition of a potent iron chelator, such as desferrioxamine, to the system to determine its effect on lipid peroxidation.

Frequently, iron-catalyzed lipid peroxidation is actually considered to be lipid hydroperoxide-dependent lipid peroxidation. That is, lipid peroxidation is often thought to be dependent on the presence of preexisting lipid hydroperoxides (20). This may indeed be the case *in vivo* and in some *in vitro* situations. Lipid hydroperoxides are produced *in vivo*, for example, by prostaglandin synthase. These hydroperoxides may be involved in lipid hydroperoxide-dependent lipid peroxidation. It is quite easy to study lipid or organic hydroperoxide-dependent lipid peroxidation. Lipid hydroperoxides or organic hydroperoxides, such as cumene hydroperoxide, can be used to test for hydroperoxide-dependent lipid peroxidation. Also, hydroperoxides can be simply mixed directly with the TBA reagent rather than the lipid peroxidation system to determine whether MDA arises from the original hydroperoxide. Second, TBA assays should be conducted with or without BHT. Without BHT the results will include hydroperoxide-dependent lipid peroxidation that occurs during the assay with the remaining added hydroperoxide as well as with the lipid hydroperoxides formed as intermediates in the lipid peroxidation. With BHT added the assay only detects preformed MDA. The difference is that due to hydroperoxides.

There is another somewhat different subject that must be addressed when considering the mechanism of lipid peroxidation. This has to do with whether lipid peroxidation actually involves some form of partially reduced species of oxygen such as $O_2^{\overline{\cdot}}$, H_2O_2, or the hydroxyl radical ($^{\cdot}OH$). In some cases these species are combined into a term called reactive oxygen intermediates, metabolites or species. This also provides for the inclusion of species such as, the ferryl ion (FeO^{2+}), in which it is difficult to clearly discern the difference between $^{\cdot}OH$ and the ferryl ion. The hydroxy radical is often stated to result from an iron-catalyzed Haber–Weiss reaction. However, if this were true, it is still important to understand the source of the iron. Iron is well controlled in biology, perhaps much better than in the laboratory, and therein lies a problem. The subject is probably best exemplified by oxygen toxicity, although it could also be discussed in relation to ischemia/reperfusion, paraquat toxicity, etc. It is possible to demonstrate the effect of all of these on lipid peroxidation, and to show that they cause lipid peroxidation. But it is still impossible to know how. In the case of hyperoxia, it is often stated that hyperoxia causes the overproduction of reactive oxygen species. That is, they are overproduced in relation to the activity of protective enzymes such as superoxide dismutase, catalase, and glutathione peroxidase. The reactive oxygen species are often said to arise by excess oxygen reduction by mitochondria or the endoplasmic reticulum. We have studied microsomal NADPH oxidation as a measure of the ability to reduce molecular oxygen to either $O_2^{\overline{\cdot}}$ or H_2O_2 and can demonstrate little NADPH oxidation. The microsomal reductase, NADPH–cytochrome P-450 reductase, produces little or no $O_2^{\overline{\cdot}}$, and the addition of cytochrome P-450 results in little additional $O_2^{\overline{\cdot}}$ (45). However, $O_2^{\overline{\cdot}}$ production is dramatically affected by iron and activity is affected by the iron chelator (46). This can probably best be demonstrated for EDTA-chelated iron (47). NADPH–cytochrome P-450 reductase rapidly reduces EDTA-chelated iron, causing rapid NADPH oxidation and $O_2^{\overline{\cdot}}$, H_2O_2 and $^{\cdot}OH$ production. The production of the latter (a partially reduced species of oxygen) results from rapid autooxidation of the EDTA-chelated ferrous iron. However, EDTA is an excellent inhibitor of microsomal lipid peroxidation (48,49). Thus, increased production of reactive oxygen species does not necessarily result in lipid peroxidation. It is true that the hydroxyl radical is an excellent initiator of lipid peroxidation (47). However, it may not always do so. For every publication presenting evidence or some mechanism for the production of reactive oxygen species and their involvement in toxicity or pathology, there is a very high probability that there is another concluding that there is no evidence for such. This subject was very well reviewed by Jamieson (50).

APPLICATION OF THE TBA ASSAY TO *IN VITRO* LIPID PEROXIDATION STUDIES

The vast majority of *in vitro* lipid peroxidation studies involving cells in culture have been done with primary cultures of hepatocytes. Generally, this has been because the studies have been a study of either the mechanism of toxicity of some chemical, or the mechanism of cell death by oxidative stress or some other treatment, condition, or stress. There have also been some studies on parameters that might indirectly affect lipid peroxidation. Hepatocytes are frequently used because they are active in the metabolism of the toxins in question (i.e., CCl_4, Adriamycin, diquat, and menadione) and the liver is a principal target tissue of toxicity. It is also possible to isolate and study hepatocytes from animals after they have been treated with chemicals or diets that might affect lipid peroxidation. A classic example is the use of vitamin E-deficient hepatocytes isolated from animals fed a vitamin E-deficient diet (51,52).

There are other reasons that the hepatocyte is an excellent model for studying factors affecting lipid peroxidation. It would appear that the majority of the MDA formed in the cell appears in the extracellular media (53). This provides samples that are relatively free of potentially interfering substances, and samples can be taken repeatedly. The disadvantage is that hepatocytes can only be kept in primary culture. For this reason many investigators use cell lines instead of primary cultures to study lipid peroxidation in cultures. In addition, sometimes it is important to study tissue-specific toxins with cells from the target tissue. In this case it is sometimes necessary to use established cell lines. Some studies have been done with tumor cell lines from a specific tissue. In these cases one can always question whether the results are relevant to the *in vivo* situation, as tumor cell lines may be quite different from what exists in the normal tissue. In other cases, however, investigators have been interested in tumor cells themselves, as lipid peroxidation may be of interest in tumors. However, again, one must consider the difference between tumors and cell lines established from tumors.

METHOD: TBA REAGENT

The TBA reagent is prepared along with trichloroacetic acid (TCA) to precipitate protein in the sample and HCl to acidify the reaction mixture. The reagent is usually 15% (w/v) TCA and 0.375% (w/v) TBA in 0.25 N HCl (20.8 ml of concentrated HCl per liter). The solution must be mildly heated (~70°C) to assist in dissolution of the TBA. The reagent is stable for months, until a precipitate forms.

If BHT is to be included in the assay, we add 0.03 vol of 2% BHT in absolute ethanol (the solution is stored in the dark) to the TBA reagent just prior to use. The BHT will form in a fine precipitate that must be kept in suspension by constant stirring.

PROCEDURE

The sample is mixed with 2 vol of the TBA reagent to terminate the process of lipid peroxidation and to initiate the assay. The solution is heated for 15 min in a boiling water bath. After cooling, any precipitate present is removed by centrifugation at 1000–2000 *g* for 10 min. The absorbance of the sample is determined at 535 nm against a blank that contains the reagent with the sample replaced by an equal volume of water (or buffer, media, etc.). The MDA concentration of the sample can be determined using an extinction coefficient of $1.56 \times 10^5\ M^{-1}\ cm^{-1}$ (54). However, it is advisable to prepare a standard curve using 1,1,3,3-tetramethoxypropane (which gives MDA upon hydrolysis) during the assay. The MDA adduct can also be extracted and analyzed by HPLC (28).

COMMENTS

There are a number of problems with use of the TBA assay for MDA and they are more or less important when the assay is applied to cells in culture. The first is the fact that MDA may be metabolized (21). Thus, the relationship of the values obtained to the actual amount of MDA is unknown. Second, MDA can be produced from lipid hydroperoxides during the TBA assay. As mentioned earlier, this can be eliminated by the inclusion of the antioxidant BHT in the reagent. As also mentioned earlier, if assays are conducted both with and without BHT added to the reagent, it is possible to get two values, and the difference reflects the amount of lipid hydroperoxides in the sample. Thus, this can actually, in turn, be of advantage in providing more information. In any case it is necessary to be careful when comparing values for MDA production in various experimental conditions, assays, etc., especially when comparing different values from the literature. It is necessary to very carefully consider the manner in which experiments and assays are conducted.

Perhaps the most often cited criticism of the TBA assay in that it is not specific. Sometimes this can be a problem and sometimes it can be useful. For example, the degradation of deoxyribose can give rise to MDA. Thus, samples containing significant amounts of DNA which can be oxidized either in the experiment or in the assay (which can be blocked by BHT) can give misleading results if one is only interested in MDA arising from lipid peroxidation. On the other hand, the assay can actually be used to study the oxidation of DNA or deoxyribose (29), or even as an assay for ˙OH production using deoxyribose, as it is generally thought that deoxyribose oxidation is rather specific for ˙OH (55).

Another source of what might be considered interference in the TBA assay is other aldehyde products of lipid peroxidation. There are two solutions. One is to carefully determine the absorption maximum of the adduct produced, as other aldehydes give different absorption maxima and extinction coefficients (27). The second solution, which is more common, is to simply report the data as TBA-reactive material if the other aldehydes are also products of lipid peroxidation.

A third type of interference is other substances, not related in any way to lipid or any other type of oxidation, that also react with TBA to absorb in the region of 535 nm. A classic example is sucrose (27,56). Sucrose must be removed if used, for example, for subcellular fractionation. Sucrose can be quite easily removed from cells and subcellular fraction by resuspension in saline or buffer and centrifugation.

In summary, the TBA assay for MDA can be very useful to assess lipid peroxidation, especially in *in vitro* experiments. There are some precautions to be taken, but these are quite reasonable and simple.

REFERENCES

1. S. Orrenius, *Trends. Pharmacol. Sci.* **6,** S15 (1985).
2. D. J. Reed and M. W. Fariss, *Pharmacol. Rev.* **36,** 25S (1984).
3. A. F. Casini, A. Pompella, and M. Comporti, *Am. J. Pathol.* **118,** 225 (1985).
4. A. Wendel, S. Feuerstein, and K. H. Kony, *Biochem. Pharmacol.* **28,** 2051 (1979).
5. L. F. Prescott, R. N. Illingworth, J. A. J. H. Critchley, M. J. Stewart, R. D. Adams, and A. T. Procedfoot, *Br. Med. J.* **2,** 1087 (1979).
6. M. R. Landauer, H. D. Davis, J. A. Dominitz, and J. F. Weiss, *Pharmacol. Ther.* **39,** 97 (1988).
7. B. H. Lautenbury, G. B. Corcoran, and J. R. Mitchell, *J. Clin. Invest.* **71,** 980 (1983).
8. S. D. Aust and B. A. Svingen, *in* "Free Radicals in Biology" (W.A. Pryor, ed.), Vol. 5, pp. 29–64. Academic Press, New York, 1982.
9. C. E. Thomas and S.D. Aust, *J. Biol. Chem.* **261,** 13064 (1986).
10. D. W. Reif, I. L. P. Beales, C. E. Thomas, and S. D. Aust, *Toxicol. Appl. Pharmacol.* **93,** 506 (1988).
11. E. Baysal, H. P. Monteiro, S. G. Sullivan, and A. Stern, *Free Radic. Biol. Med.* **9,** 5 (1990).

12. S. Sadrzadeh, E. Graf, S. S. Panter, P. E. Halloway, and J. W. Eaton, *J. Biol. Chem.* **259,** 14354 (1984).
13. E. D. Wills, *in* "Oxidative Stress" (H. Sies, ed.), pp. 197–218. Academic Press, Orlando, Florida, 1985.
14. S. N. Chatterjee and S. Agarwal, *J. Free Radic. Biol. Med.* **4,** 51 (1988).
15. K. Yagi, N. Ishida, S. Komura, and N. Ohishi, *J. Clin. Biochem. Nutr.* **9,** 179 (1990).
16. B. Halliwell and J. M. C. Gutteridge, *in* "Methods in Enzymology" (L. Packer and A. N. Glazer, eds.), Vol. 186, pp. 1–85. Academic Press, San Diego, 1990.
17. T. P. Ryan and S. D. Aust, *CRC Crit. Rev. Toxicol.* **22,** 119 (1992).
18. R. A. Floyd, *FASEB J.* **4,** 2587 (1990).
19. J. T. Salonen, K. Nyyssonen, H. Korpeld, J. Tuomilehto, R. Seppanen, and R. Salonen, *Circulation* **86,** 803 (1992).
20. J. M. C. Gutteridge and B. Halliwell, *Trends Biochem. Sci.* **15,** 130 (1990).
21. D. R. Janero, *Free Radic. Biol. Med.* **9,** 515 (1990).
22. H. Ohkawa, N. Ohishi, and K. Yagi, *Anal. Biochem.* **95,** 351 (1979).
23. W. A. Pryor and J. P. Stanley, *J. Org. Chem.* **40,** 3615 (1975).
24. T. C. Pederson, J. A. Buege, and S.D. Aust, *J. Biol. Chem.* **248,** 7134 (1973).
25. J. A. Buege and S.D. Aust, in "Methods in Enzymology" (K. Moldave and L. Grossman, eds.), Vol. 30, pp. 302–310. Academic Press, New York, 1978.
26. H. Kosugi, T. Kato, and K. Kikugawa, *Anal. Biochem.* **165,** 456 (1987).
27. T. F. Slater, "Free Radical Mechanisms of Tissue Injury," p. 34. Pion, London, 1972.
28. C. Largilliene and S. B. Melancon, *Anal. Biochem.* **170,** 123 (1988).
29. M. F. Janieck, W. A. Haseltine, and W. D. Henner, *Nucleic Acids Res.* **13,** 9011 (1985).
30. P. Hochstein and L. Ernster, *Biochem. Biophys. Res. Commun.* **12,** 388 (1963).
31. P. Hochstein, K. Nordenbrand, and L. Ernster, *Biochem. Biophys. Res. Commun.* **14,** 323 (1964).
32. A. Beloff-Chain, R. Catanzaro, and S. Serlupi-Crescenzi, *Nature (London)* **198,** 351 (1963).
33. J. L. Poyer and P. B. McCay, *J. Biol. Chem.* **246,** 263 (1971).
34. B. Halliwell and J. M. C. Gutteridge, *Biochem. J.* **219,** 1 (1984).
35. J. R. Bucher, M. Tien, and S. D. Aust, *Biochem. Biophys. Res. Commun.* **111,** 777 (1983).
36. J. M. Braughler, L. A. Duncan, and R. L. Chase, *J. Biol. Chem.* **261,** 10282 (1986).
37. G. Minotti and S. D. Aust, *J. Biol. Chem.* **262,** 1098 (1986).
38. A. Puppo, G. Herrada, and J. Rigand, *Plant Physiol.* **96,** 826 (1991).
39. S. D. Aust, L. A. Morehouse, and C. E. Thomas, *J. Free Radic. Biol. Med.* **1,** 3 (1985).
40. G. Minotti and S. D. Aust, *Lipids* **27,** 219 (1992).
41. G. R. Buettner, *Free Radic. Res. Comm.* **1,** 349 (1986).
42. G. R. Buettner, *J. Biochem. Biophys. Methods* **16,** 27 (1988).
43. D. M. Miller, G. R. Buettner, and S. D. Aust, *Free Radic. Biol. Med.* **8,** 95 (1990).
44. D. M. Miller and S. D. Aust, *Arch. Biochem. Biophys.* **271,** 113 (1988).
45. L. A. Morehouse and S. D. Aust, *Free Radic. Biol. Med.* **4,** 269 (1988).
46. L. A. Morehouse, C. E. Thomas, and S. D. Aust, *Arch. Biochem. Biophys.* **232,** 366 (1984).
47. M. Tien, L. A. Morehouse, J. R. Bucher, and S. D. Aust, *Arch. Biochem. Biophys.* **218,** 450 (1982).
48. D. J. Kornbrust and R. D. Mavis, *Mol. Pharmacol.* **17,** 400 (1980).

49. M. A. Trush, E. G. Mimnaugh, E. Ginsburgh, and T. E. Gram, *Toxicol. Appl. Pharmacol.* **60,** 279 (1981).
50. D. Jamieson, *Free Radic. Biol. Med.* **7,** 87 (1989).
51. G. A. Pascoe, K. Olafsdottin, and D. J. Reed, *Arch. Biochem. Biophys.* **256,** 150 (1987).
52. M. S. Sandy, D. DiMonte, and M. T. Smith, *Toxicol. Appl. Pharmacol.* **93,** 288 (1988).
53. M. W. Fariss, *Free Radic. Biol. Med.* **9,** 333 (1990).
54. E. D. Wills, *Biochem. J.* **113,** 325 (1969).
55. K. H. Cheeseman, A. Beavis, and H. Esterbauer, *Biochem. J.* **252,** 649 (1988).
56. C. T. Huber, H. H. Edwards, and M. Morrison, *Arch. Biochem. Biophys.* **168,** 463 (1975).

31 Volatile Hydrocarbons

Hermann Kappus

INTRODUCTION

The formation of ethane and *n*-pentane has been related to lipid peroxidation of n3- and n6-unsaturated fatty acids (see Fig. 1). The reaction scheme shown demonstrates that this pathway is only part of the whole lipid peroxidation process. However, because of the high volatility of ethane and *n*-pentane, these hydrocarbons can be used for the measurement of lipid peroxidation *in vivo,* because they are found in the expiratory air. After the first report (1) on *in vivo* exhalation of ethane by animals after treatment with CCl_4, numerous studies have been performed which used this noninvasive method to evaluate lipid peroxidation *in vivo.*

For *in vitro* studies a number of convenient methods to determine lipid peroxidation are available, and therefore the measurement of ethane and *n*-pentane has not been carried out so extensively. Furthermore, *in vitro* measurements of these hydrocarbons are relatively difficult when applied *in vitro.* Nevertheless, ethane and/or *n*-pentane formation has been applied for incubations with enzyme systems, cell particles, whole cells, tissue slices, and isolated perfused organs (2). It became obvious that there is no principal difference between hydrocarbon formation *in vitro* and the *in vivo* situation. But the experiments performed *in vitro* demonstrated organ specificity and elucidated the underlying mechanism of lipid peroxidation. On the other hand, the *in vitro* experiments resulted in detection of a number of other hydrocarbons which could not yet be definitely related to lipid peroxidation (3,4).

In general, during studies *in vitro* ethane and *n*-pentane formation are much easier to detect and quantify as compared to analysis of the exhaled air of animals.

PROCEDURES

Incubation of Isolated Cell Particles or Cells

All of these experiments have been carried out in incubation vials equipped with various caps. Mostly glass vials are used and incubated at 37°C under various conditions. In liver microsomes, for example, lipid peroxidation is induced

METHODS IN TOXICOLOGY, Volume 1B

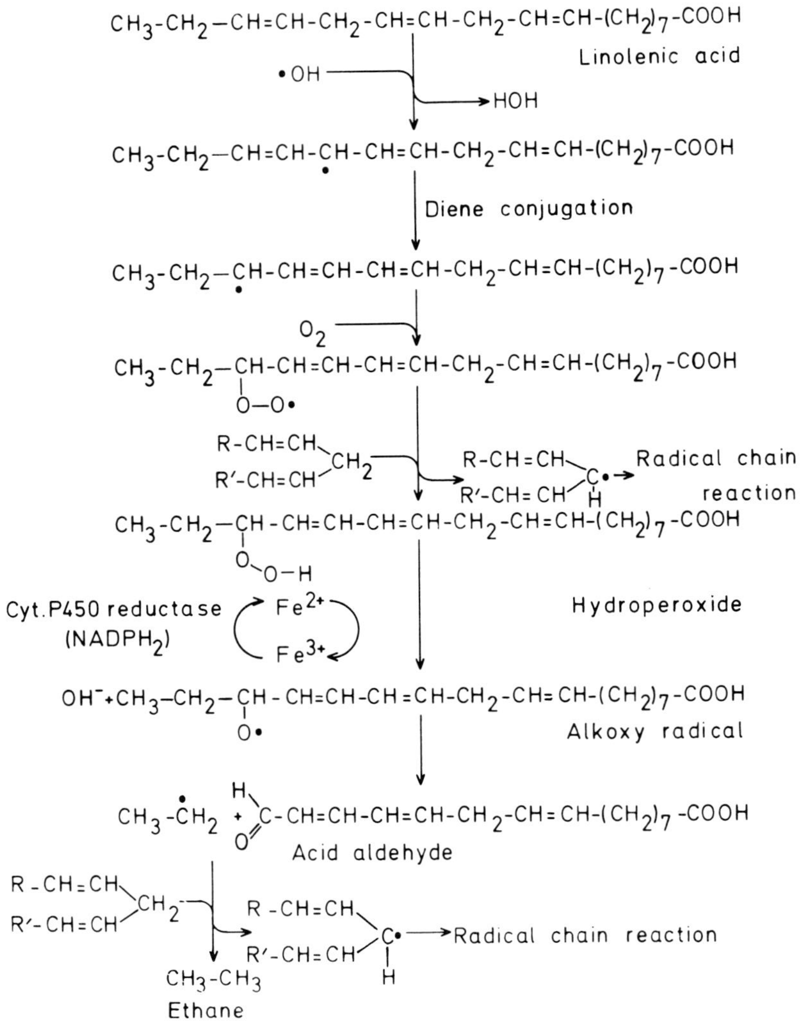

Figure 1 Ethane formation from an n3-unsaturated fatty acid during lipid peroxidation. n6-Unsaturated fatty acids result in *n*-pentane formation. The steric configuration of the lipid molecules is not shown. (Modified from Ref. 20.)

by iron complexes or by halogenated hydrocarbons such as CCl_4 (3). The head space volume of the flasks is generally much greater than the incubation suspension. With ongoing lipid peroxidation the hydrocarbons are mainly present in the head space air due to their volatility.

The main difficulty is the collection of this head space air. Wendel and colleagues (5) used a glass syringe for the incubation of liver microsomes. The incubation volume was 2 ml and the head space volume was 7 ml. After some

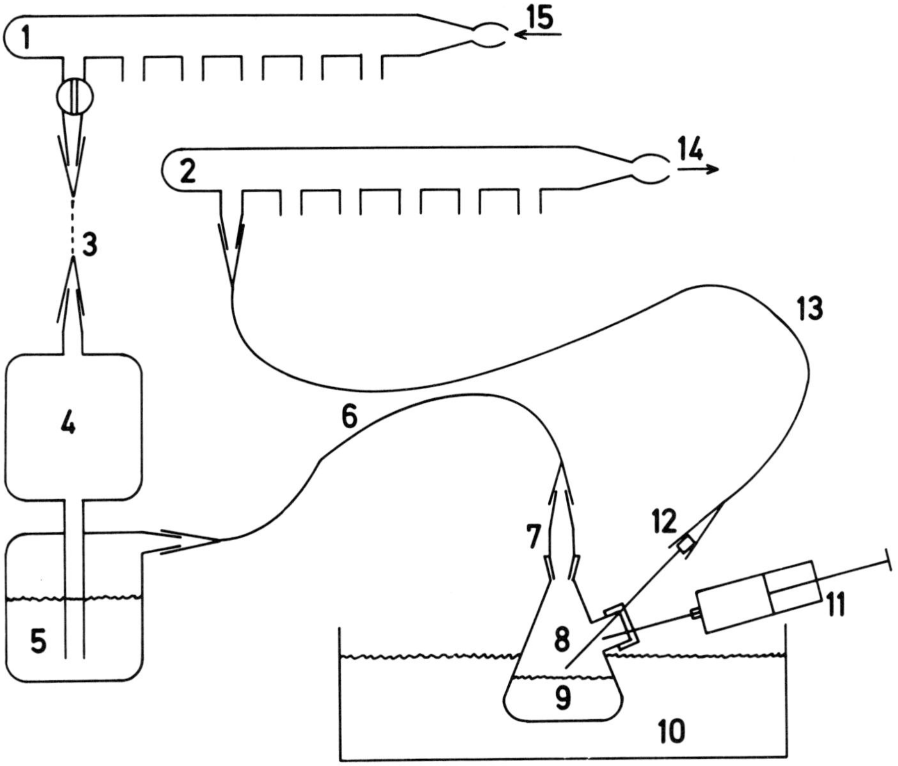

Figure 2 System used for incubations of isolated cell particles or cells and sampling of volatile hydrocarbons (e.g., ethane and/or *n*-pentane). The design shown allows six independent simultaneous incubations. All glass parts shown will have to be custom made by a glass blower. (1 and 2) All-glass systems (each about 20 cm long) with stopcocks and tube connections, respectively; (3) Teflon tube (~5 cm long); (4) specially made glass flask (33 ml); (5) water (15 ml) as a barrier fluid; (6 and 13) Teflon tubes (~50 cm long); (7) ground glass stopper; (8) Erlenmeyer flask (22 ml) with side arm, screw cap, and Teflon-coated silicon septum (0.8-cm width); (9) incubation mixture (5 ml or less); (10) water bath (37°C), shaking at the normal rate for the cell type or preparation used; (11) gastight syringe (10 ml) with a needle for gas sampling of the head space air of the Erlenmeyer flask; (12) long stainless steel needle (gauge 1; ~10 cm long) for degassing of the head space and the incubation mixure; (14) vacuum pump; and (15) hydrocarbon-free gas (e.g., synthetic air or O_2/N_2 mixtures). (Modified from Ref. 3.)

time the total head space gas was directly injected into a gas chromatograph. Using this technique, no change in volume or pressure occurred. But in this system measurement of continuous accumulation of ethane and *n*-pentane with time is impossible and therefore the sensitivity cannot be increased by increasing the incubation time.

In other studies the head space volume was chosen large enough to allow removal of air without much change in pressure (6,7). We developed a system (3) in which the removed head space air is replaced by an identical volume of the respective gas and the air sample is diluted before removal of the sample (see Fig. 2). This system allows one to sample air for a long incubation period without change in pressure and without the risk of taking up air from outside the incubation flask, which could be contaminated with the hydrocarbons studied. In this system the air removed is replaced by hydrocarbon-free gas which is identical to the head space air of the flask. This allows the incubation of cells or cell particles under different atmospheres (e.g., different oxygen concentrations) (8).

Use of Cultured Cells

Cultured cells cannot be transferred to another flask and must therefore be analyzed for hydrocarbon formation directly in the cell culture flasks. This has also been applied in a number of studies on cellular lipid peroxidation (9–11). Cell culture flasks can be gassed with 95% O_2/5% CO_2 or with other oxygen concentrations through the cap. At the start of the experiment the culture flask can be made gastight by closing the cap, and compounds which may initiate lipid peroxidation can be added to the cells via the cap by sticking a needle through it. At various time intervals air samples can be removed from the head space, allowing fresh air to penetrate via the second needle (comparable to 12 in Fig. 2). The air samples are taken using a gastight syringe. The disadvantage of this method is the fact that only one sample can be taken from one cell culture flask due to change in air pressure by which laboratory air is taken up. This might be contaminated with hydrocarbons. This results not only in the need for a greater amount of flasks and therefore of cells, but also leads to a higher variability. Nevertheless, this is the only method to measure lipid peroxidation without disturbing the culture itself, because after sampling culturing can be continued and measurements of other parameters can be performed later.

Use of Isolated Perfused Organs

Mainly isolated perfused liver has been used to measure drug-induced lipid peroxidation and alkane production. The system has been described in detail elsewhere (2,12). In principle, the perfused organ is placed in a Plexiglas chamber with gastight inlets and outlets similar to those described above. The amounts of alkanes diffused into the surrounding air are measured. However, they are relatively low compared to the total amounts produced and vary depending on the organ as well as on the experimental conditions due to different tissue absorption and metabolism. Therefore, these systems cannot yet be recommended for *in vitro* studies of lipid peroxidation.

A relatively recent approach has been applied by using air-ventilated isolated perfused lung (13). But in this system no alkanes could be produced or measured under oxidative stress conditions in which they were expected to be. Therefore, this is also not yet a standardized model.

Analysis of Hydrocarbons

Ethane and *n*-pentane are quantified by gas chromatography. In most of the methods applied the other hydrocarbons formed (e.g., ethene, propane, butane, and isobutene) are separated simultaneously.

Because of the relatively high concentration of ethane and *n*-pentane in *in vitro* experiments the head space air of incubation or cell culture flasks can be directly injected into a gas chromatograph. Most authors use sample valves for this purpose. For example, we used 8 ml of head space air and injected it into a 5-ml valve (3). Others injected low volumes of air (0.5–1 ml) directly onto the column of the gas chromatograph (4,6,14,15). Another method involves concentrating the hydrocarbons in the sample either by freezing them in liquid nitrogen or by adsorbing them on particular phases such as activated charcoal followed by a heating step which transfers the hydrocarbons to the gas chromatograph (16–18). While this method is mainly applied during the measurement of ethane and *n*-pentane *in vivo,* when the concentrations are much lower, it might be adaptable for *in vitro* studies if additional sensitivity is desired.

A great number of different chromatographic columns and materials to separate the alkanes has been used, including silica gel, aluminium oxide (alumina), porasil C, porapack N, porapack Q, and others. Either stainless steel columns or capillary glass columns are used for gas chromatography. Here, the details cannot be given for all techniques applied and the reader is referred to the particular references, including our own (see below).

We have used in our recent experiments 2-m stainless steel columns (0.25 inch) filled with aluminum oxide (Sigma, Munich, Germany) which has specially been treated (filtering, acid treatment, and drying) (19). The carrier gas was N_2 (2.6 bar) and the oven temperature was 90°C for ethane or 170°C for *n*-pentane. The retention times of the two hydrocarbons were 0.9 and 2.9 min, respectively. They were detected by flame ionization. All other methods used the same detector. With our method using 5-ml head space gas, concentrations of 10 vpb ethane or *n*-pentane, respectively, could be detected.

COMMENTS

The major pitfalls of hydrocarbon measurements to study lipid peroxidation are the following.

1. Ethane and *n*-pentane originate from specific unsaturated fatty acids and their amount formed during lipid peroxidation can change due to different fatty acid composition (20).

2. Ethane and *n*-pentane are only minor products of lipid peroxidation and therefore may not reflect the total process (20).

3. The formation of ethane and *n*-pentane is dependent on oxygen; that is, high oxygen concentrations inhibit their formation, whereas another parameter malondialdehyde increases with increasing oxygen concentrations (8,21).

4. The alkanes ethane and *n*-pentane can be bound to various tissues and biological molecules and therefore mostly only an aliquot produced is measured in the head space air. This is more relevant for *n*-pentane because of its lower volatility (2,10) and therefore the amount formed may be underestimated.

5. *n*-Pentane can be metabolized by cytochrome P-450, but this effect is not constant and depends on the cell system used as well as the conditions applied (2,19,20,22,23). Therefore, it may not be as reliable or sensitive as ethane.

6. Sampling of the head space air is changing the incubation conditions. This leads to a change in the equilibrium between the cell suspension or incubation mixture and the head space air. Taking smaller gas volumes would minimize this change, but would also decrease the sensitivity of the measurement.

7. If the system described here is not used and airtightness of the flasks during incubation and sampling is not guaranteed, it can often not be avoided that hydrocarbons present in the surrounding air are taken up during sampling.

8. When the hydrocarbons produced are concentrated on an adsorbent, the results can be too low due to incomplete adsorption or release during the heating step.

Although especially ethane and *n*-pentane are easily measurable and can be quantified simply, the results obtained with this method must be interpreted with much caution. The technology has been satisfactorily developed, but the biological meaning of the results, especially in regard to quantitative aspects of hydrocarbon formation, is not completely understood. For qualitative measurements in toxicology, hydrocarbon formation is a good indicator for lipid peroxidation. But no one should rely on this method alone.

REFERENCES

1. C. Riely, G. Cohen, and M. Lieberman, *Science* **183,** 208 (1974).
2. A. Müller and H. Sies, *in* "Methods in Enzymology" (L. Packer, ed.), Vol. 105, p. 311. Academic Press, Orlando, Florida, 1984.
3. H. Kappus and H. Muliawan, *Biochem. Pharmacol.* **31,** 597 (1982).
4. M. R. Clemens, H. Remmer, and H. D. Waller, *Biochem. Pharmacol.* **33,** 1715 (1984).
5. R. Reiter and A. Wendel, *Biochem. Pharmacol.* **32,** 665 (1983).

6. M. T. Smith, H. Thor, P. Hartzell, and S. Orrenius, *Biochem. Pharmacol.* **31,** 19 (1982).
7. N. H. Stacey and H. Kappus, *J. Toxicol. Environ. Health* **9,** 277 (1982).
8. J. Kostrucha and H. Kappus, *Biochim. Biophys. Acta* **879,** 120 (1986).
9. N. de Ruiter, H. Muliawan, and H. Kappus, *Toxicology* **17,** 265 (1980).
10. N. de Ruiter, H. Ottenwälder, H. Muliawan, and H. Kappus, *Arch. Toxicol.* **49,** 265 (1982).
11. N. H. Stacey, H. Ottenwälder, and H. Kappus, *Toxicol. Appl. Pharmacol.* **62,** 421 (1982).
12. S. Dutta, A. Müller, T. Ishikawa, M. Zimmer, and H. Sies, *Toxicol. Lett.* **44,** 55 (1988).
13. W. Seeger, N. E. M. Remy, and H. Neuhof, *Exp. Lung Res.* **14,** 387 (1988).
14. V. C. Gavino, C. J. Dillard, and A. L. Tappel, *Arch. Biochem. Biophys.* **233,** 741 (1984).
15. J. G. Goddard, D. Basford, and G. D. Sweeney, *Biochem. Pharmacol.* **35,** 2381 (1986).
16. G. A. A. Kivits, M. A. C. R. Ganguli-Swarttouw, and E. J. Christ, *Biochim. Biophys. Acta* **665,** 559 (1981).
17. G. D. Lawrence and G. Cohen, *in* "Methods in Enzymology" (L. Packer, ed.), Vol. 105, p. 305. Academic Press, Orlando, Florida, 1984.
18. O. M. Pitkänen, M. Hallman, and S. M. Andersson, *Lipids* **24,** 157 (1989).
19. J. G. Filser, H. M. Bolt, H. Muliawan, and H. Kappus, *Arch. Toxicol.* **52,** 135 (1983).
20. H. Kappus, *in* "Oxidative Stress" (H. Sies, ed.), p. 273, Academic Press, Orlando, Florida, 1985.
21. R. Reiter and R. F. Burk, *Biochem. Pharmacol.* **36,** 925 (1987).
22. H. Remmer, T. Hintze, H. Frank, and M. Müh-Zange, *Xenobiotica* **14,** 207 (1984).
23. S. R. B. Allerheiligen, T. M. Ludden, and R. F. Burk, *Drug Metab. Dispos.* **15,** 794 (1987).

32 Electronically Excited State Formation

Enrique Cadenas, Cecilia Giulivi, Fulvio Ursini, and Alberto Boveris

INTRODUCTION

Lipid hydroperoxides are the primary products of lipid peroxidation (see Refs. 1 and 2) originating upon attack of polyunsaturated fatty acids by species which can circumvent the spin barrier between the singlet multiplicity of polyunsaturated fatty acids and the triplet multiplicity of ground state O_2 (i.e., by $^1O_2$ or free radicals). Lipid peroxide formation during polyunsaturated fatty acid autoxidation entails the well-known sequence of initiation and propagation reactions (3). The divinyl methane structure (—CH=CH—CH_2—CH=CH—), present in all polyunsaturated fatty acids, is particularly susceptible to H abstraction, resulting in the formation of a lipid alkyl radical ($R^{\cdot}$), which reacts at diffusion-controlled rates with O_2 to form lipid peroxyl radicals ($ROO^{\cdot}$). Subsequent propagation reactions ($ROO^{\cdot} + RH \rightarrow ROOH + R^{\cdot}$) yield lipid peroxides. Conversely, the most likely chain-initiating reactions involving lipid hydroperoxides may be their metal-catalyzed homolytic scission leading to alkoxyl radical formation ($ROOH + M^n \rightarrow RO^{\cdot} + HO^- + M^{n+1}$); this reaction is of particular importance in a nonpolar medium in which the fatty acid chains would be located and in which the chelated metal ions could be dispersed (4).

Thus, lipid peroxyl and alkoxyl radicals are obligatory intermediates in the progression steps leading to lipid hydroperoxide formation. These electrophilic radicals are also formed during reactions other than those involved in fatty acid oxidation, such as lipoxygenase-catalyzed reactions, conversion of lipid hydroperoxides to different products mediated by hematin or organic peroxide/hematin mixtures, and hemoprotein-mediated peroxide breakdown.

Regardless of the process leading to the formation of secondary peroxyl and alkoxyl radicals, their recombination—within the context of termination reactions—is likely to be a major source of electronically excited states of singlet and/or triplet multiplicity. The relaxation of an excited state (P^*) to the ground state with emission of a photon [$P^* \rightarrow P + h\nu$], a process often observed in connection with certain oxidative biological reactions, is termed low-level chemiluminescence, dark chemiluminescence, or ultraweak chemiluminescence, thus named to differentiate this phenomenon from the photoemission of the luciferin–luciferase systems, which is 10^3-10^6-fold brighter. Therefore, for the

METHODS IN TOXICOLOGY, Volume 1B

systems referred to here, low-level chemiluminescence is a functional manifestation of free radical biochemical reactions encompassing electronically excited state generation.

The formation of excited species during polyunsaturated fatty acid peroxidation or peroxide breakdown is apparently a common feature to diverse forms of cellular injury (5–7). Among the electronically excited states, $^1O_2$ and triplet carbonyls seem to contribute largely to the process of biological chemiluminescence. Although there are no quantitative studies referring to the actual contribution of these species to oxidative reactions, the possibility exists that they are generated in high yields, but they are almost totally physically quenched; conversely, their generation may represent minor side reactions.

The detection of low-level chemiluminescence, stemming from oxidative free radical reactions, requires a particular methodology, which has been described previously (7–9). This survey provides a brief description of the apparatus required for the detection of low-level chemiluminescence and its manifold applications, along with a discussion on the likely mechanisms leading to the formation of electronically excited states during lipid peroxidation and peroxide breakdown.

METHODOLOGY

Single Photon-Counting Apparatus

The photon-counting apparatus used for these studies (Fig. 1) consists of a red-sensitive photomultiplier cooled to −40°C by a thermoelectric cooler (FACT 50 MKIII, EMI Gencom, Plainview, NY) in order to reduce the dark current. Suitable photomultipliers with an S-20 response (usually 300–800 nm) are EMI 9658AM (10) and 9814 (11), RCA4832 and 8852 (RCA, Lancaster, PA) (12),

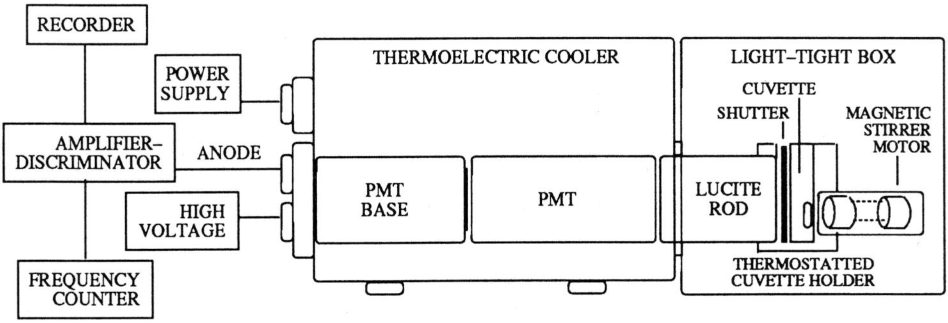

Figure 1 Single photon-counting apparatus for the measurement of low-level chemiluminescence. [Modified from Boveris *et al.* (10).]

and Hamamatsu HTV R374, R375, R550, and R878 (Hamamatsu Photonics, Hamamatsu City, Japan) (13–15). The applied potential to the photomultiplier varies between −0.9 and −1.2 kV (dark current 20–80 counts/sec.) The phototube output is connected to an amplifier discriminator (EG&G Princeton Applied Research, Princeton, NJ) adjusted for single photon counting and connected to both a frequency counter (8–10) and a recorder or oscilloscope. Efficient light gathering and thermal isolation from the sample are established by using a Lucite rod (8–10) as optical coupler or an ellipsoidal light reflector (13). A shutter allows continuous operation of the photomultiplier in order to remain dark adapted. Recently, the application of multichannel plate and position sensitive detector to studies of ultraweak light emission of biological materials permitted the first observation of tissue-specific localization of photon emission *in situ* as well as the first well-resolved spectra of some ultraweak emission processes (16). The two-dimensional photon counting may considerably amplify the potential of single photon-counting imaging in chemiluminescence research inasmuch as it provides a means to obtain information about the spatial distribution of ultraweak emission intensity in tissues (16).

Photoemissive Systems

The single photon-counting apparatus shown in Fig. 1 can be adjusted easily to monitor continuously photoemission from several *in vitro* and *in vivo* experimental models. Thus, placed inside a lighttight box and facing the optical coupler could be (8–10): (a) a thermostatted cuvette equipped with a magnetic stirrer to maintain homogeneous suspensions (Fig. 1); the cuvette lid contains ports for an oxygen electrode—thus allowing simultaneous monitoring of oxygen uptake and low-level chemiluminescence—and for required tubings which facilitate gas exchange or injection of reactants to the reaction mixture without interruption of the measurements. This operating mode permits experiments with isolated cells, subcellular organelles, enzymic reactions, etc. (b) Perfused organs [e.g., liver (10,17), heart (18–20), or lung (21,22)] can be placed as close as possible to the end of the Lucite rod/optical coupler. In general, oxidative stress conditions are imposed on the perfused organs and chemiluminescence is monitored continuously for extended periods. (c) A similar approach as above is used for studies of exposed organ surfaces *in situ*. In the latter instances excited species could be detected from a 0.05-mm thickness of the organ surface (value observed for 50% transmittance against tissue thickness), and hence, total area exposed as well as minimization of dark current values are critical for ample evaluation of organ chemiluminescence. The spontaneous photoemission from the *in situ* perfused liver is a linear function of the exposed organ area (23).

Identification of Excited States

The detection of photoemission in the conditions described above only indicates that the formation of electronically excited states is a functional manifestation of oxidative conditions. However, in order to understand the molecular mechanisms underlying the formation of excited species, three approaches—whose applicability depends on the experimental models—are desirable: (a) to establish a correlation between electronically excited state formation and accumulation of stable molecular products (24); (b) by evaluating sensitized emission, that is, assessing the feasibility of energy transfer to different acceptors to gather knowledge on the nature and mechanisms of formation of excited carbonyl compounds (25,26) and (c) to identify the wavelength(s) of maximal chemiluminescence emission, which could be attributed to a particular excited state.

For spectral analysis of emitted light, optical filters are placed into the light path and, according to the type of filter used, a broad or rather resolved spectral distribution of photoemission can be obtained. Thus, interference filters, having a narrow bandwidth (8–22 nm), are expected to allow for a more resolved spectral analysis of chemiluminescence. However, because of their low transmission value (usually 45–55%), their use would be restricted to those systems with high chemiluminescence yield. Alternatively, cutoff filters, consisting of colored glass (Toshiba Electric, Minato-ku-Tokyo, Japan, or Jenaer Glaswerke Schott, Mainz, Germany) or gelatin filters (Wratten gelatin filters, Eastman-Kodak, Rochester, NY), provide a 1–99% transmission range. The use of cutoff filters does not provide a satisfactory spectral resolution, but it offers a rather valuable clue as to the maximal wavelength of photoemission. The difference between the spectral characteristics of two successive cutoff filters [i.e., $\Delta F_{1,2}(\lambda) = F_1(\lambda) - F_2(\lambda)$] is corrected for the transmittance characteristics of the filters and for the photomultiplier tube quantum efficiency at that particular wavelength (27).

Although low-level chemiluminescence, if aided by spectral analysis, can point to the involvement of a particular excited species, the task becomes much more problematic with increasing complexity of the biological system. Photoemission from living systems exhibits an intricate spectral distribution, thus revealing that light emission might be more complex than that observed in the relaxation of a sole excited state to the ground state. Therefore, the unambiguous identification of the main excited species, whose relaxation yields chemiluminescence, is likely to require the assistance of the technical approaches described above, along with those pertaining to the particular chemistry with which the excited state is endowed, such as its chemical reactivity and specific quenching.

FORMATION OF ELECTRONICALLY EXCITED STATES DURING LIPID PEROXIDATION

The low-level chemiluminescence accompanying the autoxidation- or lipoxygenase-catalyzed oxidation of fatty acids along with the decomposition of lipid hydroperoxides by hematin or the high oxidation state of hemoproteins has been generally interpreted in terms of the radiative decay of two electronically excited states: triplet carbonyls and/or singlet oxygen. The following is a survey of the molecular mechanisms leading to the generation of these excited species and their contribution to the overall process of unsaturated fatty acid oxidation.

Excited Carbonyls

Excited carbonyls can originate (a) from free radical recombination reactions involving peroxyl or alkoxyl radicals generated during the free radical chain propagation of polyunsaturated fatty acid autoxidation and (b) from the breakdown of a dioxetane intermediate.

Peroxyl and Alkoxyl Radical Recombination

Sources of peroxyl radical include the propagation steps of polyunsaturated fatty acid oxidation, that is, the quenching of the carbon-centered radical by molecular O_2 [reaction (1)]. Alternative pathways involve H abstraction of a lipid hydroperoxide

$$R^{\cdot} + O_2 \longrightarrow ROO^{\cdot} \qquad (1)$$

by (a) an oxoferryl complex ($Fe^{IV} = O$) [reaction (2a)], the ubiquitous nature of which—even at relatively low levels—implies that it could be a quantitatively important catalyst of hydroperoxide metabolism in mammalian cells or an Fe^{III} complex [reaction (2b)], and (b) alkoxyl radicals [reaction (3)]. The latter radicals are produced during the metal ion- and lipoxygenase-catalyzed breakdown of

$$ROOH + [Fe^{IV}{=}O] \longrightarrow ROO^{\cdot} + Fe^{III} + H_2O \qquad (2a)$$

$$ROOH + Fe^{III} \longrightarrow ROO^{\cdot} + H^{+} + Fe^{II} \qquad (2b)$$

$$ROOH + RO^{\cdot} \longrightarrow ROO^{\cdot} + ROH \qquad (3)$$

peroxidized fatty acids by one-electron reductive cleavage of hydroperoxides [reaction (4)] (28).

$$ROOH + Fe^{II} \longrightarrow RO^{\cdot} + HO^{-} + Fe^{III} \quad (4)$$

Alkoxyl radicas can undergo a number of competing reactions (28), including H abstraction from hydroperoxides or fatty acids to yield peroxyl radicals [reaction (3)] or carbon-centered radicals [reaction (5)], respectively.

$$RO^{\cdot} + RH \longrightarrow ROH + R^{\cdot} \quad (5)$$

Peroxyl radicals, formed by any of the mechanisms outlined above, can participate in recombination reactions, which proceed via a tetroxide intermediate with elimination of a ketone, an alcohol, and O_2. The disproportionation of peroxyl radicals is concerted (29): (a) Since the reaction exothermicity is ~115–150 kcal and the energy of the carbonyl is commonly 75–80 kcal (S_1 and T_1 state of acetone), a concerted reaction is virtually required to concentrate the energy in the ketone fragment, at least for those events leading to chemiluminescence; (b) the termination rate constant for secondary peroxyl radicals is 10^3-fold faster than for tertiary peroxyl radicals, in which there is no α-hydrogen, and it decreases by a factor of 1.9 with deuteration. A rationalization of this sequence of events can be explained by the accompanying Russell diagram (30) in Fig. 2.

To obtain an excited state, the reaction exothermicity must be concerted in the carbonyl fragment. The concerted fragmentation then gives singlet ground-state alcohol and triplet ground-state O_2. To satisfy selection rules, the excited carbonyl must be of triplet multiplicity (29). The product distribution resulting from secondary peroxyl radical recombination is conventionally written as in reaction (6). The annihilation of alkoxyl radicals is an additional source of triplet ketones (31), according to reaction (7).

$$ROO^{\cdot} + ROO^{\cdot} \longrightarrow ROH + {}^3[RO]^* + {}^3O_2 \quad (6)$$

$$RO^{\cdot} + RO^{\cdot} \longrightarrow {}^3[RO]^* + ROH \quad (7)$$

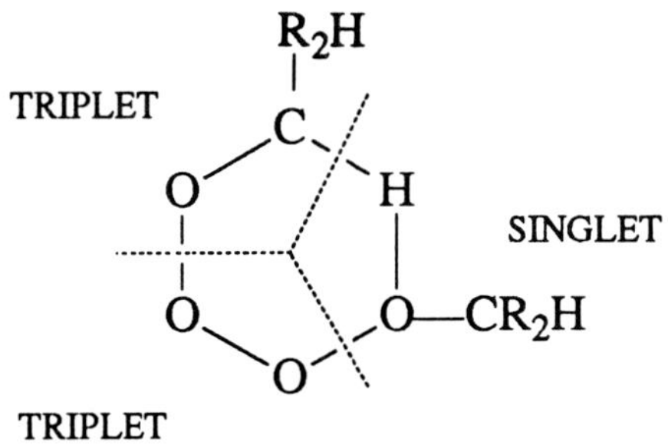

Figure 2 Russell diagram.

Cleavage of Dioxetane Intermediates

An alternative route for excited carbonyl formation during lipd peroxidation was proposed to encompass dioxetane thermolysis as in reaction (8). Although

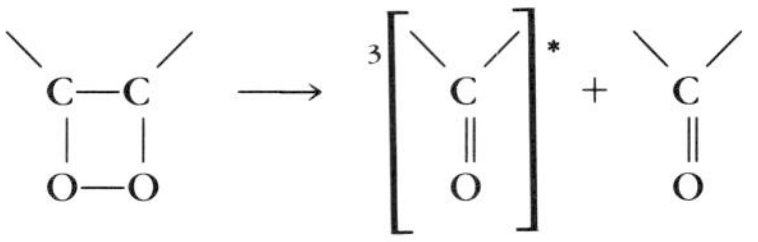

(8)

in several instances excited carbonyls are expected to be formed through the cleavage of a hypothetical dioxetane intermediate, the occurrence of the latter during lipid peroxidation is questionable (32), for the (2 + 2) cycloaddition of singlet oxygen to electron-poor olefins, such as unsaturated fatty acids [reaction (9)], is an unlikely event. The main product following the photooxygenation of lionoleate is the corresponding allylic hydroperoxide, which undergoes the so-called Hock cleavage upon treatment with Lewis acids to yield the same carbonyl fragments as those obtained from the thermolysis of a dioxetane [reaction (8)], but in the ground state (32).

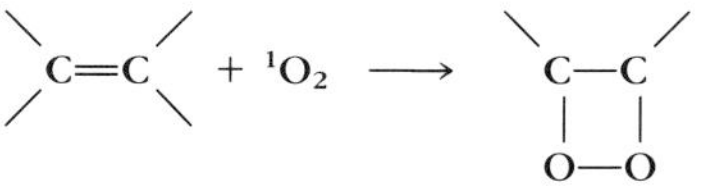

(9)

Despite this, excited carbonyls of different energy levels are formed during lipid peroxidation, as attested by the energetic requirements for excitation of different acceptors (33). The triplet excited carbonyls generated during the peroxidase/oxidase activity of soybean lipoxygenase are possibly formed from a transition-state analog to a 1,2-dioxetane (34).

The relative value of triple carbonyl yield from the sources described above was reported to decrease in the order of precursor dioxetane [reaction (8)] > alkoxyl pair [reaction (7)] > peroxyl pair [reaciton (6)] (35).

Triplet carbonyls can abstract H from fatty acid moieties in lipid structures [reaction (10] (36) in

$$^{3}[>C{=}O]^{*} + RH \longrightarrow >C^{\cdot}OH + R^{\cdot} \qquad (10)$$

a fashion similar to alkoxyl radicals [reaciton (5)] (36) and related to the number secondary, allylic, and doubly allylic H atoms in the fatty acids. The fate of the fatty acid radical ($R^{\cdot}$) formed as in reaction could be envisaged in terms of its rapid quenching by O_2 [reaction (1)], thus suggesting that triplet species—generated during the termination reactions of lipid peroxidation—could contribute to the propagation steps of this process. Of note, the rates of chemical quenching of $^1O_2$ by these fatty acids (37) are significantly smaller than the rates of H-abstraction by triplet carbonyls (38).

Singlet Oxygen

The formation of $^1O_2$ during recombination of peroxyl radicals can be further explained by a more efficient quenching of the triplet carbonyl by the O_2 eliminated in the reaction and retained in the solvent cage [reaction (11)]. The rate of triple–triplet transfer quenching in the solvent cage has been estimated as $\sim 10^{11}$ sec^{-1} (29). However, the yield of $^1O_2$ from reaction (12) amounts to ~4–14% (39,40), whereas triplet carbonyls are the predominant excited state originating from the annihilation of secondary peroxyl [reaction (6)] or alkoxyl radicals [reaction (7)]. The overall formation of $^1O_2$ during peroxyl radical disproportionation is usually written as in reaction (12).

$$^3[RO]^* + {}^3O_2\,[cage] \longrightarrow RO + {}^1O_2 \qquad (11)$$

$$ROO^{\cdot} + ROO^{\cdot} \longrightarrow ROH + RO + {}^1O_2 \qquad (12)$$

LIPID PEROXIDATION AND LOW-LEVEL CHEMILUMINESCENCE

After the pioneering work of Howes and Steele (41) on chemiluminescence associated with microsomal lipid peroxidation, the selective use of specific quenchers and sensitizers and spectral analysis led other investigators to draw attention to two excited species formed during the process: singlet molecular oxygen ($^1O_2$) and triplet carbonyls. However, spectral analysis of chemiluminescence arising from systems involving unsaturated fatty acid oxidation reveals a complex structure, which suggests the contribution of a variety of excited species of different multiplicities as well as distinct mechanisms for their generation.

Excited triplet carbonyls—generated during lipid peroxidation by the mechanisms outlined above—can emit phosphorescence in the visible region [reaction (13)]. Conversely, singlet oxygen ($^1\Delta O_2$) emits in the infrared [reaction (14)] and red [reaction (15)] regions, encompassing its monomol and dimol (a one-photon two-molecule collisionally induced process) emissions, respectively.

$$^3[>C{=}O]^* \longrightarrow\ >C{=}O + h\nu_{380-450\ nm} \qquad (13)$$

$$^1\Delta O_2 \longrightarrow {}^3\textstyle\sum O_2 + h\nu_{1270\ nm} \qquad (14)$$

$$2\ {}^1\Delta O_2 \longrightarrow 2\ {}^3\textstyle\sum O_2 + h\nu_{633\ nm} \qquad (15)$$

The weak emission arising from triplet or singlet carbonyls on decaying to the ground state takes place around 380–450 nm. This excitation can be emitted directly [reaction (13)] or transferred to a fluorophor. In some systems the formation of triplet species might be reasonably postulated to occur, although the presence of O_2 (an efficient quencher of triplet species with a cellular concentration of $\sim 10^{-4}$ *M*) makes the identification of these triplet species difficult.

Alternatively, the occurrence of excited carbonyl compounds can be attested by excitation upon energy transfer to adequate acceptors (24–26): Molecules with heavy atoms, such as 9,10-dibromoanthracene (DBA), are capable of accepting excitation energy of a chemienergized triplet carbonyl product and release it in the form of fluorescence. The overall mechanism can be considered a triplet–singlet energy transfer that leads to the observed fluorescence, although it presumably involves the intermediate formation of a T_2 state of the fluorophor, which decays to the S_1 state by intersystem crossing. Triplet–singlet energy transfer would be the dominant mechanism in the case of "heavy atom"-substituted anthracenes [e.g., DBA or its water-soluble adduct, 9,10-dibromoanthracene-2-sulphonate (DBAS)] [reactions (16) and (17)], whereas singlet–singlet

$$^{3}[{>}C{=}O]^{*} + DBA \longrightarrow {>}C{=}O + {}^{1}DBA^{*} \qquad (16)$$

$$^{1}DBA^{*} \longrightarrow DBA + h\nu_{fl} \qquad (17)$$

energy transfer predominates in the case of non-heavy atom-substituted anthracenes (e.g., diphenylanthracene). Thus, the triplet nature of a carbonyl compound could be further attested by the failure to excite acceptors which lack the "heavy" atom necessary for spin exchange (24–26).

The DBA and chlorophyll *a*-sensitized emission from the arachidonate/lipoxygenase is $\sim 10^3$-fold higher than in the absence of sensitizers (33). Since both acceptors have different energy requirements to populate their fluorescence state, two possible mechanisms for the generation of triplet carbonyl can be envisaged. First, free radical interactions yielding conjugated carbonyl compounds (Fig. 3) have enough energy to promote chlorophyll *a*-sensitized emission [$\Delta E(S_1)_{\text{chlorophyll } a} = 41.5$ kcal/mol] (42).

Second, the excited carbonyls formed during the lipoxygenase-catalyzed oxidation of arachidonate are able to excite DBAS [$\Delta E(S_1)_{DBAS} = 70.2$ kcal/mol] (33). This suggests the formation of excited carbonyls with energy higher as those formed during the recombination of peroxyl radicals [reaction (12)] (Fig. 3). The peroxidase/oxidase activity of soybean lipoxygenase would account for this finding in terms of a mechanism comprising the ferric and ferrous states of the enzyme in a catalytic cycle and leading to the formation of a transient state analog to a 1,2-dioxetane, which cleaves to generated unconjugated carbonyls (34).

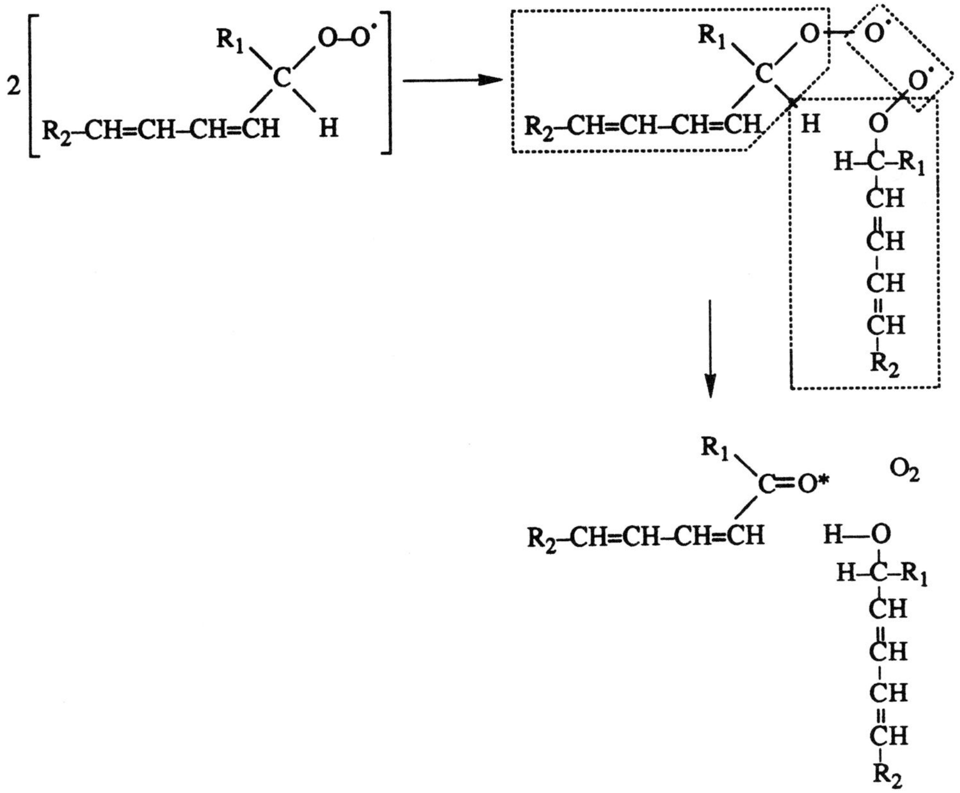

Figure 3 Generation of conjugated triplet carbonyls upon recombination of lipid peroxyl radicals.

In addition, the sensitization of diphenylanthracene, DBAS, eosin, and rose bengal during microsomal lipid peroxidation (42,43) and the lipoxygenase-catalyzed oxidation of linoleate (42) suggest that singlet carbonyls are also formed. Of note, if lipoxygenase also has a weak secondary peroxidase/oxidase activity, the nonconjugated aldehyde may react to yield the next lower aldehyde in the triplet state (34). These findings point to a variety of excited species of different multiplicity formed during the fatty acid oxidation (42).

The generation of $^1O_2$ during microsomal lipid peroxidation (43) and during the degradation of a mixture of 13-hydroperoxylinoleate and linoleate by soybean lipoxygenase-3 (44) has been confirmed spectroscopically in terms of dimol [reaction (15)] and monomol [reaction (14)] emission, respectively. $^1O_2$ generation was explained in both instances in terms of the bimolecular reaction of peroxyl radicals within termination reaction [reaction (12)].

Table I Lipid Peroxidation and Low-Level Chemiluminescence

System	Initiator/catalyst	Reference
Unsaturated fatty acids		
Arachidonic, linolenic, and linoleic	Soybean lipoxygenase	33,34,42
Linoleic and oleic	Hemoprotein/H_2O_2	47
13-Hydroperoxylinoleate/ 15-hydroperoxyarachidonate	Fe^{III}–bleomycin/methemoglobin	48
13-Hydroperoxylinoleate/linoleate	Soybean lipoxygenase	44
Microsomal membranes	NADPH	41,49,50
	NADPH/ADP–Fe	46,51,52
	Ascorbate/ADP–Fe	53
	Organic hydroperoxides	42,54–57
	Indole acetate/horseradish peroxidase	58
Mitochondrial membranes	Ascorbate/ADP–Fe	59
	Organic hydroperoxides	60
	Acetaldehyde/Cu^{2+}	61
Cells		
Hepatocytes	Hyperoxia	62
Erythrocytes	Xanthine/xanthine oxidase	63
Tissue homogenates		
Liver	Lipid hydroperoxides	64,65
	Organic hydroperoxides	66
	CCl_4	67
Brain	Hyperoxia	66,68
	Organic hydroperoxides	66
	Ascorbate/hemoglobin	69
	2,2′-Azi-bis-(2-amidinopropane)	70
Lymphoid	Methyl linoleate hydroperoxide	71

The molecular mechanisms summarized above would be operative in different cellular oxidative situations associated with lipid peroxidation and have been inferred (to a different extent) in a variety of biological chemiluminescence models. Table I lists some of these models in terms of oxidative impairment of phospholipids in microsomal and mitochondrial membranes, cell suspensions, and tissue homogenates caused by metal complexes in the presence of NADPH or ascorbate, enzymatically generated triplet species, during the heterolytic or homolygic cleavage of organic hydroperoxides by cytochrome P_{450} and other hemoproteins, and other oxidative conditions, such as hyperoxia and metabolism of CCl_4.

A correlation between the formation of electronically excited states—detected as low-level chemiluminescence—and other parameters for lipid peroxidation, such as the formation of thiobarbituric acid-reactive material, diene conjugates, lipid peroxides, and fluorescent pigments, is difficult to establish and certainly cannot be accounted for by a single molecular mechanism. An attempt to present some correlations between low-level chemiluminescence and other parameters of lipid peroxidation has been presented (9,45,46) and appears to be dependent on the type of lipid peroxidation model with emphasis on the catalyst or initiator. More detailed discussions regarding particular peroxidation models can be found in the pertaining references in Table I (33, 34, 41, 42, 44, 46–71).

COMMENTS

The oxidative impairment of membrane phospholipids is associated with the formation of electronically excited states. Several aspects of this phenomenon need further comments.

First, these excited states may be generated in low yields, representing a small part of the product of free radical termination reactions. In addition, the detection of low-level chemiluminescence during lipid peroxidation processes may reflect only one of several decay pathways of the excited states (i.e., radiative decay). Alternatively, the excited species could be totally or partially physically quenched, transfer energy to adequate acceptors, or—depending on their chemical reactivity—react with different cellular constituents. In the latter instances the H-abstraction reactivity of triplet carbonyls toward polyunsaturated fatty acids (38) [reaction (10)] may be of significance to the overall process of lipid peroxidation, for these species, which are formed int he termination steps [reactions (6) and (7)], could subsequently act as chain carriers within the propagation reactions.

Second, since oxidative impairment of membrane phospholipids is a feature often encountered in several forms of oxidative stress, it is conceivable that the photoemission from tissue homogenates and exposed organs originates at least partly from excited states formed by the free radical chain oxidation of polyunsaturated fatty acids. However, the photoemission associated with redox cycling of quinones (72), mitomycin C (73), and paraquat (74) as well as that originating from the interaction of several oxene donors with microsomes or isolated cytochrome P_{450} (75) is not accompanied by lipid peroxidation. Whether the photoemission arising from perfused or *in situ* organs and tissue homogenates during treatment with doxorubicins (76,77) shares similar characteristics remains to be evaluated.

Third, the apparent occurrence of oxy-radicals in several pathological disorders led to the development of *in vivo* (or closely related) experimental models, which permit the examination of cellular oxidative changes and the test of different drugs. In this regard low-level chemiluminescence offers noninvasive and continuous monitoring of electronically excited state formation and, hence, "indirectly," an assessment of oxy-radical recombination reactions. Thus, the allopurinol- and superoxide dismutase-sensitive spontaneous chemiluminescence (78) or sensitized chemiluminescence (79) from intestine or liver (80) following reperfusion indicates the requirement of O_2 to observe photoemission and the participation of $O_2^{\overline{\cdot}}$ in some step leading to the formation of an excited product. The increased ultraweak chemiluminescence from rat heart during postischemic reoxygenation was sensitive to the tissue content of α-tocopherol (81). Also, the increase in tissue spontaneous chemiluminescence from intact animals fed a diet containing lipid hydroperoxides (82–84) and during chronic alcoholism treatment (85) as well as the effect on it of dietary antioxidants, such as ascorbate and vitamin E (86), suggests some relationship of this parameter to lipid peroxidation.

However, when oxidative stress conditions are not imposed on cells, spontaneous chemiluminescence might not reflect a base level of lipid peroxidation, but the steady-state concentration of H_2O_2. Thus, the spontaneous photoemission from isolated rat hepatocytes treated with aminotriazol (an inhibitor of catalase) is related to the square concentration of the intracellular steady-state concentration of H_2O_2 (87). The latter was calculated, taking into account that the extent of inhibition of catalase activity by aminotriazol corresponded to a H_2O_2 concentration equal to the reciprocal of remaining activity (the relationship chemiluminescence = K $[H_2O_2]^2$ yielded an experimental K value of 7×10^{-9} M^{-1} S^{-1}, similar to the theoretical value [$K = 3.5 \times 10^{-9}$ M^{-1} s^{-1}] (87).

Monitoring luminescence from *in vivo* or *in vitro* models has shown that this technique is useful for the noninvasive evaluation of cellular oxidative stress, as indicated by the increased emission in tumor-bearing mice (88), from α-tocopherol- and selenium-deficient rat liver (89), from *in situ* liver upon chloroform anesthesia (90) and actue (91) and chronic (92) ethanol intoxication, form betamethasone effects on paraquat lung toxicity (93), and by the decreased emission of *in situ* liver by certain flavonoid antioxidants (94).

REFERENCES

1. F. Ursini and A. Sevanian, *in* "Oxidative Stress: Oxidants and Antioxidants" (H. Sies, ed.), p. 319. Academic Press, San Diego, 1991.
2. S. D. Aust and B. A. Svingen, *in* "Free Radicals in Biology" (W. A. Pryor, ed.), Vol. 5, p. 1. Academic Press, New York, 1982.
3. N. Porter, *in* "Membrane Lipid Oxidation" (C. Vigo-Pelfrey, ed.), Vol. 1, p. 33. CRC Press, Boca Raton, Florida, 1990.
4. J. F. Mead, *in* "Free Radicals in Biology" (W. A. Pryor, ed.), Vol. 1, p. 51 Academic Press, New York, 1976.
5. E. Cadenas, *Photochem. Photobiol.* **40,** 823 (1984).
6. D. Slawinska and J. Slawinski, *Photochem. Photobiol.* **37,** 709 (1983).
7. E. Cadenas, A. Boveris, and B. Chance, *in* "Free Radicals in Biology" (W. A. Pryor, ed.), Vol. 6, p. 212. Academic Press, Orlando, Florida, 1984.

8. E. Cadenas and H. Sies, *in* "Methods in Enzymology" (L. Packer, ed.), Vol. 105, p. 221. Academic Press, Orlando, Florida, 1984.
9. M. E. Murphy and H. Sies, *in* "Methods in Enzymology" (L. Packer and A. N. Glazer, eds.), Vol. 186, p. 595. Academic Press, San Diego, 1993.
10. A Boveris, E. Cadenas, and B. Chance, *Fed. Proc., Fed. Am. Soc. Exp. Biol.* **40,** 1985 (1981).
11. R. Barsacchi, P. Camici, U. Bottigli, P. A. Salvadori, G. Pelosi, M. Maiorino, and F. Ursini, *Biochim. Biophys. Acta* **762,** 241 (1983).
12. C. F. Deneke and N. I. Krinsky, *Photochem. Photobiol.* **25,** 299 (1977).
13. H. Inaba, Y. Shimizu, Y. Tsuji, and A. Zamagishi, *Photochem. Photobiol.* **30,** 169 (1979).
14. H. Inaba, *Experientia* **44,** 550 (1988).
15. H. Inaba, A. Yamagishi, C. Takyu, B. Yoda, Y. Goto, T. Miyazawa, T. Kaneda, and A. Saeki, *Optics Lasers Eng.* **3,** 125 (1982).
16. R. Q. Scott and H. Inaba, *J. Biolumin. Chemilumin.* **4,** 507 (1989).
17. H. Wefers and H. Sies, *Arch. Biochem. Biophys.* **224,** 568 (1983).
18. R. Barsacchi, G. Pelosi, P. Camici, L. Bonaldo, M. Maiorino, and F. Ursini, *Biochim. Biophys. Acta* **804,** 356 (1984).
19. F. Ursini, R. Barsacchi, G. Pelosi, and A. Benassi, *J. Biolumin. Chemilumin.* **4,** 241 (1989).
20. F. Ursini, G. Pelosi, G. Tomassi, A. Benassi, M. Di Felice, and R. Barsacchi, *Biochim. Biophys. Acta* **919,** 93 (1987).
21. E. Cadenas, I. D. Arad, A Boveris, A. B. Fisher, and B. Chance, *FEBS Lett.* **111,** 413 (1980).
22. E. Cadenas, I. D. Arad, A. B. Fisher, A. Boveris, and B. Chance, *Biochem. J.* **192,** 303 (1980).
23. B. Gonzalez-Flecha and A. Boveris, unpublished observations (1992).
24. G. Cilento, N. Durán, K. Zinner, C. C. C. Vidigal, O. M. M. Faria Oliveria, M. Haun, A. Faljoni, O. Augusto, R. Casadei de Baptista, and E. J. H. Bechara, *Photochem. Photobiol.* **28,** 445 (1978).
25. G. Cilento, *in* "Chemical and Biological Generation of Excited States" (W. Adam and G. Cilento, eds.), p. 278. Academic Press, New York, 1982.
26. G. Cilento, *Pure Appl. Chem.* **56,** 1179 (1984).
27. B. R. Andersen, T. F. Lint, and A. M. Brendzel, *Biochim. Biophys. Acta* **542,** 527 (1978).
28. J. Terao, *in* "Membrane Lipid Oxidation" (C. Vigo-Pelfrey, ed.), Vol. I, p. 219 CRC Press, Boca Raton, Florida, (1990).
29. R. E. Kellog, *J. Am. Chem. Soc.* **91,** 5433 (1969).
30. G. S. Russell, *J. Am. Chem. Soc.* **79,** 3871 (1957).
31. D. Phillips, V. Anissimov, O. Karpukhin, and V. Shliapintokh, *Nature (London)* **215,** 1163 (1967).
32. P. Di Mascio, L. H. Catalani, and E. J. H. Bechara, *Free Radical Biol. Med.* **12,** 471 (1992).
33. T. Schulte-Herbrüggen and E. Cadenas, *Photobiochem. Photobiophys.* **10,** 35 (1985).
34. T. Schulte-Herbrüggen and H. Sies, *Photochem. Photobiol.* **49,** 697 (1989).
35. G. D. Mendenhall and X. C. Sheng, *J. Am. Chem. Soc.* **113,** 8977 (1991).

36. R. D. Small, J. C. Scaiano, and L. K. Patterson, *Photochem. Photobiol.* **29,** 49 (1979).
37. F. H. Doleiden, S. R. Fahrenholtz, A. A. Lamola, and A. M. Trozzolo, *Photochem. Photobiol.* **20,** 519 (1974).
38. D. Z. Markovic and L. K. Patterson, *Photochem. Photobiol.* **49,** 531 (1989).
39. Q. J. Niu and G. D. Mendenhall, *J. Am. Chem. Soc.* **114,** 165 (1992).
40. Q. Niu and G. D. Mendenhall, *J. Am. Chem. Soc.* **112,** 1656 (1990).
41. R. M. Howes and R. H. Steele, *Res. Commun. Chem. Pathol. Pharmacol.* **2,** 619 (1971).
42. E. Rivas, D. Mira, G. Cilento, and A. Boveris, *in* "Superoxide and Superoxide Dismutase in Chemistry, Biology, and Medicine" (G. Rotilio, ed.), p. 108. Elsevier, Amsterdam, 1986.
43. K. Sugioka and M. Nakano, *Biochim. Biophys. Acta* **423,** 203 (1976).
44. J. R. Kanofsky and B. A. Axelrod, *J. Biol. Chem.* **261,** 1099 (1986).
45. M. Nakano, *in* "Membrane Lipid Oxidation" (C. Vigo-Pelfrey, ed.), Vol. 1, p. 181. CRC Press, Boca Raton, 1990.
46. T. Noll, H. de Groot, and H. Sies, *Arch. Biochem. Biophys.* **252,** 284 (1987).
47. E. Cadenas, A. Boveris, and B. Chance, *Biochem. J.* **188,** 577 (1980).
48. J. R. Kanofsky, *J. Biol. Chem.* **261,** 13546 (1986).
49. R. M. Howes and R. H. Steele, *Res. Commun. Chem. Pathol. Pharmacol.* **3,** 349 (1972).
50. A. R. Shoaf and R. H. Steele, *Biochem. Biophys. Res. Commun.* **61,** 1363 (1974).
51. M. Nakano, T. Noguchi, K. Sugioka, H. Fukuyama, M. Sato, Y. Shimizu, Y. Tsuji, and H. Inaba, *J. Biol. Chem.* **250,** 2404 (1975).
52. H. Wefers and H. Sies, *Eur. J. Biochem.* **174,** 353 (1988).
53. E. Cadenas, M. Ginsberg, U. Rabe, and H. Sies, *Biochem. J.* **223,** 755 (1984).
54. E. Cadenas and H. Sies, *Eur. J. Biochem.* **124,** 349 (1982).
55. E. Cadenas, H. Sies, H. Graf, and V. Ullrich, *Eur. J. Biochem.* **130,** 117 (1983).
56. B. S. Gonzalez Flecha, M. Repetto, P. Evelson, and A. Boveris, *Xenobiotica* **21,** 1013 (1991).
57. V. Narayanaswami and H. Sies, *Free Radical Res. Commun.* **10,** 237 (1990).
58. N. Durán, A. Campa, L. C. C. Leite, G. Cilento, and E. Cadenas, *Photobiochem. Photobiophys.* **11,** 281 (1986).
59. V. Narayanaswami and H. Sies. *Biochem. Pharmacol.* **40,** 1623 (1990).
60. E. Cadenas, A. Boveris, and B. Chance, *Biochem. J.* **186,** 659 (1980).
61. R. H. Steele, J. Sabic, R. R. Benerito, and S. W. O'Dea, *Arch. Biochem. Biophys.* **267,** 125 (1988).
62. E. Cadenas, H. Wefers, and H. Sies, *Eur. J. Biochem.* **119,** 531 (1981).
63. H. Yasuda, M. Miki, Y. Takenaka, H. Tamai, and M. Mino, *Arch. Biochem. Biophys.* **272,** 81, (1989).
64. T. Miyazawa, T. Kaneda, C. Takyu, A. Yamagishi, and H. Inaba, *Agric. Biol. Chem.* **45,** 1597 (1981).
65. T. Miyazawa, A. Nagaoka, and T. Kaneda, *Agric. Biol. Chem.* **47,** 1333 (1983).
66. E. Cadenas, A. I. Varsavsky, A. Boveris, and B. Chance, *Biochem. J.* **198,** 645 (1981).
67. T. Miyazawa, K. Tuschiya, and T. Kaneda, *Nutr. Rep. Int.* **29,** 157 (1984).
68. E. A. Lissi, T. Cáceres, and L. A. Videla, *J. Free Radical Biol. Med.* **2,** 63 (1986).
69. A. G. Pratt and J. F. Turrens, *Free Radical Biol. Med.* **8,** 319 (1990)

70. M. Faure, E. A. Lissi, and L. A.Videla, *Biochem. Int.* **21,** 357 (1990).
71. M. Oarada, E. Ito, Terao, T. Miyazawa, K. Fujimoto, and T. Kaneda, *Biochim. Biophys. Acta* **960,** 229 (1988).
72. H. Wefers and H. Sies. *Arch. Biochem. Biophys.* **224,** 568 (1983).
73. S. Napetschnig and H. Sies, *Biochem. Pharmacol.* **36,** 1617 (1987).
74. J. F. Turrens, C. Giulivi, C. R. Pinus, C. Lavagno, and A. Boveris, *Free Radical Biol. Med.* **5,** 319 (1988).
75. E. Cadenas, H. Sies, H. Graf, and V. Ullrich, *Eur. J. Biochem.* **130,** 117 (1983).
76. S. F. Llesuy, J. Milei, B. S. Gonzalez Flecha, and A. Boveris, *Free Radical Biol. Med.* **8,** 259 (1990).
77. J. Bustamante, M. Galleano, E. E. Medrano, and A. Boveris, *Breast Cancer Res. Treat.* **17,** 145 (1990).
78. J. F. Turrens, C. Giulivi, C. Pinus, E. Roldán, C. Lavagno, and A. Boveris, *in* "Oxygen Radicals in Biology and Medicine" (M. G. Simic, K. A. Tayulor, J. F. Ward, and C. von Sonntag, eds.), p. 239. Plenum, New York, 1988.
79. J. B. Morris, G. B. Bulkley, U. Haglund, E. Cadenas, and H. Sies, Proc. *Int. Congr. Oxygen Radicals, 4th* p. 67 (1987) (abstr.).
80. P. J. Cohen, *Ann. N. Y. Acad. Sci.* **625,** 821 (1991).
81. R. Barsacchi, M. Coassin, M. Maiorino, G. Pelosi, C. Simonelli, and F. Ursini, *Free Radical Biol. Med.* **6,** 573 (1989).
82. T. Miyazawa, T. Kaneda, C. Takyu, and H. Inaba, *J. Nutr. Sci. Vitaminol.* **29,** 53 (1983).
83. T. Miyazawa, C. Sato, and T. Kaneda, *Agric. Biol. Chem.* **47,** 1577 (1983).
84. T. Miyazawa, A. Nagaoka, and T. Kaneda, *Agric. Biol. Chem.* **47,** 1333 (1983).
85. A. Boveris, C. G. Fraga, A. I. Varsavsky, and O. R. Koch, *Arch. Biochem. Biophys.* **227,** 534 (1982).
86. T. Miyazawa, T. Ando, and T. Kaneda, *Agric. Biol. Chem.* **50,** 71 (1986).
87. C. Giulivi, Ph.D. dissertation. School of Pharmacy and Biochemistry, Universtiy of Buenos Aires, 1988.
88. A. Boveris, S. F. Llesuy, and C. G. Fraga, *J. Free Radical Biol. Med.* **1,** 131 (1985).
89. C. G. Fraga, V. S. Martino, G. E. Ferraro, J. D. Coussio, and A. Boveris, *Biochem. Pharmacol.* **36,** 717 (1987).
90. P. J. Cohen and B. Chance, *Biochim. Biophys. Acta* **884,** 517 (1986).
91. L. A. videla, C. G. Fraga, O. R. Koch, and A. Boveris, *Biochem. Pharmacol.* **32,** 2822 (1983).
92. V. D. Antonenkov and S. V. Pirozhkov, *Int. J. Biochem.* **23,** 153 (1991).
93. C. Lavagno, C. Giulivi, and A. Boveris, *Xenobiotica* **21,** 1003 (1991).
94. C. G. Fraga, R. F. Ariasf, S. F. Llesuy, O. R. Koch, and A. Boveris, *Biochem. J.* **242,** 383 (1987).

33 Spectrophotometric Detection of Lipid-Conjugated Dienes

Eric A. Glende, Jr., and Richard O. Recknagel†

Within the context of the study of basic mechanisms of cell injury, the possible occurrence of lipid peroxidation has attracted a great deal of attention. This is due in part to the wide range of toxicological and pathological situations in which lipid peroxidation is known to play a role. By way of example, lipid peroxidation is known to be involved in the toxicological mechanism of action of many xenobiotics (1); see Table 9-1 of Ref. 2 for a list of 30 xenobiotics known to initiate peroxidative decomposition of liver lipids. Lipid peroxidation is also known to play a role in the cell injury associated with inflammatory processes, shock, and spinal cord injury, in the liver injury associated with iron overload, and in the tissue injury occasioned by ischemia followed by reflow (2). Lipid peroxidation has also been implicated in the biochemistry of the aging process, and in certain instances of carcinogenesis.

From an operational point of view, an important point is that once it can be established for a particular instance of cell injury that lipid peroxidation is involved, the investigator is provided with a range of new opportunities, not only for further analysis of the mechanisms of the cell injury, but also for possible pharmaceutical intervention. For these and related reasons there naturally has been a continuing interest in the availability of methods for the detection and quantitative estimation of the extent of lipid peroxidation in cells and tissues. These methods include the thiobarbituric acid (TBA) reaction for detection of malonic dialdehyde, chromatographic methods for detection of 4-hydroxyalkenals, detection of volatile hydrocarbon breakdown products of peroxidized lipids, chemiluminescence, gas chromatographic–mass spectrophotometric detection of lipid hydroperoxide intermediates, and detection of lipid-conjugated dienes. Obviously, these methods all rest on the basic chemistry of the lipid peroxidation reactions, which are complex (3–5).

The appearance of conjugated dienes in peroxidized unsaturated fatty acids is due to resonance following free radical attack on the bis-allelic hydrogens of methylene groups separating double bonds in these compounds. Generation of

† Deceased December 2, 1991.

METHODS IN TOXICOLOGY, Volume 1B

lipid-conjugated dienes can take place in the absence of molecular O_2. For example, conjugated dienes appear in the lipids of rat liver microsomes that have been incubated anaerobically in the presence of NADPH and CCl_4 (6). However, the extremely rapid reaction of lipid organic radicals with O_2 will ensure that peroxidation reactions, in the strict sense of formation of peroxyl functions, will occur in aerobic systems in which polyenoic fatty acids are attacked by radicals; see Ref. 2 for the basic chemistry. It is for this reason that the shift of the double bond, which does not itself involve peroxide formation, is nevertheless a clear sign that lipid peroxidation has occurred, if molecular O_2 is present.

Lipid-conjugated dienes can be detected by three methods. Two of these methods depend on UV spectrophotometry. The first of these two methods, the difference spectrum method, is described in this chapter. It is based on the determination of simple UV absorption spectra of peroxidized lipids as compared to simple UV absorption spectra of control nonperoxidized lipids (6,7). The second method, discussed in Chapter 35, is based on taking the second derivative of the UV absorption spectra of the peroxidized lipids (8,9). It does not depend on comparison of UV spectra of peroxidized lipids relative to control samples. The third method for detection and quantitation of lipid conjugated dienes involves use of [^{14}C]tetracyanoethylene in a Diels–Alder reaction (see Chapter 34).

DIFFERENCE SPECTRUM METHOD

Basic Principles

Naturally occurring lipids exhibit simple end absorption in UV light as the wavelength is lowered toward 200 nm. The spectra of peroxidized lipids, however, are characterized by an intense K band near 233 nm, with a lesser secondary absorption maximum due to ketone dienes in the 260- to 280-nm region. See Fig. 1 and Ref. 8 for typical spectra. Since samples of peroxidized lipids encountered in biological work will usually be mixtures of peroxidized and nonperoxidized lipids, the absorption of the K band near 233 nm due to the peroxidized lipids will be superimposed on the end absorption of the nonperoxidized lipids present in the sample being analyzed. It is for this reason that a key aspect of the method being described here involves determination of the difference between the 233-nm absorption of the peroxidized lipid sample and the 233-nm absorption of a corresponding sample of nonperoxidized lipid serving as a control. Since the difference spectrum depends on two measured quantities, error in the difference spectrum will be greater than for each of the measured quantities alone. Because of this tendency for greater error in the difference spectrum, we routinely obtain a mean difference spectrum, with samples from at least three control and three experimental animals. (Replication of individual spectra

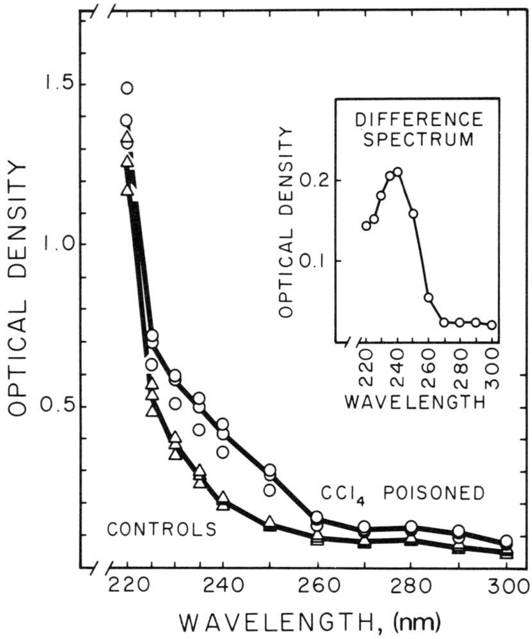

Figure 1 Conjugated diene absorption in rat liver microsomal lipids 5 min after intragastric administration of carbon tetrachloride (CCl_4). The lower trace is end absorption of nonperoxidized microsomal lipids from untreated rats. (From Ref. 13, reproduced with permission.)

should reproduce with an error of measurement of less than 5%.) Finally, since the raw spectrophotometric readings are adjusted to a final concentration of 0.1 g/dl (see below), the mean difference spectrum is multiplied by 10 to obtain the convenient mean difference spectrum at a concentration of 1%. This yields the so-called "mean $\Delta E^{1\%}_{1cm}$" value (7).

In some cases tissue samples are passed through aqueous phase procedures preparatory to lipid extraction (e.g., homogenization of the tissue followed by centrifugation procedures.) All such aqueous phase procedures should be carried out in the presence of suitable iron-chelating agents to avoid possible lipid peroxidation prior to lipid extraction. Total lipids of tissue samples can be extracted conveniently with chloroform:methanol (2:1), according to Folch *et al.* (11), with slight modifications (see below for details). Extracted lipids in chloroform are eventually recovered by removing the chloroform under a stream of absolutely oxygen-free nitrogen or in suitable evaporation devices. (Note: If oxygen is present during the dry-down step, the lipids will peroxidize.) The dried-down and chloroform-free lipid is dissolved in spectrophotometric-grade cyclohexane for spectrophotometric analysis. (Note: It is important to remove all traces of chloroform, since chloroform absorbs strongly below 260 nm.) The final concentration of lipid in cyclohexane can be determined according to Chiang *et al.* (12); see below for details.

Reagents

Chloroform
Methanol
Chloroform : Methanol [2 : 1 (v : v)]: Commercially available reagent grades of these solvents are satisfactory without further purification
Cyclohexane, spectrophotometric grade
Nitrogen, oxygen free: Final traces of oxygen, present in even highest grades of nitrogen, can be effectively removed by use of oxygen traps originally designed for purifying carrier gases for gas–liquid chromatography, such as the high-capacity gas purifier available from Supelco (Bellfonte, PA)

Procedure

The following procedure has been written for possible detection of conjugated dienes in lipids extracted from isolated rat liver microsomes. It is equally applicable to any isolated subcellular fraction, isolated cells, tissue samples, etc.

1. Final sedimentation of the microsomes is carried out in plastic centrifuge tubes made of polyallomer or polypropylene copolymer that resist methanol. Discard the final supernatant fraction and any fat clinging to the walls of the centrifuge tube. Transfer the sedimented microsomes (usually from 2–3 g of whole liver) quantitatively with 7 ml of methanol to a graduated 40-ml stoppered glass centrifuge tube (Kimax Cat. No. 45201-40, Kimble/Kontes, Vineland, NJ).
2. Add 14 ml of chloroform, stopper, and vortex to mix thoroughly. Allow the mixture to stand at room temperature for ~10 min, with occasional mixing.
3. Centrifuge the mixture at ~260 *g* for 10 min at room temperature to sediment the insoluble material. Decant the supernatant fraction into another 40-ml graduated stoppered centrifuge tube. Adjust the final volume of the lipid extract to 30 ml by the addition of chloroform : methanol [2 : 1 (v : v)]. Alternatively, insoluble material in the original chloroform : methanol extract can be removed by filtration (e.g., through a medium-porosity fritted-disk glass Buchner funnel).
4. Add 10 ml of water. Mix gently but completely by inversion. Too-vigorous mixing at this point results in emulsions which sometimes are difficult to break.
5. Centrifuge for 10 min at approximately 260 *g*.
6. By means of aspiration remove the upper methanol–water phase and any insoluble material at the interface between the two phases. (Note: At this stage

additional traces of methanol–water can be removed by placing the tubes in an ice bath for 5 min, recentrifuging, and aspirating off any remaining methanol-water droplets.)

7. Transfer 2-ml aliquots of the chloroform phase into clean tubes, place in a water bath or block heater at 40–50°C, and evaporate the chloroform under a stream of oxygen-free nitrogen. All traces of chloroform must be removed.

8. Dissolve the extracted chloroform-free lipid in 3 ml of cyclohexane and record the absorbance (1-cm light path) from 300 to 220 nm, against a cyclohexane blank with a scanning spectrophotometer. Alternatively, read the absorbance manually at periodic wavelength intervals and plot the results. See Fig. 1 for an example of the latter method.

9. After the absorbance measurements have been recorded, remove 0.25-ml aliquots from each sample for analysis of the total lipid content (see below).

10. Correct all absorbance density measurements to a uniform base of 1 mg of lipid per 1 ml of cyclohexane.

11. After rationalization of the raw absorbance values to a common base of 1 mg of lipid per 1 ml of cyclohexane, the average absorbance at each of several selected wavelengths for three experimental samples is now calculated, as well as the average absorbance at corresponding wavelengths for three control samples. In this case the control samples would be liver microsomal lipids from otherwise untreated rats brought through the same isolation procedure. The difference between these average absorbance values plotted against wavelength is the mean difference spectrum; see Fig. 1 for a typical result. The mean difference spectrum will peak near 235–240 nm. The maximum, or peak, absorbance of the mean difference spectrum, multiplied by 10, is considered the mean $\Delta E^{1\%}_{1cm}$ value (7).

For analysis of isolated hepatocytes in suspension, use at least 10×10^6 hepatocytes (~0.1 g of cells containing ~3 mg of phospholipid) for extraction of lipids according to the above procedures, using 20 times the volume (in milliliters) of chloroform : methanol (2 : 1) than the weight (in grams) of hepatocytes [e.g., for 0.3 g of hepatocytes extract lipids with 6.0 ml of chloroform : methanol (2 : 1)]. In any case, adjust conditions to obtain a final concentration of lipid in cyclohexane for spectroscopy approaching 1 mg of lipid per 1 ml of cyclohexane.

See Chapter 35 by Corongiu *et al.* for additional analysis of lipid-conjugated dienes by second-derivative UV spectroscopy.

ANALYSIS FOR CONCENTRATION OF LIPID

The following method is based on that of Chiang *et al.* (12).

Basic Principle

Lipid extracted from biological material, or lipid standards, usually dissolved in a solvent such as $CHCl_3$, is recovered by evaporation and then oxidized in potassium dichromate and concentrated H_2SO_4. The optical density of the green color of the chromate ion is determined at 600 nm.

Reagents

The oxidizing reagent is 2% $K_2Cr_2O_7$ in concentrated H_2SO_4 [American Chemical Society (ACS) grade]. To prepare this reagent, add 5 g of $K_2Cr_2O_7$ (ASC grade) to 10 ml of water; then concentrated H_2SO_4 is added to a final volume of 250 ml. All $K_2Cr_2O_7$ must be completely dissolved. (Note: This reagent is hygroscopic and it will react with dust, etc. In our experience, if kept clean and well stoppered to prevent absorption of atmospheric water, no detectable change will occur in the properties of the reagent for at least several months. The ultimate test is reproducibility of results on standards, and constancy of results on standards over time.)

Lipid Standard

Corn oil *stock solution*: 2.00 mg of corn oil per 1 ml of $CHCl_3$
Corn oil *working standard:* 100 μg of corn oil per 1 ml of $CHCl_3$ made from the stock solution

Store these standards at 0–4°C in polyethylene-stoppered glass containers. Also, the *working standard* is held in an ice bath during sampling to avoid possible errors in aliquoting due to the fact that $CHCl_3$ has a rather high coefficient of thermal expansion.

Procedure for Standard Curve

1. To prepare a standard curve within the linear absorbance range pipette aliquots of *working standard* containing 50–1000 μg of corn oil into 16 × 125-mm glass tubes.
2. Remove chloroform by evaporation with a stream of nitrogen.
3. Add 2 ml of oxidizing reagent. Vortex to mix thoroughly.
4. Heat for 15 min in a boiling water bath.
5. Cool to room temperature in a water bath.
6. Add 2 ml of water and vortex to mix thoroughly.
7. Read the absorbance at 600 nm against a water blank in a colorimeter or a spectrophotometer.

Procedure on Unknowns

The procedure on unknowns is the same as for the corn oil standard as above. Pick aliquots containing 100–1000 μg of total lipid.

REFERENCES

1. H. Kappus, *Chem. Phys. Lipids* **45,** 105 (1987).
2. R. O. Recknagel, E. A. Glende, Jr., and R. S. Britton, *in* "Hepatoxicology" (R. G. Meeks, S. D. Harrison, and R .J. Bull, eds.), p. 401. CRC Press, Boca Raton, Florida, 1991.
3. N. A. Porter, *in* "Methods in Enzymology" (L. Packer, ed.), Vol. 105, p. 273. Academic Press, Orlando, Florida, 1984.
4. H. Kappus, *in* "Oxidative Stress" (H. Sies, ed.), p. 273. Academic Press, Orlando, Florida, 1985.
5. M. Simic and K. A. Taylor, *in* "Flavor Quality of Fresh Meats: Warmed-Over Flavor" (A. J. St. Angelo and M. E. Bailey, eds.), p. 69. Academic Press, Orlando, Florida, 1987.
6. C. L. Wood, A. J. Gandolfi, and R. A. Van Dyke, *Drug Metab. Dispos.* **4,** 305 (1976).
7. R. O. Recknagel and A. K. Ghoshal, *Exp. Mol. Pathol.* **5,** 413 (1966).
8. R. O. Recknagel and E. A. Glende, Jr., *in* "Methods in Enzymology" (L. Packer, ed.), Vol. 105, p. 331. Academic Press, Orlando, Florida, 1984.
9. F. P. Corongiu, G. Poli, M. U. Dianzani, K. V. Cheeseman, and T. F. Slater, *Chem.–Biol. Interact.* **59,** 147 (1986).
10. S. Banni, R. E. Basford, F. P. Corongiu, and B. Lombardi, *Adv. Biosci.* **76,** 187 (1989).
11. J. Folch, M. Lees, and G. H. Sloane-Stanley, *J. Biol. Chem.* **226,** 497 (1957).
12. S. P. Chiang, C. F. Gessert, and O. H. Lowry, *in* "Research Report 56-113," Colorimetric Determination of Extracted Lipids, Air University School of Aviation Medicine, U.S. Air Force, Texas, 1957.
13. K. S. Rao and R. O. Recknagel, *Exp. Mol. Pathol.* **9,** 271 (1968).

34 Quantitation of Conjugated Dienes by a Diels–Alder Reaction

D. A. G. Mickle

INTRODUCTION

This method is essentially that of Waller and Recknagel (1). After purification and measurement of phospholipid content of the sample, the fatty acids are removed by hydrolysis and purified. The essence of this procedure is a Diels–Alder condensation reaction between either [1,2-^{14}14C]tetracyanoethylene or tetra-[^{14}C]cyanoethylene (designated [^{14}C]TCNE) and a fatty acid-conjugated diene bond in a 1 : 1 ratio (Fig.1). Quantitation of the radiolabeled fatty acid-conjugated diene bonds is through a standard curve established for the [^{14}C]TCNE–hexadiene adduct formed between *trans*-2,*trans*-4-hexadiene which has one conjugated diene bond and [^{14}C]TCNE.

The method is precise with a within-batch precision of ~5%. The analytical recovery of the assay using hexadiene is between 75% and 80%. Tissue requirements are less than those required by the high-performance liquid chromatography–gas chromatography (HPLC–GC) mass spectrometry technique (2). As little as 10–50 mg wet weight of myocardium, liver (3), or cultured cells can be processed with success. Serum samples can also be analyzed, but may require additional purification of the extracted phospholipids.

Compared to the HPLC–GC mass spectrometry method, the TCNE method is more easily performed and more precise. A technologist can analyze 30 specimens every 5 working days using the TCNE method, but would require 7 working days to process five specimens by the HPLC–GC mass spectrometry tech-

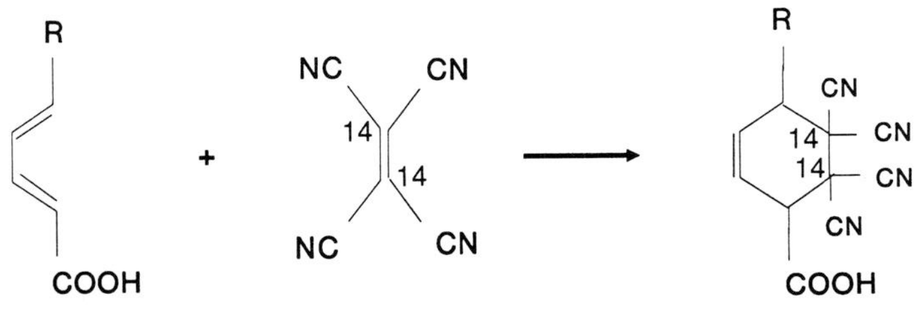

Figure 1 Diels–Alder condensation reaction between a fatty acid containing a conjugated diene bond and [1,2-^{14}C]tetracyanoethylene.

nique. Interpretation and quantitation of the HPLC peaks are not precise compared to quantitation of the [^{14}C]diene adducts. The TCNE method does not require sophisticated and expensive equipment. The analysis can be done in most routine research laboratories. The major disadvantage of the TCNE method is the expense of purchasing [^{14}C]malononitrile.

MATERIALS AND REAGENTS

Acid reagent [water: sulfuric acid: perchloric acid 5 : 2.5 : 2 by volume]
Bromine, American Chemical Society (ACS) grade, Fisher, Fairlawn, NJ)
Chloroform [HPLC grade, British Drug House (BDH), Toronto, Ontario, Canada]
Chloroform : Methanol [2 : 1 (v : v)]
Copper powder (ACS grade, BDH)
1,2-Dichloroethane (ACS grade BDH)
Diethyl ether (dry, glass distilled, BDH)
Dipalmitoylphosphatidylcholine (99+%, Sigma, St. Louis, MO)
Hydrochloric acid (1 *M*)
Lithium aluminum hydride, (J. T. Baker, Toronto, Ontario, Canada)
[2-^{14}C] – or [1,3-^{14}C]malononitrile (synthesized by Sigma)
Methanol, (HPLC grade, BDH)
Molecular sieve (4A, four to eight mesh, Aldrich, Milwaukee, WI)
Molybdate reagent [1.6 m*M* ammonium molybdate (99+%, BDH) 22 m*M* Triton X-100 (Calbiochem-Behring, San Diego, CA), and 0.5 *M* sulfuric acid]
Neutral aluminum (activated, column chromatography grade, Bio-Rad, Richmond, CA)
Nitrogen (oxygen free)
Silicic acid (activated, 200–325 mesh, Clarkson Chemical Co., Williamsport, PA)
Sodium acetate (saturated solution, 100 ml
Sodium bicarbonate (5% solution 1 liter)
Sodium chloride (ACS grade, 0.9%, 1liter)
trans-2,*trans*-4-Hexadiene (99%, Aldrich)

EQUIPMENT

Vortex mixer
Glass tissue homogenizer
Centrifuge (IEC Centra-7R refrigerated centrifuge, Fisher, Pittsburgh, PA)
Freezer (−86°C)
Dryer (Reacti-ThermIII Heating Nodule, Pierce, Rockford, IL)
ISO TEM oven (Model 338F, Fisher)

Spectrophotometer (DU-40, Beckman, Fullerton, CA)
Distillation system (Wheaton Kit 24/40, Mandel Scientific, Guelph, ONT, Canada)
Liquid scintillation counter
Balance

EXTRACTION OF LIPID FROM TISSUE

1. Weigh 10–500 mg of tissue and add a volume of chloroform : methanol [2 : 1 (v : v)] equivalent to 10 times the weight of the tissue.
2. Homogenize the tissue at 0–4°C in a glass tissue grinder for 3 min.
3. Separate the chloroform : methanol fraction from the insoluble material by centrifugation at 4°C and 875 *g* for 10 min, and transfer to a clean methanol-rinsed glass tube with a Teflon-lined cap (also methanol prerinsed). (At this point the chloroform : methanol extracts may be stored at −80°C overnight.)
4. Add normal saline (0.9% NaCl) equal to 20% of the total volume of chloroform : methanol. (Allow −80°C-stored samples to warm to room temperature before adding the saline solution.)
5. Vortex the mixture briefly and centrifuge at 4°C and 875 *g* for 10 min.
6. Discard the upper aqueous methanol phase and transfer the lower chloroform phase to a methanol-washed screw-cap tube.
7. Evaporate the chloroform to dryness at room temperature with a gentle stream of oxygen-free nitrogen. (The procedure may be stopped at this stage by redissolving the lipid residues in methanol and storing at −80°C. The tubes must be dry; evaporate off the methanol with a nitrogen stream before proceeding to separate the phospholipid from the total lipid.)

SEPARATION OF PHOSPHOLIPID FROM TOTAL LIPID

1. Transfer 1 g of silicic acid to a 20-ml screw-cap tube. Cover the tube lightly with foil. Place the tube in an oven at 200°C overnight to activate the silicic acid.
2. Remove the tube from the oven and allow to cool.
3. Add 2 ml of chloroform to the silicic acid and vortex well. A gel is formed.
4. Add 1 ml of chloroform to the tube containing the dried lipid, vortex briefly, and transfer to the silicic acid gel by pipetting. Repeat the process with another 1–2 ml of chloroform and add to the gel. Sufficient chloroform must be added to bring the final volume to 7 ml.
5. Vortex for 1 min. Centrifuge at 4°C and 875 *g* for 5 min.
6. Pipette off and discard the chloroform fraction which contains neutral lipids. Add 5 ml of chloroform to the gel, vortex well, centrifuge at 4°C and 875

g for 5 min, and discard the chloroform. Repeat this procedure using 10 ml of chloroform.

7. Add 5 ml of methanol to the silicic acid gel, vortex well for 5 min, and centrifuge at 4°C and 875 *g* for 5 min. Transfer the methanol fraction which contains the phospholipid to a methanol-rinsed tube. Repeat the extraction procedure twice more. Pool the methanol fractions.

8. Evaporate the pooled methanol fraction to dryness with oxygen-free nitrogen as above.

9. Reconstitute the phospholipid residue in 1 ml of methanol.

PHOSPHATE ASSAY FOR PHOSPHOLIPID CONTENT

1. Add 50 μl of phospholipid-containing methanol (from step 9 in the previous procedure) to a 5 mL acid-washed conical screw-cap tube. Evaporate the methanol to dryness with nitrogen as described above.

2. A phospholipid standard curve is prepared in the following manner.

a. A 1-m*M* standard phospholipid solution is made by adding 4 mg of dipalmitoylphosphatidylcholine to an acid-washed conical screw-cap tube. Add 5 ml of chloroform and vortex well

b. Pipette the following volumes of phospholipid standard (STD) into acid-washed tubes: STD 1, 10 μl; STD 2, 20 μl; STD 3, 50 μl; STD 4, 80 μl; and STD 5, 100 μl.

c. Evaporate each tube to dryness with nitrogen as described above.

3. Add 100 μl of the acid reagent (water : sulfuric acid : perchloric acid [5 : 2.5 : 2, (v : v : v)] to each dry residue.

4. Cap the tubes loosely and place in a fume hood for 1 hr in a sand bath which has been heated to ~200°C. The solutions will undergo a color change (i.e., dark brown to light brown to yellow–green.)

5. Allow the tubes to cool to room temperature.

6. Add 250 μl of saturated sodium acetate solution and vortex briefly.

7. Allow the samples to stand for ~5 min before adding 1.5 ml of molybdate solution. Mix thoroughly but gently by manual inversion.

8. Allow the color (yellow–green) to develop completely (at least 30 min).

9. Determine the absorbance at 366 nm in a spectrophotometer.

10. One nanomole of phosphate is equivalent to 1 nmol of phospholipid.

HYDROLYSIS OF PHOSPHOLIPID WITH LITHIUM ALUMINUM HYDRIDE

1. Evaporate 950 μl of phospholipid-containing methanol (i.e., remainder of 1 ml) to dryness with nitrogen.

2. Add 10 ml of diethyl ether that has first been passed through an activated neutral aluminum column to remove any peroxides. Vortex briefly.

3. Slowly add 20 mg of lithium aluminum hydride to the solution. (*Note: This is a vigorous reaction and caution should be taken by carrying out this reaction in a protected hood.*)

4. Allow this mixture to stand for 10 min.

5. Repeat steps 3 and 4 twice.

6. Add small pieces of ice to the tubes to inactivate the unreacted lithium aluminum hydride. (*Note: This is a vigorous reaction and caution should be taken.*)

7. Acidify the solution to pH 5.0 as assessed by litmus paper with 1 *M* hydrochloric acid.

8. Centrifuge the solutions and pipette the top ether layer to methanol-washed tubes. Evaporate the ether with nitrogen as above.

9. Add 1 ml of methanol to the dry residue and store capped at −80°C. This fraction contains the free (unesterified) fatty acids.

REACTION OF [^{14}C]-TCNE WITH LIPID-CONJUGATED DIENES

1. The content of phospholipid-conjugated diene is determined from a standard curve established for the reaction between a conjugated diene standard, *trans*-2,*trans*-4-hexadiene, and [^{14}C]-TCNE. (See the section below for synthesis of [1,2-^{14}C]-TCNE.) The [^{14}C]-TCNE reagent is prepared by dissolving 0.75 mg of [^{14}C]-TCNE in 10 ml of dry chloroform to yield a 585 μM solution.

2. The hexadiene standards are prepared in the following manner.

a. The 58.4-m*M* hexadiene stock solution is made by adding 20 μl of hexadiene into 2980 μl of dry chloroform in a glass test tube. (Note: The chloroform is dried over an activated molecular sieve for several hours prior to use. The molecular sieve is activated by heating at 200°C for 6 hr. It is important that the chloroform be dry, as TCNE reacts with water. The chloroform can be kept in a screw-cap glass container for 1 week.)

b. Dilute the 58.4-m*M* hexadiene stock standard with dry chloroform to make the following standard solutions:

STD	Dilution	Yield (nmol/100 μl)
1	50,000×	0.117
2	10,000×	0.584
3	500×	11.69
4	200×	29.22
5	100×	58.43
6	50×	116.9
7	10×	584.3

c. Pipette 100 μl of each standard into clean dry methanol-rinsed tubes.

3. Evaporate 1 ml of phospholipid-containing methanol saved for analysis (from step 9 under "Hydrolysis of Phospholipid with Lithium Aluminum Hydride") to dryness with nitrogen and redissolve in 100 μl of dry chloroform.

4. Add 500 μl [^{14}C]-TCNE to each tube, including a blank sample containing 100 μl of dry chloroform.

5. Allow the reaction to progress for 10 min at room temperature.

6. Wash each sample by the addition of 4 ml of a 5% sodium bicarbonate solution. Vortex the tube briefly, centrifuge at 4°C and 875 *g* for 5 min, and discard the upper aqueous layer. Repeat this three more times and once with water.

7. Transfer the chloroform, which contains the [^{14}C]-TCNE adduct, to a scintillation vial. Wash the tube twice with 0.5 ml of methanol and transfer these methanol fractions to the same scintillation vial.

8. Count the radioactivity of the sample and blank tubes.

9. Quantitation of the phospholipid-conjugated diene is based on a linear standard curve established for the disintegrations per minute of the isolated [^{14}C]TCNE adduct versus the nanomoles of conjugated hexadiene substrate. The amount of phospholipid-conjugated diene is conveniently expressed as nanomoles of conjugated diene per nanomole of phospholipid.

SYNTHESIS OF [1,2-^{14}C]TETRACYANOETHYLENE (OR TETRA-[^{14}C]CYANOETHYLENE)

The synthesis of [^{14}C]-TCNE as described by Waller and Recknagel (1) is difficult and yields a product of low specific activity. The following procedure produces [^{14}C]-TCNE with a high yield and a high specific activity which permits analysis of small biological samples. See Fig. 2 for an outline of the synthesis. This synthesis will permit ~15,000 assays. (*Note: It is imperative that an experienced chemist carry out these reactions because of the very toxic nature of the reactants and products.*)

1. Add 99 g (1.5 mol) of molten malononitrile (warmed by a heating pad) containing 10 mCi of [2-^{14}C]-malononitrile to 450 ml of ice-cold water followed immediately by 250 g of ice and then 150 ml (3.05 mol) of room-temperature bromine. The bromine is added over 5–10 min; during this addition enough ice (about 200 g) is added to maintain the reaction temperature of 10–15°C. (Note: [2-^{14}C]-or [1,3-^{14}C]malononitrile can be purchased from Sigma.)

2. With a magnetic stirrer stir the mixture for 1 hr at 20°C.

3. The heavy layer containing [^{14}C]-dibromomalononitrile is separated using a separatory funnel. The upper aqueous layer is extracted twice with 50 ml of dry 1,2-dichloroethane.

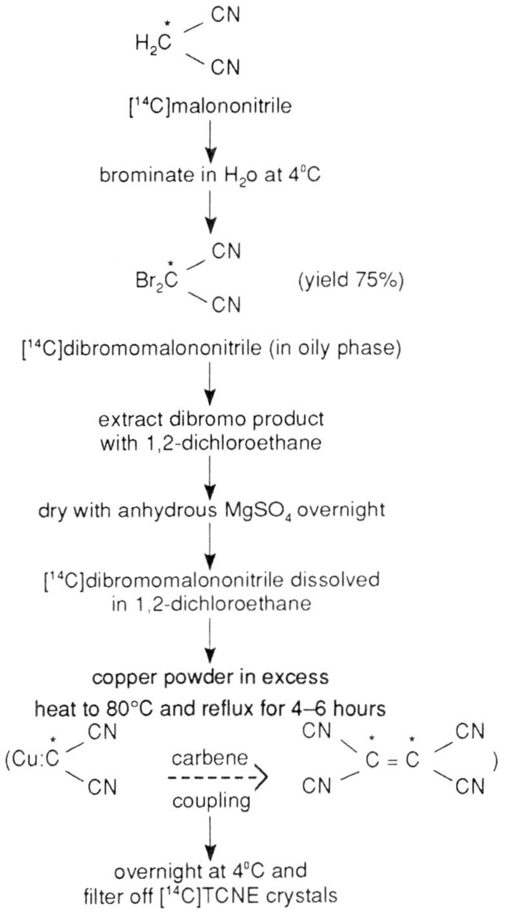

Figure 2 Outline of [1,2-^{14}C]tetracyanoethylene ([^{14}C]TCNE) synthesis.

4. Combine the [^{14}C]-dibromomalononitrile and 1,2-dichloroethane extracts, dry for 4 hr by adding 10 g of anhydrous magnesium sulfate, and add 750 ml of 1,2-dichloroethane dried by molecular sieves.

5. Add 20 g of copper powder to the [^{14}C]-dibromomalononitrile extracts and heat the mixture to a gentle reflux with stirring. After 10 min add another 20 g of copper powder. This process is repeated until a total of 120 g of copper powder is added.

6. Reflux the mixture for 4–6 hr.

7. The solids are separated by filtration with a Buchner funnel and Whatman No. 1 filter paper. Wash the filter paper with 20 ml of 50°C dry 1,2-dichloroethane and store the filtrate in a screw-cap container overnight at 0–5°C.

8. The almost colorless [1,2-^{14}C]-TCNE crystals formed overnight are separated with a Buchner funnel, washed with 10 ml of dry 1,2-dichloroethane, and dried in a vacuum desiccator for 3 hr or longer.

9. The overall yield of [1,2-^{14}C]TCNE is 30–40%, with a purity of 98%. A more purified product can be obtained by sublimation at 130–140°C at 1 mm Hg. (Note: The specific activity of the [^{14}C]-TCNE depends on the starting ratio of [^{14}C]malononitrile to "cold" malononitrile. If [1,3-^{14}C]-malononitrile is used at step 1, the resultant product will be tetra-[^{14}C]cyanoethylene.

ACKNOWLEDGMENTS

Financial support for this work was generously provided by the Medical Research Council of Canada (MT 10392) and The Heart and Stroke Foundation of Ontario (T2010).

REFERENCES

1. R. L. Waller and R. O. Recknagel, *Lipids* **12,** 914 (1978).
2 A. D. Romaschin, I. Rebeyka, G. J. Wilson, and D. A. G. Mickle, *J. Mol. Cell. Cardiol.* **19,** 289 (1987).
3 T.-W. Wu, N. Hashimoto, J.-X. Au, D. A. G. Mickle, and D. Carey, *Hepatology* **13,** 575 (1991).

35 Quantitation of Conjugated Dienes by Second-Derivative UV Spectroscopy

F. P. Corongiu, S. Banni, and B. Lombardi

INTRODUCTION

For familiarization with the principles and practice of derivative UV spectroscopy, the reader is referred to a few available sources (1–4). Derivative UV spectroscopy is particularly suited for analysis of complex mixtures in which band overlaps occur, or shoulders on slopes are present in conventional absorption spectra. In first-derivative spectroscopy the rate of change of absorbance with wavelength ($dA/d\lambda$) is measured, resulting in a reduction of the band width of individual components and, therefore, in spectra of greater resolution (2). In second-derivative spectroscopy, a differential is made of the first-derivative spectrum ($d^2A/d\lambda^2$), a treatment which is particularly effective in extracting distinct signals out of the shoulders on absorption slopes (2). As explained elsewhere in this volume (5), the latter is exactly the situation and difficulty one is confronted with in the detection and determination of conjugated dienes by means of conventional UV spectroscopy.

Figure 1 shows the conventional (lower curve) and second-derivative (upper curve) absorption spectra of a preparation of partially peroxidized cod liver oil. In the lower curve the conjugated diene shoulder on the end absorption slope of the lipid is clearly visible between 250 and 220 nm. In the upper curve, however, two distinct signals are present in the same region. In the second derivative spectral assignments are made on the basis of minimum, rather than maximum, wavelength of absorption (2). The signal with a minimum at 233 nm (*a*, Fig. 1) is due to the presence of fatty acid isomers with *trans,trans*-conjugated dienes, and that with a minimum at 242 nm (*b*) is caused by isomers with *cis,trans*-conjugated dienes (6–8). This example also illustrates well the greater resolution afforded by second-derivative UV spectroscopy. Each signal has a maximum (a', b') as well as a minimum, and the difference between the two (a'–a, b'–b) represents the signal height (h, h'). Given that in second-derivative spectroscopy the end absorption of lipids does not interfere with the conjugated diene bands, there is no longer a need to base the UV detection and quantitation of conjugated dienes on the spectrum difference between a peroxidized and a nonperoxidized preparation of the same lipid (5), greatly simplifying the

METHODS IN TOXICOLOGY, Volume 1B

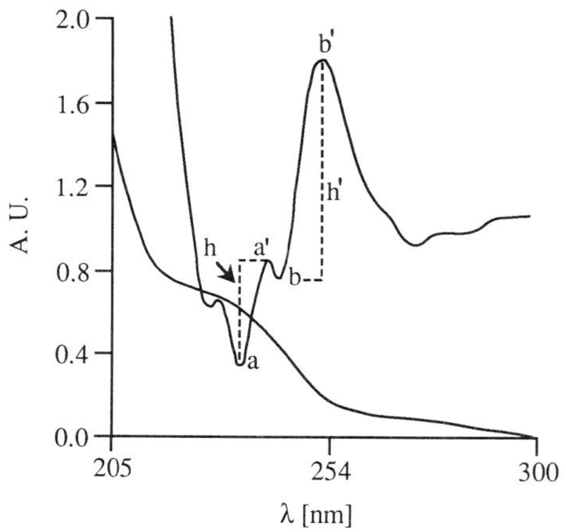

Figure 1 Conventional (lower curve) and second-derivative (upper curve) UV absorption spectra of a sample of partially peroxidized cod liver oil. For an explanation see text. Abscissa, Wavelength (λ) in nanometers; ordinate, absorption units (A. U.).

methodology. Moreover, second-derivative spectroscopy affords a more direct and precise means to quantitate conjugated dienes, since the linear relationship between sample absorption (peak height) and concentration, as governed by the Lambert–Beer law, is unaffected by differentiation (2). The conjugated diene content of a single sample of lipids can thus be determined easily with the aid of a standard curve prepared with a suitable reference compound (8–11).

CONSTRUCTION OF A STANDARD CURVE AND OPTIMIZATION OF INSTRUMENT SETTINGS

Reagents: Reagent-grade cyclohexane

Standard: A sample of as highly purified and completely peroxidized an unsaturated fatty acid as is available; we have been using (9–11) (±)-9-hydroperoxyoctadecadienoic acid (HPODE; purity >98%, Oxford Biomedical Research, Oxford, MI)

Procedure

A stock solution of the standard sample is prepared in cyclohexane at a concentration of ~100 μg/ml and placed in a small glass-stoppered flask. The flask is partially immersed in liquid N_2 to replace its air space with N_2, closed, sealed (Parafilm), and stored at −80°C. If the sample is obtained from a commercial source, it is transferred from its container into a conical glass-stoppered flask, such as Corning Cat. No. 4315 (Fisher Cat. No. 10-060-5D, Pittsburgh, PA), along with repeated washes of the container with the solvent in which the sample was delivered. The solvent, if other than cyclohexane, is dried down under vacuum, or under a stream of O_2-free nitrogen, before preparing the stock solution.

To prepare working solutions, the stock solution is thawed to room temperature, and the concentration of the sample is checked by conventional UV spectroscopy using its coefficient of extinction at the wavelength of maximum absorption, or the extinction coefficient and wavelength provided by the supplier. Working solutions are prepared at concentrations ranging from 0.5 to 15–20 μg/ml of cyclohexane, and the concentrations are checked as done with the stock solution. Triplicates of each solution are scanned between 300 and 220 nm with an instrument equipped with an electronic unit for second-derivative spectroscopy, such as are the Perkin-Elmer (Norwalk, CT), Model Lambda 15 or Hitachi (Naperville, IL), Model 557 spectrophotometers. In using these instruments, five parameters require some preliminary consideration and optimization (a–e): (a) the scan speed; (b) the bandpass (slit); (c) the response time; (d) the Δ wavelength; and (e) the ordinate scale (depending on the instrument sensitivity and height of the signals obtained). We have been using the following (a–e): (a) 60 nm/min with both of the above instruments; (b) 1 nm, with both of the above instruments; (c) 2 sec (Perkin-Elmer) and slow setting (Hitachi); (d) 4 nm with both instruments; and (e) ordinates varying from 0.05 to 0.40 absorption units. See the work of Situnayake *et al.* (8) for use of a Shimadzu double-beam scanning spectrophotometer, if that is the instrument available. Once optimized, these parameters are used throughout, except for setting the instrument baseline, in which case the scan speed is lowered; for this purpose we have been using speeds of 7.5 nm/min (Perkin-Elmer) and 15 nm/min (Hitachi). The baseline is set by scanning cyclohexane in both cuvettes.

Figure 2 shows typical conventional (lower curve) and second-derivative (upper curve) spectra of 2 μg of HPODE per 1 ml of cyclohexane. Note in the lower curve the lack of major end absorption and the shoulder due to conjugated dienes. In the upper curve two distinct signals are again present, with minima at 233 and 242 nm. After taking the second-derivative spectra, the heights of the two signals (h, h', Fig. 1) obtained with each working solution are measured and summed. A plot is then made of the sum versus concentration, to construct a standard reference curve as shown in Fig. 3. The curve is used repeatedly, as long as instrument settings 1–4 are not changed.

ANALYSIS OF BIOLOGICAL LIPID SAMPLES

The reagents and procedures described in this volume (5) for the preparation of tissue, cell, or subcellular fraction samples and the extraction, purification, and quantitation of their total lipids are fully adequate also in the present case. It is

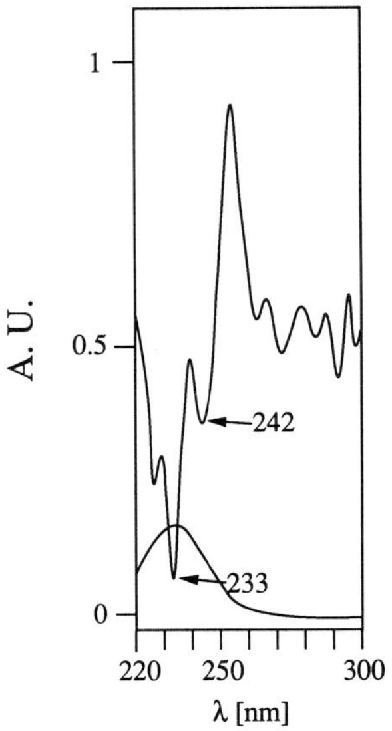

Figure 2 Conventional (lower curve) and second-derivative (upper curve) UV absorption spectra of HPODE. Note in the lower curve the lack of major end absorption and the shoulder due to conjugated dienes. In the upper curve two distinct signals are seen, with minima at 233 and 242 nm, due to the presence of *trans,trans*- and *cis,trans*-conjugated dienes, respectively. Abscissa, Wavelength (λ) in nanometers; ordinate, absorption units (A. U.).

worthy of note, however, that while conjugated diene analyses limited to total lipids are satisfactory in studies dealing with prooxidant agents, such as CCl_4, they are not when assessing whether an agent is a prooxidant. In this case initial analyses should be made on phospholipid (PL) preparations, or initial positive results should be validated by analyses of PL, since it is well established that the target of biological lipoperoxidative processes are polyunsaturated fatty acids present in cellular membrane PL (12). At least one case has been reported in the recent literature in which the presence of conjugated dienes in tissue total lipids, but not PL, was shown to result from assimilation of stable fatty acid isomers with conjugated dienes of dietary origins, rather than from a cellular lipoperoxidative process (9–11). Isolation and purification of PL, or subclasses thereof, can be satisfactorily achieved by several established chromatographic procedures (9–11). However, to obtain sufficient amounts of PL for analysis, larger (two to three times) initial samples of tissue, cells, or cellular subfractions should be used.

Once isolated, the lipids are redissolved in cyclohexane at a concentration of ~250 μg/ml [13; see also the chapter by Glende and Recknagel (5) for a description of a colorimetric determination of lipids], and their second-derivative

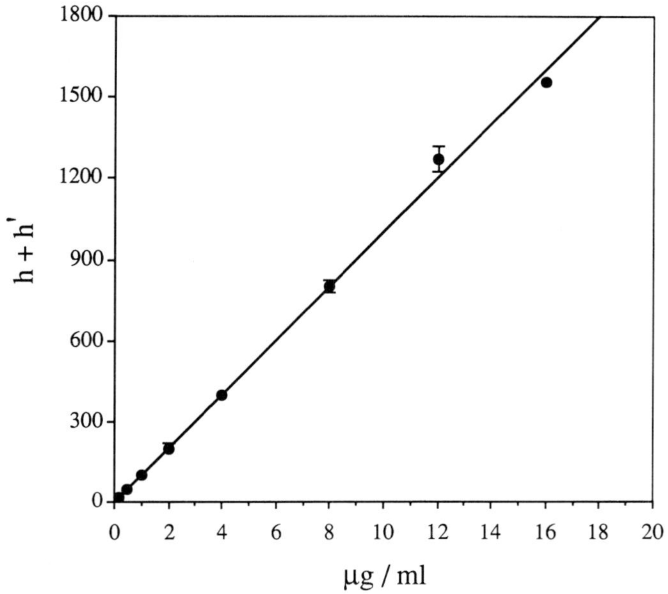

Figure 3 Standard curve prepared by plotting micrograms of HPODE per milliliter of cyclohexane (abscissa) and the height sum ($h + h'$) (ordinate, arbitrary units) of the signals at 233 and 242 nm obtained in second-derivative UV spectroscopy.

UV absorption spectrum is taken, using instrument settings as indicated for the construction of a standard curve. The heights of the signals with minima at 233 and 242 nm are measured and summed, and the concentration of conjugated dienes in the determined with reference to the standard curve. The results are expressed as micrograms of conjugated diene equivalents per milligram of lipid (9–11).

REFERENCES

1. A. Schmitt, "Applied UV Spectroscopy. Derivative Spectroscopy. An Introduction with a Practical Example," No. 1 E, pp. 3–10. Bodenseewerk Perkin-Elmer, Uberlingen, Germany.
2. D. Botten, T. Honkawa, and S. Tohyama, *Perkin-Elmer Appl. Data Bull.* **X-77,** 1 (1977).
3. J. E. Cahill, *Perkin-Elmer Appl. Data Bull.* **ADS-115,** 1 (1979).
4. J. E. Cahill, and F. G. Padera, *Perkin-Elmer Appl. Data Bull.* **ADS-122,** 1 (1980).
5. E. A. Glende, Jr., and R. O. Recknagel, this volume, Ch. 33.
6. F. P. Corongiu and A. Milia, *Chem.–Biol. Interact.* **44,** 289 (1983).
7. F. P. Corongiu, G. Poli, M. U. Dianzani, K. H. Cheeseman, and T. F. Slater, *Chem.–Biol. Interact.* **59,** 147 (1986).

8. R. D. Situnayake, B. J. Crump, A. V. Zevulka, M. Davis, B. McConkey, and D. I. Thurnham, *Ann. Clin. Biochem.* **27,** 258 (1990).
9. S. Banni, R. E. Basford, F. P. Corongiu, and B. Lombardi, *Adv. Biosci.* **76,** 187 (1989).
10. S. Banni, R. W. Evans, M. G. Salgo, F. P. Corongiu, and B. Lombardi, *Carcinogenesis* **11,** 2047 (1990).
11. S. Banni, M. G. Salgo, R. W. Evans, F. P. Corongiu, and B. Lombardi, *Carcinogenesis* **11,** 2053 (1990).
12. R. O. Recknagel, E. A. Glende, Jr., and R. S. Britton, *in* "Hepatotoxicology" (R. G. Meeks, S. D. Harrison, and R. J. Bull, eds.), p. 401. CRC Press, Boca Raton, Florida, (1991).
13. S. P. Chiang, C. F. Gessert, and O. H. Lowry, *in* "Research Report 56-113". Air University School of Aviation Medicine, U. S. Air Force, Texas, 1957.

36

A CENTRIFUGE FILTRATION SEPARATION OF CELLS, AND THE MEASUREMENT OF CONSTITUENTS

Donald J. Reed

INTRODUCTION

In toxicity studies with isolated cell suspensions, the measurement of cell viability and analysis of intracellular constituents require the separation of cells from medium. In the technique discussed here viable cells (hepatocytes) are rapidly separated from nonviable cells and medium by centrifugation through a dibutyl phthalate oil layer. This technique, based on dibutyl phthalate as the separation medium, is similar to the centrifugation filtration methods described with the use of silicon oil or brominated hydrocarbons. However, the use of dibutyl phthalate permits the separation of viable from nonviable cells. It is important to note that during a toxic challenge, regardless of the ratio of viable to nonviable cells in the suspension, more than 90% of cells centrifuged through dibutyl phthalate will be viable, while more than 90% of the cells recovered above the oil layer will not be viable (1).

The centrifugation filtration method with silicon oil or brominated hydrocarbons does not cause a separation of viable and nonviable cells because of differences in density and viscosity of these oils as well as the lower density of nonviable cells compared to viable cells. It has been shown previously that the density of viable heptocytes (d = 1.07–1.08) (2) is considerably higher than that of nonviable hepatocytes (d = 1.02–1.03) (3,4). Because the density of dibutyl phthalate is 1.046, denser viable hepatocytes would be expected to penetrate this oil. In contrast, lighter nonviable cells would not be expected to penetrate the silicon oil and brominated hydrocarbon layers, as the density of these oils is ~1.02.

An alternative method of centrifuging and washing the cells with saline somewhat lessens the effects of nonviable cells. This separation technique, however, has several disadvantages. The saline wash can mechanically damage hepatocytes, especially if they have already been injured by a chemical insult. Mechanically induced cell injury can be mistaken for chemically induced cell injury. Also, several minutes of preparation are needed before the cells are finally lysed

METHODS IN TOXICOLOGY, Volume 1B

and enzymatic activity is stopped. Alterations in cellular events during this slow inactivation period can be confused with changes resulting from a toxic insult. The major limitation of the saline wash separation method is that both viable and nonviable cells are analyzed together in the cell pellet. Consequently, the cellular events that are directly *responsible* for cell injury or death cannot be distinguished from the events that *result* from cell injury or death.

To compensate for these limitations in methodology, a centrifugation filtration separation method has been utilized in studies measuring cell viability (5,6) and intracellular constituents (7,8). Hepatocytes are forced through an oil layer and into acid, which results in the release of intracellular contents into the acid layer with minimal contamination from medium. The oils most widely used with this separation technique are silicon oil (5,6) and brominated hydrocarbons (8). Although this separation method eliminates the need for a saline wash, the separation of viable from nonviable cells has not been demonstrated. The dibutyl phthalate separation technique offers the advantage of monitoring only viable cells for changes in membrane integrity or metabolic performance during a toxic chemical insult.

Mitochondria possess enzyme systems and metabolites that are physiologically distinct and separate from the remainder of the cell. The dibutyl phthalate centrifugation separation technique, combined with the use of digitonin, makes it possible to permeabilize or remove the plasma membrane and many of the cytosolic constituents, yet retain the ability to monitor the permeabilized cell for mitochondrial constituents. For example, mitochondria possess a reservoir of reducing equivalents with a complete glutathione redox system, which consists of reduced glutathione (GSH), glutathione reductase, glutathione peroxidase, and NADPH. Because glutathione functions in intracellular compartments, defining a cellular role for glutathione requires the simultaneous measurement of intracellular, subcellular, and extracellular amounts in the reduced, oxidized, and mixed disulfide forms.

To facilitate these measurements, we have developed a rapid separation technique for hepatocytes and other cells in suspension (1). As already mentioned, this technique offers the advantage of analyzing only viable cells for changes in cellular glutathione and other thiols and disulfides, and it eliminates the measurement of cellular alterations that occur after cell death (nonviable cells). Separation of viable hepatocytes is accomplished in a microcentrifuge tube by layering a sample of hepatocyte suspension over a dibutyl phthalate oil layer, which is layered over perchloric acid (PCA), and then centrifuging. Only viable hepatocytes are forced through the oil layer into the 10% PCA, which causes the release of intracellular contents. Intracellular constituents are then measured in the 10% PCA layer. The medium above the oil layer is analyzed for extracellular constituents. Measurement of mitochondrial constituents is accomplished by alteration of the cell suspension by digitonin, a process by which

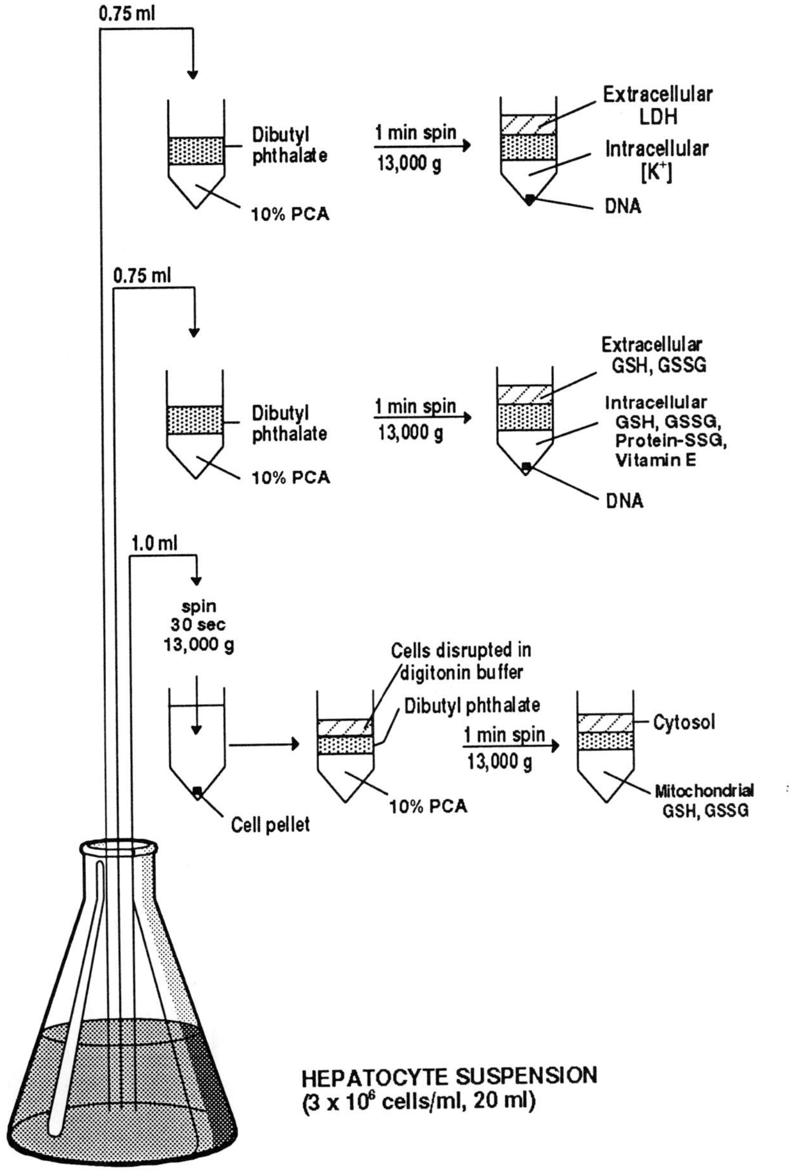

Figure 1 Analysis of intracellular contents and cell viability by the dibutyl phthalate separation method. PCA, Perchloric acid; LDH, lactate dehydrogenase; GSH, reduced glutathione; GSSG, oxidized glutathione; Protein-SSG, protein glutathione mixed disulfide.

membranes become selectively permeable; then mitochondrial constituents are measured in the PCA layer following centrifugation through the dibutyl phthalate oil layer (Fig. 1).

SAMPLE PREPARATION

Principle

The accurate measurement of intracellular constituents of viable cells, including enzyme activity levels, vitamin E, glutathione and related thiols and disulfides, and certain ions in biological specimens, relies in part on sample preparation, that is, the rapid termination of metabolic processes in fluids, cells, and tissues during the assay procedure. To satisfy these criteria, biological specimens are promptly separated into either PCA (1 *M* or 10%) containing a metal chelator such as 1 m*M* bathophenanthrolinedisulfonic acid (BPDS) or Percoll. By substituting Percoll for PCA, the separation procedure results in viable cells pelleted under the Percoll layer.

Reagents

PCA (70%) (Analytical Reagent, Mallinckrodt, St. Louis, MO)
PCA [10% (v/v) in metal-free water] (Milli-Q reagent water system, Millipore, Bedford, MA) containing 1 m*M* BPDS (G. B. Smith Chemicals)
γ-Glutamyl glutamate (15 m*M*, γ-Glu-Glu) (Vega Biotechnologies, Tucson, AZ) in 0.3%
PCA, stored at −10°C, stable at room temperature for several days, used as an internal standard
Dibutyl phthalate (*d* = 1.046) (Aldrich, Milwaukee, WI)
BPDS (15 m*M*) in metal-free water (Aldrich)
N-Morpholinopropanesulfonic acid (MOPS) buffer at pH 8.0 containing MOPS (50 m*M*) and 1,4-dithiothreitol (25 m*M*, DTT)
Percoll [36% (v/v) in Hanks' salt solution with a final density of 1.06)] (Pharmacia, Uppsala, Sweden)
Digitonin buffer at pH 7.4 containing mannitol (250 m*M*), MOPS (17 m*M*), EDTA (2.5 m*M*), and digitonin (0.8 mg/ml) (Sigma, St. Louis, MO)
α-Tocopherol (Kodak, Rochester, NY)
γ-Tocopherol (Kodak)

Separation of Cells from the Medium

In a 1.5-ml microcentrifuge tube, layer 0.45 ml of dibutyl phthalate (*d* = 1.046) over 0.50 ml of 10% PCA (*d* = 1.06) and centrifuge for 1 min at ambient temperature at 13,000 *g*. This initial centrifugation to establish a discrete boundary between the PCA and oil is not shown in Fig. 1. Rapid separation of hepatocytes from medium is accomplished by layering 0.5 ml of isolated cell suspension over the dibutyl phthalate layer and centrifuging for 1 min at ambient temperature at ~13,000 *g* in an Eppendorf Model 5412 microfuge (Brinkmann Instruments, Inc., Westbury, NY) (Fig. 1). As a result viable hepatocytes are forced through the dibutyl phthalate into 10% PCA, thus releasing intracellular contents. The number of cells lysed in the PCA layer is determined by analyzing the PCA-precipitated pellet for DNA content.

Intact hepatocytes are prepared by layering 0.45 ml of dibutyl phthalate over 0.50 ml of 36% (v/v) Percoll in Hanks' salt solution (final density = 1.06). By substituting Percoll for PCA, the separation procedure described above results in viable hepatocytes pelleted under the Percoll layer.

Cells can also be separated from the medium by centrifugation followed by a medium wash at ambient temperature. A sample (0.75 ml) of cell suspension is centrifuged for 2 sec at 13,000 *g*, and the medium is discarded. The cell pellet is resuspended in Ca^{2+}-free medium and centrifuged for 2 sec, and the supernatant fraction is discarded. The intracellular contents of the resulting cell pellet are released into 10% PCA. The number of cells contributing to the PCA extract is determined by analyzing the PCA extract for DNA content.

APPLICATION OF THE CENTRIFUGATION TECHNIQUE TO THE MEASUREMENT OF INTRACELLULAR CONSTITUENTS

Determination of Intracellular K^+

Intracellular K^+ is determined in the 10% PCA cell extracts [the lower fraction in the microcentrifuge tube (Fig. 1) or after centrifugation and medium wash]. A sample of the PCA extract is analyzed for intracellular K^+ content with a Perkin-Elmer Model 51 flame photometer (Perkin-Elmer, Norwalk, CT). Intracellular concentrations of K^+ are corrected for the number of cells in the PCA pellet as determined by the DNA content and expressed per 10^6 cells. A standard curve for K^+ is prepared with each experiment.

DNA Determination

The DNA content of the PCA precipitate is determined by the modified method of Erwin *et al.* (9). In brief, 0.5 ml of 5% trichloroacetic acid is added to the PCA pellet, and the pellet is resuspended by sonication. The trichloroacetic acid suspension is incubated at 90°C for 30 min and then cooled for 30 min at 4°C. Following centrifugation the supernatant fraction is placed in a separate test tube, and 0.2 ml of a 3,5-diaminobenzoic acid solution (200 mg/ml) is added. The resulting solution is incubated at 60°C for 60 min, followed by the addition of 2 ml of 1 *M* HCl. The fluorescence of the product is determined with a Perkin-Elmer Model 650-10S fluorescence spectrophotometer (excitation filter,

405 nm, emission filter, 520 nm). A DNA standard curve is prepared with each experiment and is linear from 2.5 to 75 μg of DNA. Stock DNA standards are prepared in 5% trichloroacetic acid from calf thymus DNA. Using an ultrapure DNA standard, the DNA content of isolated rat hepatocytes is estimated to be 14.4 $\pm$ 0.6 μg of DNA per 10^6 cells.

Determination of Lactate Dehydrogenase (LDH) Leakage

The activity of LDH is determined in a sample (0.05 ml) of medium [the upper fraction in the microcentrifuge tube (Fig. 1)] and compared to the total LDH activity present in 0.05 ml of cell suspension. The total LDH activity is determined in a sample of cell suspension after the addition of 0.025 ml of Triton X-100 (0.4%) and sonication. Samples of both cell suspension lysate and medium are diluted with saline, and the LDH activity is measured with a 96-well plate reader (Bio Kinetics Model EL 340, Bio-Tek, Winooski, VT). The plate reader measures an increase in absorbance at 340 nm, reflecting the formation of NADH and pyruvate and the presence of LDH activity.

Total Glutathione

Cells, subcellular fractions in suspension, and cell medium are treated by adding 50 μl of γ-Glu-Glu (15 m*M*), 50 μl of BPDS (15 m*M*), and 100 μl of 70% PCA. Following mixing with a vortex mixer, freezing, thawing, and centrifuging at 13,000 *g* for 1 min at ambient temperature, a portion of the 10% PCA extract (0.5 ml) is derivatized and analyzed by high-performance liquid chromatography (HPLC) by the method of Reed *et al.* (10) as modified by Fariss and Reed (11).

Total Intracellular Glutathione

To use the dibutyl phthalate separation method (1), 0.5 ml of hepatocyte suspension is layered over dibutyl phthalate that has been layered over 10% PCA with 1 m*M* BPDS (0.55 ml), and then centrifuged for 1 min (Fig. 1). Intracellular GSH, oxidized glutathione (GSSG), and related thiols and disulfides are measured in the supernatant liquid by transferring 0.45 ml of the acid to a tube containing 50 μl of γ-Glu-Glu (15 m*M*, internal standard), followed by derivatization and analysis by HPLC (10,11).

Extracellular Glutathione

If cystine is absent from the medium, efflux of GSH and GSSG can be measured directly by transferring 0.45 ml of the medium to a tube containing 50 μl of γ-Glu-Glu (15 m*M*, internal standard), followed by derivatization and analysis by HPLC (10,11). If cystine is present, a novel *in vitro* method for determining the selective efflux of GSH and GSSG from cells can be conducted (12). This method takes advantage of the thiol–disulfide reaction between cystine (0.2 m*M*) and GSH with a stoichiometric formation of cysteinyl–glutathione disulfide. Because the formation of the mixed disulfide does not affect extracellular GSSG, the cellular efflux of GSH and GSSG can be distinguished.

Protein–Glutathione Mixed Disulfides

Treatment of protein-containing samples with 10% PCA yields a protein precipitate that can be analyzed for glutathione–protein mixed disulfides by washing with 0.5 ml of cold ethanol to denature the protein and eliminate residual nonprotein thiols (13). After mixing with a vortex mixer and centrifugation, the ethanol is discarded, and 50 μl of γ-Glu-Glu (10 m*M* in water) and 0.5 μl of a MOPS–DTT buffer are added to the protein pellet. The mixture is sonicated and incubated with shaking for 60 min at 37°C. This treatment releases GSH (thiols) from glutathione (thiols)–protein mixed disulfides. At the end of the incubation period, 50 μl of BPDS (15 m*M*) and 0.1 ml of 70% PCA are added, and the sample is processed in a vortex mixer, frozen, thawed, and centrifuged. The 10% PCA extract (0.5 ml) is derivatized and analyzed by HPLC. Aliquots of a solution of GSH-derivatized bovine serum albumin are used as controls for the measurement of protein–glutathione mixed disulfides. The above procedure, adapted from the work of Livesey and Reed (13), is also applicable to the measurement of nonglutathione thiol–protein mixed disulfides.

Mitochondrial Glutathione

Mitochondrial glutathione can be measured in freshly isolated hepatocytes and other cells in suspension (14). The rapid isolation of mitochondrial glutathione from hepatocytes was adapted from the method of Meredith and Reed (15) in which hepatocytes (3×10^6 cells) are suspended in digitonin buffer to solubilize cholesterol-containing membranes (plasma membrane) while leaving mitochondrial membranes intact (Fig. 1). After a 30-sec 13,000-*g* centrifugation of 1.0 ml of hepatocyte suspension at ambient temperature, the hepatocytes are gently suspended in a digitonin buffer and layered over dibutyl phthalate that is layered over 10% PCA with 1 m*M* BPDS (0.55 ml) and centrifuged. The dense mitochondria, along with the cell skeleton, are forced through the dibutyl phthalate layer and into the 10% PCA layer, thereby releasing mitochondrial contents. A portion of the PCA layer is analyzed by HPLC for GSH, GSSG, and related thiols and disulfides (10,11). Recently, Martin and White (16) adapted the Reed *et al.* (10) method to a fluorometric determination of oxidized and reduced glutathione by derivatization with dansyl chloride and with the same column and solvent conditions. This gives ~100-fold greater sensitivity than the ultraviolet detection of the dinitrophenylglutathione derivatives.

Vitamin E Determination

The measurement of α-tocopherol in viable cells is based on the addition of internal standard, γ-tocopherol (0.6 nmol in 40 μl of ethanol), to samples of viable cells (17). The samples are diluted with 50% ethanol (0.4 ml), sonicated, and extracted twice with 0.5 ml of hexane (18). The hexane extracts are pooled and evaporated to dryness with nitrogen gas, the residue is dissolved in 0.6 ml of methanol, and 200 μl is analyzed by HPLC. Measurements of α-tocopherol are made on a Spectra-Physics 8700 chromatograph (Thermo Separation Products, Fremont, CA) equipped with a Schoeffel 970 fluorescence detector (Applied Biosystems, Foster City, CA) (excitation filter, 205 nm; emission filter, 300 nm) (18), and a Sperisorb ODS column (20 cm $\times$ 4.6 mm; 5-μm particles; Custom LC, Houston, TX). The mobile phase, 70% A (80% methanol) and 30% B (100% methanol), is run isocratically for 5 min and then for 15 min at a linear gradient to 1% A and 99% B at a flow rate of 1.5 ml/min. The HPLC retention time for γ- and α-tocopherol is ~20 and 21 min, respectively. Intracellular α-tocopherol concentrations are corrected for the number of viable cells sampled as determined by DNA content.

COMMENTS

Typical applications of this technique continue to appear in the literature. Hepatocytes from phenobarbital-treated and naive rats were used to study the status of glutathione during menadione-mediated toxicity with the dibutyl phthalate separation method to determine the glutathione content of viable cells (19). Hepatocytes and other cells in monolayer culture have been removed from culture dishes and analyzed for intracellular constituents (14). Cannon *et al.* (20) used the dibutyl phthalate centrifugation procedure to follow rat hepatocyte viability by assessing the leakage of LDH during ATP depletion and mitochondrial dysfunction. In a carbon tetrachloride/chloroform interaction study with rat hepatocytes, O'Hara *et al.* (21) measured the release of intracellular K^+ from viable cells and LDH leakage with the dibutyl phthalate centrifugation procedure.

In determining the importance of protein thiols during *N*-methyl-*N*′-nitro-*N*-nitrosoguanidine toxicity in primary rat hepatocytes, Shertzer *et al.* (22) observed that viable hepatocytes were separated from nonviable cells and from the incubation medium by centrifugation through a diisobutyl phthalate layer rather than dibutyl phthalate. They concluded that the diisobutyl phthalate ester suitably substitutes for the dibutyl phthalate ester.

In an attempt to increase the number of viable cells in cryopreserved rat and dog hepatocyte preparations, centrifugation through a dibutyl phthalate layer was investigated and found to cause some toxicity to the cells, as measured by trypan blue exclusion and 7-ethoxycoumarin dealkylation (23). Percoll colloidal silica solution was found to be satisfactory; however, Powis *et al.* concluded that the density of viable cells immediately after cryopreservation is different from that of fresh hepatocytes. After adjustment for this difference, the recovery of viable cells was substantially lower than a protocol that required freshly isolated hepatocytes.

The dibutyl phthalate centrifugation method was utilized to demonstrate a species difference in the uptake of *N*-nitrosobis(2-oxopropyl)amine by isolated rat and hamster hepatocytes (24). Mangino *et al.* reported for the first time a value for the intracellular water of hamster hepatocytes. Hamster hepatocytes and pancreatic acinar cells were compared by the dibutyl phthalate method for *N*-nitrosobis(2-oxopropyl)amine uptake rates (25).

It is necessary to establish conditions for each cell type to be evaluated by an oil-based separation procedure. Since there are appreciable differences in the densities of the phthalate esters, it should be possible to utilize these differences to select appropriate separation conditions.

ACKNOWLEDGMENTS

I would like to thank R. Bodine and B. Hommel for their help in preparing this manuscript. This work was supported by National Institute of Environmental Health Sciences grants ES00210 and ES01978.

REFERENCES

1. M. W. Fariss, M. K. Brown, J. A. Schmitz, and D. J. Reed, *Toxicol. Appl. Pharmacol.* **79,** 283 (1985).
2. H. A. Krebs, N. W. Cornell, P. Lund, and R. Hems, *in* "Regulation of Hepatic Metabolism" (F. Lundquist and N. Tygstrup, eds.), pp. 726–750. Academic Press, New York, 1974.
3. H. Pertoft, K. Rubin, L. Kjellén, T. C. Laurent, and B. Klingeborn, *Exp. Cell Res.* **110,** 449 (1977).
4. C. Dalet, M. Fehlmann, and P. Debey, *Anal. Biochem.* **122,** 119 (1982).
5. N. H. Stacey, L. R. Cantilena, and C. D. Klaassen, *Toxicol. Appl. Pharmacol.* **53,** 470 (1980).
6. H. Baur, S. Kasperek, and E. Pfaff, *Hoppe-Seyler's Z. Physiol. Chem.* **356,** 827 (1975).
7. G. M. Sainsbury, M. Stubbs, R. Hems, and H. A. Krebs, *Biochem. J.* **180,** 685 (1979).
8. N. W. Cornell, *Anal. Biochem.* **102,** 326 (1980).
9. B. G. Erwin, C. M. Stoscheck, and J. R. Florini, *Anal. Biochem.* **110,** 291 (1981).
10. D. J. Reed, J. R. Babson, P. W. Beatty, A. E. Brodie, W. W. Ellis, and D. W. Potter, *Anal. Biochem.* **106,** 55 (1980).
11. M. W. Fariss and D. J. Reed, *in* "Methods in Enzymol." (W. B. Jakoby and O. Griffith, eds.), Vol. 143, p. 101. Academic Press, Orlando, Florida, 1987.
12. M. W. Fariss and D. J. Reed, *in* "Isolation, Characterization and Use of Hepatocytes" (R. A. Harriss and N. W. Cornell, eds.), p. 349. Elsevier, New York, 1983.
13. J. C. Livesey and D. J. Reed, *Int. J. Radiat. Oncol., Biol., Phys.* **10,** 1507 (1984).

14. D. J. Reed, this series, Vol. 2, pp. 219–226.
15. M. J. Meredith and D. J. Reed, *J. Biol. Chem.* **257,** 3747 (1982).
16. J. Martin and I. N. H. White, *J. Chromatogr.* **568,** 219 (1991).
17. M. W. Fariss, G. A. Pascoe, and D. J. Reed, *Science* **227,** 751 (1985).
18. S. K. Howell and Y. Wang, *J. Chromatogr.* **227,** 174 (1982).
19. W. S. Utley and H. M. Mehendale, *Toxicol. Appl. Pharmacol.* **99,** 323 (1989).
20. J. R. Cannon, P. J. Harvison, and G. F. Rush, *Toxicol. Appl. Pharmacol.* **108,** 407 (1991).
21. T. M. O'Hara, J. F. Borzelleca, E. C. Clarke, M. A. Sheppard, and L. W. Condie, Jr. *Fundam. Appl. Toxicol.* **13,** 605 (1989).
22. H. G. Shertzer, M. Sainsbury, and M. L. Berger, *Toxicol. Appl. Pharmacol.* **105,** 19 (1990).
23. G. Powis, K. S. Santone, D. C. Melder, L. Thomas, D. J. Moore, and T. J. Wilke, *Drug Metab. Dispos.* **15,** 826 (1987).
24. M. M. Mangino, P. F. Hollenberg, and D. G. Scarpelli, *Carcinogenesis* **9,** 1763 (1988).
25. M. M. Mangino, D. G. Scarpelli, and D. M. Kokkinakis, *Carcinogenesis* **11,** 625 (1990).

37 Flow Cytometry

Jeffrey D. Laskin and Debra L. Laskin

INTRODUCTION

Flow cytometry is a laser-based technology that permits rapid and quantitative multiparameter analysis and separation of particles. In the biological and medical sciences these particles can be cells, organelles, chromosomes, large immune complexes, liposomes, fungi, bacteria, cell hybrids, cell aggregates, or small multicellular organisms. Measurements of visible and fluorescent light emission allow quantitation of antigenic, biochemical, and biophysical characteristics of individual cells. A major advantage of flow cytometry is the speed of analysis (up to 10,000 cells per second). In addition, heterogeneity within a cell population in terms of physical or functional properties can be assessed. In this chapter methods are provided for analysis of antibody binding to cells, DNA cell cycle, and intracellular oxidative metabolism. A large number of other biochemical and functional characteristics of individual cells can be measured by flow cytometry, including stimulus-induced changes in intracellular calcium, pH, and glutathione, as well as membrane potential and fluidity, DNA, RNA and chromosome content, phagocytosis, and viability. Methods and applications of a variety of flow-cytometric techniques have been reviewed elsewhere (1–3).

MEASUREMENT OF ANTIBODY BINDING BY DIRECT OR INDIRECT IMMUNOFLUORESCENCE

Expression of proteins, receptors, or antigenic markers on the cell surface or intracellularly can be measured by quantifying binding of directly or indirectly labeled fluorescent antibodies or ligands to specific cell-associated molecules. These can be used to characterize and define different cell types within heterogeneous populations or to analyze the purity of isolated cell subpopulations.

Materials and Reagents

Cells for analysis
V-bottomed 96-well microtiter dish
12 × 75-mm disposable glass tubes
Fetal bovine serum (FBS)

METHODS IN TOXICOLOGY, Volume 1B

Phosphate-buffered saline (PBS), calcium and magnesium free (Sigma, St. Louis, MO)
Hanks' balanced salt solution (HBSS), calcium and magnesium free (Sigma)
3% Paraformaldehyde: (pH 7.2)
Primary antibody, titrated prior to use
Isotypic control antibody: titrated prior to use
Secondary antibody labeled either with fluorescein isothiocyanate (FITC) or phycoerythrin (PE), titrated prior to use

Note: Primary antibodies conjugated to biotin can also be used. These are detected with fluorochrome-labeled avidin.

Procedures

Measurement of Cell Surface Antigen Expression by Indirect Immunofluorescence

1. Prepare a single cell suspension of cells to be analyzed and wash in PBS (300*g*, 8 min).
2. Resuspend to 2×10^7 cells/ml in PBS.
3. Add 50 μl of the cell suspension to each well of the microtiter dish.
4. Add 75 μl of FBS to each well.
5. Centrifuge the plates containing the cells [(Beckman, Palo Alto, CA) Beckman TJ6-R, 500*g*, 5 min at 4°C].
6. Decant the supernatant by inverting the plate and vigorously shaking it once.
7. Resuspend the cells in 50 μl of the appropriate dilution of primary antibody or irrelevant isotypic control antibody.
8. Incubate for 30 min at 4°C.
9. Add 75 μl of FBS to each well.
10. Centrifuge the plates containing the cells (300*g*, 5 min, 4°C) as above; decant the supernatants as described in step 6.
11. Resuspend the cells in 50 μl of the appropriate dilution of secondary antibody.
12. Cover with aluminum foil and incubate for 30 min at 4°C.
13. Add 75 μl of FBS to each well.
14. Centrifuge the plates containing the cells (500*g*, 5 min, 4°C) as above; decant supernatants as described in step 6.
15. Resuspend the cells in 50 μl of 3% paraformaldehyde.
16. Cover with aluminum foil and incubate overnight at 4°C.
17. Centrifuge the plates containing the cells (500 *g*, 5 min, 4°C) as above; decant the supernatants as described in step 6.
18. Resuspend the cells in 50 μl of PBS.
19. Transfer the cells to 12 × 75-mm tubes containing 1 ml of PBS for analysis.

Note: Stained samples can be stored at 4°C in the dark for analysis within 3–5 days. Samples *may* remain stable for longer periods.

Measurement of Cell Surface Antigen Expression by Direct Immunofluorescence Using Labeled Primary Antibodies or Ligands

Follow the protocol described above, omitting steps 11–14, adding fluorescently labeled antibody or ligand to the cells.

Simultaneous Analysis of the Expression of More Than One Cell Surface Antigen

This is most easily accomplished using antibodies directly conjugated to fluorochromes such as FITC or PE, which can be analyzed simultaneously since their excitation maxima are the same (488 nm), but their emission spectra are distinct (525 nm for FITC and 630 nm for PE). For dual labeling of cells with fluorescently labeled primary antibodies, follow the protocol described above omitting steps 11–14, adding both primary antibodies to the cells at the same time. If direct and indirect staining are used in the same protocol, the indirect labeling should be performed first.

Measurement of Intracellular Antigen Expression

For analysis of intracellular antigens using specific antibodies, the cells are fixed and permeabilized prior to incubation with the antibody. This is accomplished by incubating the cells overnight in 2% paraformaldehyde. The cells are then washed in PBS (300 *g*, 8 min) and permeabilized by the addition of 0.05% Triton X-100 (prepared in HBSS). After washing in PBS, the cells are stained with antibody as described above.

Note: All of the procedures described above can be performed in 15 × 75-cm tubes if microtiter dishes are not available or if fewer numbers of samples are to be analyzed. In this modified procedure, 1×10^6 cells and 200 μl of antibody or ligand are used per tube. The cells are washed with 250 μl of FBS and 500 μl of PBS.

Data Analysis

All commercially available flow cytometers have standard analytical packages for measurement of the percentage of specific antibody binding to the cells in comparison to the isotypic controls. Care should be taken in interpreting data if significant population heterogeneity in antibody binding is observed.

Comment In general, immunofluorescence staining is simple to perform, although several factors should be considered. Antibody cross-linking should be minimized, since this can lead to alterations and internalization of surface antigens. This can be accomplished by maintaining the samples at 4°C, by adding sodium azide (0.1%) to the sample buffer, or by using monovalent antibodies prepared as Fab fragments if they are available. Unstained cells should also be analyzed in each experiment to establish levels of background autofluorescence.

DNA CELL CYCLE ANALYSIS AND PLOIDY DETERMINATION USING PROPIDIUM IODIDE

As cells traverse the cell cycle, their DNA content changes. During the cell growth, or S, phase, the nuclear DNA doubles from the G_0/G_1 level (2*N*) to the G_2M level (4*N*). By staining cells with fluorochromes that specifically bind DNA, estimations can be made of the percentage of cells within a population in the different phases of the cell cycle, since cells in G_2M will be approximately two times more fluorescent than cells in G_0/G_1. Several fluorescent dyes are commercially available that can be used effectively to stain cellular DNA. These include guanine–cytosine (GC)-specific dyes such as mithramycin, adenine–thymine (AT)-specific dyes such as Hoechst 33342 (Molecular Probes, Eugene, OR), bromodeoxyuridine, and diamidinophenolindol, as well as the intercalating dye, propidium iodide (reviewed in Ref. 4). Also of use is acridine orange, a metachromatic dye that forms polymeric stacks within the DNA helix (5). This dye is particularly valuable for simultaneous analysis of single-and double-stranded nucleic acids which emit red and green fluorescence, respectively. Thus, acridine orange can be used to simultaneously quantify RNA and DNA content as well as to distinguish between cells in the G_2 and M phases of the cell cycle (5,6). In this section, methods are described to analyze cellular DNA using propidium iodide, which has excitation/emmission spectra of 488 nm/630 nm and thus can be used in most commonly available flow cytometers.

Propidium Iodide Staining for DNA Cell Cycle

Materials and Reagents

Cells for analysis (2×10^6 per sample)
Nylon mesh (35 μm): (Tetko, Lancaster, NY)
PBS
Citrate buffer: (100 ml): 4.5 g of sucrose (Sigma), 1.18 g of citrate trisodium (Sigma), and 5 ml of Dimethyl sulfoxide (Sigma); bring the volume up to 100 ml with distilled water, filter sterilize through 0.22-μm cellulose acetate membrane filter and store at 4°C
T-TBS solution (100 ml): 0.016 g of Tris-HCl (Bio-Rad, Richmond, CA); 0.88 g of NaCl; and 0.1 m of 0.1% Tween-20 (Bio-Rad); dissolve in 70 ml of distilled water by vigorously shaking; add 100,000 U of RNase A (Sigma); bring the volume up to 100 ml with distilled water, boil for 10 min, aliquot into 10-ml samples, and freeze at −20°C
Propidium iodide solution (25 ml, 10 μg/ml): 2.5 g of propidium iodide

(Sigma); bring the volume up to 25 ml with PBS, aliquot into 500-μl samples and freeze at $-20°C$

Procedure

1. Prepare a suspension of cells to be analyzed (2×10^6 per sample) in 12×75-mm tubes and wash in PBS (300 *g*, 8 min).
2. Resuspend in 500 μl of citrate buffer.
3. Freeze at $-70°C$ for 10–15 min (the sample may also be stored for several months).
4. Thaw at room temperature.
5. Centrifuge the cells at 300 *g* for 8 min at 4°C and discard the supernatant.
6. Resuspend the cells in 750 μl T-TBS solution.
7. Incubate for 60 min at room temperature.
8. Centrifuge the cells at 300 *g* for 8 min at 4°C and discard the supernatant.
9. Resuspend in 750 μl of PBS and filter the cell sample through 35 μm nylon mesh.
10. Add 7.5 μl of propidium iodide solution.
11. Cover samples tightly with foil and store at 4°C until analysis within 2 days.

Data Analysis

All commercially available flow cytometers have standard analytical packages for analysis of the percentage of cells in the different phases of the cell cycle. Several other software programs are also available. These programs, however, are based on certain models and assumptions which may change under different experimental conditions (i.e., when aneuploid cells are analyzed). Care should be taken to use the same software program for analysis of the data within one experiment, since estimations of cells within the S phase vary from program to program.

Comment Sample preparation for cell cycle analysis using propidium iodide is relatively straightforward. Since propidium iodide binds to double-stranded DNA and RNA, however, samples should be treated with RNase A to improve the resolution of the DNA analysis. In addition, cell concentrations among samples should be the same for better comparison. Propidium iodide binding to DNA is also dependent on the salt concentration. Therefore, the staining solutions should approximate those used in the cytometer during analysis.

MEASUREMENT OF INTRACELLULAR OXIDATIVE METABOLISM USING DICHLOROFLUORESCIN DIACETATE (DCFH-DA)

All cells exhibit some degree of intracellular oxidative metabolism resulting in the formation of oxygen radicals. Macrophages and neutrophils also produce reactive oxygen intermediates such as superoxide anion, hydrogen peroxide, and hydroxyl radical to destroy invading pathogens and tumor cells. DCFH-DA is a convenient and sensitive dye that can be used to quantify intracellular levels of hydroperoxy radicals such as hydrogen peroxide (7,8). DCFH-DA readily diffuses into cells. There, the diacetate groups are cleaved from the molecule by intracellular esterases, yielding a nonfluorescent product, DCFH, which is trapped within the cells. In the presence of hydroperoxides, DCFH is oxidized to the highly fluorescent molecule, dichlorofluorescein, which is excited at 488 nm and detected at 525 nm by flow cytometry. Thus, in this assay, green fluorescence intensity is proportional to hydrogen peroxide production by the cells.

Materials and Reagents

Cells for analysis
12 × 75-mm disposable glass tubes
HBSS (Sigma), as above
DCFH-DA (Molecular Probes, Eugene, OR): Prepare as a 5 m*M* stock solution in 100% ethanol; store at −20°C
Stimulus for the cells [e.g., for phagocytic cells, 100 n*M* 12-*O*-tetradecanoyl phorbol-13-acetate (LC Services, Woburn, MA), prepared as a 100× stock solution in ethanol]

Procedure

1. Collect and resuspend the cells, in HBSS at a concentration of 1×10^6/ml.
2. Add 1 ml per tube of the cell suspension to 12 × 75-mm tubes.
3. Add 10 μl of DCFH-DA solution to each tube at 5-min intervals.
4. Incubate each tube in a shaking 37°C water bath for 20 min.
5. Add 10 μl of buffer control or 100× stimulus to the tubes containing the cells.
6. Incubate the cells in a shaking 37°C water bath for 20 min.
7. Immediately analyze green fluorescence at 525 nm.

Data Analysis

Data on both basal and stimulated levels of hydrogen peroxide production by the cells should be collected and compared. Care should be taken in interpreting data if significant population heterogeneity in oxidative metabolism is observed.

Comment DCFH-DA is continuously taken up by cells and oxidized to the fluorescent product. Thus, it is important that all of the cell samples be incubated with DCFH-DA, as well as with the stimulus, for the same period. This is accomplished by staggering the addition of DCFH-DA and the stimulus or buffer to the cells by at least 5 min between samples. This will permit sufficient time to analyze cell samples on the flow cytometer.

REFERENCES

1. M. R. Melamed, T. Lindmo, and M. L. Mendelsohn (eds.), "Flow Cytometry and Sorting," 2nd Ed. Wiley–Liss, New York, 1990.
2. H. M. Shapiro (ed.), "Practical Flow Cytometry," 2nd ed. Liss, New York, 1988.
3. A. Yen (ed.), "Flow Cytometry: Advanced Research and Clinical Applications," (Vols. I and II. CRC Press, Boca Raton, Florida, (1989).
4. J. W. Gray and Z. Darzynkiewicz, (eds.), "Techniques in Cell Cycle Analysis." Humana, Clifton, New Jersey, 1987.
5. Z. Darzynkiewicz, F. Traganos, T. Sharpless, and M. R. Melamed, *Exp. Cell Res.* **110,** 201 (1977).
6. D. L. Laskin, A. A. Sirak, and J. D. Laskin, *Cell Prolif.* **24,** 341 (1991).
7. D. A. Bass, J. W. Parce, L. R. Dechatelet, P. Szejda, M. C. Seeds, and M. Thomas. *J. Immunol.* **130,** 1910 (1983).
8. T. W. McCloskey, J. A. Todaro, and D. L. Laskin. *Hepatology* **16,** 191 (1992).

38 Single-Cell Microscopic Techniques for Studying Toxic Injury

John J. Lemasters, Anna-Liisa Nieminen, Enrique Chacon, John M. Bond, Ian Harper, Jeffrey M. Reece, and Brian Herman

INTRODUCTION

In acute toxicity a sequence of events is initiated that culminates in loss of cell viability and tissue necrosis. The response of individual cells in a tissue to toxic stress is often heterogeneous, with each cell progressing at its own rate. As a consequence bulk biochemical measurements may fail to represent adequately the true cause-and-effect relationships between various toxicant-induced phenomena. An approach to circumvent this difficulty is the study of single cells. By following the progression of injury in single cells after exposure to toxicants, the timing and sequence of events leading up to cell death can be determined. Furthermore, events preceding cell killing can be distinguished from those that follow cell death. Here, we describe the application of multiparameter digitized video microscopy (MDVM) to single-cell toxicology.

EQUIPMENT

Equipment from many vendors is now available for performing MDVM. The essential elements are an inverted fluorescence microscope, a low-light video camera, and a computer system to collect, process, and store video images. For confocal microscopy a scan head and additional computer system are required. Figure 1 illustrates the basic configuration of our system. The system is built around a Nikon Diaphot inverted fluorescence microscope (Nikon, Garden City, NY) equipped with differential interference contrast (DIC) and phase optics. Two eight-position filter wheels (Metatek, Cary, NC) under computer control are used to place interference and neutral density filters in the path of excitation light from a xenon lamp. Phase, DIC, and fluorescence images are collected by an intensified charge-coupled device camera (DAGE/MTI, Michigan City, IN). Camera output goes to a Sparcstation (Sun Microsystems, Mountain View, CA) through Datacube imaging boards (Datacube, Peabody, MA) for frame averaging, background subtraction, ratioing, and other types of image processing. In some instances we record the camera output directly with a video cassette recorder.

METHODS IN TOXICOLOGY, Volume 1B

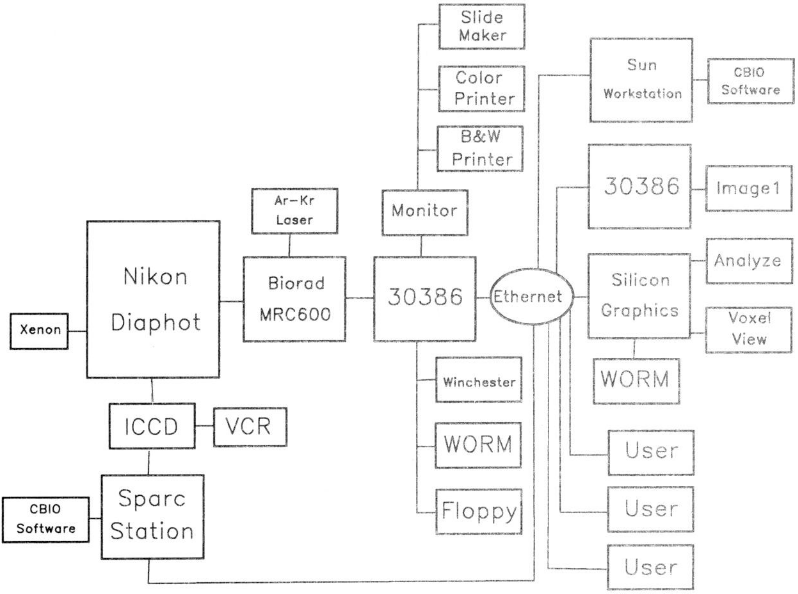

Figure 1 Multiparameter digitized video microscope system. See text for abbreviations and details.

Our microscope is also equipped with a Bio-Rad (Cambridge, MA) MRC-600 laser scanning confocal attachment operating with an argon--krypton mixed-gas laser (Ion Laser Technology, Salt Lake City, UT). Image acquisition and initial processing are controlled by a microcomputer operating Bio-Rad applications software. Dual fluorescence detectors allow simultaneous multiparameter detection. A transmitted light detector permits collection of nonconfocal bright-field images simultaneously with confocal fluorescence images.

Collection of video images rapidly consumes large amounts of computer memory, and large capacity hard (Winchester) disk drives with more than 200 Mbytes of disk space are necessary for initial storage of data. For archival storage optical disk drives storing as much as a Gbyte of data per disk are required. In practice, data sets are rarely erased and so-called Write-Once-Read-Many (WORM) drives (e.g., Model LF-5010, Panasonic, Secaucus, NJ) that are not erasable can be used. However, the price of rewritable optical drives has fallen greatly. Thus, there is at present no longer any great price advantage of WORM drives over rewritable optical drives.

The Sparcstation and 30386 microcomputer are used both to acquire images and to analyze them later. A disadvantage of this arrangement is that image analysis may compete with image collection. This is especially important in a multi-user environment in which one user performing image analysis prevents another from using the microscope to acquire data. To avoid such conflicts, we encourage users to download their images via Ethernet to one of several other computers in our facility or to their own computers. By this means users can process and analyze their images off-line using either our own software or commercial packages such as Image-1 (Universal Imaging, West Chester, PA). A Silicon Graphics 4D/310 VGX Imaging Superworkstation (Mountain View, CA) is particularly powerful for image analysis and generates three-dimensional displays of confocal image sets using VoxelView (Vital Images, Fairfield, IA) and ANALYZE (Mayo Foundation, Rochester, MN) software. An optical drive is also needed to store the processed images.

BRIGHT-FIELD MICROSCOPY

During exposure to toxic chemicals, bright-field microscopy often reveals early structural changes. In many cell types, including liver, kidney, and heart cells, the development of blisterlike protrusions of the plasma membrane, called blebs, is an early structural alteration in cell injury (Fig. 2) (1). Breakdown or rupture of one of these blebs is the event that precipitates irreversible cell death. To observe such events, we usually use phase-contrast optics for contrast enhancement. Phase contrast is relatively simple to set up and easily permits observation of fluorescence images at the same time.

FLUORESCENT PROBES

Bright-field microscopy provides general and relatively unspecific information concerning cellular responses to toxicants. For more specific information cells can be labeled with fluorophores whose fluorescence is a function of specific cellular parameters, such as ion concentration or membrane potential. By loading two or more fluorophores with nonoverlapping excitation and emission spectra, several parameters or interest can be measured quantitatively over time in single living cells through selection of appropriate excitation and emission fluorescence wavelengths. This is the basis for MDVM.

The range of useful fluorophores is large and growing rapidly. Table I lists some of the more useful probes. These fluorophores can be divided into three groups: (a) probes of general cell function, such as cell viability and membrane potential; (b) markers of specific subcellular compartments, such as lysosomes, Golgi, and mitochondria; and (c) probes of specific chemical species, such as ions and free thiol groups. An excellent and exhaustive description of commercially available fluorophore probes is found in Haugland's *Handbook of Fluorescent Probes and Research Chemicals* (2), which summarizes applications of fluorophores sold by Molecular Probes (Eugene, OR).

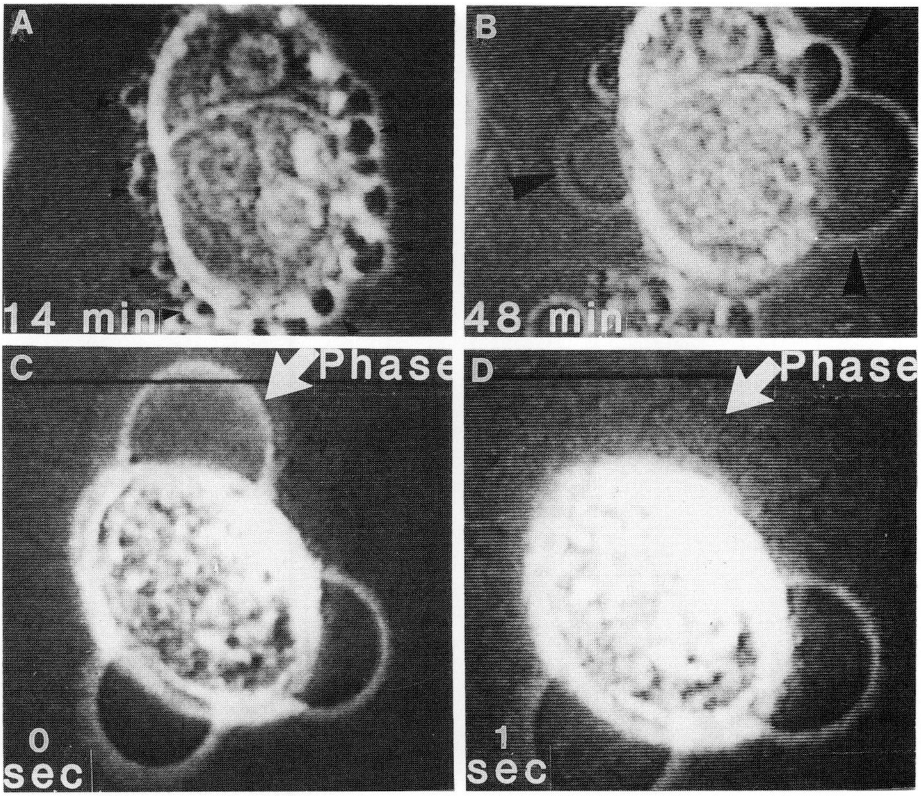

Figure 2 Bright-field microscopy of bleb formation and rupture during cell injury. Cultured rat hepatocytes were exposed to 2.5 mM KCN and 0.5 mM iodoacetate ("chemical hypoxia") and observed by phase-contrast microscopy. (A) Numerous small surface blebs developed within a few minutes. (B) Small blebs enlarged and coalesced by fusion. (C) In another cell only a few large terminal blebs remained after ~45 min. (D) The onset of cell death was initiated by the abrupt rupture of one of the blebs 1 sec later. Nuclear labeling with propidium iodide followed several seconds later (not shown).

CELL VIABILITY

The classic indicator of loss of cell viability is nuclear uptake of trypan blue. Trypan blue is a cationic chromophore that intercalates into DNA. In viable cells the plasma membrane prevents trypan blue from entering and labeling the nucleus. At the onset of cell death, the plasma membrane permeability barrier fails and trypan blue readily stains the nucleus. Fluorescent DNA intercalators, such as propidium iodide, behave identically to trypan blue in labeling nuclei of non-

Table I Fluorophores for Multiparameter Digitized Video Microscopy[a]

Cellular parameter	Fluorophore
Probes of general cell function	
Cell viability	Propidium iodide, Ethidium homodimer, PRO probes, Fluorescein diacetate, and Calcein acetoxymethyl ester
Membrane potentials	Rhodamine-123 and TMRM
Markers of subcellular compartments	
Cell volume/topography	Calcein
Endosomes	Rhodamine microspheres
Lysosomes	Rhodamine–dextran and Texas red–dextran
Golgi apparatus	BODIPY–ceramide
Endoplasmic reticulum	Carbocyanine dyes
Probes of specific chemical species	
Ca^{2+}	Fura-2, Indo-1, and Fluo-3
pH	BCECF and SNARF-1
Mg^{2+}	Mag-Fura
Na^{+}	SBFI
K^{+}	PBFI
Glutathione	Monochlorobimane
Protein thiols	Monobromobimane
Oxygen radicals	Dichlorofluorescin, Dihydrorhodamine-123, and Dihydroethidium

[a] Abbreviations are explained in the text.

viable cells (3,4). Binding is associated with an enhancement of fluorescence, and nuclei of nonviable cells are readily identified by fluorescence microscopy even at low concentrations (0.5–5μM) of fluorophore. Other probes, including ethidium homodimer and the so-called PRO probes (PO-PRO, BO-PRO, YO-PRO, and TO-PRO) from Molecular Probes, also enter the cell at the onset of cell death and label the nucleus (2,5). These fluorophores fluoresce at a variety of different wavelengths, so that a viability-indicating fluorohore can be selected that does not interfere with other parameter-specific fluorophores in use.

Cellular retention of anionic fluorophores, such as fluorescein and calcein, is also used to indicate cell viability (3). These fluorophores are loaded as their acetate or acetoxymethyl esters by incubating cells for 15–45 min with 1–10 μM of the easter derivative. However, many cells have plasma membrane carriers that catalyze the outward movement of anionic fluorophores. Thus, dye retention over long periods is not as reliable an indicator of cell viability as dye exclusion. Nonetheless, the rapid and complete loss of anionic fluorophore is surely indicative of cell death. Loss of dye occurs in just a few seconds (6). Ion-indicating probes such as Fura-2 and 2′,7′-biscarboxyethyl-5,6-carboxyfluorescein (BCECF) can also be used in this fashion by imaging them at parameter-insensitive wavelengths. By imaging at parameter-sensitive wavelengths in addition, these ion-sensitive fluorophores can measure both free ion concentration and cell viability (7,8).

Electrical Gradients inside Cells

Membrane-permeant cationic probes such as rhodamine-123 and tetramethylrhodamine methylester (TMRM) distribute into negatively charged cellular organelles in accordance with the Nernst equation:

$$\Delta\Psi = -60 \log F_{in}/F_{out} \quad (1)$$

where $\Delta\Psi$ is the electrical potential difference across the organelle's membrane, and F_{in} and F_{out} are fluorophore intensities inside and outside (9–11). According to Eq. (1), a 10 : 1 uptake ratio corresponds to a $\Delta\Psi$ of −60 mV; a 100 : 1 gradient, to −120 mV; and a 1000 : 1 gradient, to −180 mV. Since mitochondria have a $\Delta\Psi$ approaching −180 mV, rhodamine-123 and TMRM accumulate avidly into mitochondria. Since there is a 10-fold loss of fluorophore for every 60 mV of depolarization, even a relatively small extent of mitochondrial depolarization will lead to large and easily measurable decreases of fluorescence.

For excitable cells such as myocytes and neurons, a plasma membrane $\Delta\Psi$ of −90 mV will be additive with the mitochondrial $\Delta\Psi$. Thus, mitochondria inside an excitable cell are as much as 270 mV more negative than the outside the cell. This corresponds to a 30,000 : 1 gradient of fluorophore inside mitochondria to that outside the cell. With conventional video cameras and eight-bit frame memories storing only 256 gray levels for each picture element (pixel), quantitation of such concentration gradients is not possible. However, using confocal microscopy, gamma circuits can apply a logarithmic function to the image output and condense a very large signal range into the available 256 gray levels of video memory (12). In this way, mitochondrial and plasma membrane $\Delta\Psi$ can be quantified in single cells.

CELL SIZE AND SHAPE

A basic aspect to cell structure is size and shape. To determine size and shape, cells can be loaded with calcein by incubating with 3–10 μM calcein acetoxymethyl ester for 30–60 min at 37°C. Intracellular esterases cleave the ester bonds to liberate calcein free acid in the cytosol. Ester loading is a common technique for loading fluorophores with carboxyl groups, such as Fura-2 and fluorescein. Calcein, however, is unaffected by physiological changes of pH or ion concentration and simply marks the size and shape of the intracellular space. Used in conjunction with confocal microscopy (discussed below), calcein can reveal the full three-dimensional extent of individual cells (12).

ORGANELLE MARKERS

As described above, incubation of cells with rhodamine-123 or TMRM (0.1–1.0 μM for 15–30 min) brightly labels mitochondria. Rhodamine–dextran and Texas red–dextran are convenient labels of lysosomes (7,8). Incubation of cell cultures overnight with 1 μg/ml of dextran conjugate provides adequate loading, which occurs by endocytosis and subsequent segregation into lysosomes. Hepatocytes can be loaded prior to isolation by intraperitoneal injection of 20 mg of rhodamine–dextran/100 g body weight 1 day prior to the isolation procedure. Lysosomes do not appreciably digest these dextran conjugates, and fluorescence will persist for many days in culture. Cells loaded with rhodamine– or Texas red–dextran can be coloaded with rhodamine-123 *in vitro.* Mitochondria are then identified by green fluorescence using blue excitation light, and lysosomes are identified by red fluorescence using green excitation light. A growing number of other organelle-specific fluorophores have been described. For example, difluoroboradiazaindacene (BODIPY)–ceramide derivatives to label the Golgi apparatus and carbocyanine dyes to mark the endoplasmic reticulum have been used successfully (13,14).

PROBES FOR FREE THIOLS AND REACTIVE OXYGEN SPECIES

For toxicologists, cellular content of protein and nonprotein thiols may be particularly important information. Glutathione (GSH), the predominant nonprotein thiol of cells, protects cells against free radicals, oxidants, and electrophilic metabolites of toxic chemicals. Free thiols are essential for the activity of many enzymes. Protein and nonprotein thiols may be imaged after derivatization with membrane-permeant bimanes (15). Monochlorobimane reacts with nonprotein thiols, mainly GSH, catalyzed by GSH *S*-transferase. Monobromobimane reacts with all free thiols nonenzymatically. The covalent thiol adducts of both bimanes are highly fluorescent, whereas unreacted bimanes have little fluorescence. In hepatocytes 200 μM monochlorobimane and 1 mM monobromobimane are the minimum concentrations to give maximum rates of reaction. The reaction with monobromobimane is very rapid and goes to completion in 1 min. The reaction with monochlorobimane is complete after ~5 min.

The intracellular compartmentation of bimane adducts may be estimated as described below by addition of increasing strengths of detergents. In monobromobimane-labeled cells low concentrations of digitonin release 85–90% of fluorescence, which represents mostly soluble glutathione. Even after Triton X-100 extraction, nuclear staining by monobromobimane remains, indicating labeling of sulfhydryls in chromatin and the nuclear matrix. Virtually all monochlorobimane fluorescence is released by low concentrations of digitonin. This represents cytosolic glutathione. Little identifiable mitochondrial glutathione remains, evidently because mitochondria lack the GSH *S*-transferase needed to form mitochondria monochlorobimane adducts (16).

OXYGEN RADICAL PROBES

Several compounds react with reactive oxygen species to form fluorescent products that may be visualized by MDVM. Dichlorofluore*scin* reacts with organic hydroperoxides to form highly fluorescent dichlorofluore*scein* (17). In hepatocytes dichlorofluorescin is loaded as its diacetate ester (10 μM for 30 min at room temperature) (18). Low levels of excitation light must be used when imaging dichlorofluorescein, since photobleaching leads to free radical formation and autocatalytic conversion of dichlorofluorescin to dichlorofluorescein. Carboxydichlorofluorescin may be used in a similar fashion (2).

Dihydrorhodamine-123 and dihydroethidium are more robust probes that reportedly react with superoxide to form the fluorescent products rhodamine-123 and ethidium (19,20). Both have been used to follow superoxide formation during toxic injury. Their use in fluorescent imaging is limited by the fact that both reaction products will redistribute within cells: rhodamine-123 to mitochondria and ethidium to the cell nucleus.

ION-INDICATING PROBES

A variety of probes is now available to measure the concentrations of various ions inside single living cells. These include Fura-2 and Indo-1 for Ca^{2+}, biscarboxyethylcarboxyfluorescein (BCECF) and SNARF-1 for H^+, SBFI for Na^+, PBFI for K^+, and Mag-Fura for Mg^{2+} (7,8,12,21–28). The probes are loaded as their lipid-soluble ester derivatives, and endogenous esterases release the ion-sensitive free acid forms of the fluorophores in the cytosol. Alternatives to ester loading include microinjection, scrape loading, and ATP permeabilization (reviewed in Ref. 29). Fluorescence of these ion-indicating fluorophores is dependent upon the concentration of the ions they measure. However, fluorescence

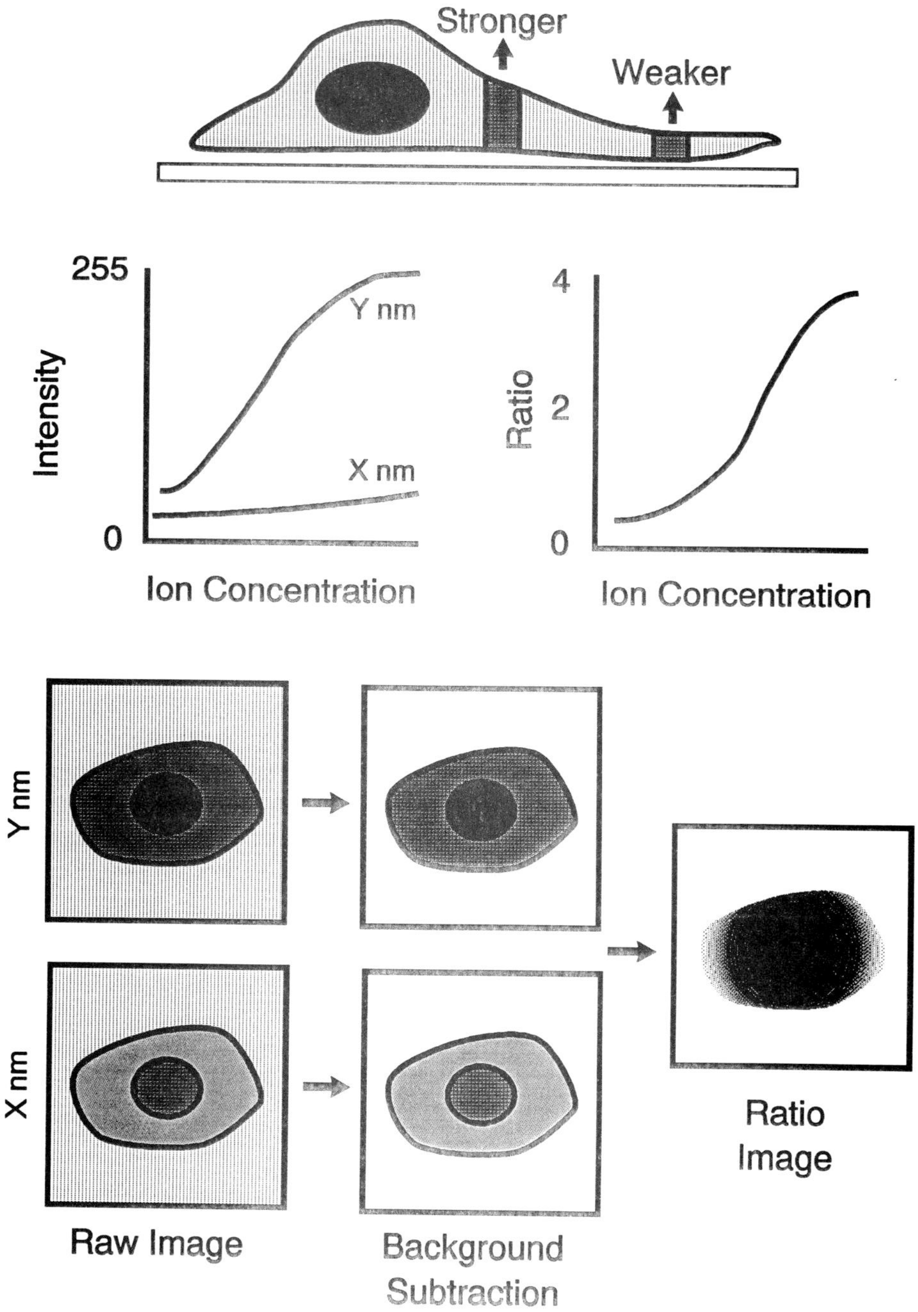
Stronger
Weaker
255
Intensity
0
Y nm
X nm
Ion Concentration
4
Ratio
2
0
Ion Concentration
Y nm
X nm
Raw Image
Background
Subtraction
Ratio
Image

will also depend on probe content in the light path and will vary due to variations of cell thickness, presence of organelles excluding the fluorophore, and variable probe loading from cell to cell (Fig. 3).

To correct for variations of fluorescence due to variable path length and fluorophore loading, a ratioing procedure can be used that takes advantage of ion-induced shifts of the excitation or emission spectra of many probes (Fig. 3) (30). Images are acquired from cells at two different excitation or emission wavelengths, one that is parameter sensitive and one that is not (or whose fluorescence changes in the opposite direction). After background subtraction the first image is divided by the second on a pixel-by-pixel basis to generate a ratio image. Standard curves are generated by imaging fluorophore-containing calibration buffers through the microscope optics or by exposing loaded cells to appropriate ionophores in the presence of various concentrations of ion. From standard curves look-up tables for converting ratios to actual ions concentrations are created. The final result is a map of the distribution of ions within single cells, which is often represented by an arbitrary color or gray scale (Fig. 4). Using this rationing procedure, errors introduced by differences of path length, regional fluorophore concentration, dye leakage over time, photobleaching, and accessible volume are corrected. Not all ion-indicating fluorophores can be ratioed in this way. Fluo-3 (31), a Ca^{2+} indicator, cannot be used for ratio imaging. However, because Fluo-3 is excited by visible light, it is a useful probe in confocal microscopy. For specific applications of Ca^{2+}-indicating fluorophores, see Chapter 25, by A. P. Thomas.

Figure 3 Principles of ratio imaging. Fluorescence of ion-indicating fluorophores is sensitive both to ion concentration and to the optical path length. As a consequence, thicker and thinner areas of cells give rise to stronger and weaker signals. Fluorescence ratioing corrects for this effect. Fluorescence of ion-indicating fluorophores is collected at two excitation or emission wavelengths (X nm and Y nm). At one wavelength fluorescence increases as the ion concentration increases. The other wavelength produces ion-independent fluorescence. The ratio of ion-dependent to ion-independent fluorescence is proportional only to ion concentration, as illustrated, and errors due to variations of cell thickness, accessible volume, and fluorophore loading are eliminated. The bottom illustrates the steps involved in making a ratio image. First, raw images of fluorophore-loaded cells are collected at the two excitation (or emission) wavelengths. Images are also collected in adjacent cell-free regions at each wavelength. These background images are then subtracted from the raw images to eliminate any nonspecific fluorescence. Finally, the images after background subtraction are divided into one another on a pixel-to-pixel basis to generate the ratio image. Actual ion concentration is then determined by comparison to the standard curve.

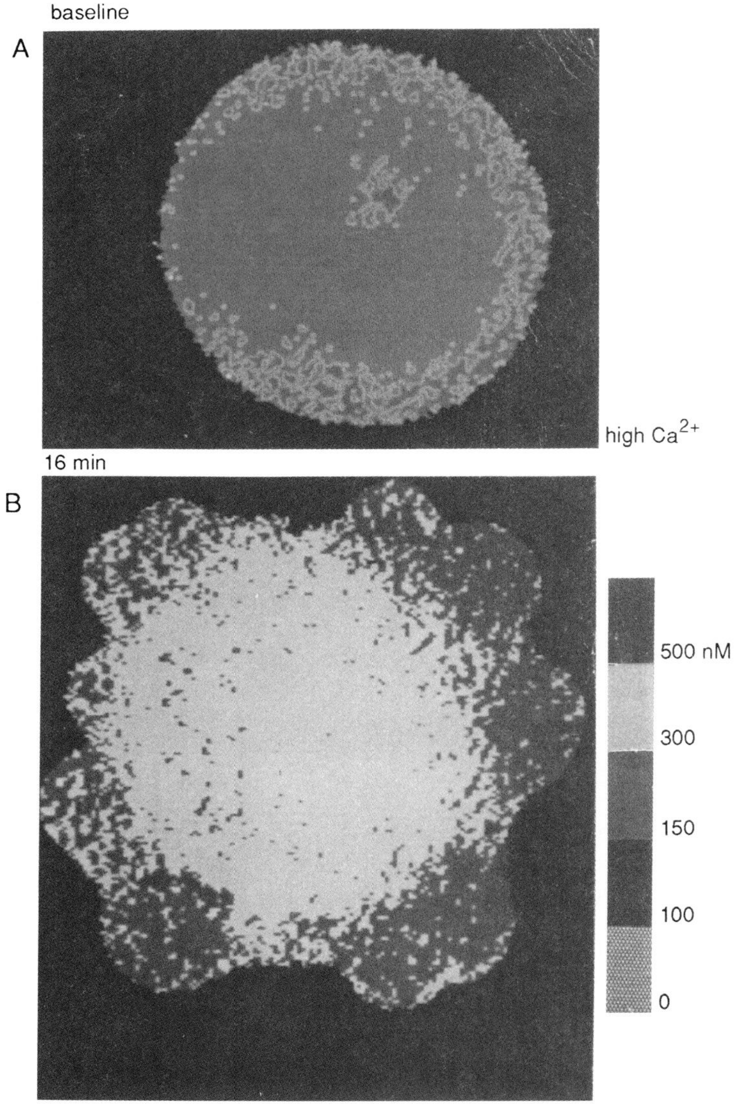

Figure 4 Cytosolic free Ca^{2+} during toxic cell injury measured by ratio imaging of Fura-2 fluorescence. A cultured rat hepatocyte was exposed to 50 μM $HgCl_2$, and cytosolic free Ca^{2+} was measured by ratio imaging of Fura-2 fluorescence. Note the increase in Ca^{2+}, which is especially marked in blebs (from a color original).

SUBCELLULAR LOCALIZATION

For fluorophores loaded as neutral membrane-permeant esters, sequestration into organelles such as mitochondria may occur. A useful approach to quantitatively assess the extent of organelle uptake is to coload cells with additional probes that are specific for various subcellular compartments, such as rhodamine-123 for mitochondria, rhodamine–dextran for lysosomes, and rhodamine microspheres (0.1-μm diameter) for the prelysosomal endocytic compartment (7,8). Specific compartments in the multilabeled cells are opened by addition of increasing strengths of detergent, as illustrated in Fig. 5. A Ca^{2+}-free succinate-containing buffer (Ca^{2+}-free Krebs–Ringer's solution containing 25 m*M* Na–HEPES buffer and 5 m*M* succinate) is used to prevent mitochondrial depolarization after permeabilization of the plasma membrane. In hepatocytes

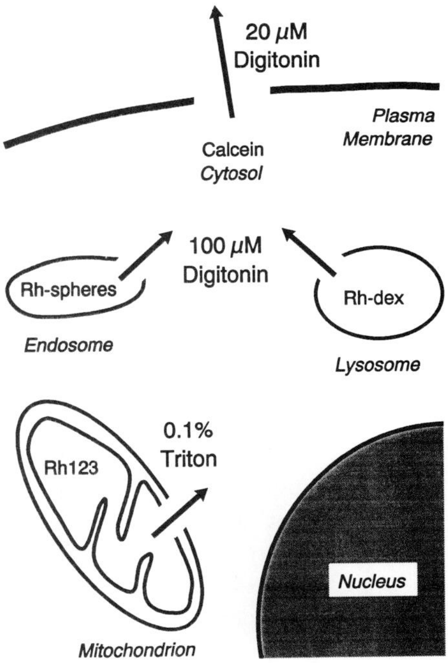

Figure 5 Release of fluorophores from subcellular compartments. Increasing strengths of detergents produce progressive opening of the subcellular compartments. The plasma membrane is permeabilized by 20 μM digitonin to cause release of calcein from the cytosol. Digitonin (100 μM) opens lysosomes and endosomes to release rhodamine–dextran (Rh-dex) and rhodamine microspheres (Rh-spheres). Triton X-100 (0.1%) is required to permeabilize mitochondrial membranes and cause the release of rhodamine-123 (Rh123).

20 μM digitonin releases fluorophores such as calcein from the cytosol within seconds, but not markers of mitochondria, endosomes, and lysosomes. Thus, retention of a fluorophore after 20 μM digitonin signifies organellar loading. Subsequent addition of 100 μM digitonin releases endosomal and lysosomal fluorophores, but not mitochondrial markers. Finally, 0.1% Triton X-100 releases mitochondrial contents. By quantifying fluorescence remaining as detergents are added, the extent of loading in noncytosolic compartments can be determined. Coloading with known markers such as rhodamine-123 and rhodamine–dextran provides a positive control which shows that specific compartments are being opened as intended. In hepatocytes organelle loading is usually negligible with most probes, although loading with high concentrations of ester derivatives can favor noncytosolic uptake. By contrast, in cardiac myocytes mitochondrial loading accounts for 30–40% of the distribution of fluorophores such as Fura-2 and BCECF. Because organelle loading varies among cell types and different fluorophores, it is essential to evaluate compartmentation for each new cell type and for each new fluorophore. Variation of time, temperature, pH, and concentrations used in ester loading may influence the extent of organelle loading.

CONFOCAL MICROSCOPY

With conventional fluorescence optics mitochondrial loading of ion-indicating fluorophores means that the investigator does not know whether measured changes are occurring in the cytosol, the mitochondria, or both. Confocal microscopy allows such discriminations to be made. In conventional fluorescence microscopy light from out-of-focus planes degrades the in-focus image. The resulting superimposition of detail prevents mitochondrial signals from being distinguished from cytosolic ones. By contrast, confocal microscopy rejects out-of-focus light and creates optical sections that are 0,5 to 1.0-μm thick for submicron resolution in three dimensions. This resolution is sufficient to distinguish mitochondria, lysosomes, and nuclei. In many respects the confocal microscope is analogous to the computerized axial tomography (CAT) scanner in radiology, and the improvement of resolution of confocal microscopy over conventional optical microscopy is similar to that for CAT scanning over conventional radiographs.

When a cell is labeled with a ion-sensitive fluorophore that labels both cytosol and mitochondria, confocal microscopy can distinguish mitochondrial from cytosolic ions (12). For example, SNARF-1 loads into both the cytosol and the mitochondria of cultured hepatocytes. The emission spectrum of SNARF-1 is pH sensitive, and it is possible to measure emitted fluorescence at two different emission wavelengths, ratio the fluorescence, and convert the ratios to pH values from a standard curve. As shown in Fig. 6, pH values from SNARF-1 fluorescence show marked heterogeneity within the cytoplasm of hepatocytes.

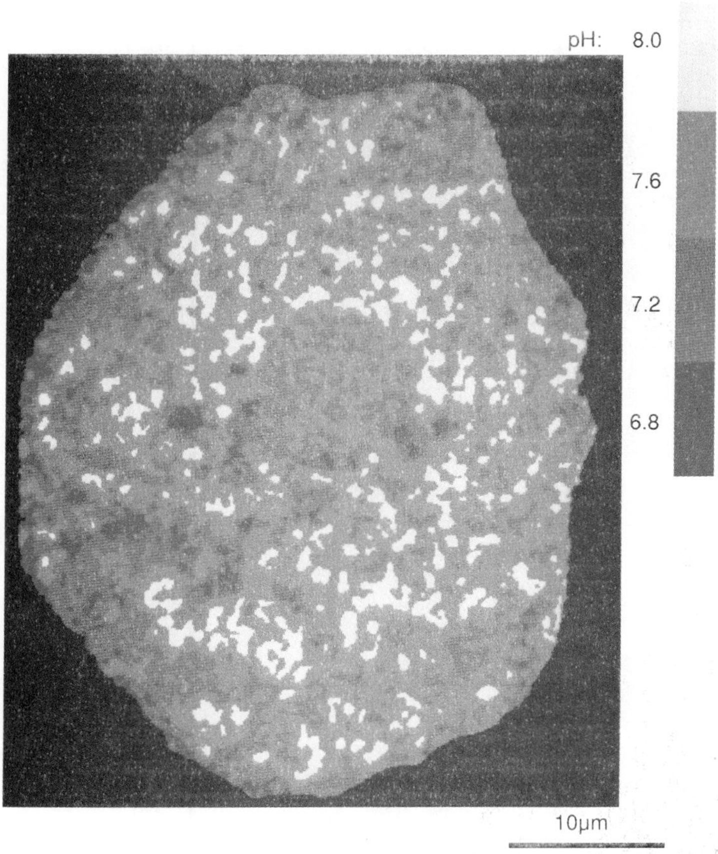

Figure 6 Confocal ratio image of intracellular pH in a cultured hepatocyte. A cultured rat hepatocyte was loaded with 5 *μM* SNARF-1 for 30 min at 37°C and imaged with a Bio-Rad MRC-600 laser scanning confocal microscope. Using 568-nm excitation light from an argon–krypton laser, fluorescence emitted at 584 ± 5 nm was divided by fluorescence at >620 nm. From an *in situ* calibration a map of intracellular pH was generated and represented by shades of gray. Note the white areas of high pH corresponding to mitochondria.

Cytosolic and nuclear areas have a pH of ~7.2, but for regions corresponding to the distribution of mitochondria, pH is 7.8–8.0. Thus, ΔpH across the mitochondrial inner membrane is 0.6–0.8 pH units.

Often the difference in ion content or other parameter is not so marked as to make obvious any differences between mitochondria and the cytosol. Under such circumstances a dual-labeling procedure may be used (32). Cells are coloaded with an ion-indicating fluorophore such as Fluo-3 for Ca^{2+} (green

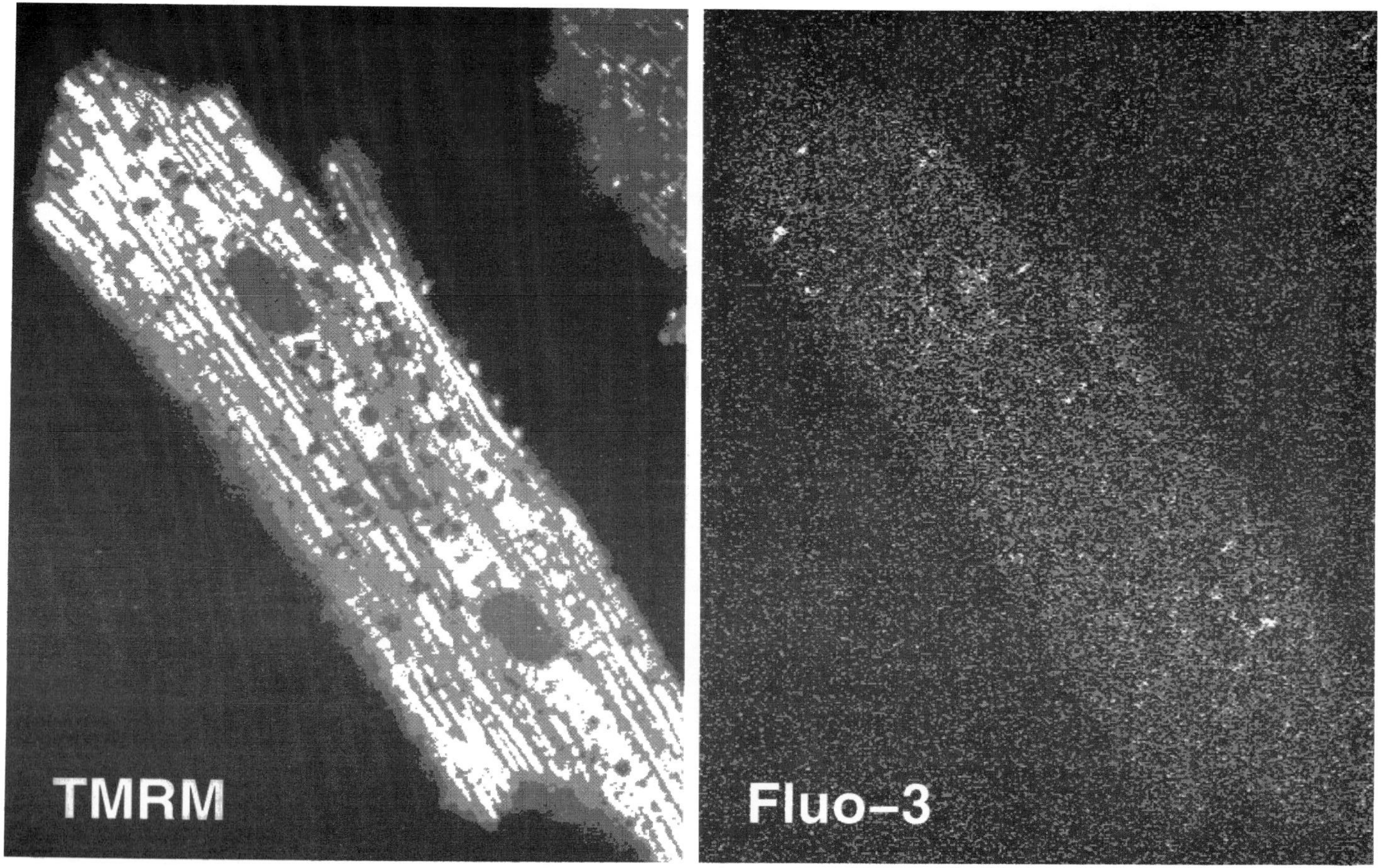
TMRM
Fluo-3

emitting) and TMRM for mitochondria (red emitting). The fluorescence of both fluorophores is imaged simultaneously using dual detectors. From TMRM images mitochondria, cytosolic, and nuclear regions are easily identified. By looking at the corresponding regions in the Fluo-3 image, relative changes in Ca^{2+} in each compartment can be examined (Fig. 7).

Simple image-processing algorithms can be used to quantify compartmental changes. The logical steps of the analysis are as follows: (1) In the TMRM image pixels of high and low intensity are identified. High-intensity pixels represent mitochondria, whereas low-intensity pixels represent cytosol and nucleus. Intermediate-intensity pixels are ignored since they may represent an overlap of cytosol and mitochondria. (2) Cytosolic regions are separated from the nucleus by outlining the nuclear area manually with a mouse. (3) In the Fluo-3 image, intensity values for pixels corresponding to mitochondria, cytosol, and nucleus are averaged to give values for relative Ca^{2+} concentration for the three regions.

COMMENTS

MDVM, together with confocal microscopy, provides a powerful new technique to study the physiology, biochemistry, and viability of single cells during toxic stress. By using nonperturbing probes, single cells can be observed repeatedly over time as injury progresses. Principal drawbacks of the approach are its expense, the degree of training required of users, and the time required to make measurements in cells one at a time. However, many systems are now available, at the cost of a good fluorometer, that perform at least some of the imaging described here. Commercially available menu- and mouse-driven software application packages are becoming easier to use and do not require extensive computer experience. For faster throughput groups of cells at lower magnification can be studied instead of a single cell. In the future it is likely that MDVM will become as common as electron microscopy in toxicological research, and just as necessary.

Figure 7 Confocal images of intracellular free Ca^{2+} and mitochondrial polarization in an adult cardiac myocyte. An adult rabbit cardiac myocyte was loaded with TMRM (600 n*M* for 30 min, then 125 n*M*) and Fluo-3 (20 μM Fluo-3 AM for 1 hr) to monitor mitochondrial membrane potential (left) and intracellular free Ca^{2+} (right), respectively. The cells were excited with the 488- and 568-nm lines of an argon–krypton laser, and confocal fluorescence images were collected at emission wavelengths of 522 ± 18 nm (Fluo-3) and >585 nm (TMRM). Pixel intensity is represented by shades of gray.

ACKNOWLEDGMENTS

This work was supported in part by grants AG-07218 and DK-30874 from the National Institutes of Health and grant J-1433 from the Office of Naval Research.

REFERENCES

1. G. J. Gores, B. Herman, and J. J. Lemasters, *Hepatology* **11,** 690 (1990).
2. R. P. Haugland, "Handbook of Fluorescent Probes and Research Chemicals," Molecular Probes, Eugene, Oregon, 1992.
3. K. H. Jones and J. A. Senft, *J. Histochem. Cytochem.* **33,** 77 (1985).
4. G. J. Gores, A.-L. Nieminen, K. E. Fleishman, T. L. Dawson, B. Herman, and J. J. Lemasters, *Am. J. Physiol.* **255,** C315 (1988).
5. A. N. Glazer, K. Peck, and R. A. Mathies, *Proc. Natl. Acad. Sci. U.S.A.* **87,** 3851 (1990).
6. B. Herman, A.-L. Nieminen, G. J. Gores, and J. J. Lemasters, *FASEB J.* **2,** 146 (1988).
7. G. J. Gores, A.-L. Nieminen, B. E. Wray, B. Herman, and J. J. Lemasters, *J. Clin. Invest.* **83,** 386 (1989).
8. A.-L. Nieminen, G. J. Gores, T. L. Dawson, B. Herman, and J. J. Lemasters, *J. Biol. Chem.* **265,** 2399 (1990).
9. L. V. Johnson, M. L. Walsh, B. J. Bockus, and L. B. Chen, *J. Cell Biol.* **88,** 526 (1981).
10. D. L. Farkas, M.-D. Wei, P. Febbroriello, J. H. Carson, and L. M. Loew, *Biophys. J.* **56,** 1053 (1989).
11. R. K. Emaus, R. Grunwald, and J. J. Lemasters, *Biochim. Biophys, Acta* **850,** 436 (1986).
12. J. J. Lemasters, E. Chacon, G. Zahrebelski, J. M. Reece, and A.-L. Nieminen, *in* "Optical Microscopy: Emerging Methods and Applications" (B. Herman and J. J. Lemasters, eds.), p. 339. Academic Press, San Diego, 1993.
13. R. E. Pagano, O. C. Martin, H. C. Kang, and R. P. Haugland, *J. Cell Biol.* **113,** 1267 (1991).
14. C. Lee and L. B. Chen, *Cell (Cambridge, Mass.)* **54,** 37 (1988).
15. A.-L. Nieminen, G. J. Gores, T. L. Dawson, B. Herman, and J. J. Lemasters, *in* "Optical Microscopy for Biology" (B. Herman and K. Jacobson, eds.), p. 323. Wiley–Liss, New York, 1990.
16. T. D. Boyer, *Hepatology* **9,** 486 (1989).
17. R. Cathcart, E. Schwiers, and B. N. Ames, *Anal. Biochem.* **134,** 111 (1983).
18. G. J. Gores, C. E. Flarsheim, T. L. Dawson, A.-L. Nieminen, B. Herman, and J. J. Lemasters, *Am. J. Physiol.* **257,** C347 (1989).
19. G. Rothe, A. Osen, and G. Valet, *Naturwissenschaften* **75,** 354 (1988).
20. G. Rothe and G. Valet, *J. Leukocyte Biol.* **47,** 440 (1990).
21. G. Grynkiewicz, M. Poenie, and R. Y. Tsien, *J. Biol. Chem.* **260,** 3440 (1985).
22. G. R. Bright, G. W. Fisher, J. Rogowska, and D. L. Taylor, *J. Cell Biol.* **104,** 1019 (1987).
23. S. Bassnett, L. Reinisch, and D. C. Beebe, *Am. J. Physiol.* **258,** C171 (1990).
24. A. Minta and R. Y. Tsien, *J. Biol. Chem.* **264,** 19449 (1989).
25. B. Raju, E. Murphy, L. A. Levy, R. D. Hall, and R. E. London, *Am. J. Physiol.* **256,** C540 (1989).

26. M. W. Roe, J. J. Lemasters, and B. Herman, *Cell Calcium* **11,** 63 (1990).
27. T. Kawanishi, A.-L. Nieminen, B. Herman, and J. J. Lemasters *J. Biol. Chem.* **266,** 20062 (1991).
28. A. W. Harman, A.-L. Nieminen, J. J. Lemasters, and B. Herman *Biochem. Biophys. Res. Commun.* **170,** 477 (1990).
29. J. J. Lemasters, G. J. Gores, A.-L. Nieminen, T. L. Dawson, B. E. Wray, and B. Herman, *Environ. Health Perspect.* **84,** 83 (1990).
30. L. Tanasugarn, P. McNeil, G. T. Reynolds, and D. L. Taylor, *J. Cell, Biol.* **98,** 717 (1984).
31. A. Minta, J. P. Y. Kao, and R. Y. Tsien, *J. Biol. Chem.* **264,** 8171 (1989).
32. E. Chacon. J. M. Reece, A.–L. Nieminen, G. Zahrebelski, B. Herman, and J. J. Lemasters, *Biophy. J.,* in press (1993).

39 Measurement of Macrophage and Neutrophil Chemotaxis

Debra L. Laskin

INTRODUCTION

Chemotaxis is the process by which macrophages and neutrophils migrate toward the site of tissue injury. It is unidirectional cell migration in response to concentration gradients of chemotactic factors released from damaged tissues and cells (1). These factors bind to specific receptors on phagocytic cells and induce directed cell migration. A number of agents have been reported to induce chemotaxis in phagocytes, including complement fragments (2,3), products involved in the kinin and coagulation pathway (4), collagen and tissue breakdown products (5,6), arachidonic acid metabolites, (particularly leukotriene B_4) (7), synthetic peptides related to bacterial-derived products such as *N*-formyl-methionine-leucine-phenylalanine (8), as well as inflammatory stimuli such as the phorbol ester tumor promoter, 12-*O*-tetradecanoyl-phorbol-13-acetate (9). During the past few years several cell-derived chemotactic factors have also been characterized (for a review see Ref. 10). These belong to a family of phagocyte chemoattractants which include macrophage inflammatory proteins, macrophage chemotactic proteins, and interleukin-8. These macrophage and neutrophil chemotactic factors are released by a variety of cell types and are thought to participate in early inflammatory responses (11,12).

In this chapter two methods are described to measure macrophage and neutrophil chemotaxis. The first method, which involves the use of microwell chemotaxis chambers, is based on the ability of cells to migrate through pores in membrane filters (2). The second method involves quantifying the number of cells and the distance they migrate under a layer of agarose toward a chemoattractant (13). Both of these methods provide useful and quantitative information on the relative ability of various agents to induce phagocyte migration and the state of activation of macrophages and neutrophils.

METHODS IN TOXICOLOGY, Volume 1B

METHOD I: MEASUREMENT OF CHEMOTAXIS IN MICROWELL CHAMBERS

Equipment

Neuroprobe 48-well Micro Chemotaxis Chamber (KIT-48, Neuro Probe Cabin John, MD)
Nucleopore membrane polycarbonate filters, 5-μm pore size (NMF-5-2580, Neuro Probe): These can be used for both macrophages and neutrophils. Chemotaxis is quantified as the number of cells that have migrated completely through and adhered to the lower side of the filter. Filters should be handled only with forceps
Two pairs of forceps (one pair reserved for staining)
Two 10-cm plastic petri dishes for staining

Materials and Reagents

Chemotaxis medium: Prepare fresh prior to use

RPMI or Dulbecco's modified Eagle's medium (DMEM) (GIBCO, Grand Island, NY), 96 ml
1 *M* HEPES, 1 ml
7.5% $NaHCO_3$, 2 ml
200 m*M* L-glutamine, 1 ml
Bovine serum albumin (Calbiochem, San Diego, CA), 0.5 g
pH medium to 7.2 with 1 N NaOH prior to use

Positive control chemoattractants for assay

For neutrophils, 5×10^{-8} *M* *N*-formyl-methionine-leucine-phenylalanine (Sigma, St. Louis, MO) (8), prepared immediately before use in chemotaxis medium from aliquots stored frozen (−20°C) as 1 m*M* stock solutions. (Note: Do not refreeze stock solutions.)
For macrophages and monocytes, 100 n*M* 12-*O*-tetradecanoyl-phorbol-13-acetate (LC Services, Woburn, MA) (9) prepared in chemotaxis medium from 1 m*M* stock solutions stored at −20°C or 0.5–10% endotoxin-activated allogeneic serum (2,3). This is prepared by incubating allogeneic serum with 10 mg/ml *Escherichia coli* lipopolysaccharide (Sigma) for 30 min at 37°C and then for 30 min at 56°C. The serum is then centrifuged at 500 *g* for 10 min (4°C) and the pellet is discarded.

Stain

Camco Quik Stain II (Baxter, McGaw Park, IL)

Cell Separation Medium

Ficoll-Paque (Pharmacia, Piscataway, NJ)
Phosphate-buffered saline (PBS) (Sigma)
6% Dextran (Sigma), 6 g in 100 ml of PBS (can be stored at 4°C)

Cells

Peripheral blood neutrophils (1–2 × 10^{-6}/ml) or monocytes (2–3 × 10^{-6}/ml) or resident or elicited tissue macrophages (2–3 × 10^{-6}/ml)

PROCEDURE

Cell Collection: Peripheral Blood Monocytes and Neutrophils

1. Collect peripheral blood in heparinized Vacutainers (Becton Dickinson, Rutherford, NJ).
2. Mix 10 ml of blood with 2 ml of 6% dextran (warmed to room temperature).
3. Allow red blood cells to sediment at room temperature for 30 min.
4. Collect the upper layer (buffy coat), wash twice in PBS (300 *g*, 8 min), and resuspend in 10 ml of PBS.
5. Layer 10-ml of the cell suspension over 4 ml of Ficoll-Paque in 15-ml conical centrifuge tubes.
6. Centrifuge at 800*g* for 25 min at room temperature.
7. Collect the mononuclear cells (~30% monocytes) at the interface of the gradient and the neutrophils in the pellet.
8. Lyse contaminating red blood cells by incubation of the cells with 10 ml of ammonium chloride buffer (1 ml of 7.5% NH_4Cl, 1 ml of 200 m*M* Tris-HCl, and 8 ml of distilled water, pH 7.2) for 10 min at 37°C in a shaking water bath.
9. Wash the cells two times in PBS (300*g*, 8 min).
10. Resuspend in chemotaxis medium at the appropriate cell concentration (see above).

Cell Collection: Macrophages

Macrophages can be obtained from various tissues using published isolation procedures. For isolation protocols involving enzymatic digestion of the tissue, the cells should be incubated overnight prior to measurement of chemotaxis.

Micropore Filter Assay

1. The microwell chemotaxis chamber is designed such that eight different test groups can be analyzed with six replicates per group. Orient the bottom of

the chamber so that the NP trademark is at the upper right. Fill each well of the bottom chamber with 25–30 μl of the positive control chemoattractant, the negative control (buffer), or various concentrations of the test compounds. The volume should be such that a slight positive meniscus is formed in each well. Be certain that there are no air bubbles in the wells. If air bubbles are present, they can be removed by puncturing with a heated needle.

2. With the shiny side facing down, cut 1 mm off the upper right corner of the membrane filter. Using forceps, carefully lower the filter onto the wells, allowing the central portion of the filter to make contact with the wells first. The upper right clipped corner should be aligned with the NP trademark on the chamber. Adjustments of the filter should be minimized once it is set in place to avoid crosscontamination among the wells.

3. Place the gasket on top of the filter with the clipped corner at the upper right, followed by the top part of the chemotaxis chamber. Screw into place securely until finger tight.

4. Cover the chamber with a 25 × 75-mm glass slide and place in a humidified 37°C CO_2 incubator for thermal equilibration (10–15 min).

5. Fill each well of the top chamber with 50 μl of cells, being careful to avoid air bubbles.

6. Incubate the chamber in a humidified 37°C CO_2 incubator, ~30 min for neutrophils, 2–3 hr for monocytes, and 3–4 hr for macrophages.

7. After the appropriate incubation time remove the chamber from the incubator, invert it, and shake it once vigorously to empty the upper chamber.

8. Dismantle the chamber, remove the filter using a forceps, and stain for 30 sec in Camco Quik stain followed by 1 min in distilled water. (Note: Although some investigators prefer to remove the cells from the top of the filter prior to staining, these cells do not interfere with counting and in fact make it somewhat easier to identify cells that have migrated through the filter in the chemotaxis chamber.)

9. Cut the filter in half and place each half, shiny side up, on a glass slide.

10. Air-dry overnight.

11. Score slides for chemotaxis microscopically under oil immersion without cover slips. Typically, 10 oil immersion fields are counted for each well. Chemotaxis is presented as the average number of cells per group that have migrated through the filter in 10 oil immersion fields (6,14).

Note: Chemotaxis chambers should be washed thoroughly in distilled water immediately after each use.

DISTINGUISHING BETWEEN CHEMOTAXIS AND CHEMOKINESIS

As indicated above, chemotaxis is directed cell migration along a concentration gradient of a chemoattractant. This is distinct from two other types of cell locomotion: random migration and chemokinesis. Random migration is spontaneous locomotion of cells in the absence of any known chemoattractant. Chemokinesis, like chemotaxis, involves stimulated cellular locomotion; however, this movement has no sustained directional component. All chemoattractants induce some degree of chemokinesis. In order to confirm the biological activity of a test agent, it is necessary to distinguish between these different types of locomotion. Random migration is measured by the level of cellular responsiveness when chemotaxis medium alone is placed in the lower wells of the chemotactic chamber. Chemotaxis and chemokinesis are differentiated by means of a checkerboard assay (6,14–16). In this assay increasing concentrations of the test reagent are placed above and below the filter in the chemotaxis chamber. If the agent is biologically active as a chemoattractant, then decreasing the concentration gradient across the filter will correspondingly decrease the extent of cell migration. A finding that cellular migration is increased over buffer alone in the absence of a chemotactic gradient (i.e., when equal concentrations are placed above and below the filter) indicates that the test agent also induces chemokinesis. An example of the experimental design for a checkerboard assay is shown in Table I.

Table I Checkerboard Assay for Distinguishing Between Chemotaxis and Chemokinesis[a]

Concentration of test reagent placed above the filter	Concentration of test reagent placed below the filter
0	100
1	100
10	100
100	100
0	10
1	10
10	10
100	10
0	1
1	1
10	1
100	1
0	0
1	0
10	0
100	0

[a] The test reagent is diluted in log increments and placed above and below the filter in the chemotaxis chamber as indicated. After the appropriate incubation period the number of cells that migrate through the filter in 10 oil immersion microscopic fields is quantified.

METHOD II: MEASUREMENT OF CHEMOTAXIS UNDER AGAROSE

Equipment

35-mm culture dishes
Pasteur pipettes

Materials and Reagents

2× RPMI or DMEM basal medium (GIBCO), 44 ml
1 *M* HEPES, 2 ml
7.5% $NaHCO_3$ 4 ml
Agarose (Calbiochem), 12 mg
Bovine serum albumin (Calbiochem), 0.5 g
Camco Quik stain
4% Paraformaldehyde

Procedure

1. Dissolve agarose in 50 ml of distilled water by heating in a boiling water bath for 10 min.
2. Cool to 48°C.
3. Mix with 50 ml of 2× medium containing 1% bovine serum albumin, HEPES, and $NaHCO_3$.
4. Pipette 1 ml into 35-mm tissue culture dishes.
5. Allow the agarose to solidify.
6. Remove the agarose covering one-half of each dish by aspiration.
7. Cut a well in the agarose (~2.4 mm in diameter, 4 mm from the center of the dish).
8. Add 30 μl of the cell suspension (5×10^5 cells) to each well.
9. Add 300 μl of chemoattractant or control reagents to the half of the dish not covered with the agarose.
10. Incubate 2–3 hr for neutrophils or 24 hr for macrophages at 37°C in a humidified CO_2 incubator.
11. Fix the cells by adding 1 ml of 4% paraformaldehyde to each dish.
12. After 30 min at room temperature or overnight at 4°C, remove the agarose by aspiration.
13. Stain the dishes with Camco Quik stain.
14. Measure cell migration as the average number of cells migrating from the edge of the cell well toward the chemoattractant (chemotaxis) and away from the chemoattractant (chemokinesis) at 0.1 mm increments (6,14). Data are expressed graphically with distance on the x-axis and number of cells on the

y-axis. Both chemotaxis and chemokinesis data should be displayed on the graph.

COMMENTS

The most frustrating aspect of chemotaxis measurements is the day-to-day variability in the responsiveness of the cells. Furthermore, even a small (5%) contamination of neutrophils in the cell preparation may adversely affect the chemotactic response of monocytes or macrophages. Phagocyte locomotion through polycarbonate filters may also vary with filter lots. In addition, there is some concern about the possibility of the cells falling off the lower surface of the filter. This difficulty can be overcome by using two filters, or by directly counting the number of cells in the fluid of the lower compartment of the chamber. In general, this is not a major problem. The under agarose assay is advantageous, since orientation and morphology can be examined in chemotactically responding cells. However, this assay is somewhat more time consuming than the micropore filter technique.

REFERENCES

1. J. Niedel and P. Cuatrecassas, *Curr. Top. Cell. Regul.* **17,** 137 (1980).
2. S. V. Boyden, *J. Exp. Med.* **115,** 453 (1962).
3. P. A. Ward and L. J. Newman, *J. Immunol.* **102,** 93 (1962).
4. A. P. Kaplan, E. J. Goetzl, and K. F. Austen, *J. Clin. Invest.* **52**, 2591 (1972).
5. C. Chang and J. C. Houck, *Proc. Soc. Exp. Biol. Med.* **134**, 22 (1970).
6. D. L. Laskin, T. Kimura, S. Sakakibara, D. J. Riley, and R. A. Berg, *J. Leukecyte Biol.* **39,** 255 (1986).
7. E. Goetzl and W. Pickett, *J. Exp. Med.* **153**, 482 (1981).
8. E. Schiffman, B. Corcoran, and S. Wahl, *Proc. Natl. Acad. Sci. U.S.A.* **72**, 1059 (1975).
9. D. L. Laskin, J. D. Laskin, I. B. Weinstein, and R. A. Carchman, *Cancer Res.* **41**, 1923 (1981).
10. M. E. Brandes and S. M. Wahl, *in* "Xenobiotic-Induced Inflammation" (L. B. Schook and D. L. Laskin, eds.), Academic Press, San Diego, 1994, In press.
11. K. Matsushima and J. J. Oppenheim, *Cytokine* **1**, 2 (1989).
12. R. M. Streiter, R. Wiggins, S. H. Phan, B. L. Warram, H. J. Showell, D. G. Remick, S. W. Chensue, and S. L. Kunkel, *Biochem. Biophys. Res. Commun.* **162**, 694 (1989).
13. R. D. Nelson, P. G. Quie and R. L. Simmons, *J. Immunol.* **115**, 1650 (1975).
14. D. L. Laskin, R. A. Soltys, R. A. Berg, and D. J. Riley, *Am. J. Respir. Cell Mol. Biol.* **2**, 463 (1990).
15. S. H. Zigmond and J. G. Hirsch, *J. Exp. Med.* **137**, 387 (1973).
16. D. L. Laskin, A. M. Pilaro, and S. Ji, *Toxicol. Appl. Pharmacol.* **86,** 216 (1986).

40

Two-Dimensional Electrophoresis as Applied to Problems of *in Vitro* and *in Vivo* Toxicology

N. L. Anderson, R. Esquer-Blasco, and N. G. Anderson

INTRODUCTION

Toxic effects frequently involve changes in the abundance or structure of specific proteins in affected cells. Since most proteins are believed to carry out significant functions in the cells in which they are found, it is natural to infer that protein changes play a role in the unfolding of many toxicological mechanisms. If this is true, it would seem reasonable to include a search for such alterations among the protocols carried out in routine toxicological studies. Given the effort and cost of carrying out specific enzyme tests (e.g., cytochrome P-450 or peroxisomal enzyme measurements), and the fact that typical cells contain several thousand different proteins, it is clear that some method more general than specific assays would be required to search for such effects on a routine basis.

The most powerful quantitative technique currently available for the global analysis of protein effects is high-resolution two-dimensional gel electrophoresis (1), the subject of this chapter. More than 1000 protein species are resolved and quantitated in a single analysis and, using computerized image-processing and data base techniques, the results of hundreds of analyses can be combined and intercompared. The technique can be applied to tissue samples, body fluids, and cells grown in culture, and typically requires only 100–200 μg of protein per analysis.

In the context of this volume, two-dimensional electrophoresis offers the possibility of answering important questions in *in vitro* toxicology. First, how similar are the cells of the *in vitro* system to those of the organ from which they were derived? Second, how similar is the response of the *in vitro* system (at the protein level) to the response of analogous cells *in vivo*? Third, how similar is the response found in animal systems to the response observed in the analogous human system, when considered at the molecular level? Answers to these ques-

METHODS IN TOXICOLOGY, Volume 1B

tions will go some way toward establishing the faithfulness of a variety of *in vitro* test systems.

MATERIALS AND REAGENTS

The most critical reagents in this procedure are the ampholytes used in the first dimension to establish the pH gradient and the sodium dodecyl sulfate (SDS) used to coat the proteins for the second dimension. For any extended study it is

Table I Reagents and Vendors

Reagent	Vendor	Cat. No.
Dithiothreitol (DTT, reducing agent)	Sigma (St. Louis, MO)	D-0632
Glycerol	Sigma	G-5516
Glycine (slab gel buffer)	Sigma	G-7126
NP-40 detergent (Nonidet P-40)	Sigma	N-6507
Sec-butanol (for slab gel overlay)	Sigma	B-1888
Tris base (slab gel buffer)	Sigma	T-1503
Trizma preset, pH 7.0 (equilibration buffer)	Sigma	T-3503
Trizma preset, pH 8.1 (slab gel buffer)	Sigma	T-4878
Tetramethylethylenediamine (TEMED)	Sigma	B44308-3G
Ammonium persulfate	Sigma	B44307-3E
Acrylamide 40% T Solution (DALT)	Amresco (Solon, OH)	0254-500ml
Acrylamide grade I (ISO)	Produced by BDH, Poole, United Kingdom; available in the United States through Gallard-Schlesinger (Carle Place, NY)	B44313-2V
Bis-acrylamide (ISO)	BDH/Gallard-Schlesinger	B44300-3M
SDS (DALT)	BDH/Gallard-Schlesinger	442152
Urea (BDH)	BDH/Gallard-Schlesinger	B45204-3W
Ammonium sulfate	Fisher (Pittsburgh, PA)	A701-50
Methanol	Fisher	A412-20
Phosphoric acid, 85%	Fisher	A242-1
Ethanol	Warner-Graham (Cockeysville, MD)	200 proof, USP
Pharmalytes 3–10 (ISO ampholyte)	Pharmacia–LKB (Piscataway, NJ)	17.0456.01
Resolyte 4–8 (ISO ampholyte, two-dimensional grade)	Hoefer (San Francisco, CA)	44340
Coomassie Brilliant Blue G250	Serva, distributed in the United States by Crescent (Hauppage, NY)	17524

important to secure a uniform supply of these reagents. This is typically achieved by buying a batch large enough to complete a major body of work. In general, reagents used in the first-dimension isoelectric focusing (IEF) separation are more critical than those used in the second dimension, and should be of the best electrophoresis grade available. Other reagents are of normal laboratory reagent grade. Table I lists the source and catalog number of each of the major reagents used successfully in our laboratory.

PROCEDURE

Two-dimensional electrophoresis involves the separation of proteins by two sequential procedures carried out in acrylamide gels: IEF followed by SDS electrophoresis in a perpendicular direction. The first step separates proteins by isoelectric point (a function of amino acid composition), while the second separates primarily on the basis of size. The result, after a detection step, is a two-dimensional array of spots, each of which represents a specific protein species (Fig. 1). The following sections summarize the technique as it is currently used for the analysis of rodent liver and hepatocyte samples; a more complete description has been published in book form (2). Analyses are carried out using equipment optimized for batches of 20 gels (the ISO-DALT system, Hoefer, San Francisco, CA) in order to provide a level of gel-to-gel reproducibility not obtainable with general purpose gel equipment (two to five gels per batch).

Sample Preparation

The objectives of the sample preparation procedure are to solubilize all of the proteins, to dissociate multisubunit complexes, and to prevent protein alterations caused by processes such as proteolysis and dephosphorylation. The simplest procedure consistent with these goals is direct homogenization in a solubilizing solution of 9 *M* urea, 2% Nonidet P-40 (NP-40) detergent, 1% dithiothreitol (to reduce disulfides), and 2% high-pH-range ampholytes (e.g., pH 9–11 Ampholines, Pharmacia–LKB, Piscataway, NJ). Tissue samples such as liver can be homogenized directly in an 8-fold excess [1 : 8 (w/v)] of the solubilizer. Typically, a small piece (100–300 mg) of tissue from the apical end of the left lobe is taken, weighed, and homogenized in the appropriate volume of solubilizer using a 7-ml glass homogenizer. Samples of cultured suspension cells are first rinsed in phosphate-buffered saline (PBS), microfuged to pellet them in capillary-bottomed microfuge tubes, and resuspended in six pellet volumes of solubilizer (i.e., 200–300 μg protein in the 10 μl typically loaded per gel). Attached cells are rinsed several times in the equivalent of a media volume of PBS, the excess fluid is drained carefully by tilting the plate on edge, and the surface of the plate, well, or flask is treated with the minimum volume of solubilizer that can wet the whole surface and be recovered by pipette. The solubilizer is made

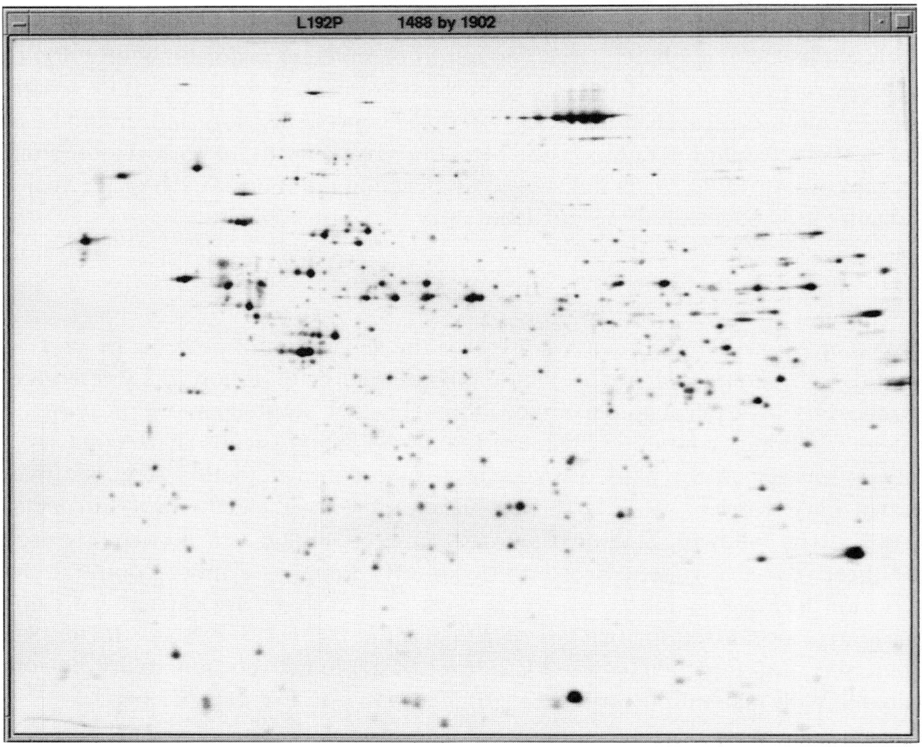

Figure 1 A two-dimensional protein pattern of human hepatocytes isolated by collagenase perfusion, plated on collagen-coated 60-mm culture dishes, and maintained in culture for 48 hr. [See F. C. Richardson, S. C. Strom, D. M. Copple, R. A. Bendele, G. S. Probst, and N. L. Anderson, *Electrophoresis* **14,** 157 (1993).]

to flow back and forth over the surface a few times (by tilting the surface) to be sure all of the cells are taken up. A dense cell layer on the surface of a plastic plate or dish will typically provide a sufficiently concentrated protein sample, when solubilized in the minimum recoverable volume of solubilizer, to yield 400–1000 two-dimensional gel spots by Coomassie Blue staining.

Isoelectric Focusing

The IEF separation is carried out in small diameter (1.5-mm) gel rods formed in glass tubes. A 20-place tube gel unit (ID125, Hoefer) is used to cast the gels (by hydrostatic displacement of the dense gel solution) and subsequently to run the IEF separation. The unit is comprised of a small upper buffer chamber, into which gel tubes are inserted through silicone rubber grommets; an outer chamber into which the upper chamber is placed, and which is filled with the lower electrode buffer during the run; a lid making electrical connections; and a casting boat which is clamped on the bottom ends of the gel tubes only during gel casting. The apparatus is assembled with 20 glass tubes which have been previously cleaned using RBS-40 detergent (Pierce, Rockford, IL) and vacuumed dry. Dilute phosphoric acid (3.26 liters of 0.010 N) is placed in the lower reservoir. A plastic casting boat is clamped to the lower ends of the tubes ready to receive the gel mixture. This is prepared by mixing 8.74 g of urea (BDH), 0.80 ml of ampholytes (40% solution; Resolyte 4–8 range), 1.68 ml of 30% acrylamide/1.8% bis-acrylamide stock solution (BDH Ltd., Poole, UK), 5.17 ml of pure water [Milli-Q (Millipore, Bedford, MA) or (Barnstead, Boston, MA)], and 1.62 ml of NP-40 detergent (20% solution, Sigma, St. Louis, MO), which is gently warmed in a microwave oven to speed dissolution of the urea. Immediately before placing the mixture in the casting boat, 100 μl each of 10% ammonium persulfate (Sigma) and 10% tetramethylethylenediamine (TEMED, Sigma) are added to the gel mixture and mixed by swirling. Once the polymerizing gel solution is placed in the casting boat, the upper gel chamber with tubes and casting boat attached is slowly lowered into the lower chamber containing the phosphoric acid lower buffer. As the casting boat is submerged, the gel solution is displaced upward into all 20 tubes hydrostatically. Polymerization is allowed to proceed for 1 hr, and then the casting boat is removed, and the upper chamber is replaced in the lower buffer reservoir. A basic "upper buffer" (200 ml of 0.020 *N* NaOH) is added to the upper chamber, and the air bubbles remaining over the IEF gels are removed using a buffer-filled Hamilton syringe. The IEF gels are prefocused for 1 hr at 200 V, after which a sample is applied to the top of each IEF gel (layered under the buffer present there) using a Hamilton syringe. Typical sample volumes are 8–20 μl. IEF is carried out for a total of 33,000 V-hr.

SDS Electrophoresis

SDS separation is carried out in 11–19%T acrylamide gradient slab gels formed in 8 × 10-inch glass cassettes. Twenty-two glass cassettes, assembled in the form of books with silicone rubber spines and permanently mounted glass spacers (ID2212-1.5, Hoefer), are placed in a gel casting box (ID220, Hoefer) with thin sheets of polycarbonate between them (to prevent gel from causing each cassette to adhere to the next), and with one or two sheets of compressible bubble-pack material at the back. A small rectangle of filter paper, on which an identifying gel number has been printed in fusible ink using a laser printer or xerographic copier, is dropped into each cassette; this number becomes polymerized into the gel and identifies it throughout the remainder of the process. An acrylamide gradient (typically 2.05 liters, of which the first 5% is 11%T acrylamide and the remainder is a linear gradient from 11 to 19%T) is pumped into the box by an Angelique computer-controlled gradient maker (Large Scale Biology, Rockville, MD), after which the feed tube is removed. The gradient maker uses peristaltic pumps to deliver a varying mixture of two acrylamide compositions (light and heavy), each of which is made up of four separately pumped components (acrylamide stock solution, buffer, ammonium persulfate, and TEMED). The slab gel buffer is 0.375 *M* Tris-HCl (same concentration and pH throughout the gel) prepared using a pH-preadjusted dry mixture (Trizma preset 8.1, Sigma). A "chaser" solution of 30% sucrose is allowed to run from a side chamber into the bottom of the casting box, thereby displacing polymerizing acrylamide from connecting tubes and providing a reservoir of liquid to make up the volume decrement (~2%) associated with acrylamide polymerization. Buffer-saturated sec-butanol (1 ml) is gently layered over the top of each gel using a pipette or an Equalizer 22-place automatic overlay device (Large Scale Biology). The gradient polymerizes from the top down (to avoid convection effects) in about ~25 min.

Following polymerization, the slab gel cassettes are removed from the casting box, rinsed to remove any adhering acrylamide, and placed in plastic dish racks. Each first-dimension IEF rod gel is carefully extruded onto the top edge of one of the glass plates of the appropriate cassette, slid down into the cassette and onto the top of the slab gel using a stream of equilibration buffer [0.125 *M* Tris-HCl, pH 6.8 (Trizma preset 7.0, Sigma), 10% glycerol, 5 m*M* dithiothreitol, 2% SDS, and sufficient bromophenol blue to yield a blue color], and fixed in position using a polyester fabric gel chock (Large Scale Biology). The cassettes are then placed in a 20-place DALT tank (ID420, Hoefer) that has been filled with 38.2 liters of 24 m*M* Tris base, 200 m*M* glycine, and 0.1% SDS, and the gels are electrophoresed for ~18 hr at 160 V and 10°C. When the bromophenol blue line reaches the end of the gels, the cassettes are removed from the DALT tank and opened and the gels are placed in fix (see below).

Staining

In order to maximize reproducibility, and hence the amount of useful quantitative data, a simple protein stain based on Coomassie Brilliant Blue G250 is used. Gels are processed in groups of 10 in plastic boxes (Rubbermaid 2220, 16 × 11 × 6 inches) and are shaken gently on a reciprocating (not orbital) shaker during all steps. Following fixation of the proteins by addition of 1.5 liters of 50% ethanol and 2% phosphoric acid for several hours, gels are washed in three successive 2-liter tap water washes (30 min each), and then treated with 1.5 liters of 17% ammonium sulfate, 34% methanol, and 3% phosphoric acid. After an equilibration period of 1 hr, ~1 g of Coomassie Blue G250 powder is added, and shaking is continued for 4 days to achieve uniform staining.

The gels are then rinsed in cold tap water to remove any adherent stain particles and stored in tap water with a little sodium azide until they are scanned.

Computer Analysis

In order to acquire quantitative data from two-dimensional gels, and thereby exploit the power of the technique for large-scale data generation, it is necessary to make use of image-processing and data base techniques implemented on graphics-oriented computer workstations. The following describes the Kepler two-dimensional software system (Large Scale Biology), which was developed for use in multisample toxicology studies and runs on systems such as VAXstation graphics workstations (Digital Equipment, Maynard, MA). Gels are scanned through an orange filter using a photodiode array scanner (Eikonix 1412, Ektron, Bedford, MA) or a laser scanner (Molecular Dynamics 300A, Sunnyvale, CA), at a final resolution of 134μm in both dimensions. The resulting images ~2000 × 1600 = 3,200,000 pixels) are processed using a sequence of digital filters to remove background and streaks and mathematical morphology operations to detect and isolate spots (procedure PROC008b, provided with the Kepler system). Spots detected in the resulting processed image are modeled by two-dimensional gaussian forms using an iterative full-matrix least-squares optimization, thus allowing accurate representation of overlapping, as well as fully resolved spots. The result is a spotfile for each image, comprising a table of x and y position, x and y halfwidth, and amplitude for each detected spot. These spotfiles can be used to render, on the workstation screen, an image of the spots on the original gel. Being much more compact than the scanned images, they can be maintained online for further analysis in large groups. Using a data base-linked experimental design program (EX2D), a series of gels is selected and assigned to experimental groups appropriate to the study at hand. In a toxicology study there is typically one control group and several treatment groups (different doses, time courses, or compounds) per segment, with multiple such segments when the experiment is too large to allow preparation of all samples in 1 day.

Prior to statistical analysis, it is necessary to match the spots in the various gels to one another through the use of a master two-dimensional pattern for the tissue and species involved. The master pattern is assembled very carefully through comparison of many gels of the same sample type, and it contains all spots seen in any of the experiments undertaken in the respective biological system (3). Its spots are numbered, and the transfer of these numbers to spots in experimental patterns constitutes matching. Initially, a series of ~50 selected spots is matched by the user in all patterns. This is done using a montage display, in which the same small region of up to 100 gels is displayed, and the spot in question is rapidly verified in all of them using the workstation mouse (the process takes ~3 hr). An automatic matching algorithm then completes the matching.

Once matched, the gels are normalized by linear scaling against the master pattern in order to remove the effects of variations in protein loaded on the gels. With reasonable care, these variations can be kept within ±15%.

While the approach used to analyze specific experiments can be quite varied, it is possible to delineate a basic scheme useful for most studies. The approach followed in the Kepler system makes extensive use of a built-in statistics software system that performs mathematical and logical calculations on all the spots of the gels in all groups simultaneously, and that displays its results by highlighting (changing to red color) spots satisfying some set of criteria. To visualize all spots having an abundance greater than 10,000 pixel-gray levels, for example, the user would type "VOL.gt.10000," and all spots meeting the criteria would turn from blue to red in all patterns displayed on the workstation screen. The system allows extended math/logic procedures to be developed rapidly to answer complex questions about two-dimensional data.

First, some basic statistics are collected to determine the quality of the data overall. These include the computation, for each group, of (a) the number of spots that occur (i.e., are matched) in all gels of the group, and (b) the number of spots for which the coefficient of variation (CV) within the group (standard deviation divided by the mean abundance) is less than 15% (spots with a CV of <15% are typically considered to be well measured). In typical studies these numbers should average at least 600 and 200 spots per group, respectively.

The next stage of the analysis involves selecting those protein spots that show a statistically significant abundance difference between the controls and some experimental group. This is typically done using the Student's t test, computed between a control group and the appropriate experimental groups. Because the number of spots (variables) is large (typically more than 1000), it is necessary to use very stringent P value limits to avoid detection of chance variations. Among 1000 variables 10 would be expected to show $P < 0.01$ effects by chance alone. Hence, it is typical to require $P < 0.001$ significance in two-dimensional studies. This requirement argues strongly for group sizes of more than five when possible.

Once sets of candidate protein spots have been selected by the t test or other criteria, including the likelihood of showing interesting effects based on results of previous studies, it is useful to reexamine each such candidate spot individually using the montage display (Fig. 2). At this stage artifacts caused by mismatching can be corrected, and genuine effects can be visually confirmed by direct examination of the primary data (the spotfiles) represented on the workstation screen. When the treatment-related effects have been reliably delineated, selected data are output in report form for the user, and stored in a rela-

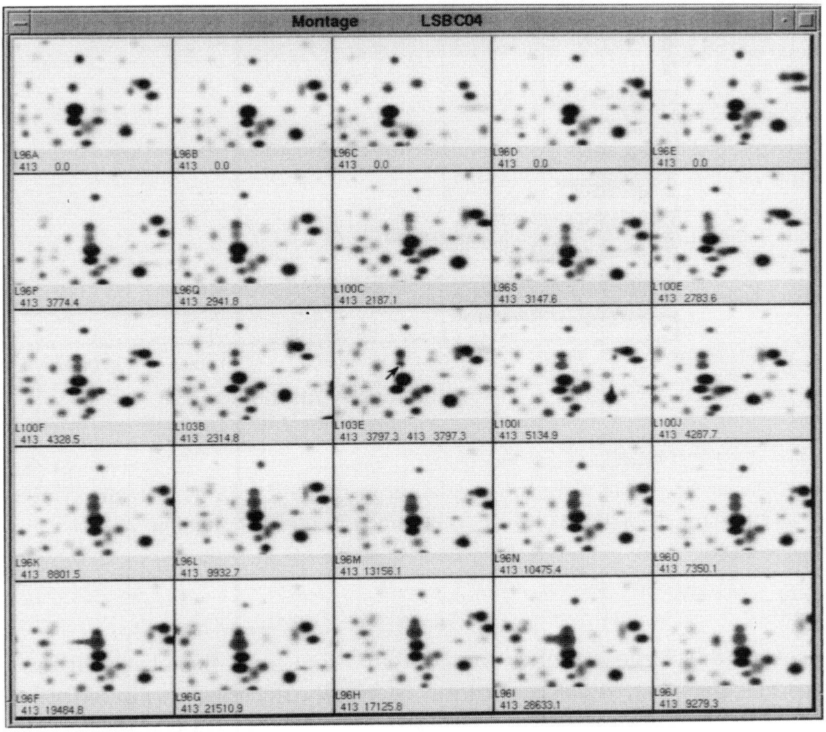

Figure 2 A montage taken from the workstation screen showing the same small region from 25 different two-dimensional gels of rat liver, centered on spot 413. Each row comprises the samples from five animals of a single experimental group. The five groups (rows) were administered diets containing (from the top): (1) 5% cholesterol, (2) no addition (controls), (3) 1% cholestyramine, (4) 0.075% lovastatin, and (5) 1% cholestyramine plus 0.075% lovastatin. Spot 413 varies strongly with treatment (the abundance in each gel is shown at the bottom of the panel). The protein has been identified as hydroxymethylglutaryl-CoA synthase, a major enzyme of cholesterol synthesis.

tional data base for use within future Kepler experiments. The data base typically receives lists of the spots found to be affected by various treatments, and the "-foldchange" associated with these effects (e.g., spot 369 increased 2.3-fold by treatment X). In addition to the numerical data, the data base supports a flexible "notes" facility which is used extensively for collecting thoughts, observations, and suspicions about individual proteins in text form. Protein abundance data are frequently presented in bar graph form (Fig. 3).

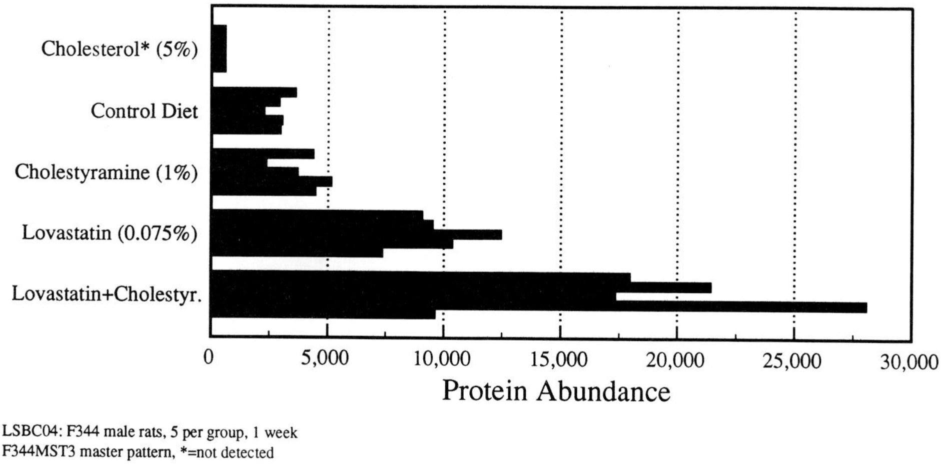

Figure 3 A bar graph showing the regulation of rat liver spot 413 (hydroxymethylglutaryl-CoA synthase, 53 kDa) with test compounds in the diet. See Fig. 2.

COMMENTS

Because of the large number of proteins that can be observed on two-dimensional gels, statistical replication is usually necessary to avoid mistaking chance quantitative variation for a significant effect: If 1000 proteins are measured, a *t* test *P* value of <0.01 between groups would yield on the order of 10 apparently significant protein differences by chance alone. Hence, it is typical to use *P* values of <0.001 to select protein spots showing genuinely significant quantitative changes due to treatment. A group size of five to 10 samples taken from identically treated animals or culture dishes usually provides good statistical power in detecting drug- or chemical-induced effects, assuming inbred strains are used. In experiments with outbred strains, significantly more samples may be necessary to avoid false detection of genetic polymorphisms as treatment-related effects. This problem can be avoided in *in vitro* studies by seeding all dishes from one (possibly pooled) preparation of cells.

Where available, it is useful to search relevant external data bases for information resulting from earlier two-dimensional and other biochemical studies. Interesting and unexpected connections result in this way: It turns out, for example, that protein 367 in the F344 rat liver master pattern was initially selected as interesting because it shows a unique antisynergistic regulation by lovastatin (Mevacor, Merck, Rahway, NJ) and cholestyramine (two agents that lower blood cholesterol by different mechanisms). Later, this fact was made more interesting by the observation that a strong peroxisome proliferator induces the same protein more strongly than any other. By following up suggestive hints of this kind (some based on identification of target proteins and some based on correlations with other chemical effects), it is frequently possible to develop and test useful hypotheses concerning the mechanism involved. However, it must be noted that two-dimensional data bases are just beginning to be collected for systems of toxicological interest (e.g., liver and hepatocytes), much early effort having been devoted to human peripheral lymphocytes, HeLa cells, REF52 rat fibroblasts, and the like.

REFERENCES

1. P. H. O'Farrell, *J. Biol. Chem.* **250,** 4007 (1975).
2. L. Anderson, "Two-Dimensional Electrophoresis: Operation of the ISO-DALT System." Large Scale Biology Press, Washington, D.C., 1991.
3. N. L. Anderson, R. Esquer-Blasco, J.-P. Hofmann, and N. G. Anderson, *Electrophoresis* **12,** 907 (1991).

Index